*Dementia
and
Communication*

# Dementia and Communication

*Editor*

Rosemary Lubinski, Ed.D.

*Associate Editors*

Joseph B. Orange, M.H.Sc.
Donald Henderson, Ph.D.
Nancy Stecker, Ph.D.

Department of Communicative Disorders and Sciences
State University of New York at Buffalo

**S** Singular Publishing Group
San Diego · London

**Singular Publishing Group, Inc.**
402 West "A" Street, Suite 325
San Diego, California 92101-7904

**Singular Publishing Ltd.**
19 Compton Terrace
London, N1 2UN, U.K.

e-mail: singpub@mail.cerfnet.com
Web site: http://www.singpub.com

©1995 by Singular Publishing Group, Inc.
Second Singular Printing November 1997

Printed in the United States of America by McNaughton & Gunn

All rights, including that of translation reserved. No part of this publication may be reproduced, stored in a retrieval system, or transmitted in any form or by any means, electronic, mechanical, recording, or otherwise, without the prior written permission of the publisher.

**Library of Congress Cataloging-in-Publication Data Available**

ISBN 1-56593-084-3

*This book is dedicated to my parents, Leo and Agnes Lubinski, for a lifetime of love, patience, prayers, and high ideals. It is also dedicated to all those individuals whose lives are enveloped by dementia.*

# *Contributors*

Nelson Butters, Ph.D.
    Professor, Department of Psychiatry
    University of California School of Medicine
    San Diego, California

    Chief, Psychological Services
    San Diego Veterans Administration Medical Center
    San Diego, California

Irene Campbell-Taylor, Ph.D.
    Assistant Professor, Faculty of Medicine
    Department of Rehabilitation Medicine
    University of Toronto
    Toronto, Ontario, Canada

    Consultant, Baycrest Centre for
    Geriatric Care
    Toronto, Ontario, Canada

    Consultant Director
    Dept. of Communication Disorders
    Surrey Place Centre
    Toronto, Ontario, Canada

Sandra Bond Chapman, Ph.D.
    Research Scientist
    Callier Center for Communication Disorders
    University of Texas at Dallas
    Dallas, Texas

Lynne W. Clark, Ph.D.
    Director, Communication Sciences Program
    Hunter College of City University of New York
    New York, New York

    Faculty Member
    Hunter/Mt. Sinai Geriatric Education Center
    New York, New York

Susan de Santi, M.S.
    Ph.D. Candidate
    Department of Communication Disorders
    City University of New York Graduate School
    New York, New York

    Speech Pathologist
    Queens College
    Queens, New York

Morris Freedman, B.Sc., M.D., FRCPC*
  Director Behavioral Neurology Program
  Staff Scientist Rotman Research Institute
  Baycrest Centre for Geriatric Care
  Toronto, Ontario, Canada

  Assistant Professor
  Faculty of Medicine
  Graduate Faculty, Institute of Medical Science
  University of Toronto
  Toronto, Ontario, Canada

  Staff Neurologist
  Staff Scientist at Mt. Sinai Research Institute
  Mt. Sinai Hospital
  Toronto, Ontario, Canada

  *Supported in part by a Career Scientist Award
  from the Ministry of Health of Ontario

Joan Goldberger, M.A.
  Speech-Language Pathologist
  Parker Jewish Geriatric Institute
  New Hyde Park, New York

Allison Grimes, M.A.
  Director of Audiological Services
  Hearing Society for the Bay Area, Inc.
  San Francisco, California

William C. Heindel, Ph.D.
  Post-Graduate Research Scientist
  Department of Neuroscience
  University of California School of Medicine
  San Diego, California

Daniel Kempler, Ph.D.
  Director of Speech Pathology
  Department of Otolaryngology
  School of Medicine
  University of Southern California
  Los Angeles, California

  Assistant Professor
  School of Medicine and
  Department of Gerontology
  University of Southern California
  Los Angeles, California

Laurie Nash Koury, M.A.
  Assistant Director and Coordinator of
  Adult Services
  Nashville Memorial Hospital
  Madison, Tennessee

Rosemary Lubinski, Ed.D.
  Associate Professor and Associate Chair
  Department of Communication Disorders and Sciences
  State University of New York at Buffalo
  Amherst, New York

D. William Molloy, M.B.
    Director of Memory Clinic and
    Director of Geriatric Consultation Services
    Henderson General Hospital
    Hamilton, Ontario, Canada

    Assistant Professor Department of Medicine and
    Director of Research Division of Geriatrics
    McMaster University
    Hamilton, Ontario, Canada

    Chairman, Health Choices for Seniors Committee
    Hamilton, Ontario, Canada

Loraine K. Obler, Ph.D.
    Professor, Department of Communication Disorders
    City University of New York Graduate School
    New York, New York

    Associate Research Professor in Neurolinguistics
    Boston University School of Medicine and
    Boston University Graduate School
    Boston, Massachusettes

Joseph B. Orange, M.H.Sc.
    Ph.D. Candidate
    Department of Communication Disorders and Sciences
    State University of New York at Buffalo
    Amherst, New York

Alicia Osimani, M.D.
    Behavioral Neurology Fellow
    Baycrest Centre for Geriatric Care
    Toronto, Ontario, Canada

    Assistant Professor of Neurology
    School of Medicine
    Neuropsychology Lecturer
    Psychology Department
    University of Ben Gurion
    Israel

    Visiting Assistant Professor
    Faculty of Medicine
    University of Toronto
    Toronto, Ontario, Canada

Marie T. Rau, M.D.
    Chief, Speech-Language Pathology Section
    Portland Veterans Medical Center
    Portland, Oregon

    Adjunct Assistant Professor
    Speech and Hearing Sciences
    Portland State University
    Portland, Oregon

    Adjunct Assistant Professor
    Speech and Hearing Department
    University of Oregon
    Portland, Oregon

Danielle Ripich, Ph.D.
    Chair and Associate Professor
    Department of Communication Sciences
    Case Western Reserve University
    Cleveland, Ohio

Ellen Bouchard Ryan, Ph.D.
    Professor of Psychiatry and
    Director of Gerontological Studies
    McMaster University
    Hamilton, Ontario, Canada

David P. Salmon, Ph.D.
    Assistant Professor
    Department of Neuroscience
    University of California School of Medicine
    San Diego, California

    Psychology Service
    San Diego Veterans Administration Center
    San Diego, California

Hanna K. Ulatowska, Ph.D.
    Professor
    Program in Communicative Disorders
    Callier Center for Communication Disorders
    University of Texas at Dallas
    Dallas, Texas

Barbara Weinstein, Ph.D.
    Associate Professor
    Speech and Hearing Center
    Lehman College, City University of New York
    New York, New York

    Faculty Member
    Hunter/Mt. Sinai Geriatric Education Center
    New York, New York

Kassie Witte, M.S.
    Director, Department of Speech Pathology and Audiology
    Hebrew Home for the Aged at Riverdale
    Bronx, New York

# *Preface*

When I was a child I wondered if Grandma was born old. I could not imagine her laughing, teasing, or being anyone's friend. My conception of her was of an old woman who spoke broken English and bound vinegar-soaked cabbage leaves around her head. I could not understand my mother's devotion to her because she wreaked such havoc on our family. There were the countless times she stood outside our back door and screamed untrue verbal abuses at my mother. So many nights were spent in vigils while Grandma prowled her house hiding things that she could not find the next morning. How did my mother balance family and career while meeting the constant demands of caring for Grandma? Why did she refuse other family members' solution of "putting Grandma away" when the alternative was her own physical and mental distress? Why did she encourage me to visit Grandma every evening and talk with her? Talking with Grandma was never easy but I realized that this was somehow significant to Grandma, Mom, and me.

Little did I realize that these experiences of a grammar-school child would generate my philosophy that communication with elderly individuals with dementia is important. Communicating with these individuals provides fertile research for better understanding the relationship between brain behavior and cognitive and communicative functioning. Verbal and nonverbal communication links us to the essence of a person's humanity. Each time we communicate with the elderly demented we are called upon to use all of our adaptive and creative skills. Although the communication of those with dementia stimulates many interesting and still unanswered questions for researchers, it represents repeated daily challenges for family and professional caregivers. Many times it seems easier avoiding talking than trying to understand and respond to the demented individual.

The purpose of this book is to provide a state-of-the-art perspective on dementia and communication. It derives from a humanistic philosophy that every person, even those with dementia, has social potential. The study of dementia and communication is at the point where aphasia research was a half century ago: Trying to understand the global nature and scope of the problem. Diagnostic methods and intervention strategies are just emerging. This book hopefully will be a seed that sprouts more questions, more alternatives, and more clinically driven research regarding dementia and communication.

The text is divided into four main sections. Section One, Bases for Communicative Changes in Dementia, focuses on the scope and definition of dementia and its physiologic, cognitive, auditory, and motor-speech characteristics. Section Two, Language Changes and Dementia, investigates the impact of aging and dementia on language and discourse abilities of those with dementia. Section Three, Social Impact of Dementia, explores the impact of dementia on the individual and caregivers. Section Four, Dementia: Diagnostic and Rehabilitative Considerations, provides a basic framework for professional services to demented individuals and their caregivers.

Each chapter has been written by a researcher or practicing clinician who has a special interest in dementia and communication. Each author defines the purposes of the chapter, provides definitions of the topic, expands on the topic, and provides clinical and research implications. Some chapters address dementia as a whole and several chapters focus specifically on Alzheimer's disease, the most common form of dementia affecting the older adult.

Perhaps after reading this text you will say "This is too much; there really isn't anything that can be done." Dementia will seem like an insurmountable slope that slides back with every step of progress. Let us as individuals and as a profession be defined not by the goals we have accomplished but by the challenges we try to meet.

ROSEMARY LUBINSKI, Ed.D.

# *Acknowledgments*

This manuscript was prepared with the generous, diligent, and continuing efforts of numerous individuals. The text was inspired by a Conference held at the State University of New York at Buffalo in March, 1989, sponsored by the Department of Communication Disorders, the Dean of Social Sciences, the Alzheimer's Disease Assistance Center, the Western New York Geriatric Center, and Conferences in the Disciplines. I am particularly grateful to Dr. Donald Henderson, Chair, Department of Communication Disorders for his encouragement, assistance, and financial support of the conference, to Dr. Ross McKinnon, Dean and to Dr. Arthur Cryns, all of the State University of New York at Buffalo, and Dr. John Edwards, of the Western New York Geriatric Center for their financial support of the conference.

I also wish to extend my deepest gratitude to the three associate editors who helped with the reading and editing of the manuscripts: Dr. Donald Henderson for his incisive comments, Mr. Joseph B. Orange for his fastidious reading and organization skills, and Dr. Nancy Stecker for her careful reading of the audiology chapters.

To each of the authors I offer my sincerest thanks for giving their knowledge, skill, patience, and time when preparing their manuscripts. Despite demanding schedules and often grave personal crises, each author gave his or her best to the book.

Special thanks to Dr. Kathryn Bayles of the University of Arizona, for offering her comments in the Foreword. Her scholarship has been an inspiration for this book.

Appreciation is also presented to several individuals for their critical reading of manuscripts: Dr. Elaine Stathopolous and Dr. Joan Sussman of the University of Buffalo and Dr. Deanie Vogel of the Reno, Nevada, Veterans Administration Hospital.

I am also deeply indebted to Mrs. Sandra Mundier and Mrs. Delores Sciandra of the Department of Communication Disorders at the University of Buffalo for all the personal assistance and support they so generously offered me throughout the conference and book preparation.

Thanks also to Kimberly A. LoDico and the staff at B.C. Decker for their editorial assistance.

Sincere thanks to Halli Lind, who volunteered to help with library work.

Kudos go to my student, Carolyne Simpson, who typed, retyped, alphabetized, numbered, inserted, deleted, xeroxed, and even learned new word processing programs to help me.

Finally, sincerest thanks to my father, Leo, who encouraged me every day along the way.

A number of authors wish to offer their appreciation to those who helped in the preparation of their chapters.

Dr. Loraine Obler, Ms. Susan de Santi, and Ms. Joan Goldberger offer their thanks to Helene Sabo-Abramson for testing subjects in Yiddish and for help in analysis of data. Their thanks are also given to the Parker Jewish Geriatric Institute for their help in carrying out this project. Their chapter was supported in part by grants (#6-67453) and (#6-66213) from the City University of New York Research Foundation and by the Veterans Administration grant 001 "Language in the Aging Brain."

Mr. J.B. Orange acknowledges those individuals with dementia of the Alzheimer's type who were recruited for his study from the practices of Dr. Lawrence Jacobs, of the Dent Neurological Institute affiliated with Millard Fillmore Hospital, Buffalo, New York and Dr. William Molloy and Linda Reese of the Henderson Hospital, Hamilton, Ontario. Their contributions to this study are most gratefully acknowledged. The assistance of Wenfan Yan is also deeply appreciated.

Dr. Alicia Osimani and Dr. Morris Freedman gratefully acknowledge Dr. Edith Kaplan for her helpful advice and suggestions for the preparation of this manuscript, and Vicki Giardino for secretarial assistance.

Dr. Danielle Ripich wishes to acknowledge the contribution of Colleen Visconti in the preparation of her manuscript.

Dr. David Salmon, Dr. Nelson Butters, and Dr. William Heindel are grateful for the funds received from the Medical Research Service of the Veterans Administration and by NIA grant AG-05131 to the University of California at San Diego.

Dr. Hanna Ulatowska and Dr. Sandra Chapman wish to express their appreciation to Dr. Myron Weiner and Mrs. Doris Svetlick from the Alzheimer's Unit at the Southwestern Medical School, to Mrs. Mary Link from the Dallas Chapter of the National Alzheimer's Association for their help in selecting patients for the study, to Dr. James Bartlett for his valuable help in designing the experiment, to graduate students Jean Ford, Belinda Reyes, Sue Byrd, Jill Williams, Jeyashree Venkatesan, and Dr. Mari Hayashi in data analysis, to speech pathologists Kathryn Schopfer, Margaret Carlisle, Pam Hughes, and Laurie Long from the Baylor Rehabilitation Center for their assistance in rating subjects' language, and to all their subjects for their time and willingness to participate in the study.

# *Foreword*

In the last decade, Alzheimer's disease has emerged from obscurity. Today, it is widely known and much discussed among professional and lay persons. Because Alzheimer's disease is associated with older age, and the elderly are the fastest growing population segment, care of the Alzheimer's patient is the greatest new challenge facing health professionals. Information is needed to educate practitioners about the neurobehavioral consequences of Alzheimer's and other age-related dementing diseases. Little, if any, information on the dementia patient was included in the curriculum for most clinicians. This need for education has been recognized and competently addressed by Dr. Rosemary Lubinski and the other distinguished contributors to this book. Under Dr. Lubinski's leadership, a conference was held that brought together experts from numerous disciplines whose presentations formed the basis of the chapters of this book. The result for the reader is state-of-the-art information on the epidemiology, neurology, neuropsychology, and neurolinguistics of dementia.

Emphasized in this book is the neurobehavioral deficit of communicative impairment. Particularly noteworthy is the editor's effort to give it context. To that end, chapters are included on the functional anatomy and cognitive characteristics of the demented. Practitioners not only will learn the characteristic communication deficits of dementia patients, they also will come to appreciate their cause.

*Dementia and Communication* offers the reader more than a description of the neurobehavioral deficits of demented individuals; also included are sections on diagnostic and intervention strategies in both audiology and speech language pathology and the impact of dementia on the family. Procedures are suggested for maximizing the functional communication skills of these patients during the various stages of dementia. Techniques are described for helping families cope with the exigencies of caregiving. Then, too, suggestions are made about conducting in-service training for staff members. This interdisciplinary and clinically oriented book is comprehensive in its discussion of dementia and the information contained within it is carefully documented. The integration of information from many disciplines is hard to find in a single volume. For all of these reasons, it will be of monumental assistance to health professionals preparing to meet the challenge of caring for the dementia patient.

KATHRYN A. BAYLES, Ph.D.
*University of Arizona*
*Tucson, Arizona*

# Contents

| | | |
|---|---|---|
| SECTION ONE | **Bases for Communicative Changes in Dementia** | |
| CHAPTER 1 | Dementia: Impact and Clinical Perspectives .......................... 2<br>D. WILLIAM MOLLOY and ROSEMARY LUBINSKI | |
| CHAPTER 2 | Functional Anatomy ....................................................... 22<br>ALICIA OSIMANI and MORRIS FREEDMAN | |
| CHAPTER 3 | Patterns of Cognitive Impairment in Alzheimer's Disease<br>and Other Dementing Disorders ...................................... 37<br>DAVID P. SALMON, WILLIAM C. HEINDEL, and NELSON BUTTERS | |
| CHAPTER 4 | Auditory Changes ......................................................... 47<br>ALISON M. GRIMES | |
| CHAPTER 5 | Motor Speech Changes .................................................. 70<br>IRENE CAMPBELL-TAYLOR | |
| SECTION TWO | **Language Changes and Dementia** | |
| CHAPTER 6 | Normal Aging and Language .......................................... 84<br>ELLEN BOUCHARD RYAN | |
| CHAPTER 7 | Language Changes in Dementia of the Alzheimer Type ......... 98<br>DANIEL KEMPLER | |
| CHAPTER 8 | Discourse Studies ........................................................ 115<br>HANNA K. ULATOWSKA and SANDRA BOND CHAPMAN | |
| CHAPTER 9 | Bilingual Dementia: Pragmatic Breakdown ....................... 133<br>LORAINE K. OBLER, SUSAN de SANTI, and JOAN GOLDBERGER | |
| SECTION THREE | **Social Impact of Dementia** | |
| CHAPTER 10 | Learned Helplessness: Application to Communication<br>of the Elderly ........................................................... 142<br>ROSEMARY LUBINSKI | |
| CHAPTER 11 | Impact on Families ..................................................... 152<br>MARIE T. RAU | |
| CHAPTER 12 | Perspectives of Family Members Regarding Communication<br>Changes .................................................................. 168<br>JOSEPH B. ORANGE | |

## SECTION FOUR  Dementia: Diagnostic and Rehabilitative Considerations

**CHAPTER 13**  Differential Diagnosis and Assessment .............................. 188
DANIELLE N. RIPICH

**CHAPTER 14**  Auditory Testing and Rehabilitation of the
Hearing Impaired ....................................................... 223
BARBARA E. WEINSTEIN

**CHAPTER 15**  Nature and Efficacy of Communication Management
in Alzheimer's Disease ................................................. 238
LYNNE W. CLARK and KASSIE WITTE

**CHAPTER 16**  Environmental Considerations for Elderly Patients ................ 257
ROSEMARY LUBINSKI

**CHAPTER 17**  Effective In-Service Training for Staff Working with
Communication-Impaired Patients ................................... 279
LAURIE NASH KOURY and ROSEMARY LUBINSKI

# SECTION ONE

*Bases for Communicative Changes in Dementia*

# CHAPTER 1

# Dementia: Impact and Clinical Perspectives

### D. WILLIAM MOLLOY, M.B.
### ROSEMARY LUBINSKI, Ed.D.

The passage of Public Law 101-58 by the United States Congress launched the 1990s as the "Decade of the Brain." This legislation was aimed at increasing awareness of the need for basic and applied research into brain-related diseases and disorders, including dementia. In fact, dementia is emerging as a major public-health concern,[130] and is gaining increasing importance as the population ages. Although the primary impact is on the affected individual and family caregivers, dementia also places a large burden on society in terms of health care, disability, hospital and institutional care, and premature death. *Newsweek* magazine in 1984 labeled Alzheimer's disease, the most common form of dementia in the elderly, the "disease of the century."[21] The cover story of the December, 1989 issue of *Newsweek* again brought to the attention of the American public the enormous and multifaceted impact of Alzheimer's disease.[39]

One reason that dementia stands out as a major health and societal problem is the increasing number of older individuals in developed, industrialized nations such as Canada, the United States, and European countries. Cross and Gurland estimate that 2 to 4 million Americans suffer from dementia, and the number of cases is expected to increase dramatically as the population ages.[24] Changes in fertility, mortality, migration, and life expectancy in this century have resulted in both aging of the population and an increasing proportion of elderly in the general population.[138] Interestingly, while in 1985 those over 65 years of age constituted 12 percent of the United States population, this proportion will nearly double by 2050 to 21.7 percent.[138] The number of very old (over 85 years) is the fastest growing cohort of the elderly.[3,14,138] Further, the prevalence of one form of dementia, Alzheimer's disease, among the elderly has been estimated to be as much as 10.3 percent overall, increasing to 47.2 percent for those over age 85.[36] Thus, the problem of dementia in terms of individuals affected is enormous, and unless preventive measures are discovered and implemented, it will grow significantly. (The issues of incidence, prevalence, and cost of dementia are discussed in more detail later in this chapter.)

The increasing number of older persons with dementia does little to console the affected individuals or their families. Dementia represents a personal catastrophe to the affected individual and to family members through the eventual loss of quality interaction, the increasing demands for full-time personal care, and the multiplying financial, physical, and psychological burdens. Caring for an individual with dementia is enormously time consuming and continuously stressful for older spouses who are already burdened with their own health problems and age-related concerns. Adult children are often ensnared in a labyrinth of conflicting parental, child, professional, and personal needs.

Those with dementia are caught in the "contradictory goals of American health policy—high quality care and cost containment.[138] If we are to cope effectively and humanely with the huge strain that dementia places on our health-care resources, it is essential that empirically based investigations discover the causes of these disorders so that prevention is possible or techniques are developed to improve or maintain function. The immediate goal is, however, to provide accessible community-based health and personal-care programs that support patients and family caregivers while forestalling financially and personally costly long-term institutionalization. A secondary goal is to better understand the role of communication in the problem of dementia and to develop techniques to enhance effective communication in the home and institutional settings.

This chapter provides an overview of dementia and focuses on communication. The chapter discusses the definition, prevalence, etiology, current diagnostic and management options, public-policy issues, and research needs in dementia. This discussion is not intended to replace in-depth reviews of dementia such as those by Bayles and Kazniak,[9] Cummings and Benson,[27] Cummings and Miller,[29] Heston and White,[52] Jarvik,[60] Mayeux and Rosen,[82] Reisberg,[111] and numerous others. The reader is also referred to the annotated bibliography in *Differential Diagnosis of Alzheimer's and Other Dementing Diseases* prepared by the National Library of Medicine[97] and *Health of an Aging America: 1989 Bibliography*.[127] This chapter aims to give the reader a basic introduction to dementia and to provide references for more extensive reading.

## Definition of Dementia

Dementia is a common clinical syndrome characterized by a decline in cognitive function and memory from previously attained intellectual levels, which is sustained over a period of months or years. The deterioration is of such severity that it impairs the affected individual's ability to work and to perform activities of daily living, including communication. Cummings and Benson state that at least three of the following five areas of mental activity must be involved: (1) language; (2) memory; (3) visuospatial skills; (4) emotion or personality; and (5) cognition (e.g., abstraction, calculation, and judgment).[27]

Dementia is an umbrella term that encompasses many distinct subtypes. Table 1.1 shows that there are least 11 principal dementia syndromes: (1) degenerative disorders; (2) vascular dementia syndromes; (3) myelinoclastic disorders; (4) traumatic conditions; (5) neoplastic dementias; (6) hydrocephalic dementias: (7) inflammatory conditions; (8) infection-related dementias; (9) toxic conditions; (10) metabolic disorders; and (11) psychiatric disorders. These categories can be further subdivided into dozens of specific types. See Kiloh for further description of secondary dementias of middle and later life.[73]

It is estimated that 10 to 15 percent (and perhaps as much as 30 percent) of those with dementia have a form that is reversible or improves with treatment.[18,76] Clarfield, in a review of 34 studies (2,889 subjects), concluded that the true incidence of reversible dementias may be 11 percent (8 percent partly reversed and 3 percent fully reversed).[20] He also states that the 11 percent may be a significant overestimate. Larson et al question the whole category of reversible dementias.[76] They concluded from their study of 15 persons with "reversible dementia" that most do not reverse to normal and may continue to develop dementia symptoms, and those who showed transient improvement may not have been accurately identified. Regardless of the differences in percent of individuals who have reversible dementia, what is important is that some individuals may have symptoms amenable to treatment and some may have compounding factors such as hearing or visual difficulties that make accurate identification difficult. A second critical issue is how reversible forms are managed and whether there is relapse.[20]

Bayles and Kazniak propose that one way to distinguish many reversible from irreversible dementias is whether the cognitive deterioration has a structural basis.[9] Larson et al identified three criteria that differentiate those with a reversible dementia, shorter duration of symptoms, less severe dementia, and more frequent use of prescription drugs.[76]

The most commonly given forms of reversible dementia include those related to drugs, depression, metabolic disorders, normal-pressure hydrocephalus, subdural hematoma, and neoplasm.[20] Cummings and Benson add other categories to this list including dementias related to toxic factors, infections, inflammation, Wilson's disease, Parkinson's disease, and multi-infarct dementia.[27]

Two forms of dementia deserve special description here because of their high prevalence among the elderly: Alzheimer's disease and multi-infarct dementia. In a recent study regarding the prevalence of dementia in the community, Evans et al found that Alzheimer's disease and multi-infarct dementia accounted for the vast majority of the cases of dementia.[36] Further, AIDS (acquired immunodeficiency syndrome) deserves special attention as a possible cause of dementia because of its increasing prevalence in the population and its high association with cognitive impairment. References such as those by Cummings and Benson[27,28] and Mayeux and Rosen[82] give more complete descriptions of etiology and symptomatology of a wide variety of dementia types.

## ALZHEIMER'S DISEASE

The most common form of irreversible dementia is Alzheimer's disease (DAT), which has in many respects become synonymous with the broad category of dementia. Cummings estimated that DAT constitutes 25 to 35 percent of all dementia and up to 50 percent of chronic progressive dementias.[25] To help with the difficulties of differential diagnosis, a work group was formed by the National Institute of Neurological and Communicative Disorders and Stroke (NINCDS) and the Alzheimer's Disease and Related Disorders Association

### TABLE 1.1 Etiologic Classification of the Principal Dementia Syndromes

| | |
|---|---|
| Degenerative Disorders | Inflammatory Conditions |
|   Cortical |   Systemic lupus erythematosus |
|     Alzheimer's disease |   Temporal arteritis |
|     Pick's disease |   Sarcoidosis |
|   Subcortical |   Granulomatous arteritis |
|     Parkinson's disease | Infection-Related Dementias |
|     Huntington's chorea |   Syphilis |
|     Progressive supranuclear palsy |   Chronic meningitis |
|     Spinocerebellar degenerations |   Postencephalitic dementia syndrome |
|     Idiopathic basal ganglia calcification |   Whipple's disease |
|     Striatonigral degeneration |   Acquired immunodeficiency syndrome (AIDS) |
|     Wilson's disease |   Creutzfeldt-Jakob disease |
|     Thalamic dementia |   Subacute sclerosing panencephalitis |
| Vascular Dementias |   Progressive multifocal leukoencephalopathy |
|   Multiple large-vessel occlusions | Toxic Conditions |
|   Lacunar state (multiple subcortical infarctions) |   Alcohol-related syndrome |
|   Binswanger's disease (white matter ischemic injury) |   Polydrug abuse |
|   Mixed cortical and subcortical infarctions |   Iatrogenic dementias |
| Myelinoclastic Disorders |     Anticholinergic agents |
|   Demyelinating |     Antihypertensive drugs |
|     Multiple sclerosis |     Psychotropic agents |
|     Marchiafava-Bignami disease |     Anticonvulsant agents |
|   Dysmyelinating |     Miscellaneous agents |
|     Metachromatic leukodystrophy |   Metals |
|     Adrenoleukodystrophy |   Industrial solvents |
|     Cerebrotendinous xanthomatosis | Metabolic Disorders |
| Traumatic Conditions |   Cardiopulmonary failure |
|   Posttraumatic encephalopathy |   Uremia |
|   Subdural hematoma |   Hepatic encephalopathy |
|   Dementia pugilistica |   Endocrine disorders |
| Neoplastic Dementias |     Thyroid |
|   Meningioma (particularly subfrontal) |     Adrenal |
|   Glioma |     Parathyroid |
|   Metastatic deposits |   Anemia and hematologic conditions |
|   Meningeal carcinomatosis |   Deficiency states (vitamin $B_{12}$, folate) |
| Hydrocephalic Dementias |   Porphyria |
|   Communicating | Psychiatric Disorders |
|     Normal pressure hydrocephalus |   Depression |
|   Noncommunicating |   Mania |
|     Aqueductal stenosis |   Schizophrenia |
|     Intraventricular neoplasm | |
|     Intraventricular cyst | |
|     Basilar meningitis | |

From Cummings JL. Dementia syndromes: Neurobehavioral and neuropsychiatric features. J Clin Psychiatry 1987; 48:3-8. Copyright 1987, Physicians Postgraduate Press.

(ADRDA) to propose uniform clinical criteria for the diagnosis of DAT.[86] This set of criteria expanded on those described in the 1980 Diagnostic and Statistical Manual of Mental Disorders (DSM-III). Table 1.2 presents the clinical criteria for probable, possible, and definite Alzheimer's disease developed by the NINCDS-ADRDA Work Group.[86]

In a review of diagnostic issues and DAT, Katzman states that diagnostic accuracy of DAT has improved from a 10 to 50 percent error rate to a 90 percent assurance of accuracy.[66] Cummings cautions that despite this high rate of accuracy the category of those inaccurately identified is especially important in designing and interpreting treatment studies.[29]

### Symptomatology

The major clinical features associated with DAT include severe memory deficits.[9,27] Cummings describes memory impairment as essential for the diagnosis of DAT and the most commonly recognized symptom.[26] Bayles and Kazniak state that the memory changes associated with DAT are different from those of normal aging.[9] They found that both episodic and semantic memory are compromised. In addition DAT patients have difficulty with delayed and immediate recall of information. These memory difficulties manifest themselves in difficulties with orientation to time, place, and person as well as difficulty in learning and retaining new material.

TABLE 1.2 **Criteria for Clinical Diagnosis of Alzheimer's Disease**

I. The criteria for the clinical diagnosis of PROBABLE Alzheimer's disease include:

dementia established by clinical examination and documented by the Mini-Mental Test, Blessed Dementia Scale, or some similar examination, and confirmed by neuropsychological tests;

deficits in two or more areas of cognition;

progressive worsening of memory and other cognitive functions;

no disturbance of consciousness;

onset between ages 40 and 90, most often after age 65; and

absence of systemic disorders or other brain diseases that in and of themselves could account for the progressive deficits in memory and cognition.

II. The diagnosis of PROBABLE Alzheimer's disease is supported by:

progressive deterioration of specific cognitive functions such as language (aphasia), motor skills (apraxia), and perception (agnosia);

impaired activities of daily living and altered patterns of behavior;

family history of similar disorders, particularly if confirmed neuropathologically; and

laboratory results of:

normal lumbar puncture as evaluated by standard techniques,

normal pattern or nonspecific changes in EEG, such as increased slow-wave activity, and

evidence of cerebral atrophy on CT with progression documented by serial observation.

III. Other clinical features consistent with the diagnosis of PROBABLE Alzheimer's disease, after exclusion of causes of dementia other than Alzheimer's disease, include:

plateaus in the course of progression of the illness;

associated symptoms of depression, insomnia, incontinence, delusions, illusions, hallucinations, catastrophic verbal, emotional, or physical outbursts, sexual disorders, and weight loss;

other neurologic abnormalities in some patients, especially with more advanced disease and including motor signs such as increased muscle tone, myoclonus, or gait disorder;

seizures in advanced disease; and

CT normal for age.

IV. Features that make the diagnosis of PROBABLE Alzheimer's disease uncertain or unlikely include:

sudden, apoplectic onset;

focal neurologic findings such as hemiparesis, sensory loss, visual field deficits, and incoordination early in the course of the illness; and

seizures or gait disturbances at the onset or very early in the course of the illness.

V. Clinical diagnosis of POSSIBLE Alzheimer's disease

may be made on the basis of the dementia syndrome, in the absence of other neurologic, psychiatric, or systemic disorders sufficient to cause dementia, and in the presence of variations in the onset, in the presentation, or in the clinical course;

may be made in the presence of a second systemic or brain disorder sufficient to produce dementia, which is not considered to be the cause of the dementia; and

should be used in research studies when a single, gradually progressive severe cognitive deficit is identified in the absence of other identifiable cause.

VI. Criteria for diagnosis of DEFINITE Alzheimer's disease are:

the clinical criteria for probable Alzheimer's disease and

histopathologic evidence obtained from a biopsy or autopsy.

VII. Classification of Alzheimer's disease for research purposes should specify features that may differentiate subtypes of the disorder, such as:

familial occurrence;

onset before age of 65;

presence of trisomy-21; and

coexistence of other relevant conditions such as Parkinson's disease.

From McKhann G, Drachman D, Folstein M, et al. Clinical diagnosis of Alzheimer's disease: Report of the NINCDS-ADRDA work group under the auspices of Department of Health and Human Services Task force on Alzheimer's disease. Neurology 1984; 34:939–944.

Another major clinical feature of DAT is impairment in communication.[4,9,27,34,49,79,100,101,125] This awareness that language and communication are disturbed in DAT is relatively recent and has spurred a controversy as to the relationship of language changes in dementia versus those observed in the classic aphasia syndromes. This text helps to highlight the scope of auditory and expressive difficulties associated with dementia in general and Alzheimer's disease in particular.

Other symptoms of DAT include difficulties in the following: visuospatial skills, such as wayfinding problems; cognition, including calculation and abstraction; motor systems and neuropsychiatric or personality dysfunctions. Bayles and Kazniak provide an excellent description of cognitive and perceptual disruptions in DAT.[9]

Research reveals a wide variety of behavioral symptomatology associated with DAT. Reisberg et al, in a study of 57 outpatients diagnosed with

DAT, found that 58 percent had significant behavioral symptomatology.[113] Major behavioral disorders include: delusions (particularly of someone stealing), agitation, diurnal rhythm disturbances, motor restlessness, violence, emotional lability symptoms, suspiciousness, and hallucinations.[112,113] Similarly, Merriam et al, in an interview study of caregivers of 195 community-dwelling DAT patients, found that symptoms of depression were "virtually ubiquitous" in their population.[87] Major psychiatric disorders included dysphoria, psychomotor dysregulation (agitation), perceptual symptoms (e.g., hallucinations), and paranoia. Finally, Teri et al documented that the number of behavioral problems increased with deterioration in cognitive ability and that the types of problems varied with cognitive severity.[123]

An increasing body of research proposes that Alzheimer's disease itself is not a unitary disorder but may rather be a heterogeneous disease grouping. Mayeux, Stern, and Spanton, in a study of the records of 121 consecutive patients with DAT, found that four groups of patients could be differentiated: (1) a benign group with little or no disease progression; (2) those with myoclonus who had severe intellectual decline, frequent mutism, and younger age at onset; (3) those with extrapyramidal symptoms who showed severe intellectual and functional decline as well as psychotic symptoms; and (4) a typical group that showed gradual progression of intellectual and functional decline but without other distinguishing features.[83] Metter states that positron emission tomographic studies suggest a metabolic heterogeneity in Alzheimer's patients.[88] Jorm discusses the possibility of subtypes of DAT based on differences in the neurochemical, neuropathologic, and clinical features of the disorder as a function of age at onset.[62,63] He proposes that rather than subtypes there may be a continuous gradation of types.

## MULTI-INFARCT DEMENTIA

A second common cause of dementia among the elderly is associated with multiple infarcts. Once known as dementia associated with "hardening of the arteries," this type of dementia is caused by multiple cerebral infarctions at both cortical and subcortical levels.[27] Diseases of the extracranial arteries and the heart, particularly hypertension, may cause multiple large and small strokes resulting in this type of dementia.[47] Cummings and Benson list over 20 specific etiologies of multi-infarct dementia, including several meningovascular infections.[27]

The major symptoms of multi-infarct dementia include "abrupt onset, stepwise deterioration, fluctuating course, nocturnal confusion, relative preservation of personality, depression, somatic complaints, emotional lability, history of hypertension and strokes, atherosclerosis, and focal neurological symptoms and signs."[27] Hachinski et al specified such symptoms as slowness, weakness, dysarthria, dysphagia, and pathologic laughing and crying. Three major subgroups of multi-infarct patients have been identified based on the area of the vascular system involved: those with deep hemispheric infarctions, those with superficial infarctions, and those with combined deep and superficial infarctions.[27,117]

## AIDS DEMENTIA COMPLEX

Although not associated with the elderly, discussion of the AIDS dementia complex is timely. One of the numerous sequelae of AIDS is dementia. In a retrospective study of 70 autopsied AIDS patients, aged 29 to 40 years, 46 revealed progressive dementia accompanied by motor and behavioral disorders.[99] Navia et al found that the dementia was characterized in early stages by memory difficulties, attention problems with conversation or written language, mental slowness necessitating additional time for formulation of responses, and spatial and temporal disorientation.[99] Motor symptoms included progressive loss of balance, leg weakness, and deterioration in handwriting. Behavioral changes such as apathy, social withdrawal, and decrease in verbalization were also common. In the later stages, patients showed global cognitive decline, severe motor abnormalities including severe ataxia, hypertonia, incontinence, leg weakness, and a confused, indifferent state. Navia et al noted that the AIDS dementia complex was the only presenting sign of overt AIDS in 25 percent of their sample.[99] The presence of intellectual, verbal, communication, and motor changes may be important clinical signs in the early diagnosis of the disorder. The symptoms appear to resemble subcortical dementias in the early stages and cortical dementias in the later stages.

# Definition of Prevalence and Incidence

Prevalence refers to the number of cases of a disease that exist at a specified instant in time or during some period of time. Incidence refers to the number of new cases of the disease that develop during some specified time interval. Incidence data require documentation of onset and longitudinal follow-up. Collecting and interpreting prevalence and incidence data on dementia are complicated by numerous factors: e.g. (1) difficulty in defining the target disorder and differentiating it from similar disorders; (2) extent and reliability of testing methodology; (3) co-existence of two types of dementia; (4) variability in diagnostic criteria for various disorders; (5) problems in identification of early cases; (6) difficulty in following cases over time; (7) participation rate; (8) sampling bias of urban versus rural populations; (9) age, sex, and racial differences of study populations; and (10) complication of other physical, sensory, and psychological disorders. In addition, prevalence for institutional- versus community-based individuals shows vast differences in number of individuals affected.

## PREVALENCE

The latest prevalence study on Alzheimer's disease in the community was conducted on 3,623 persons over age 65 years in a geographically defined United States community of East Boston, Massachusetts. Results indicate that the prevalence of this disorder may be far greater than previously reported.[36] Evans et al found that of those 65 to 74 years of age and older 10.3 percent had probable Alzheimer's disease.[36] The prevalence rose to 18.7 percent for those 75 to 84 years and to 47.2 percent for those over 85 years of age. They reported that Alzheimer's disease accounted for 84.1 percent of the cases of dementia, with multi-infarct dementia being the only other common cause. Further, they estimated that of those with Alzheimer's disease, 23 percent had mild, 51 percent had moderate, and 26 percent had severe cognitive impairment. A second recent study of community-dwelling seniors in Rochester, Minnesota yielded a prevalence rate of 3.5 percent for dementia.[74]

Similarly, the results of the Baltimore Longitudinal Study conducted by the Gerontology Research Center, National Institute of Aging, found that estimated prevalence of DAT was higher than expected from previous studies and that this prevalence increased at the alarming rate of a "hundred fold between the ages 60 and 100."[120] This study found that prevalence at age 95 was over 50 percent.

Previous studies such as those by Pfeffer estimated that prevalence of DAT for white, elderly individuals over 65 years of age was about 11.2 percent.[104] Mowry and Burvill, in a study of a random sample of community individuals aged 70 and older in Perth, Australia, found that 25 percent of the elderly had mild dementia.[94] Schoenberg et al found severe dementia among various racial groups in Mississippi and reported that 1 percent of those aged 40 demonstrated severe dementia, while 7 percent of those over 80 were severely demented.[121]

Close to two-thirds of nursing home patients are labeled demented.[129] Katzman, in a survey of a 500-bed geriatric nursing home in New York City, reported that 65 percent of the patients met the clinical and mental status for dementia.[66] He also found pathologic evidence for Alzheimer's disease in 55 percent of 100 consecutive autopsies performed.

Finally, Rocca et al predicted a major increase in prevalence of dementia in three countries: Italy, with an increase of 40 percent; the United States, with an increase of 42 percent; and Japan, with an increase of 76.6 percent.[116]

## INCIDENCE

Studies regarding the incidence of dementia are not as numerous as are those regarding the prevalence of the disorder, because of the need for follow-up studies and careful medical review.[9] The Baltimore Longitudinal Study estimated that the incidence of DAT at age 60 years was less than 1 per 1,000 cases and reached 54 per 1,000 cases by age 90.[120] Rocca et al reviewed various international studies on incidence and reported a range of incidences for DAT in those above age 60 from 0.74 to 5.8 percent.[116] They summarized their epidemiologic review by stating that there will be an "exponential" increase in the incidence of DAT with age and the higher overall rate in females. Gelman et al mirror that prediction by stating that there will be 14 million adults in America affected by Alzheimer's disease by the year 2050.[39]

## Mortality and Dementia

It is difficult to establish accurate mortality data for dementia, or DAT in particular, because these are not listed on death certificates as a cause of death.[116] Katzman states, however, that individuals with DAT show a marked decrease in life expectancy, related to age of onset.[67] In a review of European and United States epidemiologic studies on mortality, Hay and Ernst found that the average survival time for patients with DAT ranged from 5 to 10 years from the date of onset.[49] They also noted that when measured from the date of diagnosis, the average survival time was about 3 to 4 years. Women with DAT appeared to live about 2 years longer than men. These data indicate that symptoms may be present several years prior to actual diagnosis.

Belloni-Sonzogni et al studied 237 patients with DAT and multi-infarct dementia in a large nursing home in Milan, Italy.[10] After 4 years, 77.2 percent of the patients were dead. The primary predictors of mortality were age, level of autonomy, and type of diagnosis. The mortality rate for those with DAT was significantly higher (86.9 percent) than for those with multi-infarct dementia (57.1 percent). This study raises interesting questions regarding when patients with various dementia types are institutionalized, the severity of their disabilities, and possible referral bias of physicians.

## Overview

Several trends emerge from these epidemiologic studies. First, with age there is an increased likelihood that an individual will incur some form of dementia. Second, as increasing numbers of the population age, there will be more individuals exhibiting dementia. Third, women appear to be more likely to acquire DAT. Fourth, although there are many individuals with dementia being cared for in the community, at least half, if not more, of those in nursing homes have dementia. Fifth, most epidemiologic studies accent the present and future magnitude of the problem on health-care delivery and research priorities.[104] The economic and personal costs of dementia are discussed later in this chapter with regard to public policy and health care.

## Etiology and Risk Factors

Although several hypotheses have been suggested regarding the etiology of Alzheimer's disease and other dementias, the precise cause or complex of causes are unknown. De Estable-Puig et al state that the "mechanisms responsible for the morphologic and biochemical changes" have yet to be identified.[32] At least nine etiologic factors have been implicated: (1) neurotransmitter and neurotopic hormone deficiencies; (2) effects of viruses; (3) toxins or protein factors; (4) disturbances in metal-ion concentrations; (5) alterations in blood-brain barrier; (6) immunologic dysfunction; (7) chromosomal abnormalities; (8) genetic predisposition; and (9) factors associated with advancing chronologic age.[32] Whether these changes contribute to the dementing process, or are epiphenomena associated with dementia, is unclear at this time.

This chapter discusses the etiology and risk factors for the two most common dementias: Alzheimer's disease and multi-infarct dementia. Some suggested references for more in-depth reading on etiologic factors include Cummings and Benson and De Estable-Puig et al.[27,32]

## ETIOLOGY OF ALZHEIMER'S DISEASE

Jorm stated that the etiology of DAT is likely to be "multifactoral" rather than associated with a single cause.[62] To date, no single cause (other than possibly advancing age) has been identified, although a number of etiologies have been suggested including the genetic, toxic-exposure, environmental, biochemical, immunologic, and nutritional hypotheses. Studies of family histories suggest that there may be a genetic component in the etiology of some cases of DAT.[68] In particular, the studies of Down's syndrome and DAT indicate a genetic relationship through chromosome 21. Toxic substances have also been implicated including aluminum[62] and silicon.[66] Whalley and Halloway found that exposure to an unidentified toxic agent in certain areas of Edinburgh, Scotland appeared to increase the occurrence of Alzheimer's disease.[132] Slow viruses such as Kuru and Creutzfeldt-Jakob disease have also been implicated in DAT, as have abnormal immune reactions. Some of the most plausible etiologic factors pertain to the deficits in neurotransmitters and modulators. Katzman reported from a review of studies that there was a 40 to 90 percent decrease in the biosynthetic enzyme choline acetyltransferase in the cerebral cortex and hippocampus.[66] This theory has led to the development of pharmacologic substitution therapy for the cholinergic deficit. (Drug therapy is discussed later in the chapter.)

## PATHOPHYSIOLOGY OF ALZHEIMER'S DISEASE

Katzman summarized the pathophysiologic changes in the brains of those with DAT as evidencing cortical atrophy, loss of neurons, and neurofibrillary tangles and neuritic plaques.[66] In addition, there has been noted the "presence of cerebrovascular amyloid in the blood vessels of the meninges, cerebral cortex, and hippocampus." De Estable-Puig et al summarized the pathologic changes in dementia as including: " (1) cerebral atrophy; (2) ventricular dilation; (3) neuronal degeneration; (4) degenerating neuronal processes; (5) senile plaques; (6) neurofibrillary changes; (7) microangiopathy; (8) Simchovicz granulo vacuolar degeneration; (9) Hirano bodies; (10) sponginess; and (11) white matter alterations."[32] Most of the brain atrophy takes place in the mid-frontal areas of the brain, the gyri of the parietal-temporal association areas of the cerebral cortex, the hippocampus, and the substantia innominata.[66,77,124] Because of the consistent changes in the hippocampus of DAT patients, Ball et al proposed that Alzheimer's disease be called hippocampal dementia.[6] More recently, the olfactory bulb has been implicated as a site of changes in DAT.[35]

## RISK FACTORS FOR ALZHEIMER'S DISEASE

Jorm stated that there are five confirmed risk factors for Alzheimer's disease: old age, family history, Down's syndrome, a family history of Down's syndrome, and head trauma.[62] Another factor that has been implicated but not confirmed as a risk factor is advanced age of the mother at subject's birth.[2,62] Epidemiologic studies clearly show that Alzheimer's disease increases with age through the eighth decade but may show a leveling off in the ninth decade.[62]

Concerning family relationship, Heston et al found that the risk of DAT to parents and siblings of those with DAT was in the range of 10 to 23 percent.[50,51] Early onset (40 to 50 years of age) of DAT appears to increase the risk factor for siblings to 40 percent. Further, autopsy studies of those with Down's syndrome revealed the presence of plaques and tangles. Heston and Morris predict that there is a 100 percent risk of DAT in older Down's cases.[51] Further, they found that persons with Down's evidenced pathologic changes at a younger age than normals. Several studies show that Down's syndrome appears more common than expected among families of individuals with DAT.[53,54]

A number of studies have strongly implicated head injury as a risk factor for Alzheimer's disease. Heyman et al[53] found that 15 percent of their cases had reported head trauma, while Mortimer et al[90] found that 25.6 percent of their DAT patients had a history of head injury with loss of consciousness. In most cases, the head trauma had occurred 20 or more years prior to the onset of the dementia. Rudelli et al hypothesize that trauma may play a "permissive role" in the development of dementia.[118] Gedye et al, in a retrospective study of 148 subjects with probable Alzheimer's disease, found that those with severe head injury before age 65 showed an earlier onset of symptoms than those without trauma.[38] They concluded that head injury "influences the timing and signs of dementia but is not a necessary condition to cause DAT."

## ETIOLOGY OF MULTI-INFARCT DEMENTIA

The major cause of multi-infarct dementia is repeated strokes to the cerebrum and/or subcortical areas, most commonly associated with "hypertension, impaired cardiac functioning, diabetes, high normal hemoglobin values, elevated serum cholesterol, and cigarette smoking."[9] As stated previously, Cummings and Benson[27] outlined over 20 of the most common etiologies of multi-infarct dementia. Other factors that appear highly related to multi-infarct dementia include being over 60 years of age and male.

## Diagnostic Considerations

A differential and accurate diagnosis is necessary to rule out any factors that may contribute to cognitive impairment and to establish with as much certainty as possible the underlying pathology. The fact that perhaps as many as 20 to 30 percent of dementias are reversible or partially reversible underscores the importance of accurate diagnosis.[65] Accurate diagnosis is also crucial in appropriate patient management and family counseling. Physicians are ethically obliged to inform patients regarding their diagnosis and prognosis. Although technically a breach of confidentiality, caregivers are usually informed under the principle of benevolence.[40] Although the state of art in genetic counseling in dementia is equivocal, families will ask questions regarding this issue. Accurate diagnosis also helps families understand the course of the disease and its future management alternatives.

For most individuals with dementia and their families, the family physician or general practitioner is the first step in the diagnostic process.[62] The physician's primary goal is to distinguish dementia from normal aging and to exclude reversible or compounding factors. Other goals include early detection, description of symptomatology, staging of the disorder, and suggestions for patient management. Ideally, the evaluation should take place over time to assess validity and reliability of findings.

Jorm, in a review of physician accuracy in diagnosing dementia, found that general practitioners correctly identified between 13 and 60 percent of those individuals with dementia.[62] He stated, however, that physicians rarely misdiagnosed a normal individual as demented. Such findings suggest several implications. First, physicians missed a great number of cases with possible dementia. Second, we may need to redefine our concept of normal. Third, the evaluation, when possible, should amalgamate findings from a variety of specialists including the family physician or geriatrician, neurologist, psychiatrist, neuropsychologist, speech-language pathologist, audiologist, physical and occupational therapist, and others, as needed.

## SCOPE OF EVALUATION

The National Institute of Health stated that the "best diagnostic test is a careful history and physical and mental status examination by a physician with a knowledge of and interest in dementia. Such an evaluation is time consuming but nothing can replace it."[97] The process begins with a careful case history taken from knowledgeable family members concerning: (1) current and past illnesses; (2) family history of cognitive impairment; (3) medications; (4) premorbid intelligence; (5) personality; (6) social functioning; (7) current behavior; and (8) areas of particular difficulty.[59] The interview should investigate individual areas of strength and weakness, frequency and severity of symptoms, family perception of the problem, and identification of their coping strategies.[18] *When possible*, the patient himself or herself should participate in this information gathering, although the interviewer should be aware that patients may not accurately respond or may be acutely affected by the questions. Huppert and Tym suggest that a patient's own complaints may provide useful information about his or her mood, although they are generally not a reliable measure of competence.[59]

Further steps in the diagnostic process include: (1) systematic examination of mental state; (2) a complete physical examination; (3) laboratory investigations; and (4) radiologic investigations. In addition, referral to specialists for speech and language, hearing, vision, and neuropsychological assessments should be made.

Once the diagnosis of dementia has been made, there will be a need for a more detailed evaluation of the patient's ability to perform the activities of daily living.[59] This evaluation places the disability in a lifestyle context and provides some of the most important information for patient management.[110] The assessment focuses on self-care, instrumental tasks, social functioning, and patterns of daily living, and is usually completed by an occupational therapist specializing in geriatrics. In addition, this aspect of the diagnostic process should include a focus on the caregiver's mental and physical well-being.[18] Chui and Smith present a comprehensive list of and sources for instruments for evaluation of older persons.[18]

## NEUROPSYCHOLOGICAL EVALUATION

Referral to a neuropsychologist for an in-depth cognitive assessment of the dementia patient is important. This assessment can be used in the diagnostic process, in planning management strategies, and for measuring change.[59] The goals of the evaluation will determine what procedures are to be used and who will be the source of information. Although a complete neuropsychological battery would be ideal, a more realistic assessment will include administration of shorter instruments designed specifically for the elderly.[59] It should be remembered, however, that the shorter the test, the less likely it will completely assess a range of functions, be sensitive to mild difficulties, document change, or differentiate types of dementia. In addition to the neuropsychological batteries, dementia patients should have at least six areas of cognitive function tested in more depth: perception, attention, memory, abstraction and set maintenance, language, and visuospatial functions. Description of deficits in these areas helps to "clarify and refine the nature of cognitive functioning in dementia."[59] Complete discussion of the wide variety of neuropsychological tests available is beyond the scope of this chapter. See Salmon's chapter for discussion of possible cognitive areas of evaluation and Ripich's chapter for more detail on this type of elevation. Bayles and Kazniak,[9] Huppert and Tym,[59] Moss and Albert,[93] and Salmon and Butters[119] also discuss the neuropsychological evaluation in more depth.

## SPEECH, LANGUAGE, AND HEARING EVALUATION

The role of the audiologist and speech-language pathologist in the evaluation of dementia is frequently overlooked. A total evaluation of auditory functioning, comprehension, and expression is critical. Such an evaluation aids in differential diagnosis; identification of hearing loss, dysarthria, apraxia, and aphasia, which may confound the diagnosis; and in planning appropriate intervention strategies. At present, the only specialized communication test for dementia is the Arizona Battery for Communication Disorders of Dementia.[9] This test has undergone rigorous development and shows the best promise for comprehensive and differential diagnosis of communication problems of dementia. Selective administration of aphasia tests, including the Boston Diagnostic Aphasia Examination,[45] the Western Aphasia Battery,[70] and Communicative Abilities in Daily Living,[53] may provide additional information. Observation, recording, and analysis of discourse in routinized tasks such as interviews, monologues, story telling, and spontaneous conversations provide data on the functional communicative competency of the dementia individual. Analysis of breakdowns and repair strategies used by dementia patients and their conversational partners may provide the best management information. Ripich's chapter in this volume on diagnosis describes communication evaluation in more depth, while Kempler's details specific language diagnostic needs.

Similarly, evaluation of auditory function is vitally important in a dementia evaluation. Auditory difficulties may both mimic and mask dementia cognitive symptoms. Thus, evaluation of both peripheral and central hearing abilities helps to identify and define auditory difficulties that may contribute to comprehension difficulties. Elimination or reduction of auditory difficulties is a major step in accurate diagnosis and effective management of dementia. Grimes and Weinstein, in this volume, discuss the role of the audiologist in differential diagnosis and auditory management of dementia patients.

## DIAGNOSTIC IMAGING TECHNIQUES

Advancement in noninvasive brain-imaging techniques has led to the use of these techniques in the diagnosis of dementia. To date, four imaging studies have been used: computerized tomography (CT), magnetic resonance imaging (MRI), positron emission tomography (PET), and single photon scanning (SPECT). A comprehensive review of over 40 current studies on brain imaging and Alzheimer's disease is presented by McGeer.[85] He concludes that CT scanning and MRI proton tomography show the exacerbation of brain atrophy in dementia from normal aging. CT scanning and MRI proton tomography, however, are not sensitive to variable cortical involvement shown on postmortem pathologic studies. PET scanning may be the most appropriate imaging technique because it is more sensitive to regional cortical involvement through studies of brain metabolic function. Finally, SPECT studies appear to show particular decline in the parietal cortex, followed by declines in the temporal and frontal cortices. Also noted have been more modest declines in the caudate, cerebellum, and thalamus.[88] Metter provides a thorough discussion of imaging techniques for the elderly and DAT subjects, with emphasis on studies involving cerebral blood flow, oxygen metabolism, and cerebral glucose metabolism in individuals with DAT.[88] Albert and Stafford also review the use of CT studies in the identification of Alzheimer's disease, and the relationship of CT studies to neuropsychological test results.[1]

## Staging of Dementia

Once the diagnosis of dementia has been made and the symptomatology fully described, the patient's degree of severity should be determined. Global ratings of mild, moderate, and severe have been found useful in assessing prognosis and in family counseling.[59] Two of the most commonly used global instruments that score the severity of symptoms are the Clinical Dementia Rating[58] and the Global Deterioration Scale.[114] In addition, the Hachinski Scale is useful in defining the symptoms of multi-infarct dementia.[47] These and other available tools should be used and interpreted judiciously because of the considerable heterogeneity in individual cognitive and functional performance.[18]

## Management Considerations

To date, no effective management has been found for any of the irreversible dementias, although a variety of direct and indirect approaches continue to undergo investigation and consideration. Total management involves setting goals for the individual with dementia as well as for the family and professional caregivers. Until prevention or pharmaceutical programs are developed that eradicate or reduce symptomatology, a care plan will continue to focus on maximizing independent functioning and reducing excess disability of the dementia patient.

Of foremost concern in any management plan is the recognition and management of superimposed medical conditions that frequently accompany the aging process itself, irrespective of the dementia. Chui and Smith propose a care plan that minimizes excess disability through identification and management of coexistent illness, reduction of medication, behavioral or pharmacologic management of personality and behavioral disorders, and accident prevention.[18] Their care plan also involves maximizing independence and activity by maintaining self-esteem, developing meaningful activities, and enhancing activities of daily living. Their intervention plan focuses on enabling the caregiver through education, developing coping strategies, and exploring ethical and legal issues. Giombetti and Miller add that a management plan should include avoiding infections, diagnosing and managing swallowing difficulties, maintaining nutritional status, preventing dental complications, and creating a therapeutic environment.[42] Finally, no management plan would be complete without maximizing preserved functions. Particularly in the early stage of dementia, individuals have residual abilities that should be capitalized on. Table 1.3 presents a summary of current key principles in the management of dementia.

### TABLE 1.3 Key Principles in the Management of Dementia

Optimize the patient's function
    Treat underlying medical conditions (e.g., hypertension, Parkinson's disease)
    Avoid use of drugs with CNS side effects (unless required for management of psychological or behavioral disturbances)
    Assess the environment and suggest alterations, if necessary
    Encourage physical and mental activity
    Avoid situations stressing intellectual capabilities; use memory aids whenever possible
    Prepare the patient for changes in location
    Emphasize good nutrition
Identify and manage complications
    Wandering and other hazards
    Behavioral disorders
    Depression
    Agitation or aggressiveness
    Incontinence
Provide ongoing care
    Reassessment of cognitive and physical function
    Treatment of medical conditions
Provide medical information to patient and family
    Nature of the disease
    Extent of impairment
    Prognosis
Provide social service information to patient and family
    Community health care resources (day centers, homemakers, home health aides)
    Legal and financial counseling
Provide family counseling for
    Identification and resolution of family conflicts
    Handling anger and guilt
    Decisions on respite or institutional care
    Legal concerns
    Ethical concerns

From Kane RL, Ouslander JG, Abrass IB. Essentials of clinical geriatrics. New York: McGraw-Hill, 1984:59, with permission.

## PHARMACOTHERAPY

The use of psychopharmacologic agents in the treatment of dementia is receiving greater attention. Hollister proposed that there are two classes of pharmacotherapeutic agents that can be used in dementia: (1) supposed etiopathogenetic or specific agents and (2) symptomatic agents.[57] Table 1.4 presents a list of these drugs. Many of these drugs are undergoing clinical trials in Canada, Europe, and the United States. To date, the majority of drugs are aimed at symptomatic control, though none appear to have significantly and consistently reduced symptoms or prevented progression of dementia. Benefits that have been documented include changes in mood states, alertness, and general behavior.[75] Cummings and Miller present the most current discussion of the disease-specific pharmacotherapy approaches in their review of cholinomimetic agents, cholinergic agents, ergoloid mesylates, and nootropics, as well as a variety of unsuccessful treatments.[29]

Among the numerous methodologic difficulties in drug-control studies are the heterogeneity of dementia populations, difficulty in making large-scale observations in the early stages, diagnostic accuracy, and the need to develop methodology sensitive to changes in the broad spectrum of cognitive and behavioral domains.[56,75] Despite the present state of pharmacotherapy, advances in drug therapy and brain-behavior understanding may yield promising results in the future. Several excellent reviews of pharmacotherapy and dementia are by Cummings and Miller,[29] De Estable-Puig eg al,[39] Hollander, Kohs, and Davis,[56] Kopelman and Lishman,[75] and Narang and Cutler.[95]

## FAMILY AND COMMUNITY OPTIONS

Without doubt, maintaining dementia patients in the community is a desirable goal though fraught with strain for the family members who care for them. Rabins summarizes this concept by saying "One cannot draw a distinct dividing line between the care of the patient with dementia (DAT) who is living at home and the care of his family."[109] Brody called dementia the "most socially disruptive disorder" because of the severe burden placed on families.[43] Caring for the de-

TABLE 1.4 **Summary of Drugs Used to Treat Alzheimer's Disease**

**SYMPTOMATIC DRUGS**

Antipsychotics: thiothixene, haloperidol, thioridazine
Sedative-hypnotics: diazepam, oxazepam
Antidepressants: tricyclics, possibly MAO inhibitors

**SPECIFIC DRUGS**

Stimulants, analeptics: dextroamphetamine, methylphenidate, magnesium pemoline
Vasodilators: papaverine, cyclandelate, cinnarazine, pentoxyfylline
Metabolic enhancers: ergoloid mesylates, piracetam, nafronyl, vincamine
Special actions: Gerovital H-3 (procaine)
Augmentors of neurotransmission; levodopa (dopamine), 5-hydroxytryptophan (serotonin), choline, lecithin (acetylcholine presynaptic), physostigmine, tacrine (acetylcholine synaptic), arecoline, oxotremorine (acetylcholine postsynaptic).
Neuropeptides: $ACTH_{4-10}$, vasopressin homologs

From Hollister L. Drug therapy of Alzheimer's disease: Realistic or not? Prog Neuropsychopharmacol Biol Psychiatry 1986; 10:439–446.

mentia patient is done primarily by female members of the family, particularly wives and daughters. Given, Collins, and Given, in an article on stress among families caring for relatives with Alzheimer's disease, note that "intergenerational caregivers (adult children) are more likely to suffer role conflicts whereas intragenerational (spouse) caregivers suffer from role entrenchment and isolation."[43] (See Chapter 11 for more detail on family and gender issues.)

Wilson identified three stages that families go through in caring for a demented patient: Stage 1, "Taking It On": through self-dialogue, seeking solace and unburdening; Stage 2, "Going Through It," which entails taking care of business, selective resourcing, and protective governing; and Stage 3, "Turning It Over," which comprises coming to terms, giving up control, and entrusting care. Gruetzner presents five stages families go through in adjusting to dementia: denial, overinvolvement, anger, guilt, and acceptance.[46]

Numerous articles and books detail the sources of stress for family members and strategies for successful coping with the individual both at home and after being institutionalized. Complete review of these are not possible in this chapter and the reader is referred to the chapters by Rau and Orange in this volume as well as to the reference list.[22,64,72,81,105,107] Readings in these areas lead to the conclusion that once an individual develops symptoms of dementia and is identified as such, the family system is changed. Bonder states that "families often struggle valiantly to care for the DAT patient, giving up only when they are so exhausted and distressed that their own health may be compromised. In short, the system eventually runs out of energy and risks disintegration."[12]

The options for family support in the community include (1) competent health care; (2) Alzheimer's support groups; and (3) respite care.[102] In addition, numerous community-based services for personal, household, and financial management can be arranged. These include shop-at-home programs, cleaning and cooking services, home and gardening maintenance, and business managers.[9] Local senior-citizen and government programs are good sources of available resources in the community.

Family support groups such as those sponsored through the ADRDA offer social opportunities, information exchange, and opportunities for therapeutic communication with other families. There are also other resources for further understanding of the role of family-support groups.[7,46,78,80,102,133] Respite care involves (1) in-home care by other family members or professionals so that the primary caregiver may leave the home and (2) adult day programs for custodial and health care. Although available for over 100 years, home care has become one of the fastest growing segments of the health-care industry.[69] This growth is a result of increased need, cost-containment, and consumer preference. Home care involves the provision of a wide variety of nursing, supportive, and rehabilitation services.

Adult day-care programs within the United States are also growing in number because of the increasing need for respite care. These programs provide a range of social, medical, recreational, therapeutic, and custodial and supervision services for a varying number of hours per day. Similarly, comprehensive geriatric day hospitals based on a popular concept in Great Britain are increasing in the United States and Canada. Such programs offer patients comprehensive and centralized interdisciplinary team care, hospital ancillary services, medical-specialist consultation, and rehabilitation services in one location.[5,89] Jorm cautions that although these respite programs provide caregiver relief, there does not appear to be substantial evidence that they reduce the need for eventual residential care.[62] Such programs may, however, delay or postpone institutionalization.

In addition, some long-term care settings offer short-term respite care for dementia patients during family vacations, holidays, and during other family events. Arie states that short periods of admission act as immediate "decompression" for over-burdened families.[5] Some long-term care settings also provide "day-attendee" programs in conjunction with programs offered as part of health-related and skilled-nursing facilities.

## INSTITUTIONALIZATION

The decision to institutionalize the elderly individual with dementia is not an easy one for family members. Chenoweth and Spencer found that many families extended themselves beyond their capacities before institutionalizing the individual.[17] McDowell summarized families' feelings by stating that "There is a curious blend of grief, guilt, and sometimes relief."[84] Morycz found that desire to institutionalize a patient with DAT was greater when the caregiver experienced increased strain or burden, when a patient was widowed, when there was more physical labor involved in caregiving tasks, and when the patient lived alone.[92] Interestingly, he reported that male caregivers and blacks differed from female caregivers and whites in that their best predictors for institutionalizing a family member were related to the patient's age (older), living arrangements (alone), physical labor required, and functional deficits. Thus, the decision to institutionalize is related to the characteristics of the caregiver, the nature of the care required, and the availability of support to the caregiver. Unfortunately, families are not freed of stress once institutionalization takes place. York and Calsyn found that families tended to visit less often as the relative deteriorated physically and mentally, in particular.[134]

To meet the growing need for long-term care for older persons (over 90 days), the number of nursing homes has increased to about 20,000 homes and 1.4 million beds in 1977.[96] As expected, dementia is the principal cause of admission to long-term institutional care.[5] At least 55 percent of those in nursing homes are mentally impaired. The typical nursing-home patient is very old (average age 82), female (3:1), widowed (63 percent widows, 22 percent never married), white (96 percent), with four chronic disabilities, mentally impaired (55 percent), requiring assistance with walking and all activities of daily living (over 55 percent), and taking a large quantity of drugs (70 percent take five or more drugs per day).[96] Eighty-five percent of patients in nursing homes reside there more than 90 days, and in fact 45 percent of nursing-home-bed days are consumed by patients whose stays exceed 2 years.[103]

Nursing homes offer levels of care based on the amount of nursing and custodial care needed. Some dementia patients who require little assistance with activities of daily living and medical care may require a low level of nursing care; others may need a skilled-service facility. Nursing homes differ in their approach to patients with dementia and the specialized services available to them.

In choosing a nursing home for a person with dementia, caregivers should consider many factors in their on-site inspection of the facility and during discussion with admission counselors. Selection of a nursing home should be based on at least two carefully timed visits. These visits should allow the caregiver to sample the care and conditions throughout the facility, including the bedroom, dayroom, seating areas around the nurses' station, kitchen, dining room, and bathing and toileting area. Caregivers should carefully consider:

1. Type and extent of care needed by patient
2. Cost both monthly and for special needs or therapies
3. Location and ease of access for family members
4. Staff-patient ratio
5. Training, experience, and supervision of staff
6. Attrition of staff
7. Staff attention to patients, e.g., verbal and nonverbal communication, timeliness and attitude in meeting patient and family requests, handling of difficult situations, and responses to wandering and incontinence
8. Design for meeting the cognitive impairment, behavioral difficulties, and sensory limitations of patient
9. Attractiveness and cleanliness
10. Availability of sensory and socially stimulating activities appropriate for dementia patients
11. Availability of religious programs or counselors
12. Safety
13. Availability of therapy programs, e.g., speech-language therapy, occupational and physical therapy, recreation
14. Patient counseling
15. Family counseling and availability of primary staff to discuss patient and family concerns

16. Use of medications
17. Areas available for privacy with patient
18. Personalization of patient's own room
19. Appropriate clothing for adults and personal grooming services

Caregivers need to remember that this is likely to be the last home for the dementia patient and therefore should meet the highest though most reasonable standards for quality of life. Further, family caregivers should ask themselves if this is a place they would like to visit on a regular basis. See Bayles and Kazniak,[9] Calkins,[16] and McDowell[84] for discussion of nursing-home criteria.

McDowell reviews the decision-making process in institutionalizing a person with dementia, selection criteria for institutions, the admission process, and sources of help for families.[84] Beverley also presents an overview of how to match a facility with a patient's particular needs.[11] See also Chapter 16 of this text for environmental considerations in dementia.

## Cost of Dementia

Although the emotional cost of dementia is extremely high for the individual, family, and professional caregivers, the economic cost in terms of expenditures above normal health care expectations is also high. Hay and Ernst state that the actual costs are probably underestimated because some expenses are incurred prior to diagnosis.[49] Two recent studies have explored the direct and indirect costs incurred with pre- and post-nursing admission of dementia patients.

Hay and Ernst analyzed epidemiologic projections and cost information for the United States population in 1983.[49] They found that the net annual expected costs for a patient with DAT, excluding the value of lost productivity, are $18,517 in the first year and $17,643 in later years. Medical and social services accounted for about half of the costs. Depending on the patient's age at onset, total costs for each patient ranged from $48,544 to $473,277. Projecting these costs of the total population yielded a cost to the nation of about $30 billion dollars (in 1983).

Coughlin and Liu reported on the results of the 1981 National Long-Term Channeling Demonstration Project.[23] They estimated a cost of about $18,500 annually per capita for home and institutional care for cognitively impaired adults. They also found that the annual cost of community care for dementia patients was about $11,700, whereas the cost of nursing-home care was on the average $22,300. Pawlson noted that over 50 percent of long-term care is financed by the elderly and their families, 40 percent by Medicaid, 5 percent through Medicare, and 5 percent from other sources, including 1 percent from private long-term care insurance.[103] Seventy-five percent of nursing-home patients who stay for more than 6 months are dependent on Medicaid.

## Policy Issues

The number of governmental, financial, social, and caregiving issues facing those with dementia, their caregivers, and society in general is far too great for the scope of this chapter. The federal report entitled *Losing a Million Minds—Confronting the Tragedy of Alzheimer's Disease and Other Dementias* identified seven areas of public policy that need attention: (1) support for biomedical research; (2) support for health-services research; (3) education; (4) financing long-term care; (5) improving patient assessment and services; (6) increasing the range of available services; and (7) assuring quality of care.[128] Three of these issues are highlighted here as representative of the broad spectrum: financial, service delivery, and education and advocacy. Three major sources discussing public-policy issues are books by Gilhooly, Zarit, and Birren,[41] Jazwiecki,[61] and Torres-Gil and Rosenquist.[126]

### FINANCIAL CONCERNS

The major public-policy issue regarding dementia concerns the exponentially increasing costs for home and institutional care.[41] Arie made an insightful comment regarding the increasing number of elderly and demented: "The rapid increase in the numbers of the very aged and thus of the demented coincides with a crisis in the word's economy and thus in the availability of resources."[5] Government officials are faced with the dilemma of a growing constituency of dementia patients and their families and spiraling deficits.[115] Although legislators are sympathetic, there is little support for new tax credits and deductions for special populations.[115]

Thus, in the United States today, the elderly demented are faced with a shrinking financial base to cover the increasing costs of their care. For those elderly who saved for retirement, their savings cannot meet the inflation of health-care costs of the past 20 years. Many elderly people outlive their money, spouses are faced with depleting their reserves for their own current and eventual needs, and many are deprived of the life-long wish to "leave something" to their children. Yet others face accepting what they believe is charity. Families faced with institutionalization either have to deplete their savings or rely on Medicaid. The financial considerations of providing quality care are multitudinous. Currently, the United States has no coordinated national system to meet the long-term needs of dementia patients.[61,115]

In contrast, Canada provides premium-free medical care for all individuals over age 65 years who have lived in Canada for the previous 12 months. Those individuals requiring extended and chronic care are given financial assistance. Provinces differ regarding the availability of free prescription drugs.[31]

The United States Federal Advisory Panel on Alzheimer's Disease has made two policy recommendations to the Secretary of the Department of Health and Human Services.[37]
1. The establishment of an inclusive, publicly funded long-term care program for dementia patients in both eligibility and covered services
2. A federal long-term care insurance plan to replace Medicaid as its primary financial source

Weissert, in a paper exploring long-term care policy, suggests that families should be given tax incentives or subsidies for caring for the elderly and demented at home.[131] Pawlson proposed that with the skyrocketing number of baby boomers in the first half of the twenty-first century, prefunding of long-term stay in the form of self-funded medical individual retirement accounts and expansion of private long-term care insurance may be two alternatives.[103] Jazwiecki states, however, that the "greatest obstacle to development of long-term care insurance is the lack of awareness on the part of the general public about their financial vulnerability to catastrophic illness."[61] Pawlson delineates the positive and negative advantages of these and a number of other funding alternatives. Finally, Eisdorfer and Cohen call for community-oriented long-term disease management and disability prevention at funding levels similar to institutional care.[33]

## SERVICE DELIVERY

How to provide the range of quality services that meets the needs of dementia patients and their families is another major problem and policy issue. Arie notes that dementia cases require numerous services including acute general medicine; social services; institutional services on a protracted, intermittent, or permanent basis; and support services to families.[5] Little is known about the long-term benefits of home health care or what constitutes reasonable home health-care service delivery. Numerous problems exist in providing home health care to the elderly demented, including lack of physician involvement and leadership in suggesting and providing service in the home, difficulty in coordinating of home health care among various programs, and lack of appropriate standards and assessment methodology for measuring quality of care.[69]

Similarly, service delivery in long-term care settings is fraught with problems, including the establishment of standards of care, innovative programs, and measurable outcomes; and the training, retention, and morale of care providers in these settings.[5,62,106,115,131] Pynoos and Stacey strongly urge that accountability regarding quality of care be monitored not only by families but by outside groups such as ombudsmen, community members, and families who are specially trained to evaluate quality care.[106]

Of particular importance is the nursing-home reform legislation contained in the Omnibus Budget Reconciliation Act of 1987. Nursing homes must adhere to strict guidelines for admission requirements, provision of services, resident rights, and administration. Facilities must develop nursing-aide programs, competency evaluations, and improved administrator standards and resident assessments. These requirements should improve the quality of life for nursing-home residents.[61]

One large institution presently faced with major numbers of elderly demented is the Veterans Administration (VA). Rickards et al state that the VA has not established a consistent policy for servicing demented veterans.[115] This is a serious problem considering the burgeoning numbers of elderly World War II and Korean War veterans.

Another area of service delivery that should be part of an enlightened public policy is service for families of individuals with dementia. Cicirelli states that the family should be regarded as central to any policy for those with dementia.[19] For example, policies should be established that include the family as an active participant and decision maker in the care of the demented individual even when he or she is institutionalized. Cicirelli also calls for improved informational programs for family members and additional support services for home care. He concludes that if a full spectrum of services were available to families and individuals with dementia in early stages of the disease, institutionalization might be postponed to advanced stages and thus shorten the need for long-term care.

## EDUCATION AND ADVOCACY

A third major policy issue is the need for greater public and professional awareness of dementia, its effects, and possible alternatives for care.

Cutler states that although there is a meteoric increase in public concern about dementia, little is known about public attitudes or perceptions about dementia.[30] Research in this area would help form empirically based informational, educational, and counseling programs for the public at large and for families of dementia victims. Jazwiecki advocates increased public awareness concerning the financial risk associated with catastrophic disease such as dementia.[61]

Arie calls for an increase in education regarding dementia for primary care physicians in their basic and continuing-education programs.[5] Gilhooly relates this issue to the ethical obligation of physicians to care for elderly dementia patients. She states: "Elderly demented patients are generally regarded as uninteresting, and it is rare for physicians to take an active interest in the management of chronically demented patients. As a consequence, these people are abandoned by the medical profession."[40]

Similarly, other practitioners, including rehabilitation specialists such as audiologists and speech-language pathologists, need theoretic foundations in aging and dementia as well as practical training with this special population. Burnside noted that most nursing-facility staff members are not prepared educationally and psychologically to work with dementia patients.[15]

Education results not only in better service delivery but also in increased advocacy for legislative initiatives on dementia. Advocacy groups such as the ADRDA are important in increasing public and government awareness.

## Research Needs

Each chapter in this volume addresses research needs regarding the communicative functioning of dementia patients. These research needs must be placed in a broader research framework. Khachaturian, from the National Institute of Aging, recommended several themes needed in dementia research. These include the need for investigations concerning accuracy of diagnosis through longitudinal follow-up, diagnostic screening, genetics, studies of normal aging; studies of other dementia-producing diseases; and diagnostic methods and markers including neuropsychologic measures, psychopharmacologic research, electrophysiologic studies, and family pedigree studies. Khachaturian proposes that one of the greatest needs is regular information exchange among scientists of various fields, considering the volume and scope of research occurring.[71]

In addition, Rickards et al encourage the development of more research regarding clinical and research training, the development of ways to disseminate education materials and information, and more investigations of the epidemiology, etiology, pathology, diagnosis, clinical course, treatment, the family, and care provision.[115] Katzman calls for research on risk factors, cross-cultural investigations, and studies of twins.[66] Methodologic, conceptual, and future research directions in research on families and informal support systems are discussed by Ory et al,[102] Zarit and Anthony,[135] and Zarit and Toseland.[137] These authors stress the need for improved research design, sampling, measurement, goal definition, and follow-up, particularly in intervention studies.

To accomplish these research goals, continued and increased financial support of a variety of research will be needed. In 1978, 5.1 million U.S. dollars were allocated for Alzheimer's research. This allocation increased to 123.4 million dollars in 1989.[39]

Although reviews of dementia policy issues and research indicate that the area of dementia is wide open, a number of ethical issues are also raised. Examples of such cardinal ethical issues facing researchers include: Who can provide informed consent for research studies? Who will receive or be denied therapy? What type and extent of care should be provided to advanced dementia patients who have coexisting medical problems? What are the incentives, and conversely the penalties, for participating or not participating in research studies, particularly in institutional settings?[40,44] Continuing consideration of ethical issues and interdisciplinary exchange are crucial if dementia is to be understood and effectively treated.

## Concluding Remarks

This chapter has broadly reviewed the field of dementia as a foundation for this text, which concentrates on communication and dementia. One of the themes that should emerge is the importance of communication to the elderly demented, their caregivers, and among those doing basic and applied research in this area. Communication is important in the identification and diagnosis of symptoms, in the interaction between caregivers and patient in home or institution, in the education of specialists, in convincing legislators and other decision makers of the needs of the demented, and in the exchange of information by researchers in various fields. Perhaps in understanding how persons with dementia communicate, we will learn how to communicate better as individuals, professionals, and as a society.

# References

1. Albert M, Stafford J. Computed tomography studies. In: Albert M, Moss M, eds. Geriatric neuropsychology. New York: Guilford Press, 1988:211.
2. Amaducci LA, Fratiglioni L, Rocca WA, et al. Risk factors for clinically diagnosed Alzheimer's disease: A case-control study of an Italian population. Neurology 1986; 36:922–931.
3. American Association of Retired Persons (AARP). A profile of older Americans. Washington, D.C.: AARP, 1985.
4. Appell J, Kertesz A, Fisman M. A study of language functioning in Alzheimer's patients. Brain 1982; 17:73–91.
5. Arie T. Management of dementia: A review. Br Med Bull 1986; 42:91–96.
6. Ball MJ, Fisman M, Hachinski V, et al. A new definition of Alzheimer's disease: A hippocampal dementia. Lancet 1985; 1:14.
7. Barnes RF, Raskind MA, Scott M, Murphy C. Problems of families caring for Alzheimer patients: Use of a support group. J Am Geriatr Soc 1981; 29:80–85.
8. Bayles K. Communication in dementia. In: Ulatowska H, ed. The aging brain: Communication in the elderly. San Diego, CA: College-Hill Press, 1985: 157.
9. Bayles K, Kazniak A. Communication and cognition in normal aging and dementia. Boston: College-Hill Press, 1987.
10. Belloni-Sonzogni A, Tissot A, Tettamanti M, Frattura L, Spagnoli A. Mortality of demented patients in a geriatric institution. Arch Gerontol Geriatr 1989; 9:193–197.
11. Beverley EV. Nursing homes: Matching the facility to the patient's needs. Geriatrics 1976; 31:100–110.
12. Bonder BR. Family systems and Alzheimer's disease: An approach to treatment. Phys Occup Ther Geriatr 1986; 5:13–24.
13. Brody EM. Women in the middle and family help to older people. Gerontologist 1981; 21:471–480.
14. Brotman H. Population projections: Part I Tomorrow's older population to 2000. Gerontologist 1977: 17:203–209.
15. Burnside IM. Care of the Alzheimer's patient in an institution. Generations 1982; 7:22–23.
16. Calkins M. Design for dementia. Owings Mills, MD: National Health Publishing, 1988.
17. Chenoweth B, Spencer B. Dementia: The experience of family caregivers. Gerontologist 1986; 26:267–272.
18. Chui HC, Smith B. Rehabilitation of persons with dementia. In: Kemp B, Brummel-Smith K, Ramsdell J, eds. Geriatric rehabilitation. Boston: College-Hill Press, 1990:389.
19. Ciricelli V. Family relationships and care/management of the dementing elderly. In: Gilhooly M, Zarit S, Birren J, eds. The dementias: Policy and management. Englewood Cliffs, NJ: Prentice-Hall, 1986:93.
20. Clarfield AM. The reversible dementias: Do they reverse? Ann Intern Med 1988; 104:476–486.
21. Clark M, Gosnell M, Witherspoon D, Huck J, Hager M, Junkin D, King P, Wallace A, Robinson TL. A slow death of the mind. Newsweek December 3, 1984.
22. Cohen D, Eisdorfer C. Depression in family members caring for a relative with Alzheimer's disease. J Am Geriatr Soc 1988; 36:885–889.
23. Coughlin TA, Liu K. Health care costs for older persons with cognitive impairments. Gerontologist 1989; 29:173–181.
24. Cross PS, Gurland BJ. The epidemiology of dementing disorders: A report on work performed by and submitted to the U.S. Congress, Office of Technology Assessment. New York: Columbia University Center for Geriatrics, Gerontology and Long-Term Care, 1985.
25. Cummings JL. Clinical diagnosis of Alzheimer's disease. In: Cummings JL, Miller BL. Alzheimer's disease treatment and long-term management. New York: Marcel Dekker, 1990:3–20.
26. Cummings JL. Dementia syndromes: Neurobehavioral and neuropsychiatric features. J Clin Psychiatry 1987; 48:3–8.
27. Cummings JL, Benson DF. Dementia: A clinical approach. Boston: Butterworth, 1983.
28. Cummings JL, Benson DF. Dementia of the Alzheimer type: An inventory of diagnostic clinical features. J Am Geriatr Soc 1986; 34:12–19.
29. Cummings JL, Miller BL, eds. Alzheimer's disease treatment and long-term management. New York: Marcel Dekker, 1990.
30. Cutler N. Public response: The national politics of Alzheimer's disease. In: Gilhooly M, Zarit S, Birren J, eds. The Dementias Policy and Management. Englewood Cliffs, NJ: Prentice-Hall, 1986:161–189
31. Davison T, Finucane T, Molloy DW, Smith K. Care of the elderly in other English-speaking countries. In: Pathy MSJ, Finucane T, eds. Geriatric medicine problems and practice. London: Springer-Verlag, 1989:367–374.
32. De Estable-Puig RF, Estable-Puig JF, Ven Murthy MR, et al. On the pathogenesis and therapy of dementia of the Alzheimer type: Some neuropathological, biochemical, genetic and pharmacotherapeutic considerations. Prog Neuropsychopharmacol Biol Psychiat 1986; 10:355–390.
33. Eisdorfer C, Cohen D. Health policy implications: Risking a serious crisis. Generations 1982; 7:36.
34. Emery O. Language and memory processing in senile dementia Alzheimer's type. In: Light L, Burke D, eds. Language, memory and aging. Cambridge: Cambridge University Press, 1988:221–243.
35. Esiri MM, Wilcock GK. The olfactory bulbs in Alzheimer's disease. J Neurol Neurosurg Psychiatry 1984; 47:56–60.
36. Evans DA, Funkenstein HH, Albert MS, et al. Prevalence of Alzheimer's disease in a community population of older persons: Higher than previously reported. JAMA 1989; 262:2551–2556.
37. Federal Advisory Panel on Alzheimer's makes recommendations to HHS. Geriatr Care News 1989; 14:1453.
38. Gedye A, Beattie B, Tuokko H, Horton A, Korsarek E. Severe head injury hastens onset of Alzheimer's disease. J Am Geriatr Soc 1989; 37:970–973.
39. Gelman D, Hayer M, Quade V. The brain killer. Newsweek December 19, 1989, 54–56.
40. Gilhooly M. Legal and ethical issues in the management of the dementing elderly. In: Gilhooly M, Zarit S, Birren J, eds. The dementias: Policy and management. Englewood Cliffs, NJ: Prentice-Hall, 1986:137.
41. Gilhooly M, Zarit S, Birren J, eds. The dementias: Policy and management. Englewood Cliffs, NJ: Prentice-Hall, 1986.
42. Giombetti RJ, Miller BK. Recognition and manage-

ment of superimposed medical conditions. In: Cummings JL, Miller BL, eds. Alzheimer's disease treatment and long-term management. New York: Marcel Dekker, 1990:253.
43. Given CW, Collins CE, Given BA. Sources of stress among families caring for relatives with Alzheimer's disease. Nurs Clin North Am 1988; 23:69-81.
44. Goldberg MA. Ethics of treatment. In: Cummings JL, Miller BL, eds. Alzheimer's disease treatment and long-term management. New York: Marcel Dekker, 1990:267.
45. Goodglass H, Kaplan E. The Boston diagnostic aphasia examination. In: Goodglass H, Kaplan E, eds. The assessment of aphasia and related disorders. rev. ed. Philadelphia: Lea & Febiger, 1983.
46. Gruetzner H. Alzheimer's: A caregivers guide and sourcebook. New York: John Wiley & Sons, 1988.
47. Hachinski VC, Lassen NA, Marshall J. Multi-infarct dementia: A cause of mental deterioration in the elderly. Lancet 1974; 2:207-210.
48. Hart S. Language and dementia: A review. Psychol Med 1988; 18:99-112.
49. Hay JW, Ernst RL. The economic costs of Alzheimer's disease. Am J Public Health 1987; 77:1169-1175.
50. Heston L, Mastri A, Anderson V, White J. Dementia of the Alzheimer type: Clinical genetics, natural history and associated conditions. Arch Gen Psychiatry 1981; 30:1085-1090.
51. Heston LL, Morris ML. Family studies of Alzheimer's dementia: Results and prospects. Can J Neurol Sci 1986; 12:432-434.
52. Heston L, White J. Dementia: A practical guide to Alzheimer's disease and related illnesses. New York: W.H. Freeman and Co., 1983.
53. Heyman A, Wilkinson WE, Hurwitz B, et al. Alzheimer's disease and associated clinical disorders. Ann Neurol 1983; 14:507-515.
54. Heyman A, Wilkinson WE, Stafford JA, et al. Alzheimer's disease: A study of epidemiological aspects. Ann Neurol 1984; 15:335-341.
55. Holland A. Communicative abilities in daily living. Baltimore: University Park Press, 1980.
56. Hollander E, Kohs RC, Davis KL. Cholinergic approaches to the treatment of Alzheimer's disease. Br Med Bull 1986; 42:97-100.
57. Hollister L. Drug therapy for Alzheimer's disease: Realistic or not? Prog Neuropsychopharmacol Biol Psychiatry 1986; 10:439-446.
58. Hughes CP, Berg L, Danziger WL, Cohen LA, Martin RL. A new clinical scale for the staging of dementia. Br J Psychiatry 1982; 140:566-572.
59. Huppert FA, Tym E. Clinical and neuropsychological assessment of dementia. Br Med Bull 1986; 42:11-18.
60. Jarvik LF, Winograd CH, eds. Treatments for the Alzheimer patient. New York: Springer Publishing, 1988.
61. Jazwiecki T. Future policy directions. In: Cummings JL, Miller BL, eds. Alzheimer's disease: Treatment and long-term management. New York: Marcel Dekker, 1990:371-380.
62. Jorm AF. Alzheimer's disease. In: Howells JG, ed. Modern perspectives in clinical psychiatry. New York: Brunner/Mazel, 1988:261-301.
63. Jorm AF. Subtypes of Alzheimer's dementia: A conceptual analysis and critical review. Psycho Med 1985; 15:543-553.
64. Kahan J, Kemp B, Staples FR, Brummel-Smith K. Decreasing the burden in families caring for a relative with a dementing illness: A controlled study. J Am Geriatr Soc 1985; 33:664-670.
65. Kane RL, Ouslander JG, Abrass IB. Essentials of clinical geriatrics. New York: McGraw-Hill, 1989.
66. Katzman R. Medical progress in Alzheimer's disease. N Engl J Med 1986; 314:964-973.
67. Katzman R. The prevalence and malignancy of Alzheimer's disease. Arch Neurol 1976; 33:217-218.
68. Kay DWK. The genetics of Alzheimer's disease. Br Med Bull 1986; 42:19-23.
69. Keenan JM, Fanale JE. Home care: Past and present, problems and potential. J Am Geriatr Soc 1989; 37:1076-1083.
70. Kertesz A. Western aphasia battery. New York: Grune and Stratton, 1982.
71. Khachaturian ZS. Progress of research on Alzheimer's disease: Research opportunities for behavioral scientists. Am Psychol 1985; 40:1251-1255.
72. Kiecolt-Glaser JK, Glaser R, Shuttleworth EC, et al. Chronic stress and immunity in family caregivers of Alzheimer's disease victims. Psychosom Med 1987; 49:523-535.
73. Kiloh LG. The secondary dementias of middle and later life. Br Med Bull 1986; 42:106-110.
74. Kokmen E, Beard M, Offord KP, Kurland LT. Prevalence of medically diagnosed dementia in a defined United States population: Rochester, Minnesota, January 1, 1975. Neurology 1989; 39:773-776.
75. Kopelman MD, Lishman WA. Pharmacological treatments of dementia (non-cholinergic). Br Med Bull 1986; 42:101-105.
76. Larson E, Reifler B, Featherstone H, English D. Dementia in elderly outpatients: A prospective study. Ann Intern Med 1984; 100:417-423.
77. Lauter H. What do we know about Alzheimer's disease today? Dan Med Bull 1985; 31:1-21.
78. Lazarus LW, Stafford B, Cooper K, Cohler B, Dysken M. A pilot study of an Alzheimer's patients' relatives discussion group. Gerontologist 1981; 21:353-358.
79. Lebrun Y, Devereux F, Rousseau JJ. Disorders of communication behavior in degenerative dementia. Folia Phoniatr 1987; 39:1-8.
80. Mace N, Rabins P. The 36-hour day. Baltimore: Johns Hopkins University Press, 1981.
81. Maletta GJ, Hepburn K. Helping families cope with Alzheimer's: The physician's role. Geriatrics 1986; 41:81-90.
82. Mayeux R, Rosen WG, eds. Advances in neurology: The dementias. v. 38. New York: Raven Press, 1983.
83. Mayeux R, Stern Y, Spanton S. Heterogeneity in dementia of Alzheimer type: Evidence of subgroups. Neurology 1985; 35:453-461.
84. McDowell FH. Choosing a nursing home for the person with intellectual loss. White Plains, New York: Burke Rehabilitation Center, 1980.
85. McGeer PL. Brain imaging in Alzheimer's disease. Br Med Bull 1986; 42:24-28.
86. McKhann G, Drachman D, Folstein M, et al. Clinical diagnosis of Alzheimer's disease: Report of the NINCDS-ADRDA work group under the auspices of Department of Health and Human Services task force on Alzheimer's disease. Neurology 1984; 34:939-944.
87. Merriam AE, Aaronson MK, Gaston P, Wey SL, Katz I. The psychiatric symptoms of Alzheimer's disease. J Am Geriatr Soc 1988; 36:7-12.
88. Metter J. Positron emission tomography and cerebral blood flow studies. In: Albert M, Moss M, eds. Geri-

89. Morishita L, Siu AL, Wang RT, et al. Comprehensive geriatric care in a day hospital: A demonstration of the British model in the United States. Gerontologist 1989; 29:336–340.
90. Mortimer JA, French LR, Hutton JT, Schuman LM. Head injury as a risk factor for Alzheimer's disease. Neurology 1985; 35:264–267.
91. Mortimer JA, Schuman LM, French LR. Epidemiology of dementia: Overview and prospects. In: Mortimer JA, Schuman LM, eds. The epidemiology of dementia. New York: Oxford University Press, 1981:173.
92. Morycz RK. Caregiving strain and the desire to institutionalize family members with Alzheimer's disease. Res Aging 1985; 7:329–361.
93. Moss M, Albert M. Alzheimer's disease and other dementing disorders. In: Albert M, Moss M, eds. Geriatric neuropsychology. New York: Guilford Press, 1988:145.
94. Mowry B, Burvill P. A study of mild dementia in the community using a wide range of diagnostic criteria. Br J Psychiatry 1988; 153:328–334.
95. Narang PK, Cutler NR. Pharmacotherapy in Alzheimer's disease: Basis and rationale. Prog Neuropsychopharmacol Biol Psychiatry 1986; 10:519–531.
96. National Health Survey. Characteristics of nursing home residents, health status and care received: National nursing home survey. Hyattsville, MD: U.S. Dept. of Health and Human Services National Center for Health Statistics, 1981.
97. National Institutes of Health Consensus Development Conference Statement. Differential diagnosis of dementing diseases. Washington, D.C.: U.S. Government Printing Office, 1987; 6:109.
98. National Library of Medicine Literature Search No. 87-6. Differential diagnosis of Alzheimer's and other dementing diseases. Washington D.C.: U.S. Department of Health and Human Services, 1987.
99. Navia BA, Jordan BD, Price RW. The AIDS dementia complex: I. Clinical features. Ann Neurol 1986; 19:517–524.
100. Obler L. Language and brain dysfunction in dementia. In: Segalowitz S, ed. Language functions and brain organization. New York: Academic Press, 1983:267.
101. Obler LK, Albert ML. Language in the elderly aphasic and in the dementing patient. In: Sarno M. ed. Acquired aphasia. New York: Academic Press, 1981:385.
102. Ory MG, Williams TF, Emr M, et al. Families, informal supports and Alzheimer's disease. Current research on future agendas. Res Aging 1985; 7:623–643.
103. Pawlson LG. Financing long-term care. J Am Geriatr Soc 1989; 37:631–638.
104. Pfeffer RI, Afifi AA, Chance JM. Prevalence of Alzheimer's in a retirement community. Am J Epidemiol 1987; 125:420–436.
105. Powell L, Courtice K. Alzheimer's disease: A guide for families. Menlo Park, CA: Addison-Wesley, 1983.
106. Pynoos J, Stacey C. Specialized facilities for senile dementia patients. In: Gilhooly M, Zarit S, Birren J, eds. The dementias: Policy and management. Englewood Cliffs, NJ: Prentice-Hall, 1986:111.
107. Quayhagen MP, Quayhagen M. Alzheimer's stress: Coping with the caregiving role. Gerontologist 1988; 28:391–396.
108. Rabins PV. Establishing Alzheimer's disease units in nursing homes: Pros and cons. Hosp Community Psychiatry 1986; 37:120–121.
109. Rabins PV. Family-directed therapy. In: Cummings JL, Miller BL, eds. Alzheimer's disease treatment and long-term management. New York: Marcel Dekker, 1990:225.
110. Ramsdell J. A rehabilitation orientation in the work up of general medical problems. In: Kemp B, Brummell-Smith K, Ramsdell J, eds. Geriatric rehabilitation. Boston: College-Hill Press, 1990:23.
111. Reisberg B. Alzheimer's disease: The standard reference. New York: Free Press, 1983.
112. Reisberg B, Borenstein J, Frassen E, Shulman E, Steinberg G, Ferris SH. Remediable behavioral symptomatology in Alzheimer's disease. Hosp Community Psychiatry 1986; 37:1199–1201.
113. Reisberg B, Borenstein J, Salob SP, et al. Behavioral symptoms in Alzheimer's disease: Phenomenology and treatment. J Clin Psychiatry 1987; 48:9–15.
114. Reisberg B, Ferris SH, DeLeon MJ, Crook T. The global deterioration scale of assessment of primary degenerative dementia. Am J Psychiatry 1982 139:1136–1139.
115. Rickards LD, Zuckerman DM, West PR. Alzheimer's disease current congressional response. Am Psychol 1985; 40:1256–1261.
116. Rocca WA, Amaducci LA, Schoenberg BS. Epidemiology of clinically diagnosed Alzheimer's disease. Ann Neurol 1986; 19:415–424.
117. Rogers RL, Meyer JS, Mortel KF, Mahuri RK, Judd BW. Decreased cerebral blood flow precedes multi-infarct dementia but follows senile dementia of the Alzheimer's type. Neurology 1986; 36:1–6.
118. Rudelli R, Strom JO, Welch PT, Ambler MW. Posttraumatic premature Alzheimer's disease. Arch Neurol 1982; 39:570–575.
119. Salmon D, Butters N. Neuropsychological assessment of dementia in the elderly. In: Katzman R, Rowe J, eds. Geriatric neurology: Principles and practice. Philadelphia: F.A. Davis (in press).
120. Sayetta RB. Rates of senile dementia—Alzheimer's type in the Baltimore longitudinal study. J Chronic Dis 1986; 39:271–286.
121. Schoenberg BS, Anderson DW, Haerer AF. Severe dementia. Prevalence and clinical features in a biracial U.S. population. Arch Neurol 1985; 42:740–743.
122. Subcommittee on Long Term Care of the Special Committee on Aging. U.S. Senate. Nursing home care in the U.S.: Failure in public policy. Washington D.C.: U.S. Government Printing Office, 1974:16.
123. Teri L, Larson EB, Reifler BV. Behavioral disturbance in the dementia of the Alzheimer's type. J Am Geriatr Soc 1988; 36:1–6.
124. Terry R. Clues to the cause of senile dementia. Science 1981; 211:1032.
125. Thompson I. Language in dementia. Int J Geriatr Psychiatry 1987; 2:145–161.
126. Torres-Gil F, Rosenquist LL. Public policy and geriatric rehabilitation. In: Kemp B, Brummel-Smith K, Ramsdell J, eds. Geriatric rehabilitation. Boston: College-Hill Press, 1990.
127. U.S. Department of Health and Human Services. Health of an aging America: 1989 bibliography. Hyattsville, MD: Public Health Service, 1989.
128. U.S. Office of Technology Assessment. Losing a million minds: Confronting the tragedy of Alzheimer's disease. Washington, D.C.: U.S. Government Printing Office, 1984.
129. U.S. Office of Technology Assessment. Technology and aging in America OTA-BA-264. Washington, D.C.: U.S. Government Printing Office, 1985.
130. Weiler P. The public health impact of Alzheimer's disease. Am J Public Health 1987; 77:1157–1158.

131. Weissert WG. Long-term care: Current policy and directions for the 1980s. In: Tedrich T, ed. Aging: Issues and policies for the 1980s. New York: Praeger Publishers, 1985:61.
132. Whaley L, Halloway S. Non-random geographical distribution of Alzheimer's presenile dementia in Edinburgh. 1953-76. Lancet 1985; 1:578.
133. Wilson HS. Family caregiving for a relative with Alzheimer's dementia: Coping with negative choices. Nurs Res 1989; 38:94-98.
134. York J, Calsyn R. Family involvement in nursing homes. Gerontologist 1977; 17:500-505.
135. Zarit S, Anthony C. Interventions with dementia patients and their families. In: Gilhooly M, Zarit S, Birren J, eds. The dementias policy and management. Englewood Cliffs, NJ: Prentice-Hall, 1986:66-92.
136. Zarit S, Orr NK, Zarit J. The hidden victims of Alzheimer's disease: Families under stress. New York: New York University Press, 1985.
137. Zarit SH, Toseland RW. Current and future direction in family and caregiving research. Gerontologist 1989; 29:481-483.
138. Zopf PE. Number and distribution of older people. In: Zopf PE, ed. America's older population. Houston: Cap and Gown Press, 1986:1.

# CHAPTER 2

# Functional Anatomy

ALICIA OSIMANI, M.D.
MORRIS FREEDMAN, B.Sc., M.D., FRCPC*

Advances in modern medicine, combined with a low birth rate, have resulted in a significant increase in the proportion of older persons in our society. Because dementia affects mainly the elderly, this disorder has become an increasingly prevalent medical and social problem. It has been estimated that approximately 5 percent of the population over age 65 years are severely demented, and that an additional 10 percent have mild to moderate intellectual impairment.[25]

According to the revised third edition of the Diagnostic and Statistical Manual of Mental Disorders,[32] dementia is defined as a loss of intellectual abilities of sufficient severity to interfere with social or occupational functioning. Diagnostic criteria include memory impairment and at least one of the following: (1) impairment of abstract thinking; (2) impaired judgment; (3) other disturbances of higher cortical function (e.g., aphasia, agnosia, apraxia); and (4) personality change (alteration or accentuation of premorbid traits). The report of the NINCDS-ADRDA Work Group defines dementia as "a decline of memory and other cognitive functions in comparison with the patient's previous level of function as determined by a history of decline in performance and by abnormalities noted from clinical examination and neuropsychological tests."[78] This report stresses that the diagnosis is based on behavioral criteria and cannot be determined by computerized tomography, electroencephalography, or other laboratory techniques, although specific causes of dementia may be identified by these means. These definitions indicate that dementia is a clinical neurobehavioral syndrome, in which memory impairment constitutes a central and early symptom. The underlying neuroanatomy and neuropathology vary with the specific disease process and determine the profile of cognitive deficits. The neuroanatomic mechanisms underlying dementia, however, are still far from being understood.

Because a discussion of the anatomic bases of all of the many different dementing diseases is beyond the scope of this chapter, we will focus on two of the most common types of neurodegenerative dementia, i.e., Alzheimer's disease and Parkinson's disease. First, the controversial distinction that has been applied to the dementias of Alzheimer's and Parkinson's diseases is mentioned briefly, i.e., subcortical versus cortical dementia. The term subcortical dementia was first used by Albert et al in 1974 to describe the intellectual deterioration of progressive supranuclear palsy.[2] Four characteristic features were identified: forgetfulness; slowness of thought process; altered personality with apathy, depression, or irritability; and impaired ability to manipulate acquired knowledge. A remarkable finding was the lack of aphasia, apraxia, and agnosia, features that have traditionally been considered "cortical." McHugh et al also described subcortical dementia in patients with Huntington's disease.[77] Since its introduction over a decade ago, the concept of subcortical dementia has been applied to several types of dementia, including those associated with Parkinson's disease, Wilson's disease, multiple sclerosis, Binswanger's disease, and spinocerebellar degeneration. Although a classic picture of subcortical dementia with prominent frontal signs is frequently found in lacunar states,[58] multi-infarct dementia may show a profile of either cortical or subcortical dementia, depending on the site of the infarcts.[49]

During the past two decades there have been many developments that have had an impact upon our understanding of the mechanisms underlying dementia. Of note is that neurochemical cholinergic deficits have been identified in a subcortical structure (i.e., the basal forebrain) in Alzheimer's

---

*Dr. Freedman is supported in part by a Career Scientist Award from the Ministry of Health of Ontario.

disease, which is the prototypical example of cortical dementia. A similar deficit is also associated with the subcortical dementia of Parkinson's disease.[116] Moreover, both Alzheimer's disease and Parkinson's disease with dementia are associated with neurofibrillary tangles and senile plaques in the cerebral cortex.[10] The terms "cortical" and "subcortical" have thus become controversial. The anatomical overlap between subcortical and cortical dementia was put forth as a strong argument against these concepts being considered distinct entities. This argument, however, tended to ignore the fact that the terms subcortical and cortical dementia, although not strictly accurate from an anatomic point of view, are useful to differentiate behavioral syndromes that are distinctly dissimilar clinically.[25,39]

There are several approaches to the study of the anatomy of dementia. Neurobehavioral studies provide useful information because many of the cognitive functions have traditionally been associated with specific brain regions on the basis of focal-lesion studies. Neurochemical studies have contributed valuable knowledge about neurotransmitters and neural pathways. Neuroanatomic studies integrating the clinical data, anatomy, neuropathology, and modern neuro-imaging techniques [e.g., computerized tomography (CT), positron emission tomography (PET), single photon scanning (SPECT), and magnetic resonance imaging (MRI)] constitute another important source of information. Figures 2.1 and 2.2 have been included to orient the reader to the anatomy of the lobes of the cerebral hemispheres and selected subcortical structures. During the last decade, the use of experimental paradigms adopted from animal models (comparative neuropsychology) has proven to be a valuable approach to the study of the functional neuroanatomy of dementia.[90,114]

The following sections summarize relevant findings based on these approaches. First, the most salient clinical findings in dementia are discussed, as well as their possible relationships to specific areas of the brain. Emphasis is placed on clinical differences between cortical and subcortical dementia, suggesting that they represent different entities, with different anatomical substrates. The section on neurochemistry and experimental studies reviews the current knowledge on neurotransmitters and neuromodulators, and the theories about their role in dementia. A section on neuroanatomic perspective summarizes recent theories on the structures involved in dementia and the processes involved. Finally, some relevant experiments in comparative neuropsychology are highlighted. These suggest involvement of certain pathways and areas of the brain in cortical and subcortical dementias, again indicating different clinical and anatomical entities.

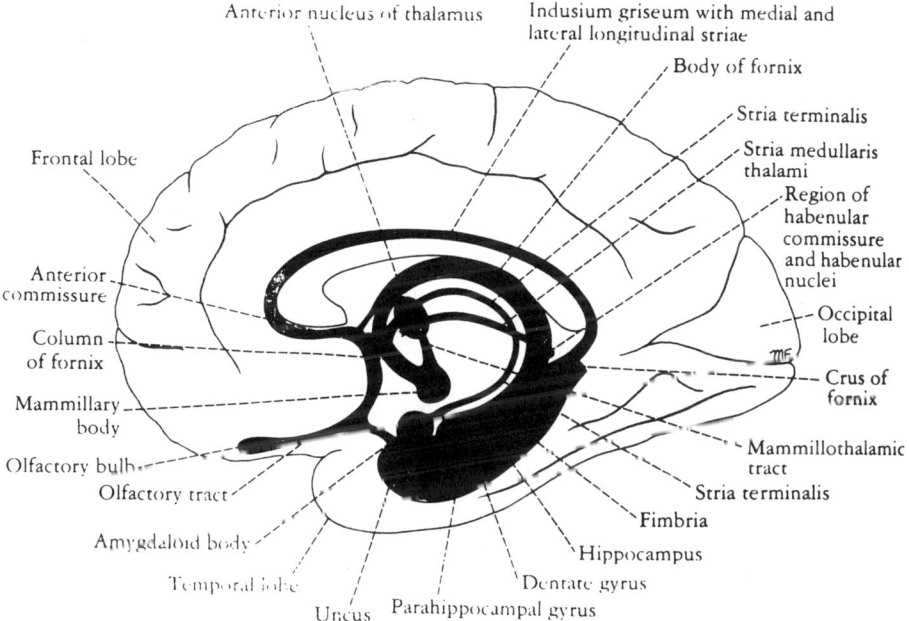

**Figure 2.1** Medial aspect of right cerebral hemisphere, showing structures that form the limbic system. From Snell R. Clinical neuroanatomy for medical students. Boston: Little, Brown & Co., 1980:276.

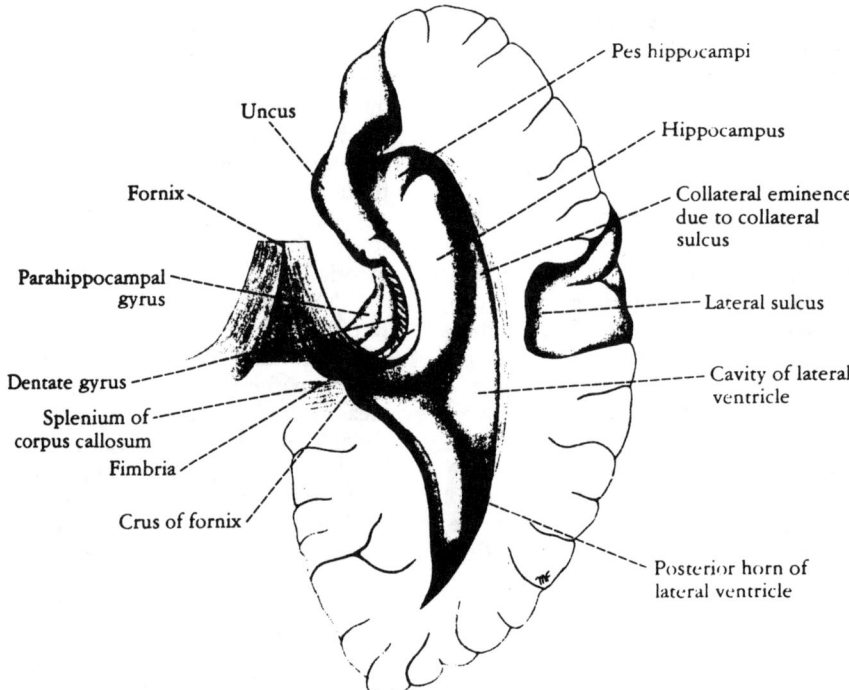

**Figure 2.2** Dissection of the right cerebral hemisphere exposing the cavity of the lateral ventricle. This shows the hippocampus, the dentate gyrus, and the fornix. From Snell R. Clinical neuroanatomy for medical students. Boston: Little, Brown & Co., 1980:277.

## Neurobehavioral Approach

The diagnosis of dementia is based on the impairment of a variety of cognitive functions. Among these, memory, language, praxis, gnosis, visuospatial performance, and manipulation of acquired knowledge have been found to be, on the one hand, most relevant anatomically, and on the other hand, most useful for the differentiation of dementia syndromes.

### MEMORY

Memory loss is an early feature of dementia. Different amnestic patterns, however, distinguish the cortical and subcortical dementias. Episodic memory is defined as "knowledge of a specific stimulus and its location in relation to other stimuli in a given situation and in relation to the perceiver."[28] It is impaired early in most dementias and affects both anterograde memory (ability to form new memories) and retrograde memory (ability to recall memories formed prior to the illness), although anterograde memory is more severely impaired.

Sagar et al studied retrograde amnesia in patients with Parkinson's and Alzheimer's disease.[97] They found that memory for both public events and personal events was impaired in the two groups and that retrograde amnesia showed a temporal gradient, that is, the more remote events were better preserved than the more recent ones. The latter finding is in contrast to those of other studies.[3,43,118] Parkinson's patients, however, differed from Alzheimer's patients in that they showed a more significant impairment for recalling dates than for recalling events, i.e., they could recall some events, but they could not place them in the correct temporal order.

The impairment in recall of temporal order is similar to that described in the amnestic syndrome following frontal and basal forebrain lesions.[29] For example, patient HW had a frontal-lobe syndrome with amnesia following extensive bilateral infarction of the frontal lobes following clipping of an aneurysm of the anterior communicating artery.[85] He showed poor recall of the temporal order of both public and autobiographic events. He was presented with 10 events of his life and 15 from history and was asked about each event itself and its date or temporal order.

Recall of temporal order was extremely impaired, although he could recall the events themselves. Others have described the same impairment of temporal order in frontal-lobe-syndrome patients.[35] Frontal-system involvement may, therefore, underlie at least some components of the memory disorder of Parkinson's disease, i.e., the deficit in recall of the temporal order of events.

Moss et al reported significant differences in performance on recall tasks between patients with Alzheimer's disease and Huntington's disease (another form of subcortical dementia).[86] Both groups were equally impaired with a shorter delay (15 sec). When tested after longer delays, however, the Alzheimer's patients performed significantly worse than the Huntington's patients. In other words, they showed a more rapid rate of forgetting.

Semantic memory, a term proposed by Tulving, denotes knowledge of the basic properties, category, and function of a stimulus.[109] For example, semantic memory refers to the knowledge that a dog is a domestic animal of a certain size and shape. It is far more complex than episodic memory, for it requires the integration of several cognitive functions. It is consistently impaired in dementia.

Procedural memory refers to the ability to acquire a perceptual motor or pattern-analyzing skill that is based on rules.[24] Procedural memory has been reported to be preserved in patients with Alzheimer's disease. For example, they were able to learn a pursuit rotor task as well as controls.[34] In sharp contrast, patients with Parkinson's disease have impaired procedural memory, as tested on a simplified version of the Tower of Hanoi puzzle.[98]

Although the anatomic structures subserving memory are still poorly understood, several studies of amnesic patients have contributed some interesting facts. Huppert and Piercy have provided evidence to suggest that amnesia resulting from combined damage to the amygdala and hippocampus,[55] such as in patient HM,[100] might produce a more rapid rate of forgetting than amnesia attributed to medial diencephalic structures (alcoholic Korsakoff syndrome). The rapid rate of forgetting in Alzheimer's disease could be attributed to involvement of the hippocampus and amygdala (see Figs. 2.1 and 2.2). The impairment of semantic memory, however, cannot be explained by this mechanism because patients with severe hippocampal involvement (e.g., patient HM) have intact semantic memory. Patients with extensive frontal-lobe lesion infarctions of the anterior communicating-artery territory (e.g., patient HW) usually have a well-preserved semantic memory as well. Van Hoesen et al postulate that semantic memory deficits in Alzheimer's disease result from damage to the network that includes the higher order intermodal association cortices located in posterior temporal and inferior parietal regions (Brodmann's areas) (Fig. 2.3).[35-37,39,112]

In summary, although memory loss is a constant sign in almost all dementias, different etiologies seem to show some distinguishing features. Temporal location of past memories seems to be especially affected in Parkinson's disease; Alzheimer's disease is characterized by a more rapid rate of forgetting than some cortical dementias; procedural memory is intact in Alzheimer's disease and impaired in Parkinson's disease. A comparison of the neurobehavioral profiles characterizing dementia resulting from different pathologies may contribute to a better understanding of the anatomic structures involved in the memory loss.

## LANGUAGE IMPAIRMENT

Language impairment is an important feature differentiating cortical from subcortical dementias. In subcortical dementias, there is often an early dysarthria (see Chapter 5 on motor speech disorders), whereas aphasia occurs rarely. There may be a more selective deficit in work-finding difficulty and impaired naming to visual confrontation.[26,43,47] Cummings et al carried out an extensive examination of language impairment in Parkinson's patients with and without dementia and in Alzheimer's patients.[26] They were able to distinguish the different groups on the basis of their speech and language characteristics. Parkinson's patients showed more motor speech and writing difficulties, whereas Alzheimer's patients were more impaired in information content of spontaneous speech, word-list generation, and naming. These findings were in agreement with previous reports.[6,54] Furthermore, Cummings et al found that in Alzheimer's disease, the impairment of naming, as tested by the Boston Naming Test, did not correlate with severity of dementia.[67] Patients with significant naming deficits could show mild degrees of dementia. Parkinson's patients, on the contrary, showed a clear correlation, so that the more severe naming deficits corresponded to the more advanced stage of dementia. This suggests that the language impairment in Parkinson's disease may reflect an overall cognitive decline, whereas the language deficits in Alzheimer's disease may represent instrumental-linguistic dysfunction associated with pathologic changes in the primary language areas of the cerebral cortex (Fig. 2.4).

In Alzheimer's disease, there is a progressive language impairment but no dysarthria. It usually manifests early in the disease as a word-finding difficulty with frequent circumlocutions, and progresses to a severe naming deficit. Semantic

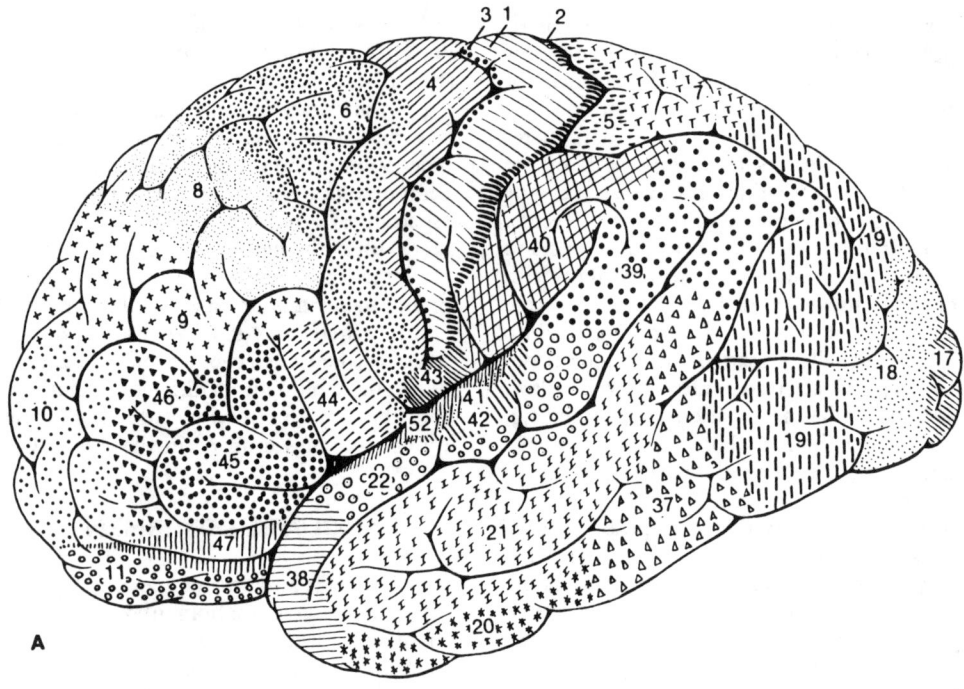

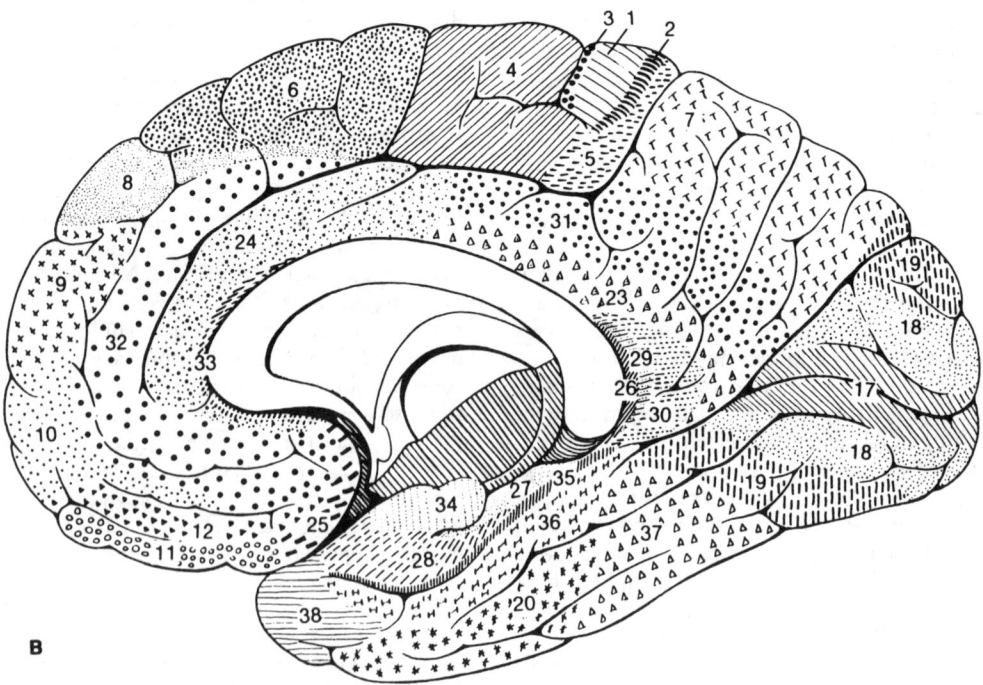

**Figure 2.3** Areas of the cerebral cortex, each of which possesses a distinctive structure. A: Lateral surface. B: Medial surface. From De Jong R. The neurological examination. New York: Harper & Row, 1979:306.

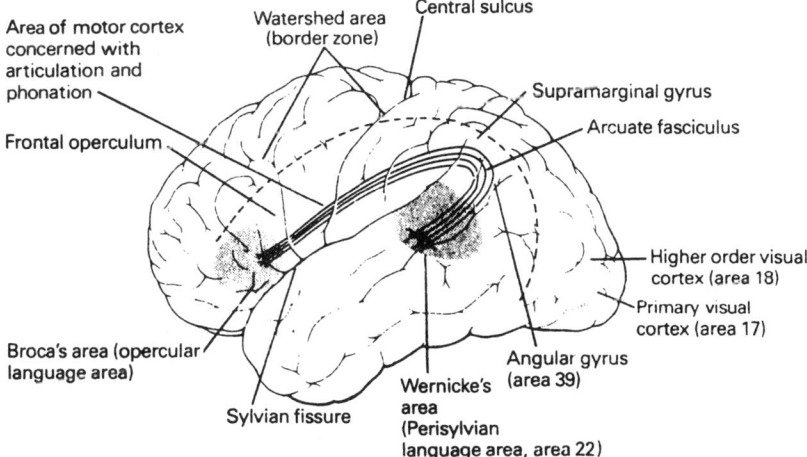

Figure 2.4 Primary language areas of the brain. From Kandel E, Schwartz J. Principles of neuroscience. New York: Elsevier, 1985:693. Copyright 1985 Elsevier Science Publishing Co.

paraphasias are also detected early in the disease. At this stage, speech is fluent and repetition and comprehension are relatively intact. The speech is similar to that of anomic aphasia. Comprehension then becomes progressively impaired, and the resulting language profile begins to resemble that of a transcortical sensory aphasia. At a later stage, repetition becomes impaired. The speech profile then approximates that of a Wernicke's aphasia. In advanced Alzheimer's disease, speech becomes nonfluent, with paraphasias and poor comprehension. In some cases mutism occurs in the terminal stage.[25]

Micrographia is a distinct sign of Parkinson's disease. Cummings et al found a higher prevalence of motor writing disorders in Parkinson's patients than in Alzheimer's patients, in whom there was more linguistic impairment.[26] In Alzheimer's disease, agraphia is present in the form of lexical agraphia with relative sparing of phonologic spelling.[95]

Reading is impaired early in Alzheimer's disease.[112] Recent reports, however, indicate that comprehension for written material is better preserved than what may be expected from the results of traditional testing. When semantic ability was tested by oral reading of sentences containing homographs, Alzheimer's patients showed relatively intact reading comprehension. Thus, reading aloud may be a useful tool in managing Alzheimer's patients.[20]

The previously mentioned patterns of language impairment point to different neural substrates. In Parkinson's disease (i.e., subcortical dementia) there are prominent motor speech problems that may result from basal ganglion involvement. In contrast, prominent language deficits are seen in Alzheimer's disease and may reflect the temporal-parietal cortical involvement that occurs early in this disorder.[15,21,27] The initial naming deficits with paraphasic output may be the result of dysfunction in the posterior temporal and inferior parietal regions (Brodmann's areas 37 to 39) (see Fig. 2.3.)[112]

## PRAXIS

Apraxia is a characteristic feature of Alzheimer's disease that has traditionally been considered to be present in the cortical dementias but not in the subcortical dementias. It is important to stress that there are different forms of apraxia and that the type of apraxia must be specified in any discussion of this condition. In *ideomotor apraxia*, the patient is impaired in performing movements to command and to imitation, but not when using real objects. There may be some improvement in performance to imitation. The apraxia may involve the limbs, buccofacial structures, or midline body structures. Following focal lesions in the left hemisphere, praxis for midline body (axial) commands is usually spared.[46] Conversely, *ideational apraxia* refers to an inability to carry out a series of motor actions in the correct sequence with the actual object.[31]

Rapcsak et al studied ideomotor and ideational apraxia in patients with Alzheimer's disease.[96] They found that the Alzheimer's patients had significant ideomotor apraxia affecting primarily limb transitive movements (e.g., comb your hair). Limb intransitive (e.g., wave goodbye), buccofacial, and axial movements were relatively spared. The patients were also significantly impaired on tests of ideational apraxia. They suggested that the praxic deficits resulted from posterior left-hemisphere cortical involvement.

## GNOSIA

Agnosia is a characteristic feature that occurs late in Alzheimer's disease and, like apraxia, is traditionally thought to differentiate cortical and subcortical dementias. Focal lesions that produce agnosia in nondemented individuals are situated in the temporo-occipital and parieto-occipital association cortices.[51] Although further study is required, involvement of these posterior regions may underlie the agnosia characteristic of Alzheimer's disease as well.

## VISUOSPATIAL FUNCTIONS

Impairment of visuospatial function has traditionally been related to posterior right-hemisphere lesions, particularly the posterior temporal and parietal lobes.[1,50] Left-hemisphere lesions may also produce visuospatial problems, with different characteristics.[66] Patients with frontal-lobe lesions, however, also show some degree of impairment both in visuoperceptive and visuoconstructive tasks.[9,68,70,75] The visuospatial disorders found in frontal-lobe patients are, however, of a different quality than those seen with right posterior lesions.[66] Visuoperceptual and visuoconstructive deficits have been documented in frontal patients by means of complex tasks.[7,76,101,106,107]

In clinical practice, when a patient with frontal-lobe damage is required to draw some relatively complex figure, such as a cube or a clock, the performance is often deficient. There is often perseveration and a lack of a planned strategy. Yet, when the patient is given a model to copy, performance improves. Stuss and Benson[104] described the visuospatial deficit of frontal patients as a function-dependent impairment. If the tasks involve selection, initiation, direction, planning flexibility, and monitoring, performance may be significantly impaired. They claim that visuospatial tasks frequently demand sensory-motor coordination. The frontal lobes predict and anticipate, presetting sensory mechanisms with a corollary discharge so that the result of the motor output can be evaluated and changed if necessary. Damage to the frontal lobe prevents this feedback control mechanism.

It seems clear that normal performance on visuospatial tasks requires intact function and integration of several sensory modalities and their further integration to motor activities, in both hemispheres. Multimodal integration is related to the highly associative areas in the temporal, parieto-occipital, and prefrontal cortices. Damage to these areas or to their projection systems could result in derangement of visuospatial tasks.

In dementia, visuospatial function is often impaired. The impairment of Alzheimer's patients on visual-perceptual and visual-constructional tasks is well established.[25] In Parkinson's disease, performance on these tasks has been repeatedly documented: difficulty with angle matching;[11] figure ground discrimination and perception of spatial position, perception of constancy of shape and size, and perception of spatial relationships;[113] judgment of the visual vertical and horizontal;[30,94] route walking based on a visual map;[14] touching their own body parts corresponding to those designated on a diagram;[13] and tracing tasks.[103]

The visuospatial deficits of Alzheimer's patients may be accounted for by the bilateral involvement of the parietal and frontal lobes. In Parkinson's patients, the related pathology still requires further investigation but may be related to the involvement of subcortical structures, such as the head of the caudate, which receives topographic projections from the frontal cortex (see Fig. 2.5).[63]

## MANIPULATION OF ACQUIRED KNOWLEDGE

One of the first symptoms of dementia is the reduction in the ability to manipulate acquired knowledge. Patients lose their ability to abstract, to solve problems, to plan on the basis of previous experiences, and to adapt to new tasks. These cognitive features are often described following lesions of the highly associative cortex of the prefrontal lobes.[104]

The mechanisms of cognitive disruption underlying this impairment remain to be determined in detail. It is evident that the impairment of memory is strongly related to these deficits. A demented patient cannot judge reality properly if he does not have the necessary memories of past experiences. Neuropsychological tests, however, reveal a much more complex set of interfering phenomena: inability to shift set, perseveration, and stimulus-bound behavior, all of which are related to prefrontal dysfunction.[44,104] Distinction between cortical and subcortical dementia, however, cannot be made on these grounds.

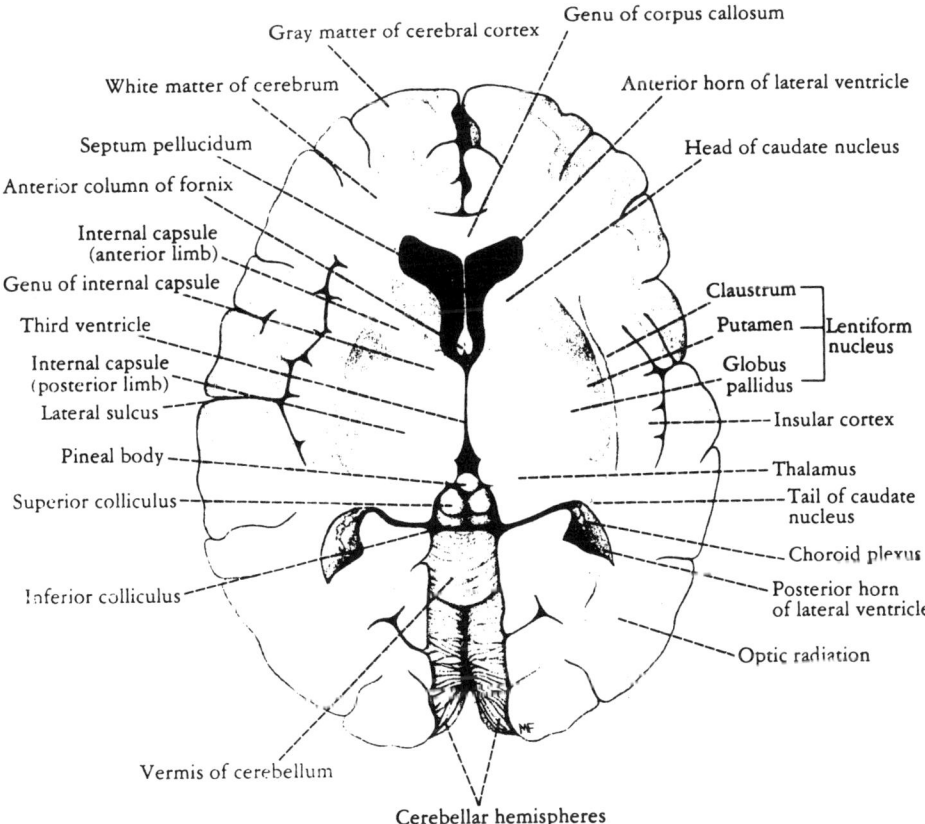

**Figure 2.5** Horizontal section of the cerebrum showing the relationship between the lentiform nucleus, the caudate nucleus, the thalamus, and the internal capsule. From Snell R. Clinical neuroanatomy for medical students. Boston: Little, Brown & Co., 1980:240.

## Neurochemistry and Experimental Studies

With the development of newer techniques to study neurotransmitters and neuromodulators, it has been possible to distinguish specific neurochemical pathways. The cholinergic and dopaminergic systems have been the object of intense research and appear to have an important role in dementia.

### CHOLINERGIC SYSTEMS

Cholinergic neurons have been detected in the striatal complex, the basal forebrain, and the pontomesencephalic reticular formation.[80-82] In the striatal complex, these large cells are more densely packed in the olfactory tubercle and the nucleus accumbens (ventral striatum) than in the caudate and putamen. In the basal forebrain, these neurons are found in the septal area, the diagonal band of Broca, and the substantia innominata, forming a continuum that extends from the medial septum to the lateral geniculate nucleus. On the basis of cytochemical and connectivity patterns, these neurons are subdivided into four major sectors (Ch1 to Ch4). The most anterior group (Ch1) is in the medial septal region, with relatively small round neurons, 10 percent of which are actually cholinergic. The second group (Ch2), with large, fusiform neurons, is embedded within the vertical limb of the diagonal band of Broca. It is continued by a collection of smaller neurons, ventral to the nucleus basalis of Meynert. These cells appear as a horizontal extension of the diagonal band of Broca and constitute the Ch3 group. The most conspicuous group of large neurons is that of the nucleus basalis of Meynert (Ch4), dorsal to Ch3. Its neurons extend from septal levels to the level of the lateral geniculate nucleus, always in juxtaposition with the globus pallidus, the internal capsule, the anterior commissure, and the stria terminalis.

In the upper brainstem, cholinergic neurons can be subdivided into two subgroups, Ch5 and Ch6. Ch5 is mostly within the pedunculopontine nucleus of Olchewsky and Baxter; Ch6 occupies a lateral position that corresponds to that of the dorsolateral tegmental nucleus.

Not all of the cells of these groups are cholinergic; only some of the magnocellular elements of each group give positive choline acetyltransferase (ChAT) staining and are rich in acetylcholinesterase (AChE). ChAT is an enzyme that synthesizes acetylcholine; AChE is the enzyme that degrades it after it has acted on the synapse. To determine that a cell is cholinergic, it must give positive reactions to these two enzymes. Ch1 contains only 10 percent of cholinergic cells, Ch2 70 percent, Ch3 2 to 3 percent, Ch4 90 percent, Ch5 50 percent, and Ch6 90 percent. Taking into consideration the absolute number of cells in each group, it becomes evident that the most important part of this cholinergic system, at least quantitatively, is the nucleus basalis.

The ventral striatum has predominantly limbic affiliations.[52] It receives inputs from the hippocampus, amygdala, olfactory cortex, and limbic cortex. The striatal cholinergic neurons are mainly local circuit neurons. The cholinergic cells of the basal forebrain and brainstem reticular formation, on the contrary, have long ascending projections to the cortex and the thalamus.[64,81]

The hippocampal cortex receives its major cholinergic input from Ch1 and Ch2, the olfactory bulb from Ch3, and the thalamus from Ch5 and Ch6. Ch4 provides cholinergic input to the entire neocortex, in a topographically organized fashion. Hence, the anteromedial division of Ch4 projects to the cingulate and medial fronto-parietal areas; the anterolateral division projects to the frontoparietal opercular cortex and amygdala; the intermediate division projects to the lateral frontoparietal, orbito-insular, lateral peristriate, and inferotemporal cortices; and the posterior division projects to the superior temporal and temporo-polar areas.

The evidence in nonhuman primates for cortical cholinergic input from the nucleus basalis is impressive.[33,65,69,102] In 1984 Perry et al demonstrated that these neurons receive input from the prepyriform cortex, orbitofrontal cortex and insula, temporal pole, entorhinal cortex and medial temporal cortex, and from some subcortical sectors, mainly the septal nuclei, ventral pallidum, and hypothalamus.[81] This suggests that the Ch4 complex is in a position to act as a cholinergic relay for transmitting predominantly limbic and paralimbic information to the neocortical surface.

It has long been claimed that the cholinergic system plays a key role in cognition, mainly in memory and learning. Human subjects receiving scopolamine (an anticholinergic drug) show impairment of memory that cannot be attributed to an altered sensorium alone.[8,17] Therapeutic trials using cholinergic drugs, however, have not been successful in Alzheimer's patients.

The cholinergic deficits found in some dementias have led several authors to focus attention on the nucleus basalis of Meynert and its pathologic changes. Marked neuronal loss and gliosis have been well documented in the nucleus basalis of Meynert in both Alzheimer's and Parkinson's diseases.[115,116] In addition, there are also neurofibrillary tangles and senile plaques in the cerebral cortex in both disorders. A recent report on acetylcholinesterase-rich pyramidal neurons opens a new field of research. These neurons, pyramidal in shape, were found to be abundant in layers III, V, and VI of the cerebral cortex of the temporal lobes and at the CA1-subicular junction within the hippocampal complex. The interesting fact in this finding is that these neurons are only found in humans. They are virtually absent in childhood and become established by adolescence. Their density increases during adulthood and perhaps in senescence. They are markedly vulnerable to degeneration in Alzheimer's disease. They do not seem to be cholinergic because the adult primate cerebral cortex has never been shown to contain the necessary enzymes to synthesize acetylcholine. They may synthesize somatostatin, a neuropeptide that has been reported to coexist with AChe in human cortical neurons.[88] Somatostatin is decreased in Alzheimer's disease and Parkinson's disease but not in other forms of dementia.[36]

The pathologic significance of the above findings is not yet clear. Whether the cortical changes are purely a reflection of, or secondary to, the subcortical changes of the cholinergic system is still controversial. Perry et al found that the cholinergic deficit correlated with the number of plaques and postulated that plaques may be the result of degenerative changes of the dying cholinergic axons.[92] This hypothesis is supported by the fact that in Gerstmann-Sträussler dementia (familial spino-cerebellar degeneration and dementia), as well as in Alzheimer's disease, there is a significant decrease of ChAT. This decrease correlates with the presence of plaques. It must be remarked, however, that the neuronal loss of the nucleus basalis of Meynert and the decrease of ChAT have also been reported in Korsakoff's patients, in whom no senile plaques have been described.[4]

There still remains the question of the relationship between changes in the nucleus basalis and cognitive impairment. Neuropathologic studies and ChAT content of the brain of four members of a family known to suffer from olivopontocerebellar atrophy showed a neuronal loss of 70 percent in the nucleus basalis, and a 50 to 80 percent decrease of ChAT activity in all examined cortical subdivisions, with sparing of the hippocampus and amygdala.[72] There were no senile plaques or neurofibrillary tangles. These patients had only mild cognitive impairment that was predominantly frontal in nature. The cognitive deficits in Alzheimer's disease, however, are much more widespread. Because both Alzheimer's disease and olivopontocerebellar atrophy have a similar cortical cholinergic deficit, the inference is that the cortical cholinergic deficit alone is not sufficient to produce the cognitive deficit in Alzheimer's disease.

Furthermore, the fact that alterations of the nucleus basalis have been documented in diseases of very different pathophysiology, such as Alzheimer's disease, Korsakoff's syndrome, and Gerstmann-Sträussler syndrome, raises the question whether these changes are secondary to more fundamental lesions in the brain.

In summary, the cholinergic system of the nucleus basalis of Meynert is known to be severely affected in some dementias. This is typically the case in Alzheimer's disease. Because of its wide neocortical projections and its intricate feed-forward–feed-backward pathways, it may have an important role in dementia. There is evidence, however, to conclude that it cannot account for the entire dementia syndrome in disorders such as Alzheimer's disease.

## DOPAMINERGIC SYSTEM

In Parkinson's disease there is a severe reduction in dopamine, which is most marked in the nigro-striatal system. In the head of the caudate, the most severe reduction is found in the anterodorsal sector.[71,73] It is of note that this is the region of the caudate head to which the dorsolateral frontal cortex primarily projects.[63] This may account for the frontal-lobe deficits that are seen in Parkinson's dementia.

In addition to the dopamine loss in the nigro-striatal system in Parkinson's disease, there is severe cell loss in the ventral tegmental area, which is the source of the majority of the mesolimbic-mesocortical dopaminergic fibers. These fibers project to the frontal cortex as well as to other areas including the nucleus accumbens and entorhinal cortex.[53,62,110] Dopamine levels have been documented to correlate with intellectual impairment in Parkinson's disease.[26,103]

Finally, the documented data on neurotransmitters in Parkinson's disease suggest that there is a relationship between cognitive impairment and dopamine loss in the frontal-subcortical systems. Further documentation in animal and human studies is necessary to unravel this relationship.

## Neuroanatomical Perspective

Regional cortical pathology studies have documented changes in the occipital, parietal, temporal, and frontal cortex in Alzheimer's disease,[15,16,25,108] and in the frontal and temporal cortex in Pick's disease.[25] In the subcortical regions, changes have been noted in the substantia nigra and the ventral tegmental area in Parkinson's disease.[22] Cell loss has also been documented in the nucleus basalis of Meynert in Alzheimer's disease, Parkinson's disease, olivopontocerebellar atrophy, and Gerstmann-Sträussler syndrome.[5,45,89,115,116] No cell loss has been found in the nucleus basalis of Meynert in Huntington's disease.[23,105] In Pick's disease, some authors report depletion of cells up to 30 percent,[87] some report a moderate cell loss,[111] and others found no significant reduction of neurons.[105]

Blood-flow studies in patients with Parkinson's have shown reduced flow in the frontal mesocortex.[91] PET studies reveal abnormalities in the basal ganglia and also in the cerebral cortex.[91] Kuhl et al evaluated cerebral blood flow in 13 patients with Huntington's disease and found that there was significant hypometabolic activity in the caudate and putamen, but not in the cerebral cortex.[74]

Different areas of the brain are connected by means of intricate multisynaptic networks. Among them, and of utmost importance in the dementias, are the networks relaying sensory information. The sensory modalities (auditory, visual, and somato-sensory) reach the primary sensory cortices [areas 40, 1, 2, 3, and 17 (see Fig.2-3)] and initiate a complex feed-forward system of intrahemispheric projections towards adjacent sensory-association areas, many of which are multimodal.[112] As stated by Van Hoesen et al, new projections from the sensory association areas disseminate sensory information to other areas of the cerebral cortex.[112] Much of the information disseminated and integrated in the cerebral cortex converges towards the entorhinal cortex, area 28 of Brodmann. The main input to area 28 is formed by projections from the neighboring cortical regions, which are known to be highly associative areas. Area 28 gives rise to the perforant pathway, a major neural system of the temporal lobe that terminates in the hippocampus. In fact, the entorhinal cortex and its perforant pathway constitute the strongest input to the hippocampus and form its exclusive link to the remainder of the cerebral cortex.

The output of the hippocampus arises from the subiculum and the CA1 part. Through a long multirelay pathway, the hippocampus projects back to the associative cortices, so that the feed-forward–feed-backward system is completed. The circuit includes sensory areas in different parts of the brain and important relays in the limbic system.

The prefrontal-subcortical system is another example of a multisynaptic pathway of great importance in the understanding of the dementias. The prefrontal cortex receives afferent fibers from numerous structures of the diencephalon, the mesencephalon, the limbic system, and even the cerebellum. Projections to the prefrontal cortex from the thalamus originate mainly in the dorsomedial nucleus but also in the anterior ventral and anterior intralaminar nuclei. They convey input from the brainstem, cerebellum, and limbic structures. Direct afferents from the hypothalamus, the midbrain, the amygdala, and the limbic cortex have also been demonstrated. In addition, fibers from various neocortical areas implicated in higher sensory functions converge on the prefrontal cortex.

The connections between the prefrontal cortex and subcortical structures are topographically organized, forming systems of multisynaptic pathways. Hence, the orbitofrontal cortex is primarily connected to the medial thalamus, hypothalamus, ventrolateral caudate, and amygdala; the dorsolateral prefrontal cortex is connected to the lateral thalamus, anterodorsal caudate, hippocampus, and neocortex.

In Alzheimer's disease, the characteristic degenerative changes (i.e., neuronal loss, senile plaques, and neurofibrillary tangles) have been found to selectively affect specific cell groups in certain areas. Hence, Alzheimer's disease affects layers III and V in the isocortex of the association areas (frontal, parietal, temporal, and occipital) and spares the primary sensory and motor cortices. Layers III and V give rise to the long projection systems to other parts of the cortex. The most constant pathology in Alzheimer's disease is, however, the severe compromise of layers II and III of the entorhinal cortex, i.e., the layers that give rise to the perforant pathway. The neural system conveying cortical association input to the hippocampus is therefore destroyed. Moreover, the subiculum, the CA1 part of the hippocampus, and layer IV of the entorhinal cortex, which are the cells of output of the hippocampus, are also heavily affected. In other words, it seems that the hippocampus becomes functionally isolated in Alzheimer's disease.[56,57,112]

These findings, in addition to the clinical course of the disease, have led Van Hoesen et al to postulate the theory that there is a single early focus that resides in the temporal lobe, particularly the parahippocampal gyrus (entorhinal cortex) and hippocampal formation.[112] The condition then progresses to affect the association cortices and their pathways in a selective fashion.

In the subcortical dementia of Parkinson's disease, the underlying neuroanatomic substrates producing cognitive impairment are still unclear. The constancy of the findings in the basal ganglia and the predominance of frontal lobe symptoms in this disorder strongly suggest involvement of the prefrontal-subcortical systems.[38] It is noteworthy that within the caudate nucleus in Parkinson's disease it is the anterior position of the caudate head that undergoes the most severe loss of dopamine concentration.[71] This part of the caudate head is the area in which dorsolateral frontal cortex primarily projects and may be important in the pathophysiology of dementia in Parkinson's disease.[63]

## Comparative Neuropsychology

Animal models have long been used to study cognitive function. The use of experimental neuropsychological tasks adopted from animal models to study cognitive function in brain-damaged humans is a recent approach and has been termed comparative neuropsychology.[90,114]

Freedman and Oscar-Berman have reported distinct neuroanatomic and neurobehavioral mechanisms differentiating Alzheimer's and Parkinson's dementia.[40,42] They used experimental paradigms that have been validated for the demonstration of deficits leading to damage in the prefrontal cortical-subcortical system and parietal system in animal models. They compared a group of Parkinson's patients with dementia to a group of equally demented patients with Alzheimer's disease. Nondemented Parkinson's patients and normals served as controls.

The first experiment was designed to identify impairment related to two different prefrontal cortical-subcortical systems: the dorsolateral frontal system and the orbitofrontal system. The tasks initially used were delayed alternation (DA) and delayed response (DR). These tasks have been reported to be impaired in nonhuman primates with bilateral frontal-lobe lesions,[59-61] and in humans with bilateral frontal-lobe lesions documented by CT.[39] Both tasks measure spatial mnemonic factors.[19,48] In addition, DA is sensitive to perseveration.[84] Dorsolateral lesions result in severe impairment of DA and DR; DA may also be affected following orbitofrontal damage.[18,83]

The results of the initial experiment showed that only the Alzheimer's patients, not the Parkinson's patients, were found to be significantly impaired on the DA task, whereas both groups were impaired on the DR task. Freedman and Oscar-Berman concluded that the impairment of DR suggested dorsolateral frontal damage in both groups of patients and postulated that the orbitofrontal damage may have produced the deficits on DA in Alzheimer's patients. Freedman, therefore, administered an object alternation (OA) task to patients with Alzheimer's and Parkinson's disease.[37] This task is a measure of perseveration and is more sensitive to orbitofrontal than to dorsolateral frontal system lesions in nonhuman primates. Although both groups were impaired compared to controls, the Alzheimer's patients showed a significantly worse performance than the Parkinson's patients. An error analysis revealed that the performance of the Alzheimer's patients was characterized by response perseveration. This suggested that the significant perseverative deficits in Alzheimer's disease were caused by the presence of orbitofrontal system dysfunction, and that the milder, qualitatively different deficits in Parkinson's disease may reflect dorsolateral frontal-system involvement.

In another experiment, Freedman and Oscar-Berman used a spatial and visual discrimination learning problem that included original learning of a new problem and reversals of the original learning.[41] In nonhuman primates, these tasks show well-documented profiles of impairment of the frontal lobes, temporal lobes, and fornix, respectively.[90] Alzheimer's patients were significantly more impaired on the visual learning task than were Parkinson's patients with dementia, both in original learning and in reversal of this learning. An error analysis of the subject responses revealed that there were qualitative differences: perseverative errors were significantly more common in the Alzheimer's patients than they were in the demented Parkinson's patients. The performance profile on the visual tasks suggested that disturbance in orbitofrontal system function contributed to deficits in Alzheimer's disease. With regard to the spatial tasks, both groups were unimpaired on the original spatial discrimination problem, whereas both groups showed significant deficits on reversals of the original learning. This profile of normal performance on spatial original learning and impaired performance on spatial reversal learning has been documented following lesions in the hippocampus, anterior inferotemporal area, and fornix.[90] Further studies are required to determine the corresponding anatomic substrates involved in these tasks and their relation to Alzheimer's and Parkinson's dementia.

Freedman and Oscar-Berman also assessed the parietocortical/subcortical system in Alzheimer's and Parkinson's disease, using a tactile original learning (TOL) and tactile reversal learning (TRL) paradigm. The former is sensitive to bilateral parietal-lobe lesions in nonhuman primates.[117] In this task, Alzheimer's patients were significantly impaired compared to Parkinson's patients with dementia. These findings support the concepts discussed in previous sections about an early involvement of the parietal lobes in the degenerative process of Alzheimer's disease.

TRL provides a measure of perseveration with touch as the input modality. Both groups of patients were impaired in this task. An analysis of error patterns of the two groups showed that there was a difference in the types of errors that were made. Perseveration was a significantly greater factor in contributing to the deficits in the Alzheimer's patients compared to all other groups. Because perseveration is associated with frontal-lobe lesions, this tendency in the Alzheimer's patients is likely to be the result of the known orbitofrontal pathology in this disorder.[99,108]

## Concluding Remarks

Dementia is a neurobehavioral syndrome characterized by personality changes and widespread cognitive impairment. Recent studies lend strong support to the concept that there are important differences in the cognitive deficits associated with Alzheimer's disease as compared to Parkinson's disease. From a behavioral point of view, the data suggest that there are qualitative and quantitative differences in performance on measures of memory, learning, and language.

Neuroanatomical data suggest that in Alzheimer's disease, the most common and well-studied cortical dementia, there is specific early involvement of certain layers and cells of the associative cortices and their pathways connecting them to the hippocampus and entorhinal cortex. The involved associative areas are frontal, parietal, temporal, and occipital. This may account for cognitive deficits that have long been related to these regions in studies of the effects of focal lesions. Whether the disease is multifocal in these several sites from the beginning or whether there is an initial hippocampal-entorhinal locus, as has been suggested, requires further research.[112]

In Parkinson's disease, the most thoroughly studied form of subcortical dementia, the clinical features suggest frontal-subcortical involvement. There are indications that involvement of the dorsolateral-frontal system, which includes the anterodorsal sector of the head of the caudate, contributes to the neuropsychological deficits. Conversely, in Alzheimer's disease, the findings suggest damage of both dorsolateral and orbitofrontal systems, as well as parietal and temporal systems.

The anatomy of dementia still has many unanswered questions. A multi-disciplinary approach is most likely to find the answers.

# References

1. Adams RD, Victor M. Principles of neurology. 3rd ed. New York: McGraw-Hill, 1985.
2. Albert ML, Feldman RG, Willis AL. "The subcortical dementia" of progressive supranuclear palsy. J Neurol Neurosurg Psychiatry 1974; 37:121–130.
3. Albert MS, Butters N, Brandt J. Patterns of remote memory in amnesic and demented patients. Arch Neurol 1981; 38:495–500.
4. Arendt T, Bigl V, Arendt A. Loss of neurons in the nucleus basalis of Meynert in Alzheimer's disease, paralysis agitans and Korsakoff's disease. Acta Neuropathol (Berl) 1983; 61:101–108.
5. Arendt T, Bigl V, Arendt A. Neurone loss in the nucleus basalis of Meynert in Creutzfeldt-Jakob disease. Acta Neuropathol (Berl) 1984; 65:85–88.
6. Bayles KA, Tomodea CK. Confrontation naming impairment in dementia. Brain Lang 1983; 19:98–114.
7. Benson DF, Barton MI. Disturbances in constructional abilities. Cortex 1970; 6:19–46.
8. Besson J. Dementia: Biological solution still a long way off. Br Med J 1983; 287:926–927.
9. Black FW, Bernard BA. Constructional apraxia as a function of lesion locus and size in patients with focal brain damage. Cortex 1984; 20:111–120.
10. Boller F, Mizutani T, Roessmann U, Gambetti P. Parkinson's disease, dementia and Alzheimer disease: Clinicopathological correlations. Ann Neurol 1980; 7:329–335.
11. Boller F, Passafiume D, Keefe NC. Visuospatial impairments in Parkinson's disease: Role of perceptual and motor factors. Arch Neurol 1984; 41:485–490.
12. Botez M, Leiner HC, Leiner AL, Dow RS. Does the cerebellum contribute to mental skills? Behav Neurosci 1986; 100:443–454.
13. Bowen FP, Burns MM, Brady EM, Yahr MD. A note on alterations of personal orientation in Parkinsonism. Neuropsychologia 1976; 14:425–429.
14. Bowen FP, Hoehn MM, Yahr MD. Parkinsonism: Alterations in spatial orientation as determined by a route-walking task. Neuropsychologia 1972; 10:355–361.
15. Brun A, Englund E. Regional pattern of degeneration in Alzheimer's disease: Neuronal loss and histopathological grading. Histopathology 1981; 5:549–564.
16. Brun A, Gustafson L. Distribution of cerebral degeneration in Alzheimer's disease. Acta Psychiatr Nervenkr 1976; 223:15–33.
17. Bruno G, Mohr E, Gillespie M, Fedio P, Chase TN. Muscarinic agonist therapy of Alzheimer's disease. Arch Neurol 1986; 43:659–661.
18. Brutkowsky S, Mishkin M, Rosvold HE. In: Gutmann E, Hnik P, eds. Central and peripheral mechanisms of motor function. Prague: Czechoslovak Academy of Sciences, 1963:133.
19. Butters N, Rosvold HE. Effect of septal lesions on resistance to extinction and delayed alternation in monkeys. J Comp Physiol Psychol 1968; 66:389–395.
20. Campbell-Taylor I, Behrmann M. Semantics and reading ability in Alzheimer's disease. (Submitted.)
21. Chase TN, Foster NL, Fedio P, et al. Regional cortical dysfunction in Alzheimer's disease as determined by positron emission tomography. Ann Neurol 1984; 15:(suppl. S170–S174).
22. Chui HC, Morlimer JA, Slager U, et al. Pathologic correlates of dementia in Parkinson's disease. Arch Neurol 1986; 43:991–995.
23. Clark AW, Parhad IM, Folstein SE. The nucleus basalis in Huntington's disease. Neurology 1983; 33:1262–1267.
24. Cohen NJ, Squire L. Preserved learning and retention of pattern-analyzing skill in amnesia: Dissociation of knowing how and knowing what. Science 1980; 210:207–210.
25. Cummings JL, Benson DF. Dementia: A clinical approach. Boston: Butterworth, 1983.
26. Cummings JL, Darkins A, Mendez M, Hill MA, Benson DF. Alzheimer's disease and Parkinson's disease: Comparison of speech and language alterations. Neurology 1988; 38:680–684.
27. Cutler NR, Haxby JV, Duara R, et al. Brain metabolism as measured with positron emission tomography: Serial assessment in a patient with familial Alzheimer's disease. Neurology 1985; 35:1956–1961.
28. Damasio AR, Eslinger PJ, Damasio H, Van Hoesen HW, Cornell S. Multimodal amnesic syndrome following bilateral temporal and basal forebrain damage. Arch Neurol 1985; 42:252–259.
29. Damasio AR, Graaf-Radford N, Eslinger PJ, Damasio H, Kassell N. Amnesia following basal forebrain lesions. Arch Neurol 1985; 42:263–271.
30. Danta G, Hilton RC. Judgment of the visual vertical and horizontal in patients with Parkinsonism. Neurology 1975; 25:43–47.
31. De Renzi E, Lucheli F. Ideational apraxia. Brain 1988; 111:1173–1185.
32. Diagnostic and statistical manual of mental disorders. 3rd ed. Washington D.C.: American Psychiatric Association, 1980.
33. Divac I. Magnocellular nuclei of the basal forebrain project to neocortex, brainstem and olfactory bulb: Review of some functional correlates. Brain Res 1975; 93:385–398.
34. Eslinger PJ, Damasio AR. Preserved motor learning in Alzheimer's disease. J Neurosci 1986; 6:3006–3009.
35. Eslinger PJ, Damasio AR. Severe cognitive disturbance following bilateral frontal lobe ablation. Patient EVR. Neurology 1985; 35:1731–1741.
36. Ferrier IN, Cross AJ, Johnson JA, et al. Neuropeptides in Alzheimer type dementia. J Neurol Sci 1983; 62:159–170.
37. Freedman M. Delayed alternation and orbitofrontal system dysfunction in Alzheimer's and Parkinson's disease. (Submitted.)
38. Freedman M. Parkinson's disease and dementia: Functional anatomy and neuropsychological mechanisms. In: Cummings JL, ed. Subcortical dementia. New York: Oxford University Press. (In press.)
39. Freedman M, Oscar-Berman M. Comparative neuropsychology of cortical and subcortical dementia. Can J Neurol Sci 1986; 13:410–414.
40. Freedman M, Oscar-Berman M. Selective delayed response deficits in Alzheimer's and Parkinson's disease. Arch Neurol 1986; 43:886–890.
41. Freedman M, Oscar-Berman M. Spatial and visual reversal learning in Alzheimer's and Parkinson's disease. Brain Cogn 1989; 11:114–126.
42. Freedman M, Oscar-Berman M. Tactile discrimination learning deficits in Alzheimer's and Parkinson's disease. Arch Neurol 1987; 44:394–398.
43. Freedman M, Rivoira P, Butters N, Sax DS, Robert G. Retrograde amnesia in Parkinson's disease. Can J Neurol Sci 1984; 11:297–301.

44. Fuster JM. The prefrontal cortex: Anatomy, physiology and neuropsychology of the frontal lobe. New York: Raven Press, 1980.
45. Gaspar P, Gray F. Dementia in idiopathic Parkinson's disease. Acta Neuropathol (Berl) 1984; 64:43-52.
46. Geschwind N. The apraxias: Neural mechanisms of disorders of learned movement. Am Scientist 1975; 63:188-195.
47. Globus M, Mildworf B, Melamed E. Cerebral blood flow and cognitive impairment in Parkinson's disease. Neurology 1985; 35:1135-1139.
48. Goldman PS, Rosvold HE. Localization of function within the dorsolateral prefrontal cortex of the rhesus monkey. Exp Neurol 1970; 27:291-304.
49. Hachinsky VC, Lassen NA, Marshall J. Multiple infarct dementia, a cause of mental deterioration in the elderly. Lancet 1978; 2:207-210.
50. Hecaen H. Introduction à la neuropsychologie. Paris: Larousse, 1972.
51. Heilman K, Valenstein E. Clinical neuropsychology. Oxford: Oxford University Press, 1985.
52. Heimer L, Wilson RD. The subcortical projections of the allocortex: Similarities in the neural associations of the hippocampus, the piriform cortex and the neocortex. In: Santini M, ed. Golgi centennial symposium. New York: Raven Press, 1975:177.
53. Hornykiewicz O, Kish SJ. Biochemical pathophysiology of Parkinson's disease. In: Yahr MD, Bergmann KJ, eds. Advances in neurology. New York: Raven Press, 1986.
54. Huber SJ, Shuttleworth EC, Paulson GW, Bellchambers MJG, Clapp LE. Cortical vs subcortical dementia: Neuropsychological differences. Arch Neurol 1986; 43:392-394.
55. Huppert FA, Piercy M. Normal and abnormal forgetting in organic amnesia: Effect of locus of lesion. Cortex 1979; 15:385-390.
56. Hyman BT, Damasio AR, Van Hoesen GW, Barnes CL. Alzheimer's disease: Cell specific pathology isolates the hippocampal formation. Science 1984; 225:1168-1170.
57. Hyman BT, Van Hoesen GW, Kromer LJ, Damasio AR. The subicular cortices in Alzheimer's disease: Neuroanatomical relationships and the memory impairment. Soc Neurosci Abstr 1985; 11:458.
58. Ishii N, Nishihara Y, Inamura T. Why do frontal lobe symptoms predominate in vascular dementia with lacunes? Neurology 1986; 36:340-345.
59. Jacobsen CF. Function of the frontal association area in primates. Arch Neurol Psychiatry 1935; 33:558-569.
60. Jacobsen CF. Studies of cerebral function in primates: I. The functions of the frontal association areas in monkeys. Comp Psychol Monogr 1936; 13:3-60.
61. Jacobsen CF, Niessen HW. Studies of cerebral function in primates: IV. The effects of frontal lobe lesions on the delayed alternation habit in monkeys. J Comp Physiol Psychol 1937; 23:101-112.
62. Javoy-Agid F, Agid Y. Is the mesocortical dopaminergic system involved in Parkinson's disease? Neurology 1980; 30:1326-1330.
63. Johnson TN, Rosvold HE, Mishkin M. Projections of behaviorally defined sectors of the prefrontal cortex to the basal ganglia, septum and diencephalon in the monkey. Exp Neurol 1968; 21:20-34.
64. Johnston MV, McKinney M, Coyle CT. Evidence for a cholinergic projection to neocortex from neurons in basal forebrain. Proc Nat Acad Sci USA 1978; 76:5392-5396.
65. Jones EG, Burton H, Saper CB, Swanson LW. Midbrain, diencephalic and cortical relationships of the basal nucleus of Meynert and associated structures in primates. Comp Neurol 1976; 167:385-420.
66. Kaplan E. A process approach to neuropsychological assessment. In: Boll T, Bryant BK, eds. Clinical neuropsychology and brain function, research, measurement and practice. Washington, D.C.: American Psychological Association, 1988:121.
67. Kaplan E, Goodglass H, Weintraub S. The Boston naming test. Philadelphia: Lea and Febiger, 1983.
68. Kertesz A, Dobrowolski S. Right hemisphere deficits, lesion size and location. J Clin Neuropsychol 1981; 3:283-299.
69. Kievit J, Kuypers HGJM. Basal forebrain and hypothalamic connections to frontal and parietal cortex in the rhesus monkey. Science 1975; 187:660-662.
70. Kim Y, Morrow L, Passafiume D, Boller F. Visuoperceptual and visuomotor abilities and locus of lesion. Neuropsychologia 1984; 22:177-185.
71. Kish SJ, Rajput A, Gilbert J, et al. Elevated aminobutyric acid level in striatal but not extrastriatal brain regions in Parkinson's disease: Correlation with striatal dopamine loss. Ann Neurol 1986; 20:26-31.
72. Kish S, Robitaille Y, Freedman M, et al. Cerebral cortical cholinergic reduction in dominantly inherited olivopontocerebellar atrophy: Implications for the cholinergic hypothesis of dementia. Soc Neurosci 1988; 14(2):1221.
73. Kish SJ, Shannak K, Hornykiewicz O. Uneven pattern of dopamine loss in the striatum of patients with idiopathic Parkinson's disease. Pathophysiologic and clinical implications. N Engl J Med 1988; 318:876-880.
74. Kuhl DE, Phelps ME, Markham CH, et al. Cerebral metabolism and atrophy in Huntington's disease determined by FDG and computed tomographic scan. Ann Neurol 1982; 12:425-434.
75. Luria AR. Higher cortical functions in man. New York: Basic Books, 1980.
76. Luria AR. The working brain: An introduction to neuropsychology. Translated by B. Haigh, New York: Basic Books, 1973.
77. McHugh PR, Folstein MF. Psychiatric syndromes of Huntington's disease: A clinical and phenomenological study. In: Benson DF, Blumer D, eds. Psychiatric aspects of neurological disease. New York: Grune and Stratton, 1975:267-286.
78. McKhann G, Drachman D, Folstein M, et al. Clinical diagnosis of Alzheimer's disease. Report of the NINCDS-ADRDA workgroup under the auspices of Department of Health and Human Services Task Force on Alzheimer's disease. Neurology 1984; 34:939-944.
79. Mesulam MM, Changiz G. Acetylcholinesterase-rich pyramidal neurons in the human neocortex and hippocampus: Absence at birth, development during the life span and dissolution in Alzheimer's disease. Ann Neurol 1988; 24:765-773.
80. Mesulam MM, Muffson EJ, Levy A, Wainer BH. Cholinergic innervation of cortex by the basal forebrain: Cytochemistry and cortical connections of the septal area, diagonal band nucleus basalis (substantia innominata) and hypothalamus of the rhesus monkey. J Comp Neurol 1983; 214:170-197.
81. Mesulam MM, Muffson EJ, Levy AI, Wainer BH. Atlas of cholinergic neurons in the forebrain and upper brainstem of the macaque based on monoclonal choline acetyltransferase immunohistochemistry and acetylcholinesterase histochemistry. Neuroscience 1984; 12:669-686.
82. Mesulam MM, Volicer L, Marquis JK, Muffson EJ,

Green RC. Systematic regional differences in the cholinergic innervation of the primate cerebral cortex: Distribution of the enzyme activities and some behavioral implications. Ann Neurol 1986; 19:144–151.
83. Mishkin M. A re-examination of the effects of frontal lesions on object alternation. Neuropsychologia 1969; 7:357–363.
84. Mishkin M. Perseveration of central sets after frontal lesions in monkeys. In: Warren JM, Akert K, eds. The frontal granular cortex and behavior. New York: McGraw-Hill Book Company, 1964:219.
85. Moscovitch M. Confabulation and the frontal system: Strategy vs associative retrieval in neuropsychological theories of memory. In: Roediger HL, Craik FIM, eds. Festschrif for Endel Tulving. Hillsdale, NJ: Erlbaum (In press.)
86. Moss MB, Albert MS, Butters N, Payne M. Differential patterns of memory loss among patients with Alzheimer's disease, Huntington's disease and alcoholic Korsakoff's syndrome. Arch Neurol 1986; 43:239–246.
87. Munoz-Garcia D, Ludwin SR. Classic and generalized variants of Pick's disease. A clinicopathological, ultrastructural and immunocytochemical comparative study. Ann Neurol 1984; 16:467–480.
88. Nakamura S, Vincent SR. Acetylcholinesterase and somatostatin immunoreactivity coexist in human neocortex. Neurosci Lett 1985; 61:183–187.
89. Nakano I, Hirano A. Parkinson's disease: Neuron loss in the nucleus basalis without concomitant Alzheimer's disease. Ann Neurol 1984; 15:415–418.
90. Oscar-Berman M, Zola-Morgan SM. Comparative neuropsychology and Korsakoff's syndrome. I. Spatial and visual reversal learning. Neuropsychologia 1980; 18:499–512.
91. Perlmutter JS. New insights into the pathophysiology of Parkinson's disease: The challenge of positron emission tomography. Trends Neurosci 1988; 11:203–208.
92. Perry EK, Tomlinson BE, Blessed G, et al. Correlation of cholinergic abnormalities with senile plaques and mental test scores in senile dementia. Br Med J 1978; II:1457–1459.
93. Perry RH, Sandy JM, Perry EK. The substantia innominata and adjacent regions in the human brain: Histochemical and biochemical observations. J Anat 1984; 138(4):713–732.
94. Proctor F, Riklan M, Cooper IS, Teuver HL. Judgement of visual and postural vertical by parkinsonian patients. Neurology 1964; 14:287–293.
95. Rapcsak SZ, Arthur SA, Bliklen DA, Rubens AB. Lexical agraphia in Alzheimer's disease. Arch Neurol 1989; 46:65–68.
96. Rapcsak SZ, Croswell S, Rubens AB. Apraxia in Alzheimer's disease. Neurology 1989; 39:664–668.
97. Sagar HJ, Cohen NJ, Sullivan EV, Corkin S, Growdon JH. Remote memory function in Alzheimer's disease and Parkinson's disease. Brain 1988; 111:185–206.
98. Saint-Cry JA, Taylor AE, Lang AE. Procedural learning and neostriatal dysfunction in man. Brain 1988; 111:941–959.
99. Sandson JS, Albert ML. Varieties of perseveration. Neuropsychologia 1984; 6:715–732.
100. Scolville WB, Milner B. Loss of recent memory after bilateral hippocampal lesions. J Neurol Neurosurg Psychiatry 1957; 20:11–21.
101. Semmes J, Weinstein S, Ghent L, Teuber HL. Correlates of impaired orientation in personal and extrapersonal space. Brain 1963; 86:747–772.
102. Shute CD, Lewis PR. The ascending cholinergic reticular system: Neocortical, olfactory and subcortical projections. Brain 1967: 90:497–520.
103. Stern Y, Langston JW. Intellectual changes in patients with MPTP-induced Parkinsonism. Neurology 1985; 35:1506–1509.
104. Stuss DT, Benson DF, eds. The frontal lobes. New York: Raven Press, 1986:194.
105. Tagliavini F, Pilleri G. Basal nucleus of Meynert: A neuropathological study in Alzheimer's disease, simple senile dementia, Pick's disease and Huntington's chorea. J Neurol Sci 1983; 62:243–260.
106. Taylor LB. Psychological assessment of neurosurgical patients. In: Rasmussen T, Marino R, ed. Functional neurosurgery. New York: Raven Press, 1979:165.
107. Teuber HL. The riddle of frontal lobe function in man. In: Warren JM, Akert K, ed. The frontal granular cortex and behavior. New York: McGraw-Hill, 1964:410.
108. Tomlinson BE. The pathology of dementia. In: Wells CE, ed. Dementia. Philadelphia: FA Davis, 1977:113.
109. Tulving E. Elements of episodic memory. Oxford: Clarendon Press, 1983.
110. Uhl GR, Hedreen JC, Price DL. Parkinson's disease: Loss of neurons from the ventral tegmental area contralateral to therapeutic surgical lesions. Neurology 1985; 35:1215–1218.
111. Uhl GR, Hilt DC, Hedreen JC. Pick's disease (lobar sclerosis): Depletion of neurons in the nucleus basalis of Meynert. Neurology 1983; 33:1470–1473.
112. Van Hoesen GW, Damasio AR. Neural correlates of cognitive impairment in Alzheimer's disease. In: Montcasle V, Plum F, eds. Handbook of physiology volume on "Higher functions of the nervous system." American Physiological Society, Bethesda, MD, 1986:871.
113. Villardita C, Smirni P, Le Pira F, Zappala G, Nicoletti F. Mental deterioration, visuoperceptive disabilities and constructional apraxia in Parkinson's disease. Acta Neurol Scand 1982; 66:112–120.
114. Weiskrantz LA. A comparison of hippocampal pathology in man and in other animals. In: Weiskrantz LA, ed. Functions of the septo-hippocampal system. Ciba Foundation Symposium 58. New York: Elsevier, 1978:373–406.
115. Whitehouse PJ, Hedreen JC, White CL III, Price DL. Basal forebrain neurons in the dementia of Parkinson's disease. Ann Neurol 1983; 13:243–248.
116. Whitehouse PJ, Price DL, Clark AW, Coyle JT, DeLong MR. Alzheimer's disease: Evidence for selective loss of cholinergic neurons in the nucleus basalis. Ann Neurol 1981; 10:122–126.
117. Wilson M. Effects of circumscribed cortical lesions upon somesthetic and visual discrimination in the monkey. J Comp Physiol Psychol 1957; 50:630–635.
118. Wilson RS, Kasziak AW, Fox JH. Remote memory in senile dementia. Cortex 1981; 17:41–48.

# CHAPTER 3

# *Patterns of Cognitive Impairment in Alzheimer's Disease and Other Dementing Disorders*

DAVID P. SALMON, Ph.D.
WILLIAM C. HEINDEL, Ph.D.
NELSON BUTTERS, Ph.D.

Dementia of the Alzheimer type (DAT) is a chronic disorder distinguished by a global and progressive deterioration of memory, cognition, and personality that results from the destruction of critical cortical and subcortical brain areas.[25,61,84] This most common form of dementing illness in the elderly particularly affects cortical association areas and the primary subcortical source of cholinergic input to the cortex—the nucleus basalis of Meynert.[46,48,49,80,85]

Over the past decade, the behavioral manifestations of DAT have become the focus of considerable research interest. In particular, the patterns of behavioral impairment exhibited by patients with DAT on neuropsychological tests have been examined in order to better characterize the disease and to improve diagnostic accuracy. Because memory impairment is a hallmark of DAT, most of this research effort has been directed toward examining the breakdown in memory processes. However, there has recently been a growing interest in the deficits of language and communication, abstraction and problem solving, and visuoperceptual and constructional functions that are commonly observed in DAT.

The initial portion of the present chapter will briefly describe some of the cognitive impairments of DAT other than memory and will focus on language, abstract thinking, and visuospatial functions. The subsequent section will review recent research concerning the breakdown of memory processes in DAT and will particularly emphasize the differences in the memory impairment exhibited by DAT patients and by patients with other dementing disorders. Although dementia has been described in the past as a ubiquitous syndrome, recent research has demonstrated the heterogeneous nature of the cognitive impairment associated with DAT and other dementing disorders. Much of this recent work focuses on the difference in the memory deficits observed in DAT and in Huntington's disease, a genetically transmitted disorder that results in chorea and dementia caused by atrophy of the basal ganglia (particularly the caudate nucleus).

The final section of the chapter will discuss the implications of our current understanding of the neuropsychological characteristics of DAT and other dementing disorders for future clinical applications and research.

## Cognitive Processes

### LANGUAGE PROCESSES

A prominent disturbance in language functions is a commonly observed feature of the cognitive impairment associated with DAT. In the typical case, the DAT patient's spontaneous speech is characterized by word-finding difficulties that result in phrases that are circumlocutory, indefinite, and empty of content.[5,66] Such language disturbances are also evident on formal tests of language, particularly those assessing confrontation naming and verbal fluency.

Confrontation-naming deficits may or may not be evident early in the course of DAT, but are invariably present by the later stages.[6,37] When asked to name real items or items that are pictured in outline drawings, DAT patients often are completely unable to name them, or they commit semantic errors, such as producing the name of the superordinate category to which the item belongs (e.g., animal for horse) or an incorrect name from the same semantic category (e.g., cow for horse). This impairment in naming ability becomes more severe as dementia progresses.[12] In contrast to DAT, confrontation naming remains relatively unaffected in some other dementing disorders. For example, Butters and his colleagues[21] and Bayles and Tomoeda[7] reported that both mildly and moderately demented HD patients were unimpaired on the Boston Naming Test, a widely used test of confrontation naming.

A number of investigators have reported that patients with DAT have an impaired ability to verbally generate words beginning with a particular letter (e.g., F, A, or S), or words belonging to a particular category (e.g., animals).[18,57,67,68,83] Several studies have demonstrated that in the earliest stages of DAT, the impairment of category fluency is greater than that of letter fluency.[18,83] For example, Butters and his colleagues found that DAT patients who performed equivalently to age-matched controls on the letter-fluency task were impaired relative to these control subjects on the category-fluency task.[18] As dementia progresses and patients become moderately impaired, this letter-category fluency discrepancy becomes less prominent and patients perform equally poorly on both tasks.[67]

Despite the DAT patient's deficits in these semantic aspects of language, grammatical and syntactic processes remain relatively preserved until the later stages of the disease.[4,5,42,66] Mild-to-moderately impaired DAT patients make few syntactic errors and are similar to normals in the grammatic complexity of their speech.[51] Because the language dysfunction evident in DAT appears to result primarily from semantic rather than grammatical deficits, the impaired confrontation naming and fluency exhibited by DAT patients early in the course of the disease have important implications for the nature of their semantic memory disorder (see section on semantic memory later). The nature of the language dysfunction in DAT is discussed in greater detail in Chapters 7 and 8. Several recent reviews of research concerned with the breakdown of language functions in DAT and other dementing disorders are also available.[14,37,65]

## ABSTRACTION AND PROBLEM-SOLVING PROCESSES

An impairment of abstract thinking and problem solving and a deficient ability to shift or maintain set are often prominent clinical features of DAT.[27] These deficits are usually ascribed to the neuropathologic changes that occur in the prefrontal association cortex of patients with DAT. Although these deficits may emerge at different stages in various patients, they are invariably present by the middle stages of the disorder.

To date, there have been very few systematic studies of the abstraction and problem-solving impairment of DAT patients. However, Freedman and Oscar-Berman have reported that DAT patients are impaired on several tests that seem to depend on the integrity of the frontal lobes of the brain.[31] Patients with DAT were impaired on a tactile reversal learning test in which they had to reverse a previously learned tactile discrimination problem (i.e., learn to choose a previously unreinforced item), and on a delayed alternation test in which they were required to find a penny in one of two covered reinforcement wells by learning that the location of the penny was being alternated by the experimenter from side to side after each correct response. The impaired performance of the DAT patients on these tasks presumably results from a deficiency in cognitive flexibility that is required to alternate responses and shift mental sets. Additional systematic research is necessary to better characterize the higher order abstraction and problem-solving disabilities of patients with DAT. (See Chapter 2 for further discussion of this topic.)

## VISUOSPATIAL PROCESSES

Although not as extensively studied as other forms of cognitive impairment, visuospatial dysfunction is also a prominent feature of DAT.[11,29,62] Patients with DAT appear to suffer a selective impairment of visuospatial processing independent of lower level visual functioning. For example, Schlotterer and his colleagues demonstrated that DAT patients exhibit normal age-related changes in low-level visual functions such as spatial frequency and contrast sensitivity, but are impaired on a higher level visuoperceptual-processing task, backward visual pattern masking.[74] In the backward visual masking task, the onset of a briefly presented visual target (i.e., letters of the alphabet) preceded the onset of an interfering visual mask (i.e., overlapping letters). Although target perception may be perfect without the mask, the target may be imperceptible when followed by the mask, even though a short temporal interval separates the two. In the particular procedures employed by Schlotterer et al, backward visual masking most likely depends on higher order visual association cortices. Thus, their results are consistent with neuropathologic findings of greater deficiencies in temporal-parietal brain regions than in the striate cortex of patients with DAT.[50]

The higher level visuospatial dysfunction of patients with DAT is most evident on tests of constructional apraxia, including tests such as the Block Design subtest from the Wechsler Adult Intelligence Scale-Revised (WAIS-R) and drawing tasks.[10,12,13,23,28,55,63] The Block Design subtest requires patients to reproduce pictured red-and-white designs with three-dimensional blocks that are red on two sides, white on two sides, and half red and half white on two sides. Drawing tests usually involve spontaneously drawing to command or copying abstract complex figures, clocks, and two-dimensional representations of a cube. In addition, patients with DAT often have difficulty in visual-discrimination and visual-matching tests.[10,13,56] The progressive nature of the visuospatial impairment of DAT patients is revealed in a recent longitudinal study by Becker and his colleagues.[10]

There is evidence that subgroups of DAT patients exhibit either primarily verbal or visuospatial deficits when tested clinically, and that these differential patterns correlate with greater glucose hypometabolism in the left or right hemisphere, respectively.[10,30,38,54,55] Indeed, some DAT patients present initially with visuospatial impairment as their primary symptom.[26,55] However, little is known about how visuospatial functions are affected in the developmental progression of DAT and other dementing disorders, or about the effect of distinct visuospatial deficits on performance of visual memory tasks.

## MEMORY PROCESSES

Although DAT involves significant deficits in a number of cognitive abilities, memory impairment is usually the most prominent feature throughout the course of the disease.[45,55] Patients with DAT exhibit significant anterograde (i.e., retention of new information) and retrograde (i.e., recall of information acquired in the past) memory deficits that become progressively worse over time.[10,24,27,33,79,86] Although memory impairment has traditionally been considered to be pervasive and global in DAT, several recent studies indicate that there are at least some preserved memory capacities in these patients, and that the pattern of impaired and preserved memory processes may be useful for differentiating DAT from other forms of dementing illnesses. It is not known whether the specific characteristics of the memory deficits of early DAT patients (described below) retain their diagnostic utility as the disease progresses.

Recent studies of memory processes in demented patients have focused upon *explicit* and *implicit* memory.[73] Explicit memory refers to information that the subject specifically attempts to retain and subsequently recall or recognize, or to particular knowledge that can be consciously retrieved from an existing store. In contrast, implicit memory refers to information that does not require conscious recollection; rather, it is knowledge that is expressed through the performance of the specific operations comprising a particular task. In many tests of implicit memory, the subject's performance is unconsciously facilitated by the presentation of previous stimulus materials (e.g., priming) or by repeated experience with a motor task. The use of implicit memory tests with demented patients was spurred by recent demonstrations of preserved memory capacities in patients with circumscribed amnesia (i.e., memory disorder with no concomitant cognitive deficits). Patients with severe anterograde and retrograde amnesia demonstrate the ability to acquire and retain certain kinds of information when retention is tested implicitly. For example, these patients show normal classical conditioning of the eyeblink response, psychophysical biasing, acquisition of motor and visuoperceptual skills, and lexical and semantic priming.[73,78]

### Explicit Memory

The preponderance of available knowledge concerning the memory disorder of Alzheimer's disease has been acquired with tests of explicit memory in which the patient consciously attempts to retain and retrieve information. Explicit memory tests can be further subdivided into those that assess *episodic* or *semantic* memory.[82] Episodic memory consists of information for events and episodes that remain tightly linked to the spatial and temporal context in which they were originally acquired. Examples of episodic memory include remembering the score of last night's baseball game and remembering a list of words in a traditional verbal-memory test. Semantic memory, on the other hand, comprises general knowledge, rules and procedures that are highly overlearned and essentially context-free. For example, knowledge of the alphabet, rules of arithmetic, and the words that make up one's vocabulary are all part of semantic memory.

Tests of episodic memory are very sensitive to memory impairment of any etiology including DAT, other forms of dementia, and circumscribed amnesic syndromes. Accordingly, episodic memory tests are often used to differentiate patients with dementia from nonimpaired elderly individuals.[15,52,53]

For example, in a recent study of recognition memory,[71] an abbreviated form of Moss et al's Recognition Span Test (RST)[64] was administered to patients with mild or moderate DAT and to intact control subjects. This test requires subjects to retain increasingly longer strings of verbal, spatial, or complex visual information in memory. In the various forms of the test, disks containing the appropriate information are placed one at a time in various locations on a test board. The subject must point to an added new disk on each trial. Thus, the subject must retain the information contained on each additional disk with each successive trial. Recognition span is the number of new disks correctly identified prior to the first error. Memory spans for verbal (words), spatial, and configurational (faces) information were assessed. Delayed recall (15 seconds and 2 minutes) of the words used on the verbal recognition span was also determined. The results showed that both DAT patient groups were impaired on the three recognition tasks relative to normal control subjects, and that the spatial and verbal forms of the task differentiated the mild from the moderately demented patients. The mean overall recognition span scores (spatial + verbal + facial) differentiated between DAT patients and intact controls to a high degree, with 37 of 39 patients falling beyond the 95 percent confidence limits derived from the control subject's scores. On the delayed verbal recall portion of the test, both the mild and moderately demented patients were severely impaired and evidenced a rapid rate of forgetting between the 15-second and 2-minute recall attempts. These findings suggest that the RST is not only highly sensitive to memory disorders in the early stages of DAT, but also effective in discriminating among various stages of the disorder.

Patients with DAT are also impaired on explicit tests of semantic memory. A number of recent studies have demonstrated that DAT patients often evidence difficulty in retrieving specific information from their general store of knowledge when searching for a particular word in a naming task[5,6] or when attempting to generate rapidly words from a particular lexical category (e.g., words that begin with F) or semantic category (e.g., supermarket items).[57,67,68,83] As discussed later, these results may indicate a breakdown in the structure and organization of semantic memory in DAT.

In addition to discriminating between demented and normal individuals, neuropsychological tests that explicitly assess episodic and semantic memory have proven useful in differentiating among various forms of dementia. Recent studies demonstrate that both patients with DAT and patients with Huntington's disease (HD) are impaired on explicit memory tests, but they fail for distinctly different reasons. Although the capacity to store new verbal information seems relatively preserved in HD, these patients are deficient in initiating systematic retrieval strategies when asked to recall information from either episodic or semantic memory.[18,20] Conversely, patients with DAT encounter unusual difficulty in consolidating new information, are highly sensitive to proactive interference (i.e., make numerous intrusion and perseverative errors), and endure a disruption of the structure of semantic knowledge.[18,40,76] These characteristics of the memory disorders of DAT and HD patients are illustrated in a series of studies examining performance on explicit memory tests.

In an initial investigation, episodic and semantic memory tasks were administered to DAT, HD, and alcoholic Korsakoff (AK) patients matched for overall severity of dementia with the Mattis Dementia Rating Scale (DRS).[18,60] Episodic memory was assessed with a task that required the recall of four short, auditorily presented passages. The semantic-memory task was a fluency test in which the patient generated words beginning with a particular letter (e.g., F, A, or S), or from a particular category (e.g., animals), as quickly as possible, for 1 minute. All three patient groups were severely and equally impaired on recall of the four passages. However, only the DAT and AK patients were highly sensitive to proactive interference. Both of these groups emitted numerous prior-story and extra-story intrusion errors. That is, more than 50 percent of the DAT and AK patients' total recall of the short stories represented intrusions from previous passages and other materials. In contrast, less than 10 percent of the HD patients' total recall involved such intrusion errors.

The performances of the early-stage DAT patients were also distinguishable from those of the other two patient groups on the test of semantic memory. The HD and AK patients demonstrated severe and moderate deficits, respectively, on both the letter and category fluency tasks, whereas the early DAT patients were impaired *only* on the category fluency task (i.e., examples of animals). As with the episodic memory test, the DAT and AK patients were more susceptible to proactive interference than were the HD patients. The DAT and AK patients made more perseverative errors (i.e., repetition of words) than did the HD patients on the letter-fluency task.

The results of this study suggest that DAT and HD patients' impairments on episodic- and semantic-memory tasks reflect different underlying processes. The performance of patients with DAT is affected by their language dysfunction and an increased sensitivity to proactive interference. The severe impairment of the HD patients in recalling the four passages and in generating words in both the letter- and category-fluency tasks is consistent with the notion that they are unable to initiate systematic retrieval strategies for accessing episodic or semantic memory.[16,22] The findings that the early DAT patients were impaired on category, but not letter fluency, suggests that their language and semantic memory problems involve a reduction in the number of exemplars comprising an abstract category and not a general retrieval deficit. It has been noted that such reductions may be the result of a breakdown in the hierarchical organization of semantic knowledge and memory.[57] The similarities in the error patterns of DAT and AK patients are consistent with the suggestion that the two disorders may share some common neuropathologic (i.e., basal forebrain) and neurochemical (i.e., cholinergic) dysfunctions.[16,17,69]

The DAT patients' propensity to make prior-item intrusion errors, as observed in the previously described study, has been considered a pathognomonic sign of the disease. Indeed, Fuld and her colleagues have reported a significant correlation between intrusion errors and certain neuropathologic indices of Alzheimer's disease (e.g., neuritic plaques).[32] The occurrence of prior-item intrusion errors is not limited to the verbal modality, but also occurs in figural memory tasks. In a study designed to assess frequency of prior-item intrusion errors in figural memory (using the Visual Reproduction Test from the Wechsler Memory Scale), Jacobs, Salmon, Troster, and Butters found that DAT patients made numerous intrusions from one figure into another, whereas HD patients produced only slightly more of these errors than did intact middle-aged subjects.[47] The findings also demonstrated that the diagnostic utility of intrusion errors may be limited to the early stages of dementia. Mildly demented DAT and HD patients differed in their production of intrusion errors, but moderately demented patients with these two disorders made similar numbers of these errors. This loss of clinical utility was the result of a significant increase in intrusion errors as the dementia of HD progressed.

The difference in the processes that underlie the semantic memory deficits of DAT and HD patients was the focus of another recent study that compared the associative encoding and retrieval abilities of these patients with Thomson and Tulving's encoding specificity paradigm.[34,81] When compared to age- and education-matched control subjects, both DAT and HD patient groups were severely and equally impaired on overall memory for word lists. However, the patient groups showed differential improvements in recall performance with the introduction of associated cues during stimulus presentation and recall. Although the HD patients, like intact subjects, were able to benefit from semantic retrieval cues (strong and weak) that were presented during input, the performance of the patients with DAT improved only with the introduction of strong cues at output (i.e., during recall), whether the cues were present or absent during initial presentation. These results suggest that DAT patients failed to encode the semantic relationship between the to-be-recalled and cue words and simply generated free associations to the cue during retrieval. The inability to utilize the semantic relationship between words as an effective cue provides further evidence that, unlike HD patients, patients with DAT suffer a breakdown in the organization of semantic memory.

The episodic memory impairment of DAT patients has been attributed, at least in part, to a failure to consolidate new information. In contrast, HD patients appear to have intact consolidation but are unable to effectively retrieve successfully stored information. The DAT and HD patients' differential capacity to consolidate new information is reflected by differences in their rates of forgetting. In studies of patients with circumscribed amnesia, rapid rates of forgetting have been associated with damage to the mesial portions of the temporal lobes. Huppert and Piercy reported that an amnesic patient with bilateral mesial temporal-lobe damage forgot pictorial materials more rapidly than did intact controls and other amnesics with mesial diencephalic lesions, even when the subjects' initial levels of recognition were made equivalent by increasing stimulus exposure for the amnesic patients.[43,44] Based on comparisons of the rates of forgetting of depressed patients receiving ECT and of alcoholics with Korsakoff's syndrome, Squire also concluded that rapid forgetting of learned materials is a consequence of damage to mesial temporal-lobe structures (e.g., hippocampi).[77]

Because the mesial temporal regions of the brain are prominently affected in DAT but not in HD, one might anticipate that DAT patients would exhibit an unusually rapid rate of forgetting that would differentiate them from HD and other basal ganglia disorders.[46] A study by Martone, Butters, and Trauner employing the Huppert and Piercy paradigm did demonstrate normal rates of forgetting in HD patients with severe memory disorders.[58] Several recent reports of rapid forgetting of verbal and visual (figural and pictorial) information in relatively early DAT patients also confirm this expectation.[19,35,36,64,71] In two of these studies HD patients were also included and were found to have relatively normal retention abilities.[19,64] In contrast to these positive findings from several different laboratories, other studies have failed to demonstrate rapid forgetting in DAT patients.[9,53] Because these published investigations of forgetting rates in DAT have varied greatly in the type of stimuli and testing paradigms employed, it is possible that the link between rapid forgetting and DAT may at least partially depend on how remembering is assessed.

In a related study, the ability of the newly revised Wechsler Memory Scale (WMS-R) to differentiate various forms of dementia and amnesia was examined.[19] The findings showed that amnesics could be distinguished from demented patients and control subjects on the basis of the differences between the Attention/Concentration and General Memory Indices (AC-GM) and between the General and Delayed Memory Indices (GM-DM). More specifically, the amnesic patients exhibited greater differences on these two measures than did the other subjects. Consistent with previous reports, savings scores calculated from the Logical Memory and Visual Reproduction tests showed that the amnesic and the DAT patients forgot verbal and figural materials more quickly than did the HD patients and normal control subjects.

The unique characteristics of the memory deficits of DAT and HD patients on explicit episodic and semantic memory tests are not limited to the acquisition and retention of new information, but are also evident in the groups' ability to retrieve information from the past. In a study of retrograde amnesia (RA),[8] patients with DAT or HD were administered an updated version of the remote-memory battery originally developed by Albert, Butters, and Levin.[1] Regardless of whether remote memory was measured by unaided recall or cued recall, HD patients exhibited deficits that were equally severe across decades. RA was more severe in DAT than in HD patients, and the DAT patients recalled significantly more items from the 1940s and 1950s than from the 1960s, 1970s, and 1980s. These findings, like recent reports focusing on these patients' abilities to learn new information and to search semantic memory, indicate that the processes underlying DAT and HD patients' memory failures are distinct.

The results of the numerous studies examining the memory processes of DAT and HD patients with explicit episodic- and semantic-memory tests demonstrate that these patients produce unique impairment profiles. Patients with DAT have a severe memory impairment that is characterized by a breakdown in the organization of semantic memory, an abnormally rapid rate of forgetting of episodic information, a temporally graded remote memory loss, and a high susceptibility to proactive interference. The memory impairment of HD, however, may result from the inability to establish or implement effective retrieval strategies for accessing episodic or semantic memory. Because these distinct patterns of explicit memory impairments exhibited by DAT and HD patients have been observed primarily early in the disease process, it is not known if the characteristic deficits that distinguish early DAT from early HD patients retain their discriminant properties in the middle and advanced stages of the diseases. Longitudinal comparisons of the performance of DAT patients and patients with other dementing disorders on explicit memory tests that assess a variety of different memory processes may provide this information.

**Implicit Memory**

Patients with DAT exhibit a unique pattern of impaired and preserved capacities on tests that assess *implicit* memory (for review, see article by Heindel, Salmon, and Butters).[40] As previously mentioned, implicit memory tests differ from traditional tests of recall and recognition memory that require the explicit, conscious recollection of previous experiences in that they allow knowledge to be expressed through the performance of the specific operations comprising the task. Two types of implicit memory tests, verbal priming and motor-skill learning, have been used extensively in the evaluation of the dementias. Several recent studies have demonstrated that DAT and HD patients differ greatly in their ability to perform these two types of implicit memory tasks.[40]

An investigation of verbal priming in DAT, HD, and amnesic patients (i.e., with AK) examined the status of semantic memory in each of these groups.[72] The first of two experiments assessed lexical priming with a stem-completion procedure. An earlier study suggested that DAT patients were severely impaired on such a priming task.[75] In the first experiment, subjects were exposed to a list of 10 target words (e.g., *motel, abstain*) and were asked to rate each word in terms of its "likability." Following two presentations and ratings of the entire list, the subjects were shown three-letter stems (e.g., *mot, abs*) of words that were and were not on the presentation list and asked to complete the stems with the "first word that comes to mind." Half of the stems could be completed with previously presented words, while the other half were used to assess baseline guessing rates. Other lists of words were used to assess the subjects' ability at free recall and recognition.

Although all three patient groups were severely and equally impaired on free recall and recognition of presented words, the AK and HD patients exhibited intact stem-completion priming. In comparison to the AK and HD patients, the DAT patients showed little or no tendency to complete the word stems with previously presented words. That is, for the DAT patients the presentation-rating procedure failed to generate the transient memory traces needed for this form of "implicit memory" or "memory without awareness."[73] This deficit suggests that even the lexical features of semantic memory have undergone deterioration in DAT.

In the second experiment of this investigation, DAT, HD, and intact control subjects were administered a semantic-priming test that required the subjects to "free associate" to the first words (e.g., *bird*) of previously presented (and rated), semantically associated word pairs (e.g., *bird-robin*). The results with this priming task showed that DAT patients were significantly less likely to produce the second word of the semantically related pair than were the other two subject groups. In fact, the priming score for the DAT patients did not differ from baseline guessing rates. The results of this experiment, like the first, suggest that the memory capacities of DAT patients are characterized by some deterioration in the structure of semantic memory and that this impairment is evident even on "automatic" (i.e., free association) processing tasks.

Heindel and his colleagues recently examined the ability of DAT, HD, and amnesic patients matched for overall degree of dementia to acquire the motor skills underlying a pursuit-rotor task.[39] This motor skill task has the advantage that subjects' initial levels of performance can be equated by manipulating the difficulty (i.e., speed of rotation of the disk) of the task. Equating initial performance ensures that group differences in skill acquisition *cannot* be attributed to ceiling or floor effects.

The results of this study showed that only the HD patients were impaired in the learning and retention of this motor skill. The DAT, amnesic, and intact control subjects all evidenced rapid and extensive motor learning over three test sessions, whereas the HD patients showed only a slight improvement from the first to the last session. It should be stressed that the DAT and amnesic patients did not differ from the control subjects on any measure of skill acquisition.

In a more recent study, patients with DAT, HD, and Parkinson's disease (PD) were directly compared on both the pursuit-rotor and lexical-priming tasks described above.[41] The results of this study demonstrated a double dissociation between DAT and HD patients on the two implicit memory tasks. The DAT patients were severely impaired on verbal priming but showed normal acquisition of the pursuit-rotor task; the HD patients showed the opposite relationship. The performance of the PD patients depended on whether they were demented or not. Demented PD patients were impaired on both implicit memory tasks, whereas the nondemented PD patients were intact on both tests. For both the HD and PD patients, impairments on the motor-skill learning task correlated with their degree of dementia, not with the severity of their motor deficits (i.e., chorea, bradykinesia, rigidity, and tremor).

To summarize the results of these implicit memory studies, HD patients appear severely impaired in their attempts to acquire motor skills (e.g., rotary pursuit), but perform normally on lexical (e.g., stem-completion) and semantic-priming tasks.[39,72] The opposite relationship is seen in patients with DAT. Alzheimer's patients acquire and retain motor skills with the same facility as intact controls and amnesic patients, but they perform poorly on stem-completion and semantic-priming tasks.[41] The results of these implicit memory experiments have some important implications for the neurologic basis of memory systems. Although both verbal-priming and motor-skill learning remain unimpaired in amnesic patients, the double dissociation between HD and DAT patients on the verbal-priming and pursuit-rotor tasks suggests that various types of so-called "preserved" or "procedural" memory depend on different neuroanatomic substrates.[78] While the HD patients' impairment on the pursuit-rotor task is certainly consistent with the proposed association between the acquisition of motor skills and the neostriatum,[59] the DAT patients' deficiencies on verbal priming (and semantic memory in general) may be attributable to the cortical neuropathology associated with this disorder. It should be kept in mind that the patterns of implicit memory performance described above were observed in patients in the early stages of dementia and have not been examined longitudinally in patients with dementing disorders. Thus, it is not known if the distinct patterns of implicit memory performance exhibited by DAT and HD patients retain their uniqueness in the middle and advanced stages of the diseases.

Taken together, the results of the investigations described above suggest that patients with DAT have a pattern of *explicit* and *implicit* memory deficits that differentiates them from at least some other forms of dementia. Even in their earliest stages, DAT patients' severe episodic and semantic memory disorders reflect increased sensitivity to proactive interference (i.e., appearance of intrusion and perseverative errors), severe deficits in remote memory, rapid rates of forgetting, and a deterioration of the linguistic structure underlying semantic memory. The deficiencies in semantic memory are severe enough to result in significant failures on lexical and semantic priming tasks as well as on tests of category fluency. In contrast to HD patients, and perhaps patients with other forms of basal ganglia dementia (i.e., Parkinson's disease), patients with DAT retain the ability to acquire and retain motor skills.

## Clinical and Research Implications

As the above brief review attests, dementia is a heterogeneous syndrome that can be characterized by diverse patterns of cognitive deficits. Patients with dementias arising from different etiologies may differ in the type of cognitive dysfunction they exhibit, or in the specific processes that underlie a similar cognitive impairment. Even within a single etiology such as Alzheimer's disease, patients may initially present with very disparate cognitive deficits, even though they will ultimately progress to the global dementia characteristic of the disease.

The heterogeneous nature of dementia has been taken into account in the most recent diagnostic classification schemes. For example, the American Psychiatric Associations's Diagnostic and Statistical Manual third edition diagnosis of dementia requires memory impairment and a deficit in at least one other cognitive function such as abstract thinking, judgment, language, constructional and visuospatial ability, or a personality change.[3] These cognitive changes must be severe enough to interfere with work, usual social activities, or relationships with others. Thus, a patient with normal language abilities, severe memory impairment, and a deficit in abstract thinking would be diagnosed as demented, as would a patient with only aphasia and moderate memory loss. Because of this diversity in possible cognitive presentation, the neuropsychological evaluation of the potentially demented patient should include assessment of those cognitive functions that are most often compromised in various forms of dementia: memory, attention, language, abstract thinking, and constructional and visuospatial abilities. A comprehensive neuropsychological evaluation of this nature will provide sufficiently detailed information to determine whether a patient has the deficits in two or more areas of cognition required to diagnose dementia. For a thorough discussion of neuropsychological testing procedures used with demented patients, see recent reviews by Albert and Moss[2] and by Salmon and Butters.[70]

Further research of both a clinical and experimental cognitive nature is necessary for a better understanding of the neuropsychological aspects of DAT and other dementing disorders. There are few studies that carefully characterize the attention, visuospatial, and abstraction and problem-solving deficits of patients with DAT. Of those few studies that do exist, only a handful examine how these deficient processes change longitudinally.[10,79] Description of the clinical presentation and natural history of DAT is crucial for improving diagnostic accuracy and prognostic ability.

Another important area of research will be to determine the clinical utility of the recent findings concerning differential impairment of implicit memory in patients with dementias of different etiologies. If these results are robust and generalizable, implicit memory tests may enhance the neuropsychologist's ability to clinically differentiate early-stage DAT from circumscribed amnesia, and to differentiate among various forms of dementia. Although patients with DAT and amnesic patients may present initially with very similar behavioral and cognitive dysfunctions, the inability of DAT patients to perform normally on lexical and semantic-priming tasks differs qualitatively from the intact priming capacity of amnesic patients. Similarly, patients with DAT may be distinguished clinically from patients with subcortical dementias such as Huntington's disease by impaired verbal priming coupled with a preserved ability to learn and retain motor skills. Patients with Huntington's disease demonstrate the opposite pattern of preserved priming ability and deficient acquisition of motor skill.

Additional research may also lead to greater understanding of the brain-behavior relationships underlying the various types of neuropsychological dysfunction in different dementias. To achieve this understanding, studies that attempt to differentiate neuropsychological processes in demented patients with different underlying neuropathology will be required. Some progress has already been made in this regard in the comparative studies of the implicit memory deficits of DAT, HD, and PD patients reported by Heindel and his colleagues.[41]

In conclusion, further neuropsychological research will extend our knowledge of the natural progression of DAT and of the diagnostic utility of some salient early features in the middle and advanced stages of the disease. This information will also make a substantial contribution to our understanding of the information-processing deficits underlying DAT patients' cognitive failures in all stages of the illness. It is hoped that this knowledge can be used for the very early detection of dementia in individuals at risk for DAT and in seemingly intact elderly persons. Such early detection will be critical if successful pharmacologic agents for retarding disease progression are ultimately developed.

### References

1. Albert MS, Butters N, Levin J. Temporal gradients in the retrograde amnesia of patients with alcoholic Korsakoff's disease. Arch Neurol 1979; 36:211–216.
2. Albert MS, Moss MB. Geriatric neuropsychology. New York: Guilford Press, 1988.
3. American Psychiatric Association. Diagnostic and statistical manual of mental disorders. 3rd ed. Washington, D.C.: American Psychiatric Association, 1980.
4. Appell J, Kertesz A, Fisman M. A study of language

functioning in Alzheimer patients. Brain Lang 1982; 17:73-91.
5. Bayles K. Language function in senile dementia. Brain Lang 1982; 16:265-280.
6. Bayles K, Kaszniak A. Communication and cognition in normal aging and dementia. Boston: College-Hill Press, 1987.
7. Bayles K, Tomoeda CK. Confrontation naming impairment in dementia. Brain Lang 1983; 19:98-114.
8. Beatty WW, Salmon DP, Butters N, Heindel WC, Granholm E. Retrograde amnesia in patients with Alzheimer's disease or Huntington's disease. Neurobiol Aging 1988; 9:181-186.
9. Becker JT, Boller F, Saxton J, McGonigle-Gibson KL. Normal rates of forgetting of verbal and non-verbal material in Alzheimer's disease. Cortex 1987; 23:59-72.
10. Becker JT, Huff FJ, Nebes RD, Holland A, Boller F. Neuropsychological function in Alzheimer's disease: Pattern of impairment and rates of progression. Arch Neurol 1988; 45:263-268.
11. Benton AL. Visuoperceptual, visuospatial, and visuoconstructive disorders. In: Heilman K, Valenstein E, eds. Clinical neuropsychology. New York: Oxford Press, 1985:151-185.
12. Berg L, Danzinger WL, Storandt M. Predictive features of mild senile dementia of the Alzheimer type. Neurology 1984; 34:563-569.
13. Brouwers P, Cox C, Martin A, Chase T, Fedio P. Differential perceptual-spatial impairment in Huntington's and Alzheimer's dementias. Arch Neurol 1984; 41:1073-1076.
14. Brown RG, Marsden CD. Subcortical dementia: The neuropsychological evidence. Neuroscience 1988; 25:363-387.
15. Buschke H, Fuld PA. Evaluating storage, retention, and retrieval in disordered memory and learning. Neurology 1974; 24:1019-1025.
16. Butters N. The clinical aspects of memory disorders: Contributions from experimental studies of amnesia and dementia. J Clin Neuropsychol 1984; 7:181-210.
17. Butters N. Alcoholic Korsakoff's syndrome: Some unresolved issues concerning etiology, neuropathology and cognitive deficits. J Clin Exp Neuropsychol 1985; 7:181-210.
18. Butters N, Granholm E, Salmon DP, Grant I, Wolfe J. Episodic and semantic memory: A comparison of amnesic and demented patients. J Clin Exper Neuropsychol 1987; 9:479-497.
19. Butters N, Salmon DP, Cullum CM. Differentiation of amnesic and demented patients with the Wechsler Memory Scale-Revised. Clin Neuropsychol 1988; 2:133-148.
20. Butters N, Salmon DP, Heindel WC, Granholm E. Episodic, semantic, and procedural memory: Some comparisons of Alzheimer's and Huntington's disease patients. In: Terry RD, ed. Aging and the brain. New York: Raven Press, 1988.63.
21. Butters N, Sax DS, Montgomery K, Tarlow S. Comparison of the neuropsychological deficits associated with early and advanced Huntington's disease. Arch Neurol 1978; 35:585-589.
22. Butters N, Wolfe J, Granholm E, Martone M. An assessment of verbal recall, recognition, and fluency abilities in patients with Huntington's disease. Cortex 1986; 86:11-32.
23. Como PG, Caine ED. A comparative neuropsychological study of AD and PD. J Clin Exper Neuropsychol 1987; 9:74.
24. Corkin S. Some relationships between global amnesias and the memory impairments of Alzheimer's disease. In: Corkin S, Davis FL, Growdon JH, Usdin E, Wurtman RJ, eds. Alzheimer's disease: A report of research in progress. Aging. Vol. 19. New York: Raven Press, 1982:149.
25. Corkin S, Davis KL, Growdon JH, Usdin E, Wurtman RJ. Alzheimer's disease: A report of research in progress. Aging. Vol. 19. New York: Raven Press, 1982.
26. Crystal HA, Horoupian DS, Katzman R, Jotkowitz S. Biopsy-proved Alzheimer's disease presenting as a right parietal lobe syndrome. Ann Neurol 1982; 12:186-188.
27. Cummings JL, Benson DF. Dementia: A clinical approach. Boston: Butterworth, 1983.
28. DeLeon MJ, Potegal M, Gurland B. Wandering and parietal signs in senile dementia of Alzheimer's type. Neuropsychobiology 1984; 11:155-157.
29. Eslinger PJ, Benton AL. Visuoperceptual performances in aging and dementia: Clinical and theoretical implications. J Clin Neuropsychol 1983; 5:213-220.
30. Foster NL, Chase TN, Fedio P. Alzheimer's disease: Focal cortical changes shown by positron emission tomography. Neurology 1983; 33:961-965.
31. Freedman M, Oscar-Berman M. Comparative neuropsychology of cortical and subcortical dementia. Can J Neurol Sci 1986; 13:410-414.
32. Fuld PA, Katzman R, Davies P, Terry RD. Intrusions as a sign of Alzheimer's dementia: Chemical and pathological verification. Ann Neurol 1982; 11:155-159.
33. Grady CL, Haxby JV, Horwitz B. A longitudinal study of the early neuropsychological and cerebral metabolic changes in dementia of the Alzheimer type. J Clin Exp Neuropsychol 1988; 10:576-596.
34. Granholm E, Butters N. Associative encoding and retrieval in Alzheimer's disease and Huntington's disease. Brain Cogn 1988; 7:335-347.
35. Hart RP, Kwentus JA, Harkins SW, Taylor JR. Rate of forgetting in mild Alzheimer's-type dementia. Brain Cogn 1988; 7:31-38.
36. Hart RP, Kwentus JA, Taylor JR, Harkins SW. Rate of forgetting in dementia and depression. J Consult Clin Psychol 1987; 55:101-105.
37. Hart S. Language and dementia: A review. Psychol Med 1988; 18:99-112.
38. Haxby JV, Duara R, Grady CL, Cutler NR, Rapoport SI. Relations between neuropsychological and cerebral metabolic asymmetries in early Alzheimer's disease. J Cereb Blood Flow Metab 1985; 5:193-200.
39. Heindel WC, Butters N, Salmon DP. Impaired learning of a motor skill in patients with Huntington's disease. Behav Neurosci 1988; 102:141-147.
40. Heindel WC, Salmon DP, Butters N. Neuropsychological differentiation of memory impairments in dementia. In: Gilmore G, Whitehouse P, Wykle M, eds. Memory and aging. New York: Springer Publishing, 1989:112.
41. Heindel WC, Salmon DP, Shults CW, Walicke PA, Butters N. Neuropsychological evidence for multiple implicit memory disease patients. J Neurosci 1989; 9:382-587.
42. Heir DB, Hagenlocker K, Shindler AG. Language disintegration in dementia: Effects of etiology and severity. Brain Lang 1985; 25:117-133.
43. Huppert FA, Piercy M. Dissociation between learning and remembering in organic amnesia. Nature 1978; 275:317-318.
44. Huppert FA, Piercy M. Normal and abnormal forgetting in organic amnesia. Cortex 1979; 15:385-390.
45. Huppert FA, Tym E. Clinical and neuropsychological assessment of dementia. Br Med Bull 1986; 42:11-18.

46. Hyman BT, Van Hoesen GW, Damasio AR, Barnes CL. Alzheimer's disease: Cell-specific pathology isolates the hippocampal formation. Science 1984; 225:1168–1170.
47. Jacobs D, Salmon DP, Troster AI, Butters N. Intrusion errors in the figur memory of patients with Alzheimer's and Huntington's diseases. Arch Clin Neuropsychol 1990; 5:49–57.
48. Katzman R. The prevalence and malignancy of Alzheimer's disease: A major killer. Arch Neurol 1976; 33:217–218.
49. Katzman R. Alzheimer's disease. N Engl J Med 1986; 314:964–973.
50. Katzman R, Terry RD, Bick KL. Alzheimer's disease: Senile dementia and related disorders. Aging. vol. 7. New York: Raven Press, 1978.
51. Kempler D, Curtiss S, Jackson C. Syntactic preservation in Alzheimer's disease. J Speech Hear Res 1987; 30:343–350.
52. Knopman DS, Ryberg S. A verbal memory test with high predictive accuracy for dementia of the Alzheimer type. Arch Neurol 1989; 46:141–145.
53. Kopelman MD. Rates of forgetting in Alzheimer-type dementia and Korsakoff's syndrome. Neuropsychologia 1985; 23:623–638.
54. Koss E, Friedland RP, Ober BA, Jagust WJ. Differences in lateral hemispheric asymmetries of glucose utilization between early- and late-onset Alzheimer-type dementia. Am J Psychiatry 1985; 142:638–640.
55. Martin A. Representation of semantic and spatial knowledge in Alzheimer's patients: Implications for models of preserved learning in amnesia. J Clin Exp Neuropsychol 1987; 9:191–224.
56. Martin A, Cox C, Brouwers P, Fedio P. A note on different patterns of impaired and preserved cognitive abilities and their relation to episodic memory deficits in Alzheimer's disease. Brain Lang 1985; 26:181–185.
57. Martin A, Fedio P. Word production and comprehension in Alzheimer's disease: The breakdown in semantic knowledge. Brain Lang 1983; 19:124–141.
58. Martone M, Butters N, Trauner D. Some analyses of forgetting of pictorial material in amnesic and demented patients. J Clin Exp Neuropsychol 1986; 8:161–178.
59. Martone M, Butters N, Payne M, Becker J, Sax DS. Dissociation between skill learning and verbal recognition in amnesia and dementia. Arch Neurol 1984; 41:965–970.
60. Mattis S. Mental status examination for organic mental syndrome in the elderly patient. In: Bellack L, Karasu TB, eds. Geriatric psychiatry. New York: Grune & Stratton, 1976.
61. Mohs RC, Greenwald BS, Dunn DD, Davis KL. Assessment of cognition and affective systems in dementia. In: Traber J, Gispen WH, eds. Senile dementia of the Alzheimer type. Berlin: Springer-Verlag, 1985.
62. Moore V, Wyke MA. Drawing disabilities in patients with senile dementia. Psychol Med 1984; 14:97–105.
63. Moss MB, Albert MS. Alzheimer's disease and other dementing disorders. In: Albert MS, Moss MB, eds. Geriatric neuropsychology. New York: Guilford Press, 1988:145–178.
64. Moss M, Albert MS, Butters N, Payne M. Differential patterns of memory loss among patients with Alzheimer's disease, Huntington's disease, and alcoholic Korsakoff's syndrome. Arch Neurol 1986: 43:239–246.
65. Nebes RD. Semantic memory in Alzheimer's disease. Psychol Bull 1989; 106:377–394.
66. Nicholas M, Obler KL, Albert ML, Helm-Estabrooks N. Empty speech in Alzheimer's disease and fluent aphasia. J Speech Hear Res 1985; 28:405–410.
67. Ober BA, Dronkers NF, Koss E, Delis DC, Friedland RP. Retrieval from semantic memory in Alzheimer-type dementia. J Clin Exp Neuropsychol 1986; 8:75–92.
68. Rosen WG. Verbal fluency in aging and dementia. J Clin Neuropsychol 1980; 2:135–146.
69. Salmon DP, Butters N. The etiology and neuropathology of alcoholic Korsakoff's syndrome: Some evidence for the role of the basal forebrain. In: Galanter M, ed. Recent developments in alcoholism. vol. 5. New York: Plenum Press, 1987: 27–58.
70. Salmon DP, Butters N. Neuropsychological assessment of dementia in the elderly. In: Katzman R, Rowe JW, eds. Geriatric neurology: Principles and practice. Philadelphia: F.A. Davis. (In press).
71. Salmon DP, Granholm E, McCullough D, Butters N, Grant I. Recognition memory span in mild and moderately demented patients with Alzheimer's disease. J Clin Exp Neuropsychol 1989; 11:429–443.
72. Salmon DP, Shimamura AP, Butters N, Smith S. Lexical and semantic priming deficits in patients with Alzheimer's disease. J Clin Exp Neuropsychol 1988; 10:477–494.
73. Schacter DL. Implicit memory: History and current status. J Exp Psychol [Learn Mem Cogn] 1987; 13:501–517.
74. Schlotterer G, Moscovitch M, Crapper-McLachlan D. Visual processing deficits as assessed by spatial frequency, contrast sensitivity and backward masking in normal ageing and Alzheimer's disease. Brain 1983; 107:309–325.
75. Shimamura AP, Salmon DP, Squire LR, Butters N. Memory dysfunction and word priming in dementia and amnesia. Behav Neurosci 1987; 101:347–351.
76. Smith S, Butters N. Activation of semantic relations in Alzheimer's and Huntington's disease. In: Whitaker H, ed. Neuropsychological studies of non-focal brain damage: Dementia and trauma. New York: Springer-Verlag, 1988:265.
77. Squire LR. Two forms of human amnesia: An analysis of forgetting. J Neurosci 1981; 1:635–640.
78. Squire LR. Memory and Brain. New York: Oxford University Press, 1987.
79. Storandt M, Botwinick J, Danziger WL. Longitudinal changes: Patients with mild SDAT and matched healthy controls. In: Poon LW, ed. Handbook for clinical memory assessment of older adults. Washington, D.C.: American Psychological Association, 1986.
80. Terry RD, Katzman R. Senile dementia of the Alzheimer type. Ann Neurol 1983; 14:497–506.
81. Thomson DM, Tulving E. Associative encoding and retrieval: Weak and strong cues. J Exp Psychol 1970; 86:255–262.
82. Tulving E. Elements of episodic memory. Oxford: Clarendon Press, 1983.
83. Weingartner H, Grafman J, Boutelle W, Kaye W, Martin PR. Forms of memory failure. Science 1983; 221:380–382.
84. Weingartner H, Kaye W, Smallberg SA, Ebert MH, Gillin JC, Sitaram H. Memory failure in progressive idiopathic dementia. J Abnorm Psychol 1981; 90:187–196.
85. Whitehouse PJ, Price DL, Struble RG. Alzheimer's disease and senile dementia: Loss of neurons in the basal forebrain. Science 1982; 215:1237–1239.
86. Wilson RS, Kaszniak AW. Longitudinal changes: Progressive idiopathic dementia. In: Poon LW, ed. Handbook for clinical memory assessment of older adults. Washington, D.C.: American Psychological Association, 1986.

# CHAPTER 4

# *Auditory Changes*

ALISON M. GRIMES, M.A.

Changes in the auditory system that occur with advancing age may result in substantial communication impairment, particularly if not appropriately recognized and remediated. Hearing impairment in the elderly is often confused with, or mistaken for, dementia or depression. Failure to thoroughly evaluate each of these tentative diagnoses can result in tragic consequences for the individual involved, particularly when the primary impairment is peripheral hearing loss and when such loss is amenable to rehabilitation.

The individual who is both elderly and demented, an increasingly common occurrence, presents a major challenge to the audiologist involved in diagnosing auditory dysfunction and prescribing appropriate rehabilitation. A person who develops dementia is certainly not immune to the effects of aging on the auditory system, and indeed, the cognitively impaired person may be disproportionately affected by the age-related changes of the auditory system. A person who is both elderly and demented may have impairments in understanding and processing speech that might be more easily overcome by a person with similar auditory impairment, but who is cognitively intact. Further, the presence of impaired cognition may render standard auditory rehabilitation measures difficult, if not impossible.

This chapter will focus on three interrelated areas: auditory function, aging, and dementia. First, the effects of normal aging on auditory function will be outlined. Second, examination of auditory function in the elderly person who is also demented will follow, focusing on central auditory-processing deficits in this population. Finally, suggestions for effective communication and remediation will be offered, as well as strategies for the successful evaluation of such patients.

## Scope of Problem

Hearing loss is one of the most prevalent impairments among elderly Americans.[68] Hearing impairment with advancing age is both peripheral (affecting the end-organ of hearing with resultant distortion and loss of sensitivity) and central (affecting the auditory pathways in the brainstem and cerebral hemispheres, and exerting more subtle effects on speech understanding such as slowed or impaired perception and processing of auditory information). Health-care professionals and the general public tend to think primarily of peripheral impairment when the topic of aging and auditory function is considered. Peripheral hearing loss has received far more clinical study and attention than central auditory impairment in the aged population. Further, the majority of research, particularly clinical research, has been directed toward peripheral impairment. Major studies have detailed the prevalence of hearing loss in the aging population, using sensitivity loss as the sole criterion.[61,68] As an example, Moscicki and colleagues reported audiologic studies in a cohort of approximately 2300 healthy, elderly persons.[68] The prevalence of hearing loss, defined as any pure tone threshold in the frequency range of 500 to 4000 Hz greater than 20 dB, was 83 percent. Depending on the method of study and the definition of "hearing impairment," other researchers have reported prevalence rates as low as 24 percent.

Unfortunately, far less is know about the anatomic and physiologic changes of the central auditory nervous system (CANS) in the elderly individual. There are a number of studies of functional impairments of the CANS based on results of behavioral and electrophysiologic assessments of elderly individuals. Although this body of literature has formed the basis of our understanding of aging and central auditory function, this research is not without its pitfalls. Among other factors, there is only a limited number of studies where either sophisticated radiographic or postmortem anatomic assessment of the CANS has been obtained to be compared with behavioral and electrophysiologic measures obtained prior to death.

In practical terms, this limited understanding of CANS function in both the normal and demented elderly populations has resulted in a perception that age-related hearing loss is only a loss in auditory sensitivity and, as such, is simply rehabilitated by the use of hearing aids. In situations where there is both peripheral and central impairment, however, measures that are conventionally taken to rehabilitate peripheral hearing loss may not be appropriate, nor successful. In persons who are demented, the effects of both peripheral and central impairments are exacerbated. Demented patients with peripheral auditory impairment have a double burden. The normal cognitive abilities that are called into play to perceive spoken language through impaired ears (through "fill-in-the-blanks" strategies that will be discussed in greater detail later in this chapter) are themselves impaired. Further, the ability to use visual speech information to supplement auditory information, "speechreading," may be impaired in elderly demented patients for the same reasons (impaired peripheral vision, impaired visual processing, and cognitive decline). Strategies exist to facilitate communication in such persons, but adequate recognition of the impairment(s) must first be made so that appropriate steps can be taken.

Several reports of auditory processing in the normal elderly listener have been published.[25,30,32,64,87] Although many age-related differences in the auditory processing of younger and older subjects have been identified, the issue of precisely how, why, and to what extent auditory function changes with age is not resolved. There are at least three confounding factors that exist when assessing auditory function through speech recognition and other behavioral auditory measures in the elderly individual. These may be summarized as follows:

1. Peripheral hearing loss confounds test outcome and interpretation when using speech and nonspeech measures of central auditory function. Virtually all auditory measures are affected to some degree by peripheral hearing loss. A persistent difficulty has been isolating that aspect of reduced performance that is attributable to age from that which is a result of peripheral hearing loss.[22,30,64]
2. In behavioral testing using either speech or nonspeech stimuli, a pervasive concern has been that elderly subjects use different response criteria than do younger subjects. Aged subjects may use a more conservative response criterion, that is, they may require greater certainty that a stimulus exists or that their identification of a stimulus is correct before making a response than a younger subject does.

There is not unanimity among researchers that the use of a conservative criterion truly affects older listeners' responses. Much of the earlier work demonstrated that a conservative response bias does occur in aged subjects;[13,82,83] in other studies, however, these significant differences between criteria used by older and younger subjects have not been found.[103] Further, in at least one study, speech recognition scores were not found to be significantly different among three groups of listeners that varied in response criteria, and it was concluded that conventional speech audiometric results were not significantly influenced by response criterion.[49]

Finally, in a recent paper, Gordon-Salant examined response criteria in elderly subjects and found that the elderly did not use a more conservative criterion for response and, in fact, actually used a *less* conservative criterion as compared with younger subjects when judging the accuracy of their responses on word-recognition tasks.[24] Gordon-Salant concluded that "elderly listeners may misunderstand the spoken message but respond as if they have understood the message...their own response to the message is inappropriate, and communication inefficiency is perpetuated."[24]

3. It has been postulated that central auditory-processing disorder in elderly individuals simply represents generalized cognitive decline and not a modality-specific impairment. That is, this condition, identified as a specific auditory impairment, is merely one manifestation of senility affecting all sensory and cognitive functions. In a recent report by the Committee on Hearing, Bioacoustics, and Biomechanics (CHABA) this theory was given strong support.[12] Although there certainly may be a relationship between cognitive deficits and measured central dysfunction, several studies have demonstrated that the two conditions are neither mutually exclusive nor mutually inclusive.[50]

Given this background, it is clear that performance on tests of auditory function by elderly listeners differs from performance by younger subjects. It is equally clear, however, that caution must be taken when ascribing auditory dysfunction observed in the elderly listener to aging per se. Some proportion of the observed decrement in performance in all probability is a function of peripheral hearing loss exerting an attenuating, distorting, or filtering effect on the stimulus. In the following sections of this chapter, function and dysfunction of the various levels of the auditory system in the elderly and demented person will be discussed, and implications for communication impairment will be presented.

## The Auditory System: Function and Dysfunction in Normal Aging

The auditory system may be divided into two portions: peripheral (conductive and cochlear–eighth cranial nerve) and central (Fig. 4.1). The structure, function, and methods of assessments of the several areas of the auditory system vary greatly.

### CONDUCTIVE MECHANISM (OUTER AND MIDDLE EAR)

Although age-related changes are well documented in the peripheral system, they are not generally found in the conductive mechanism. The external and middle ears are not believed to undergo substantial changes attributable to aging alone. The primary pathology occurring in the outer ear in an elderly individual is cerumen accumulation and eventual occlusion of the ear canal. This results in a blockage of sound transmission, resulting in conductive hearing loss of varying degree. Cerumen accumulation and occlusion may be exacerbated by chronic dermatitis, hairy ear canals, poor hygiene, and hearing-aid usage. In the sample of individuals from the Framingham cohort who were studied audiologically, cerumen occlusion was found to be the most frequently occurring conductive condition.[68]

Reports of age-related changes in the middle ear, primarily affecting the movement of the ossicular chain, have been reported, but these minor changes in ossicular movement have not been shown to significantly affect hearing sensitivity in the average-aged population. Eustachian-tube dysfunction and resultant otitis media may occur in elderly individuals, but there does not appear to be a significant relationship to age in these conditions. In the report on the Framingham group, there were few reports of specific middle-ear pathology, other than otosclerosis (less than 1 percent) and ear surgery (5 percent).[68] It was concluded that more study is required to delineate prevalence and etiology of conductive hearing loss in aged individuals.

### Assessment of Conductive Hearing Loss

The function of the conductive portion of the peripheral auditory system can be assessed using both behavioral (requiring conscious response from the patient) and objective (not requiring patient cooperation) measures. Behavioral tests of conductive hearing loss compare the sensitivity to pure-tone stimuli when delivered by air-conduction versus bone-conduction receivers. The physical integrity of the conductive mechanism is objectively assessed through a test battery of acoustic immittance measures, comprising tympanometry, static immittance, and assessment of the acoustic reflex (which reflects, in part, the integrity of the conductive mechanism and is affected by the cochlear and neural auditory status).

### SENSORY MECHANISM (COCHLEA)

It is in the cochlea and first-order neurons arising in the cochlea that the majority of research and clinical study of the effects of aging on audition

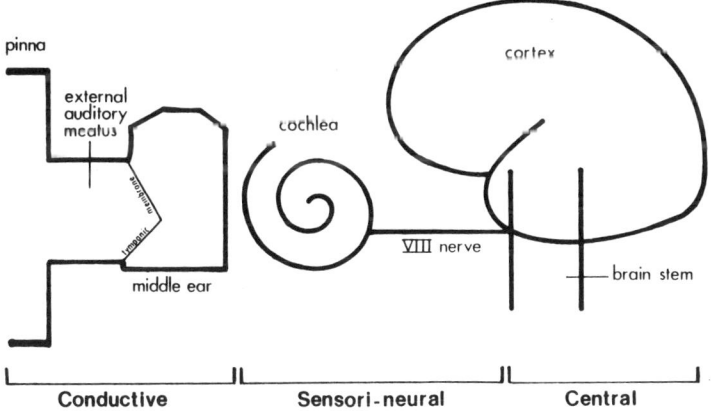

Figure 4.1 Schematic of the auditory system. From Deutsch L, Richards A, eds. Elementary hearing science. Baltimore: University Park Press, 1979:38.

has been concentrated. The cochlea is the primary site of "presbycusis" or aged hearing. Schuknecht defined presbycusis as "the classical manifestation of cochlear aging...high tone deafness caused by atrophic changes in the basal coil."[89] In this early paper, Schuknecht defined two types of presbycusis, and later refined these into the four classic types of presbycusis:[90,91]

1. *Sensory presbycusis.* Basal cochlear atrophy, characterized by a loss of hair cells and supporting structures, with secondary degeneration of neural elements (Fig. 4.2). The audiometric (sensitivity loss) pattern was defined as an abrupt, high-frequency pattern.
2. *Neural presbycusis.* A loss of spiral ganglion cells and degeneration of cochlear neurons (Fig. 4.3). This is characterized by greater distortion for speech understanding than sensory presbycusis, with disproportionately poor speech-recognition abilities considering the degree of sensitivity loss. Audiometrically, hearing loss associated with neural presbycusis decreased linearly from lower to higher frequencies.
3. *Metabolic or strial presbycusis.* Atrophy of the stria vascularis, which is a collection of blood vessels in the wall of the cochlea, affecting cochlear metabolism (Fig. 4.4). The organ of Corti and cochlear neurons are normal. Audiometrically, strial presbycusis is slowly progressive with a relatively flat audiometric configuration and good speech recognition ability.
4. *Mechanical or cochlear conductive.* Changes, primarily stiffening or loss of elasticity, of the basilar membrane (Fig. 4.5). There is limited hair-cell and neuron loss. High-frequency hearing loss typifies this type of presbycusis as well.

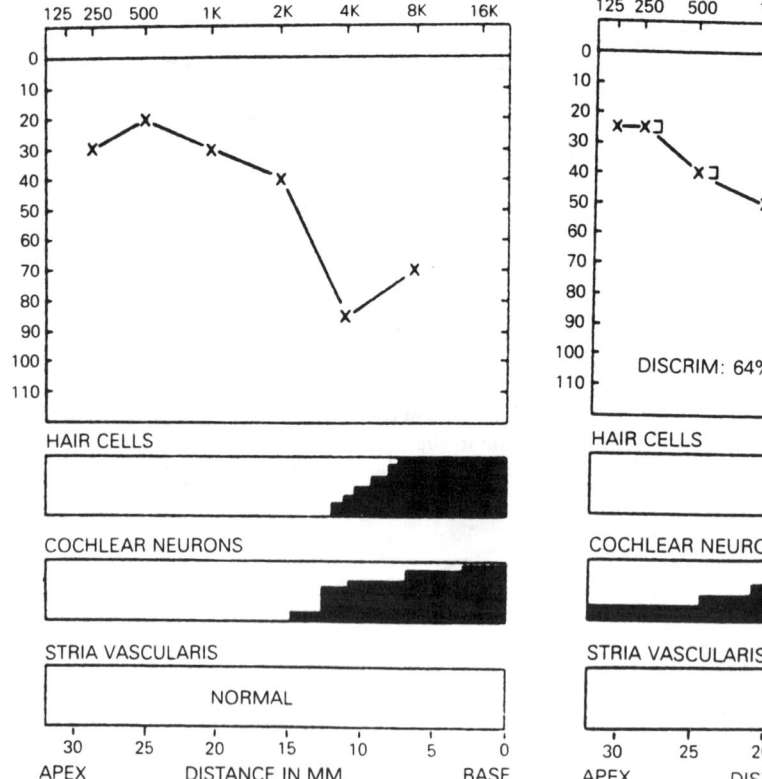

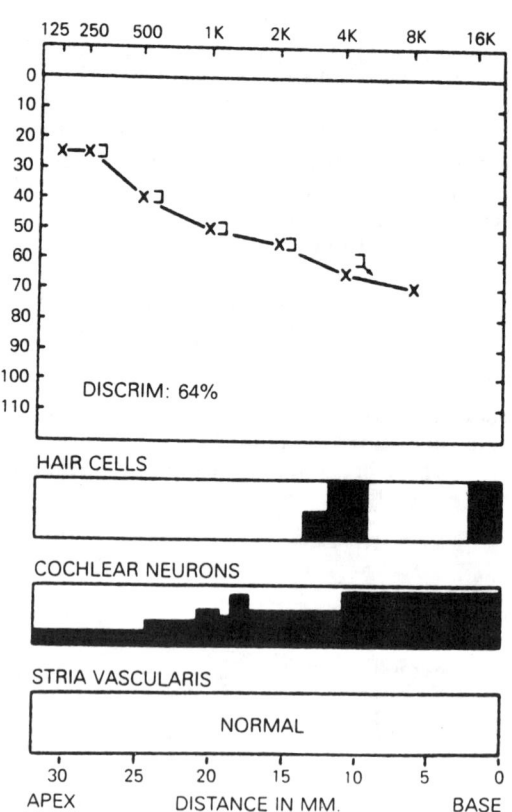

**Figure 4.2** Sensory presbycusis. Darkened areas represent loss of hair cells, cochlear neurons, and/or stria vascularis as a function of distance from the base of the cochlea. From Schuknecht H. Pathology of the ear. Cambridge, MA: Harvard University Press, 1974:56. Copyright 1974 by the President and Fellows of Harvard College.

**Figure 4.3** Neural presbycusis. Darkened areas represent loss of hair cells, cochlear neurons, and/or stria vascularis as a function of distance from the base of the cochlea. From Schuknecht H. Pathology of the ear. Cambridge, MA: Harvard University Press, 1974:57. Copyright 1974 by the President and Fellows of Harvard College.

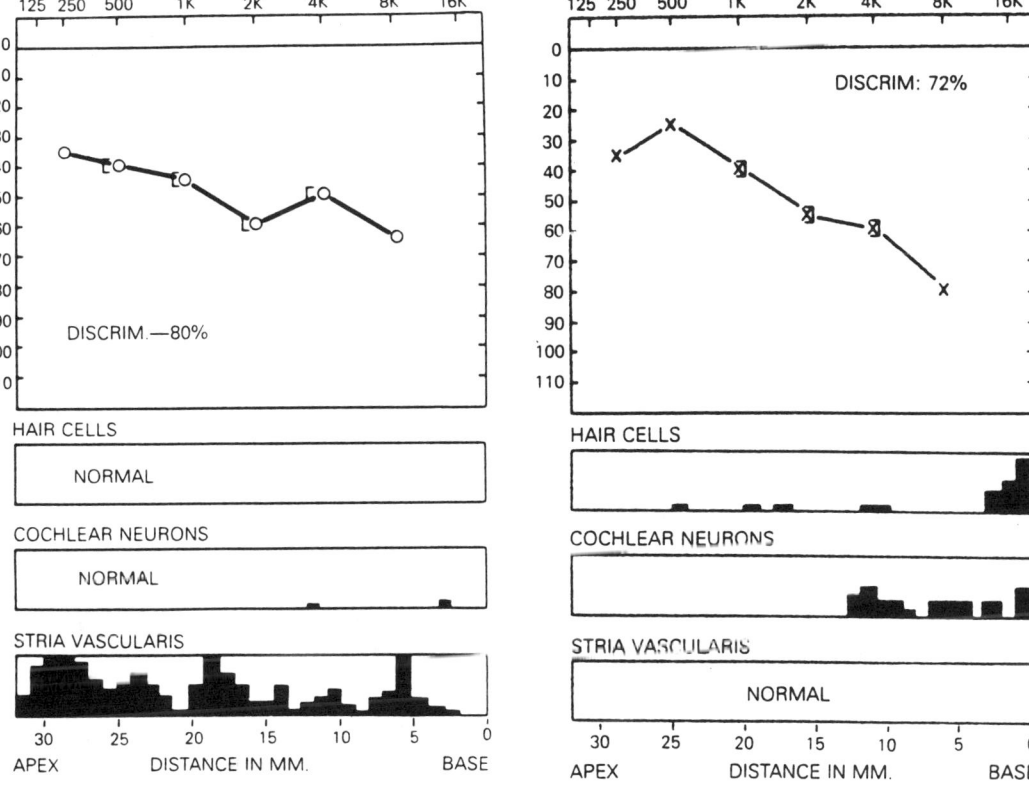

Figure 4.4 Strial presbycusis. Darkened areas represent loss of hair cells, cochlear neurons, and/or stria vascularis as a function of distance from the base of the cochlea. From Schuknecht H. Pathology of the ear. Cambridge, MA: Harvard University Press, 1974:58. Copyright 1974 by the President and Fellows of Harvard College.

Figure 4.5 Cochlear conductive presbycusis. Darkened areas represent loss of hair cells, cochlear neurons, and/or stria vascularis as a function of distance from the base of the cochlea. From Schuknecht H. Pathology of the ear. Cambridge, MA: Harvard University Press, 1974:59. Copyright 1974 by the President and Fellows of Harvard College.

These types of presbycusis do not necessarily account for all aspects of age-related changes in the cochlea, and the types and associated audiometric configurations are not rigid, mutually exclusive divisions. The entire concept of presbycusis is not without its detractors, and there are those who believe that presbycusis represents nothing more than the cumulative effects of noise, vascular disease, infection, ototoxic agents, and individual genetic susceptibility. Hawkins and Johnson note that aging alone cannot be blamed for hearing impairment in the elderly, as there are numerous exogenous and endogenous factors over one's lifetime that affect auditory structures and function.[38] Noise is the single most important exogenous factor that contributes to loss of hearing sensitivity with increasing age, and genetic predisposition is the most significant endogenous factor. These researchers studied more than 400 pairs of human temporal bones from infants to persons in their upper nineties. Most of the elderly subjects simply showed sensorineural degeneration that was most severe in the lower basal turn and was usually accompanied by vascular involution and strial atrophy. Very few cases fit the description of neural presbycusis. Further, these authors reported that mechanical presbycusis remains an "interesting but largely hypothetical concept."

Presbycusis was contrasted with both "sociocusis" (non–work-noise-induced otologic disorder) and "nosoacusis" (non–noise related otologic disorder) by Kryter, who reviewed major studies of hearing levels found in general populations to examine more closely the variables of age, sex, race, and common otologic disorders. Based on the data from combined sources representing several thousand subjects, Kryter concluded that hearing level surveys reflect the combined effects of presbycusis, nosocusis, and sociocusis, rather than "pure" presbycusis.[61]

Lowell and Paparella refer to the term "presbycusis" as "...those rare, solely age-related cases of sensorineural hearing loss" and "a vague concept of aging deafness."[62] These authors present data that support that belief that many cases of diagnosed presbycusis represented undiagnosed cases of familial or genetically related hearing loss.

It is clear that presbycusis cannot exist in a vacuum. As long as human ears are subjected to the enormous variety of noise, noxious agents, and endogenous vascular and metabolic stresses, and with the obvious factor of genetic predisposition for acquired hearing loss, presbycusis will remain a highly heterogeneous condition.

### Assessment of Sensory Hearing Loss

Cochlear lesions are evaluated behaviorally by pure-tone audiometry and tests of speech recognition, and objectively by assessment of the acoustic reflex, electrocochleography (ECoG), and auditory brainstem response (ABR) (Fig. 4.6).

Pure-tone audiometric patterns typically show impairment that is greater in the higher than in the lower frequencies, as shown in Figures 4.2 to 4.5. In speech audiometry, impairment in speech recognition can generally be predicted from the configuration of the pure-tone sensitivity loss, although in certain circumstances, speech-recognition ability is disproportionately reduced when compared with the audiometric configuration and the degree of sensitivity loss (e.g., in "neural presbycusis"). Norms for disproportionate loss in speech intelligibility were offered by Yellin et al for one speech material.[104] Although numerous studies have compared speech-recognition performance in younger and elderly subjects without reaching unanimous conclusions, it is generally believed that maximum scores on monosyllabic word lists (*PB-Max*) are no different in elderly and younger subjects when degree and configuration of sensitivity loss are held constant.[25] Speech-recognition performance greatly depends on presentation level relative to the peripheral hearing-loss configuration. Testing that does not ensure that the presentation level is sufficiently above threshold at all, or as many as possible, frequencies is unfairly biased against those subjects with peripheral hearing loss.

## NEURAL MECHANISM: EIGHTH CRANIAL NERVE AND BRAINSTEM AUDITORY NUCLEI

Age-related changes in the eighth cranial nerve have been less thoroughly studied than cochlear changes. Schuknecht's neural form of presbycusis implies degeneration of the first-order neuron.[89] Loss of myelin and hyperostosis of the internal auditory canal have been postulated to cause deterioration of the eighth nerve in aged persons. One paper reported reduction in the number of cells in the ventral cochlear, medial geniculate, and superior olivary nuclei of the auditory pathway.[57] Other researchers, however, have found no reduction in cell population in the ventral cochlear nucleus.[9] In the thalamus, Brody also found fewer neurons in elderly as compared with younger brains.[9] It has also been reported that the nucleus of the lateral lemniscus and the primary auditory projection area (Heschl's gyrus) are the two principal loci of disorder in the aging central auditory system.[43]

Mills and Ryals demonstrated that reduction in cerebrovascular circulation affected the wave V latency of the auditory brainstem response (ABR) in a group of middle-aged men.[66] Similarly, chronic hypoxemia was shown to have a deleterious effect on central auditory-processing performance in aged subjects.[15] Brainstem auditory nuclei are highly susceptible to lack of oxygen, and patients with chronic obstructive pulmonary disease are therefore susceptible to performance decrements in brainstem-level auditory tasks.

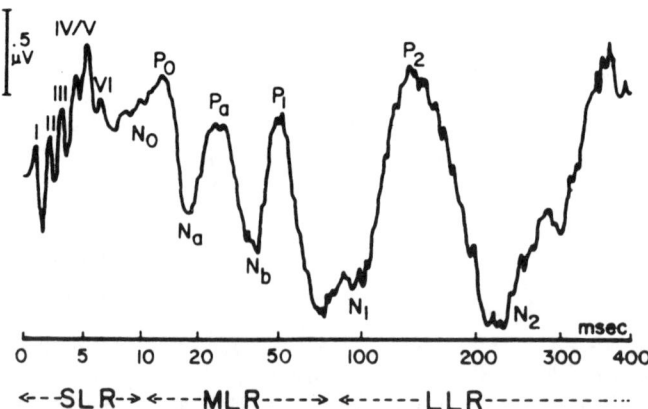

Figure 4.6 Auditory evoked potentials. Waves I–VI are the auditory brainstem response (ABR); $P_a$ is the primary component of the middle-latency response (MLR), and the $P_2$–$N_2$ is the long-latency response. Figure modified and redrawn from Michelini et al, 1982. The short latency auditory evoked potentials. In: ASHA Audiologic Evaluation Working Group on Auditory Evoked Potential Measurements. Rockville, MD: American Speech-Language-Hearing Association, 1988:29.

## Assessment of Neural Hearing Loss

Behavioral assessment of the eighth cranial nerve is generally not as successful as objective assessment measures. Impairment in pure-tone sensitivity may occur only to a small degree or not at all in a "purely" neural lesion. Assessment of speech recognition may show disproportionate impairment as compared with loss in sensitivity, but factors of test reliability may obscure this finding.[100] A more fruitful approach to assessment of neural impairment is electrophysiologic testing (acoustic reflex functions and ABR). One possible model to examine as an indication of eighth-nerve impairment is multiple sclerosis (MS), and several studies have examined the auditory function in patients with MS in whom the eighth nerve is demyelinated.[42,72] In such cases, conventional speech audiometric tests are generally unimpaired, but recognition of distorted speech materials is significantly affected. The acoustic reflex and ABR patterns observed in patients with MS and similar demyelinating pathology have been repeatedly shown to be abnormal.[28,53,84,97]

One method in which speech recognition is used in assessing neural impairment is performance-intensity functions (PIF). In this test approach, recognition of monosyllabic words is assessed at a variety of intensity levels, from slightly above threshold to just below the threshold of discomfort. In normal subjects and those with peripheral (cochlear) lesions, performance levels reach an asymptote at some level above threshold with no significant performance decrement up to the point of discomfort. However, in patients with various types of neural lesions, including aging, performance peaks at a point above threshold, and with further increases in intensity, word-recognition scores begin to decline. This is referred to as "rollover" on a PIF and is seen in cases of lesions of the eighth cranial nerve and brainstem lesions, and has been reported in normal, elderly patients. When observed in such patients, the rollover has been attributed to aging processes within the eighth cranial nerve and brainstem.[46]

Other behavioral tests have been used, with limited success, to delineate functional changes in the eighth nerve and brainstem in normal, pathologic, and aging conditions. Many behavioral tests that were once supported as sensitive and specific to neural auditory lesions have been abandoned in favor of objective measures that more efficiently and effectively diagnose neural impairments. Measures such as speech recognition in ipsilateral noise conditions and recognition of binaurally split speech or alternating speech have been found to be too greatly affected by variables of test reliability and by degree and configuration of peripheral hearing loss to be clinically useful.

One behavioral measure that is more sensitive to brainstem pathology is the masking level difference (MLD), a binaural test of tonal detection in noise in various tone-noise phase relationships. The MLD has been reported to be abnormally small in eighth nerve and brainstem pathology.[70,72] Although MLDs are known to be highly affected by peripheral hearing loss, they have been reported to be slightly abnormal in the aged subject, even when peripheral hearing sensitivity is controlled.[48] An investigation of MLD size and type of presbycusis found that those subjects with neural presbycusis had smaller MLDs than those with other types of presbycusis.[73] The data were interpreted as indicating increased internal noise levels in neural presbycusis.

The most valuable tools for assessing eighth-nerve function are the acoustic reflex and the auditory brainstem response (ABR). The acoustic reflex (Fig. 4.7) comprises the stapedius muscle of the middle ear, the cochlea, the eighth cranial nerve, the auditory brainstem nuclei (cochlear nucleus and superior olive), and the seventh cranial nerve. The acoustic reflex is affected by conductive pathology, cochlear function, eighth-nerve function, brainstem function, and seventh-nerve pathology. The research literature on the acoustic reflex is substantial, and the interested reader is referred to a summary of acoustic reflex functions in normal aging by Gordon-Salant.[25]

In examining the effects of aging on the acoustic reflex, Wilson summarized the pertinent literature as showing that:

1. Static immittance changes little until the age of approximately 60.
2. Acoustic reflex thresholds increase, decrease, or remain unchanged, depending on the study.
3. The magnitude (the immittance change that occurs between the quiescent and reflexive states) of acoustic reflex growth tends to be reduced with aging.[102]

Wilson interpreted his data that showed comparatively small magnitude of acoustic reflex in aged subjects as indicating a general decrease in the efficiency of neurophysiologic activity throughout the acoustic reflex arc. This is consistent with Schuknecht's description of deterioration in the auditory system with increasing age.

The auditory brainstem response (ABR) reflects neuronal activity from the cochlea through the brainstem and comprises the averaged evoked potential occurring in the first 10 msec following auditory stimulation. Figure 4.6 illustrates the entire auditory evoked potential, with the ABR depicted as the short-latency range potential and

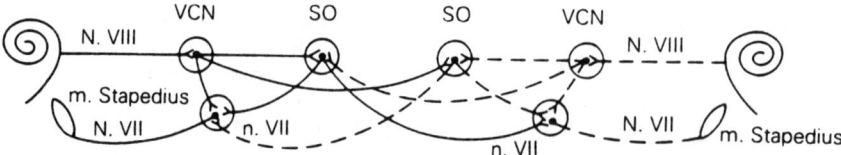

**Figure 4.7** Schematic of the stapedial reflex arc. Cranial nerve VIII is the auditory nerve; Cranial nerve VII is the facial nerve; VCN is the ventral cochlear nucleus; SO is the superior olive. From Moeller A. Auditory physiology. New York: Academic Press, 1983:34.

identified by Roman numerals I through VI. The ABR is a series of generally five vertex-positive waves, with wave I reflecting the whole-nerve action potential of the eighth cranial nerve, and subsequent waves generated by multiple sites in the brainstem. Wave I is approximately equivalent to the electrocochleogram.

Auditory brainstem responses may be abnormal in virtually any condition affecting the eighth cranial nerve and many conditions affecting the brainstem, as well as being abnormal, in qualitatively different ways, in cases of conductive and cochlear hearing impairment. Although some research has found no significant differences in ABRs between young and older subjects, the majority of the literature has reported slight absolute and interwave latency prolongations in the older groups.[75,47,88] Additionally, the replicability, amplitude, and organization of the response deteriorates in the elderly person.[86] The literature on the ABR and on the effects of aging on the ABR is substantial. For a summary, see Brewer.[6]

ABRs have been studied in patients with dementia. In a study of a small group of patients with dementia of the Alzheimer type (DAT), Harkins reported significant group differences in the wave III and wave V latencies, as well as in the I to V transmission time when comparing these patients with a normal control group.[35] Because Alzheimer's disease is believed to primarily entail gray-matter impairment, and the ABR reflects eighth cranial nerve and lower brainstem auditory-pathway conduction, Harkins' data were unexpected. To attempt to replicate these findings, Grimes and colleagues examined the ABRs of a larger group of patients with DAT.[3] ABRs were obtained in 62 patients, as well as in the age- and sex-matched controls. This design was constructed in order to avoid two possible shortcomings of the Harkins paper: small subject group (N = 6 males) and lack of sex-matching in the control group (controls were eight subjects, half of whom were female, and the control data were collapsed across sex). Mean values for absolute wave V latency and the I to V transmission time were presented in Table 4.1. No significant group differences emerged for either the absolute or interwave latencies in either of two stimulus conditions. A typical ABR from one patient is shown in Figure 4.8.

From this, it can be concluded that the lower brainstem level auditory functions as assessed using standard electrophysiologic measures are not substantially affected in persons with dementia of the Alzheimer type. Indeed, there is little in the literature that would indicate that such dysfunction should be anticipated in this disease.

## TEMPORAL LOBE

It is in the temporal lobe that the most significant changes in aging and in dementia occur. As such, investigation of auditory function using measures sensitive to the temporal lobe should be fruitful. Age-related changes in the central auditory nervous system (CANS) at the hemispheric level have been termed by some as "central presbycusis."[96] Cortical function in the CANS is generally believed to show greater changes with age than subcortical and brainstem regions. Hansen and Reske-Nielsen theorized that cortical changes are more marked than those observed in the ascending pathways.[34] Brody compared cell counts of various brain regions in younger and older brains, and found that the superior temporal gyrus showed the greatest cell loss in aging.[8] Further, it has been reported that neurofibrillary tangles have a propensity for the temporal lobe. In about 50 percent of healthy elderly subjects, the EEG is focally slowed over the left anterior temporal area, possibly reflecting neuronal degeneration and reduced cerebral metabolism in this region.[14]

### Assessment of Temporal Lobe

Audiologic approaches to the assessment of CANS function at the level of the temporal lobe are both behavioral and objective. Behavioral measures entail the recognition of distorted speech and nonspeech materials. A second behavioral test is the cognitive potential (the P300), which is an electrophysiologic potential elicited by a behavioral response to an auditory stimulus. Objective measures comprise the middle-latency response (MLR) and the long-latency responses (see Fig. 4.6).

TABLE 4.1 **Mean (+ 1 sd) ABR Values for Normal and DAT Groups, at Two Stimulus Rates**

| AT SLOWER STIMULUS RATE (11/sec)(in msec) (RIGHT AND LEFT EARS AVERAGED) | | | | | AT FASTER STIMULUS RATE (66/sec)(in msec) (RIGHT AND LEFT EARS AVERAGED) | | | |
|---|---|---|---|---|---|---|---|---|
| | n | Wave V | n | I-V Interval | | n | Wave V | Shift in V Latency from Slow to Fast |
| Normal | | | | | Normal | | | |
| Male | 18 | 6.05 (0.22) | 16 | 4.11 (0.22) | Male | 18 | 6.47 (0.25) | 9.47 (0.11) |
| Female | 17 | 5.70 (0.17) | 17 | 3.97 (0.19) | Female | 16 | 6.07 (0.20) | 0.38 (0.13) |
| DAT | | | | | DAT | | | |
| Male | 39 | 6.15 (0.36) | 26 | 4.22 (0.25) | Male | 37 | 6.50 (0.40) | 0.46 (0.25) |
| Female | 30 | 5.79 (0.25) | 13 | 3.96 (0.22) | Female | 25 | 6.13 (0.27) | 0.39 (0.13) |

*No significant group differences $p < 0.01$
From Grimes A, et al. Auditory evoked potentials in patients with dementia of the Alzheimer type. Ear Hear 1987; 8:157–161.

Behavioral testing using speech stimuli is predicated on the redundancy principle as developed and detailed by Bocca and Calearo.[5] These researchers, beginning in the mid-1950s, pioneered the techniques for using sensitized speech testing to reveal the effects of temporal-lobe pathology on speech understanding. In their work, two types of redundancy were defined: intrinsic, which refers to the multiplicity of pathways and synaptic connections of the auditory pathway, and extrinsic, referring to the redundancy inherent in a spoken message, on the phonemic, syntactic, and semantic levels. An example of internal redundancy is the enormous number and rich interconnection of neural elements in the auditory pathway, whereby some degree of neural information can be impaired or lost, and perception of speech under ideal circumstances remains possible. On the extrinsic level, Bocca and Calearo noted that a verbal message has a structure and that the presence of one element (be it phonemic, or syntactic, or semantic) in a verbal message is related to the presence of the other elements, according to certain rules of probability based on linguistic structure. This structure allows recognition of an utterance when only a portion of the information has been received.

Bocca and Calearo make the point that these two types of redundancies are reciprocal (Table 4.2), and the loss of one without the loss of the other does not necessarily result in communication breakdown. For instance, a person with a normal auditory pathway is easily able to comprehend speech information when a portion of such information is unavailable because of masking by environmental noise. In order to test the integrity of the central auditory pathways (intrinsic redundancy), the extrinsic redundancy of the speech message must be reduced. This can be accomplished in a variety of ways, including: filtering, attenua-

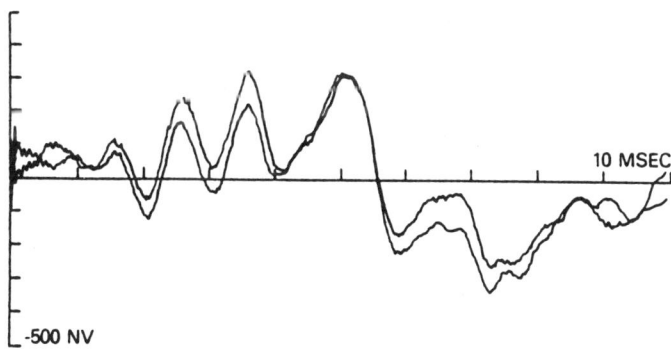

Figure 4.8 Auditory brainstem response in a patient with dementia of the Alzheimer type. From Grimes A, et al. Auditory evoked potentials in patients with dementia of the Alzheimer type. Ear Hear 1987; 8:157–161.

tion, presenting speech with some type of competing speech or noise, and altering the temporal characteristics of speech. How the extrinsic redundancy is reduced is not particularly important, as long as it is reduced to a sufficient degree that those with normal auditory function are able to perceive it and those with pathology are not.

The point is clearly made by Bocca and Calearo, although unfortunately it has not always been kept in mind in research design, that when assessing central auditory function using a reduced redundancy message, the element of phonetic recognition that occurs in the peripheral auditory system must be completely excluded as a potentially confounding variable.

Bocca and Calearo were the first to demonstrate that recognition of distorted speech (single words that were low-pass filtered or sentence material that had been time-compressed) was abnormal in the ear contralateral to a temporal-lobe lesion. This early work has formed the basis for much of the sensitized speech testing that is used today to investigate central auditory processing disorders.

The second major approach to behavioral testing of the CANS, other than presentation of monotic distorted speech, is dichotic speech recognition.[7,93-98] In dichotic presentation, a word, nonsense syllable, or sentence is presented to one ear, and simultaneously a different word, nonsense syllable, or sentence is presented to the other. The required response is either to repeat the stimulus from only one ear, or the stimuli from both ears, either in a prescribed or free-recall paradigm.

The model of dichotic listening (Fig. 4.9) of Sparks and colleagues illustrates the ipsilateral and contralateral auditory pathways from end-organ to the dominant (left) temporal lobe.[93,94] This classical model shows that generally a contralateral ear effect (decreased performance) is expected in temporal-lobe lesions, although with a left temporal-lobe lesion, both ipsilateral and contralateral effects may be observed. Dichotic stimulation requires that the two stimuli, one to each ear, compete for neural space in the left temporal lobe: the right-ear stimulus via the direct contralateral pathway and the left-ear stimulus via the indirect contralateral pathway to the right hemisphere, then via commissure pathways to the left temporal lobe.

Dichotic speech assessment has been used extensively to delineate hemispheric dominance for speech perception and to assess pathology of the temporal lobes and interhemispheric connections. In the former application, Kimura described a superiority of the right ear over the left by normal subjects in a dichotic listening paradigm.[56] This right-ear advantage for dichotically presented materials has been exhaustively studied and reported since that time. For an excellent review of the literature, see Berlin and McNeil.[4] Disclosure of temporal-lobe and interhemispheric pathologies is uniquely possible through the use of dichotic assessment. Because dichotic stimulation sets up competition for processing in the left temporal lobe, as seen in Figure 4.9, the effects of any lesion that slows input to the left temporal lobe will be revealed. For instance, a lesion in the right temporal hemisphere or corpus callosum results in impairment in the recognition of the stimulus delivered to the contralateral (left) ear. This was first reported by Kimura and has been further studied by numerous researchers (for a contemporary review, see Mueller).[44,69] Dichotic testing is generally recognized as the most sensitive speech test for detecting temporal-lobe dysfunction.

Although both monotic-degraded and dichotic speech presentations are of value in assessing temporal lobe lesions, the dichotic mode has particular advantages and increased sensitivity over the monotic mode. A major drawback of using monotic degraded speech is that it is highly sensitive to the effects of peripheral hearing loss. Hearing

TABLE 4.2 Reciprocal Relationship Between Extrinsic and Intrinsic Redundancy and Speech Processing

| | EXTRINSIC REDUNDANCY OF SPEECH | | INTRINSIC REDUNDANCY OF SPEECH | | SPEECH UNDERSTANDING | |
|---|---|---|---|---|---|---|
| 1. | IF | Normal | AND | Normal | THEN | Normal |
| 2. | IF | Normal | BUT | Impaired | THEN | Normal |
| 3. | IF | Impaired | BUT | Normal | THEN | Normal |
| 4. | IF | Impaired | AND | Impaired | THEN | ABNORMAL |

*Condition four represents the basis for central auditory processing evaluation; a person with an impaired central auditory nervous system will have abnormal understanding of speech if the extrinsic speech redundancy has been reduced

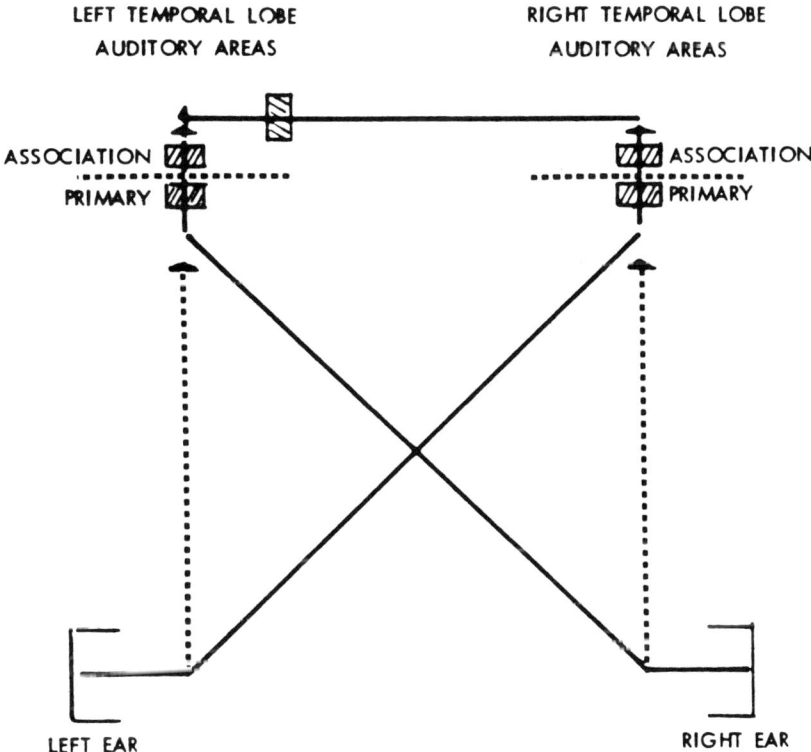

**Figure 4.9** Model of dichotic processing. The solid line represents the direct contralateral pathways, the broken line the ipsilateral routes. Note that stimuli from the left ear must travel to the left temporal lobe via the right temporal lobe and corpus callosum. The slashed boxes represent areas where lesions may cause reduced dichotic performance. From Sparks R, et al. Ipsilateral versus contralateral extinction in dichotic listening resulting from hemisphere lesions. Cortex 6:249–260.

loss, even relatively minor high-frequency impairment, is known to exert an effect on the recognition of all types of monotic degraded speech.[36,67,85] If there exists a difference in peripheral sensitivity between ears, or if there is peripheral loss in both ears that reduces performance, test interpretation is complicated. This is a particular concern when interaural comparisons are made for the purpose of determining contralateral ear effects. Although this concern is also present in dichotic presentation, a variety of test materials exists that is less affected by peripheral hearing loss (e.g., nondistorted monosyllables, bisyllables, and digits).[95]

Numerous studies have examined recognition of monotic distorted speech in the normal, aged population. Generally, performance by older listeners has been found to be lower than that of younger subjects for low-pass filtered speech and speech that has been time-compressed, interrupted, or reverberated.[3,11,57–59,77] Recognition of monosyllabic words in an ipsilateral noise environment is yet another method of reducing extrinsic redundancy of speech, and abnormal performance in aged subjects has been reported using this monotic test paradigm as well. Interpretation of word recognition in ipsilateral noise as a measure of central impairment is problematic because of a lack of standardization of speech and noise stimuli. Further, it has been noted that abnormal performance on this test may occur as a result of either peripheral hearing loss or as a result of a central lesion from any level of the auditory pathway.[74] A number of studies have reported reduced performance on speech in ipsilateral noise in aging listeners.[18,19,51,92] Although recognition of speech in ipsilateral noise is impaired in the aging person, it is clear that the cause of this reduced performance is at least partially peripheral. Further, the poor test standardization of speech in ipsilateral noise tests makes this measure "one of the most misused speech tests of CANS function."[69]

Speech in ipsilateral noise has also been used as a test of central function in normal elderly and neurologically impaired persons. Probably the most widely used application of this technique is the Synthetic Sentence Identification (SSI) in an ipsilateral-speech competition mode.[4] It has been shown that normal elderly individuals have a specific decrement in performance when the SSI in ipsilateral speech competition is compared with tests that specifically assess the peripheral mechanism. For instance, Hayes and Jerger found that elderly subjects with both "central" and "peripheral" auditory impairments perform less well with hearing aids than elderly subjects showing only a peripheral impairment.[39] In a longitudinal case study of central presbycusis, Stach and colleagues noted little change in peripheral hearing sensitivity over a 9-year period in a single individual, but substantial decline in central auditory function that paralleled this individual's progressive dissatisfaction and finally his decision to discontinue use of his hearing aids.[96] Other researchers have shown effects of aging on auditory perception using the SSI test paradigm, and it appears that as a result of the use of sentence-length materials, it is more resistant to the effects of peripheral hearing loss than other central measures.[40,96]

Dichotic speech understanding has been studied in normal aging and has also been shown to be reduced or impaired in elderly subjects.[1,2,13,21,41,65] Theories regarding the nature of the performance decrement include memory impairment, reduced storage capacity of the temporal lobe, effects of peripheral hearing loss, temporal masking, and generalized cognitive decline. Drachman and colleagues investigated the nature of dichotic processing in the elderly using scopolamine injections to mimic aging in young subjects.[17] Scopolamine had been shown in previous work to cause memory and cognition changes in young subjects similar to such changes seen in the aged. Younger subjects who had received scopolamine showed significant performance impairment as compared with young, undrugged subjects. This was interpreted as indicating that memory and cognitive decline in aging may result from impaired function in cholinergic neurons.

To assess the thesis put forth in the recent CHABA paper that central auditory dysfunction in the elderly merely reflects generalized cognitive decline,[12] Jerger et al used a dichotic sentence task (the DSI) to assess central auditory status in both normal elderly and cognitively impaired elderly individuals.[50] Central auditory status was abnormal in the presence of normal cognitive function in 23 percent of subjects and was normal in the presence of cognitive deficit in 14 percent of subjects. They concluded that decline in speech understanding in the elderly cannot be explained as the consequence of concomitant cognitive decline, but rather as a specific central auditory-processing disorder that is independent of peripheral hearing loss and cognitive status.

From this brief review, it is clear that central auditory-processing abilities are impaired in normal elderly subjects as compared with younger listeners. The exact nature of the performance decrement, whether it reflects peripheral hearing loss, response style, memory, or a specific central dysfunction, remains open to question. In all probability, all of these factors, and perhaps others as well, combine to effect this performance decrement. Careful control over nonperceptual factors such as hearing loss, cognitive status, attention, memory, and response style is necessary in research design to isolate that part of performance impairment that truly reflects central auditory processing.

## Central Auditory Function in Elderly and Demented Individuals

In persons with dementia, particularly of the Alzheimer type, significant physical and physiologic impairments of the temporal lobe are known to exist.[10,16,20,79,80] In this condition, which is characterized by bilateral temporal-lobe pathology, it is logical to examine central auditory function. One might expect that persons with dementia may demonstrate central auditory impairments similar to those seen in patients with discrete lesions of the temporal lobe.[45,63,70] An alternative hypothesis is to view dementia as a model for normal aging. It is, however, equally plausible to conclude that DAT represents a specific disease entity and not an example of "accelerated aging."[14] In any event, assessment of central auditory-processing ability is pertinent to understand better the nature of communication impairments commonly seen in demented patients.

We initiated a series of studies of auditory function in patients with dementia of the Alzheimer type (DAT). Our purpose was to evaluate CANS function through the use of dichotic and monotic degraded speech understanding, as well as the middle-latency response of the AEP, and to correlate the findings with measures of cognition and dementia.

Initally, dichotic listening was studied in a group of 38 male and female patients diagnosed as having DAT (with DSM-III criteria for primary degenerative dementia).[29] The dichotic speech recognition material was the Staggered Spondaic Word Test (SSW).[53] This test is composed of bisyllabic words in which the second syllable of the stimulus word to one ear is presented simultaneously with the first syllable of the word presented to the opposite ear. This test has the advantage of being somewhat less affected by peripheral hear-

TABLE 4.3 **Performance on the SSW in DAT and Control Groups**

| GROUP | N | | RIGHT DICHOTIC | LEFT DICHOTIC |
|---|---|---|---|---|
| Normal | 25 | | | |
| | | $\bar{x}$ | 93.7% | 90.9% |
| | | SD | 5.8 | 7.1 |
| Alzheimer | 38 | | | |
| | | $\bar{x}$ | 61.3* | 56.8* |
| | | SD | 27.2 | 26.8 |

*Significantly different from normal ($p<0.0001$)
From Grimes A, et al. Central auditory function in Alzheimer's disease. Neurology 1985; 8:352–358.

ing loss than some other dichotic speech materials.[95] Normal elderly listeners were also evaluated to provide control data. The degree and configuration of peripheral hearing losses were similar for the experimental and control groups. Any patient presenting with peripheral hearing loss that was disproportionate to their chronologic age was not included for study.

Group comparisons of the normal aged and DAT groups showed highly significant differences in correct recognition of the dichotic test stimuli (Table 4.3). As shown in Figure 4.10, the distribution of scores in the DAT group was broad, with only five subjects showing bilaterally normal performance (the level at or above which 95 percent of the normal right- and left-ear scores occurred).

To provide more specific information about the nature of the observed differences in group performance, correlations were made of dichotic test scores with a variety of measures including IQ, dementia quotient, temporal-lobe structure [through computed tomography (CT) scan] and temporal-lobe function [through position emission (PET) scan].

A neuroradiologist, who was unaware of other test results, reviewed CT scans on a 4-point scale, with 0 representing normal atrophy for chronologic aging and 3 representing atrophy that was severely increased for age. Each hemisphere was rated separately. The mean ratings are presented in Table 4.4 and indicate that it was in the temporal lobes, particularly the anterior region, where the greatest atrophy was observed.

Dichotic test scores were then compared with measures of atrophy in all eight regions studied. In Table 4.5, the mean dichotic scores, grouped ac-

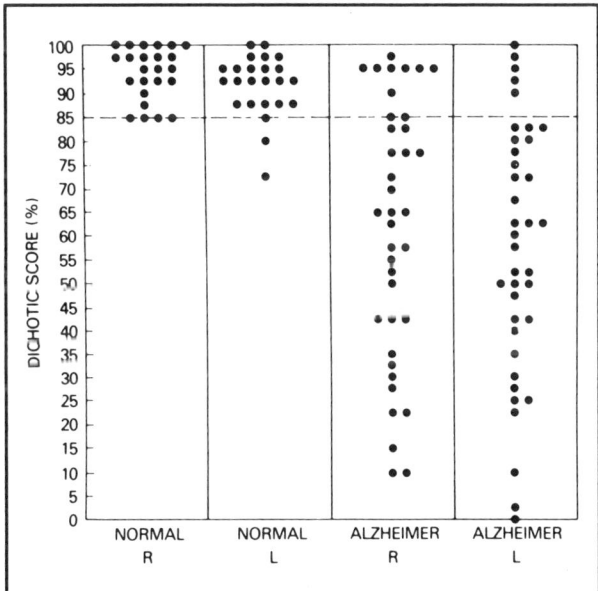

Figure 4.10 Distribution of right and left dichotic scores in patients with dementia of the Alzheimer type (N = 38) and normal controls (N = 25). Eighty-five percent value represents the lower limit of normal performance. From Grimes A, et al. Central auditory function in Alzheimer's disease. Neurology 1985; 8:352–356.

TABLE 4.4 **Mean Right and Left CT Atrophy Ratings by Lobe in Alzheimer Group (n = 37), on a Four-Point Scale (0 = Normal, 3 = Severe Atrohy)**

| FRONTAL | PARIETAL | ANTERIOR TEMPORAL | POSTERIOR TEMPORAL |
|---|---|---|---|
| 0.99*† | 1.11* | 1.72 | 1.26 |

*Significantly less than anterior temporal, $p < 0.001$. Wilcoxon Signed-Rank Test
†Significantly less than posterior temporal, $p < 0.05$. Wilcoxon Signed-Rank Test
From Grimes A, et al. Central auditory function in Alzheimer's disease. Neurology 1985; 8:352–358.

cording to each atrophy rating, are shown. For example, the mean dichotic score of all subjects with anterior temporal atrophy ratings of 2 in the right hemisphere was 53.1 percent. The effect of generalized cognition, as evidenced by IQ score, was controlled through the use of analysis of covariance, adjusting for IQ. Post-hoc analyses showed that only the temporal-lobe atrophy ratings were significantly related to dichotic scores. As atrophy rating increased (i.e., with increasing degrees of

TABLE 4.5 **Mean Dichotic Scores of Alzheimer Patients, Grouped by Atrophy Ratings, for Eight Brain Regions**

| | ATROPHY RATING | | | |
|---|---|---|---|---|
| BRAIN REGION | 0 | 1 | 2 | 3 |
| Frontal | | | | |
| R | 74.8% | 57.2% | 42.6% | 52.9% |
|  | (23.1)‡ | (23.9) | (32.6) | (19.3) |
| L | 73.3 | 58.4 | 41.8 | 52.9 |
|  | (22.7) | (24.5) | (30.2) | (19.3) |
| Parietal | | | | |
| R | 65.4 | 63.4 | 52.6 | |
|  | (21.7) | (29.4) | (25.1) | |
| L | 70.2 | 62.9 | 48.1 | |
|  | (18.5) | (28.5) | (24.5) | |
| Anterior temporal | | | | |
| R | | 70.0 | 53.1* | |
|  | | (27.9) | (23.2) | |
| L | | 84.0 | 55.6* | 37.3* |
|  | | (14.2) | (25.2) | (14.3) |
| Posterior temporal | | | | |
| R | 86.1 | 48.7† | 55.7† | |
|  | (20.0) | (24.5) | (23.5) | |
| L | 92.9 | 58.6† | 46.2† | |
|  | (5.1) | (21.4) | (23.9) | |

*Different from Group 1 $p < 0.05$
†Different from Group 0 $p < 0.05$
‡SD
From Grimes A, et al. Central auditory function in Alzheimer's disease. Neurology 1985; 8:352–358.

atrophy), dichotic scores decreased. This relationship was not observed when the atrophy in the frontal and parietal regions was compared with dichotic performance.

A subgroup of subjects, in whom atrophy was not equal in the right and left hemispheres, was then examined for performance asymmetry. There were 18 subjects in whom there was a marked difference between hemispheres in degree of atrophy. This included 8 subjects who evidenced greater atrophy in the right temporal lobe regions and 10 subjects with greater atrophy in the left temporal lobe regions. In analyzing this subset, it was seen that those with greater atrophy in the left temporal lobe had poorer overall performance, regardless of the ear affected (Fig. 4.11). Those with greater atrophy in the right temporal regions had a significant ear difference in scores. The right-ear score was significantly better than the left-ear score, and generally these subjects had higher levels of performance for both ears. This finding is consistent with the model of Sparks et al.[94] Left temporal lobe damage occurring in DAT, similar to that previously seen in temporal lobe pathology of other types, exerts an overall reduction in performance in both ears, whereas pathology of the right temporal lobe affects primarily the contralateral ear.

Positron emission tomography (PET) scans were also obtained in 21 of the subjects studied. Correlations were made of absolute metabolism in the frontal, parietal, temporal, and occipital lobes in each hemisphere, with dichotic scores. Significant relationships were found between absolute metabolism in the left temporal lobe and the right dichotic score. No other significant correlations were observed (Fig. 4.12).

As was done with the CT analyses, those subjects showing an asymmetry in metabolism between the right and left sides were analyzed separately. It was found that those subjects with greater left metabolism had higher overall dichotic performance. As the asymmetry changed (that is, as the metabolism measured on the left side decreased relative to the right side), the right dichotic score decreased (Fig. 4.13).

From this study, several conclusions emerged concerning the nature of central auditory function in older demented persons. First, it was shown that when cognition (IQ) was statistically removed as a variable, significant relationships between brain structure and performance persist. This militated against the hypothesis that central auditory impairment in elderly listeners is only a reflection of generalized cognitive decline and not a specific performance impairment. If this were attributable to impaired cognition in general, then this analysis of covariance technique would have reflected no relationship between dichotic score and atrophy when IQ was controlled.

The data from these psychophysical studies demonstrated a behavioral correlate to the observed atrophy and metabolic alteration in the temporal

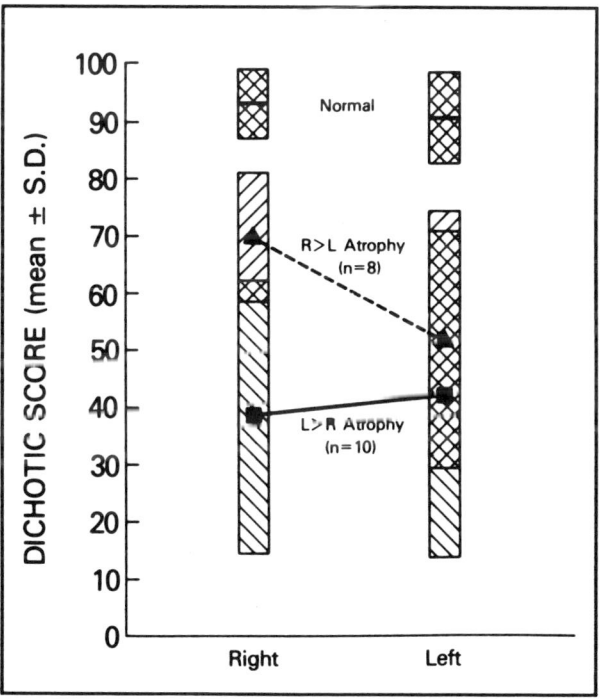

Figure 4.11 Relationship of right and left dichotic scores in three groups: normal, Alzheimer patients with greater right than left atrophy in the posterior temporal lobe, and Alzheimer patients with greater left than right atrophy in the posterior temporal lobe (mean + 1 SD). From Grimes A, et al. Central auditory function in Alzheimer's disease. Neurology 1985; 8:352–358.

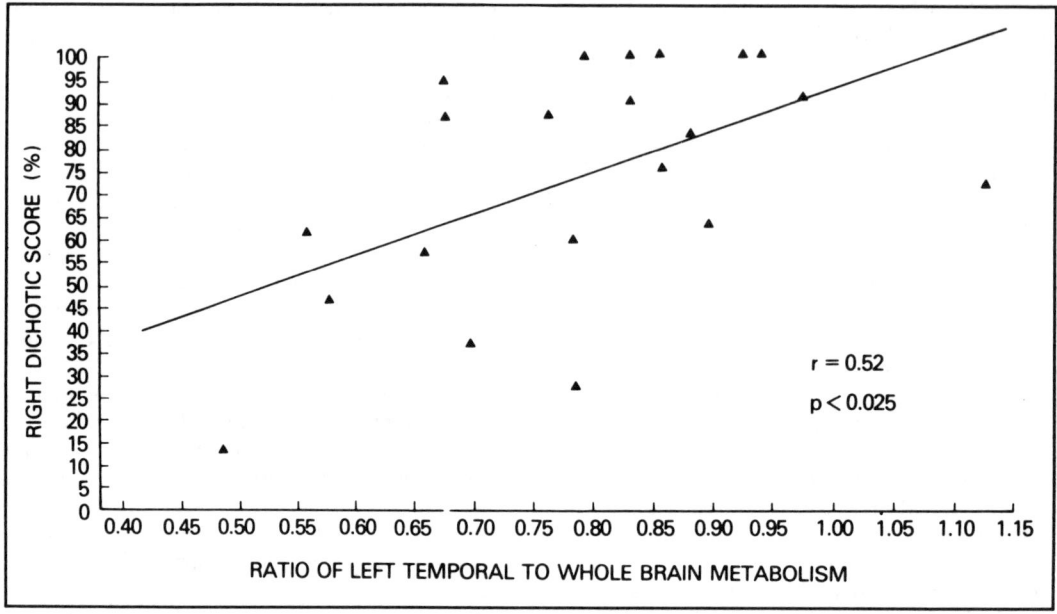

**Figure 4.12** Correlation of right dichotic score with ratio of left-temporal to whole-brain metabolism on PET scan in 21 Alzheimer's patients. From Grimes A, et al. Central auditory function in Alzheimer's disease. Neurology 1985; 8:352–358.

lobe. The presence of dysfunction, as assessed using a dichotic speech task, was significantly related to atrophy and hypometabolism only in the temporal-lobe areas. These findings can be related to the classical model of dichotic listening. It appears that the diffuse atrophy of Alzheimer's disease, when present in the left temporal lobe, exerts an overall reduction in performance for both ears, whereas pathology of the right temporal lobe affects primarily the contralateral ear. Further, it was seen that metabolic deficits also correlate with dichotic performance in the same pattern as do structural impairments.

After the initial study, it was questioned whether the relationships between auditory performance and dichotic speech processing would hold up if a monaural degraded speech were used instead. This was investigated primarily for two reasons. First, as monotic degraded speech has been reported to be abnormal in patients with other types of temporal-lobe lesions, would it also be observed in patients with DAT? Second, in persons in whom asymmetrical peripheral hearing loss precludes the use of dichotic testing, would a monotic degraded speech measure yield similar information?

To address these questions, Grady and colleagues evaluated 32 patients with DAT using a dichotic (the SSW) test and two degraded, monotic tests, time-compressed monosyllables, and low-pass filtered monosyllables.[26] Again, relationships between structure and function of the temporal lobes were investigated with both the dichotic and monotic tasks. Figure 4.14 shows the scatterplot for normals and DAT patients on the three tests (mean and one standard deviation). As can be seen, the DAT patients were significantly impaired on all three tests. Significantly more patients were impaired on the SSW than on either of the two monotic tests, and the degree of impairment on the dichotic test was greater than that on the two monotic tests.

In comparing dichotic performance with CT scans, dichotic scores were again significantly related to atrophy in both hemispheres. Those patients with more severe atrophy in the anterior temporal regions showed poorer dichotic performance than those with less atrophy. There was, however, no significant relationship between atrophy in any other region of the brain and performance on either of the monotic measures.

Similarly, two statistically significant correlations emerged between PET scans and auditory tests. The right dichotic score and the metabolism in the left anterior superior temporal region were significantly correlated, as were the right dichotic score and left posterior superior temporal region metabolism. None of the correlations between monotic test performance and PET scan values were significant.

The results of Grady et al showed that only with a dichotic or divided-attention auditory task was performance in a group of patients with DAT related to temporal-lobe structure and function.[26]

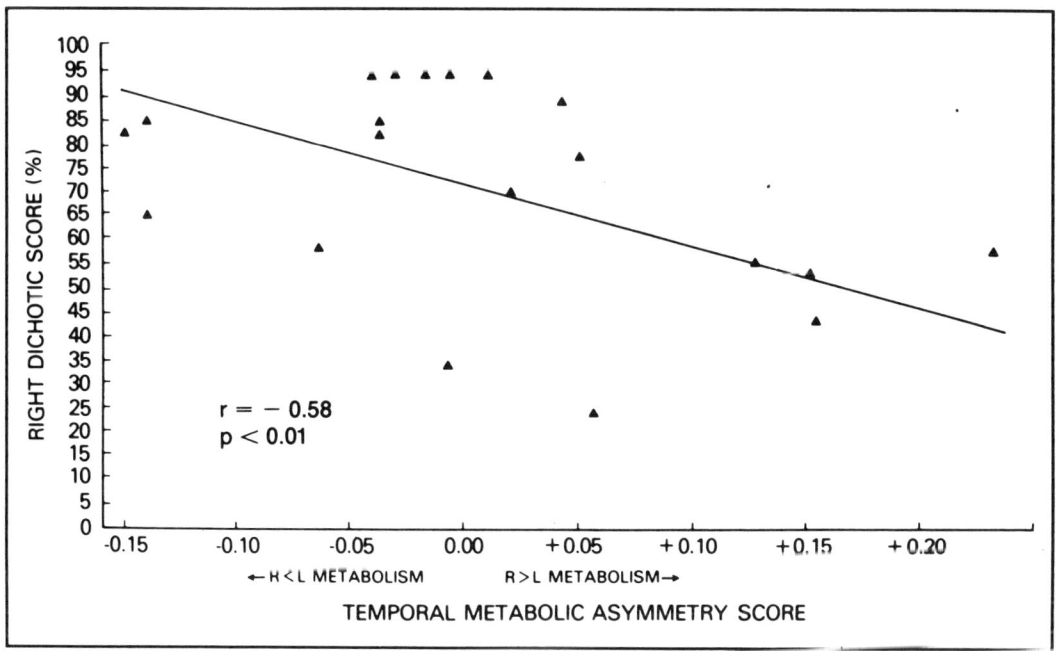

Figure 4.13 Correlation of right dichotic score with right vs left temporal-lobe metabolic asymmetry on PET scan in 13 Alzheimer's patients. From Grimes A, et al. Central auditory function in Alzheimer's disease. Neurology 1985; 8:352–358.

The disproportionately greater impairment on the dichotic measures reflected a specific deficit in divided attention. Similar difficulties in divided-attention tasks in other modalities have been demonstrated. This is a function of at least two additional variables. First, dichotic speech measures are simply more sensitive to temporal lobe dysfunction than are monotic speech measures, regardless of the temporal lobe pathology under study. Second, factors related to test variability and stabili-

TABLE 4.6 **Test Scores of DAT Patients Grouped According to Severity of Anterior Temporal Lobe Atrophy**

| | **RIGHT ANTERIOR TEMPORAL** | |
|---|---|---|
| | **Normal-Mild Atrophy (N=11)** | **Moderate-Severe Atrophy (N=20)** |
| SSW | 78 ± 18* | 59 ± 25† |
| TCS | 41 ± 15 | 41 ± 20 |
| FS | 78 ± 10 | 72 ± 16 |
| | **LEFT ANTERIOR TEMPORAL** | |
| | **Normal-Mild Atrophy (N=9)** | **Moderate-Severe Atrophy (N=22)** |
| SSW | 83 ± 8 | 59 ± 25‡ |
| TCS | 41 ± 16 | 42 ± 19 |
| FS | 77 ± 7 | 72 ± 16 |

*Mean ± SD
†Significant group difference, $p < 0.05$
‡Significant group difference, $p < 0.01$
From Grady C, Grimes A, et al. Divided attention as measured by dichotic speech performance in dementia of the Alzheimer type. Arch Neurol 1989; 46:317.

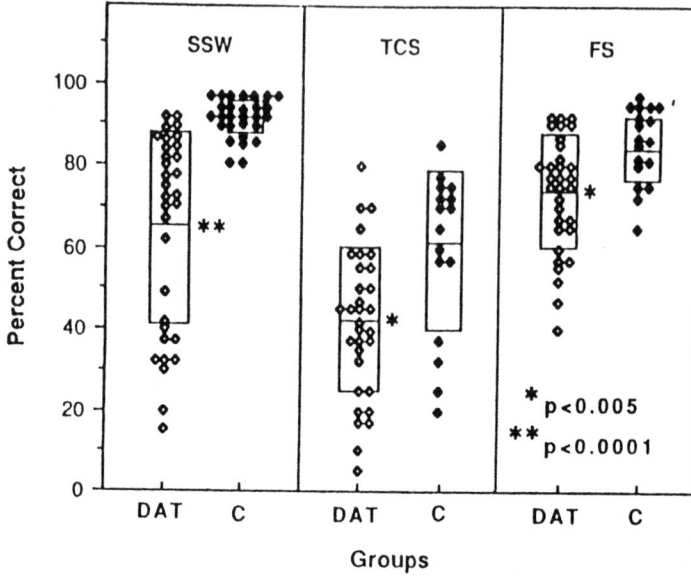

Figure 4.14 Normal distribution of performance (filled diamonds) and distribution of performance by patients with dementia of the Alzheimer type (open diamonds) on three tests of central auditory function [dichotic (SSW) and two monotic: time-compressed speech (TCS) and filtered speech (FS)]. Significant differences between normal controls and patient groups were demonstrated for all three tests. From Grady C, Grimes A, et al. Divided attention, as measured by dichotic speech performance, in dementia of the Alzheimer type. Arch Neurol 1989; 46:317.

ty, as well as effects of peripheral hearing loss, are far greater in the monotic than in the dichotic test paradigms.

Middle-latency responses (MLR) in 39 patients with DAT were also studied by Grimes et al.[30] The MLR component may be generated in the primary auditory cortex, a site where structural physiologic changes are known to occur in dementia of the Alzheimer type. For this reason, it was believed that middle-latency responses would more possibly correlate with dementia and dichotic performance than brainstem evoked potentials.

The predominant potential of the middle-latency response is a vertex-positive peak ($P_a$) at approximately 35 msec (Fig. 4.6). The specific neural generator(s) of this response has not been unambiguously defined in the literature. It may arise from the temporal lobes,[27,52,54,71,76] although there is not unanimity on this point.[60,78] The $P_a$ latency and amplitude data for the normal and DAT groups are presented in Table 4.7. There were no significant differences between groups or sexes for either measure. A typical $P_a$ response from a patient with DAT is presented in Figure 4.15. From this it appears that the bilateral temporal lobe involvement seen in patients with DAT is not generally sufficient to disrupt the generating of the $P_a$ potential.

It would be useful to go on to examine the late evoked responses, as well as the evoked poten-

TABLE 4.7 Mean (±SD) MLR Latency and Amplitude in Normal and DAT Groups*

| | | LATENCY (msec) | | AMPLITUDE (μV) | |
|---|---|---|---|---|---|
| | n | R | L | R | L |
| Normal | | | | | |
| Male | 11 | 33.6 (4.3) | 33.8 (4.9) | 1.27 (0.82) | 1.12 (0.37) |
| Female | 20 | 32.1 (3.0) | 31.4 (3.5) | 1.07 (0.59) | 1.12 (0.32) |
| DAT | | | | | |
| Male | 26 | 33.3 (4.3) | 32.0 (3.2) | 1.27 (0.66) | 1.06 (0.47) |
| Female | 13 | 31.5 (2.6) | 32.2 (3.4) | 1.50 (0.66) | 1.29 (0.65) |

From Grimes A, et al. Auditory evoked potentials in patients with dementia of the Alzheimer type. Ear Hear 1987; 8:157–161.
*No significant group differences ($p < 0.01$)

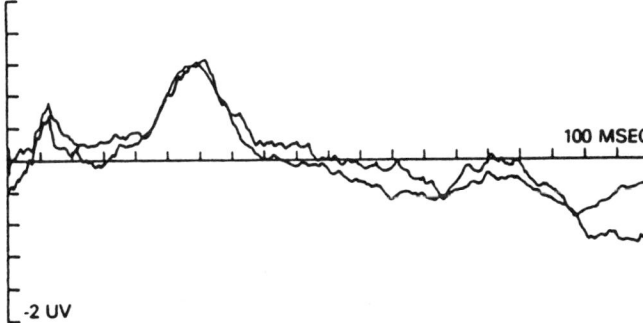

Figure 4.15 Example of a middle latency response in a patient with dementia of the Alzheimer type. From Grimes A, et al. Auditory evoked potentials in patients with dementia of the Alzheimer type. Ear Hear 1987; 8:157–161.

tial termed P300. Several researchers, primarily in the fields of neuropsychology and neurophysiology, have studied the P300 in normal aging and dementia (see reports by Goodin, Squires, and Starr and by Syndulko, Hansch, Cohen, et al[23,99]). These two reports found significant effects of dementia on the long-latency, auditory-evoked potential and the auditory evoked P300. Other researchers, however, have reported that because of the large variability of the P300 latency in the normal control group, the P300 was not conclusively demonstrated to yield diagnostic information in a demented patient group.[81]

As the understanding of the neural substrates of the later auditory-evoked potentials becomes clearer, some aspect of the MLR and slow-vertex response that has not been thoroughly studied (for instance, phase, spectral analysis) may yield a correlation with behavioral measures of central auditory function.

## Central Auditory Function in Non-Alzheimer's Dementias

Few studies of auditory function in other dementias are widely available. In our studies of patients with DAT, many patients were tested who had subsequent diagnoses of dementias other than DAT, and these patients were not included in the analysis groups. Many of these patients with other dementing conditions, however, also had impaired CANS performance, as would be expected with any condition that affects the temporal lobe. These diagnoses included multi-infarct dementia, Jakob-Creutzfeldt disease, and Pick's disease.

Recently, it has become apparent that many individuals in the last stages of acquired immunodeficiency syndrome (AIDS) become demented. It is reasonable to suspect that in this condition, as in other dementias, specific CANS impairments could be demonstrated. In a recent single-case study, peripheral and central auditory impairment in a man with AIDS were studied.[37] In this case, both brainstem dysfunction, as evidenced by abnormal ABRs, and hemisphere-level dysfunction (assessed using the SSI-CCM, a bilateral competing-speech measure) were found. AIDS differs from DAT in that both white- and gray-matter impairment is known to occur. On autopsy there was found to be temporal lobe involvement, as well as abnormalities in the inferior colliculi and throughout the pons.

## Implications: Diagnostic and Rehabilitative

Several implications and inferences can be drawn from the information presented in this chapter. Of greatest importance is that the aging auditory system in normal and demented persons exerts a tremendous influence on the ability to synthesize and process speech information. Diagnostic and rehabilitative strategies that fail to consider this factor run the risk of failure. The historic preoccupation with peripheral hearing loss to define the nature of the aging auditory system is inappropriate given the wealth of information that is available through the use of behavioral, electrophysiologic, and neuroradiologic measures of the central auditory nervous system.

### DIAGNOSTIC IMPLICATIONS

The diagnostic evaluation of the demented elderly individual forms an important basis for necessary rehabilitation and communication assistance. Traditional audiologic evaluation is usually accomplished easily with the mildly or moderately demented individual, with some modification of procedure if necessary. This might include substituting live-voice speech recognition assessment for the normally used recorded stimulus material. Also, investing additional time in conditioning responses to pure-tone threshold assessment, using pantomime as well as verbal directions, will increase accuracy and decrease testing time. Use of positive reinforcement after responses to stimuli, particularly those near threshold, will often improve test accuracy. Finally, the rate of testing may need to be slowed, particularly in the pure-tone assessment. In the more severely demented patient, it may not be possible to assess sensitivity to pure-tone stimuli, because of their lack of meaning. Threshold for speech may be the only behavioral measure of sensitivity that can be obtained with some patients. Electrophysiologic measures may be required to supplement or supplant behavioral evaluation [use of electrocochliography and/or ABR to assess threshold, for example] in more involved patients who are unable to respond appropriately to behavioral tests. See Chapter 14 for further diagnostic considerations.

## REHABILITATIVE IMPLICATIONS

A major concern centers on the appropriateness of hearing-aid fitting in the demented individual with peripheral hearing loss. Although no audiologist would advocate withholding amplification from an individual who, if not demented, would ordinarily be a candidate for hearing-aid use, it must be recognized that severely demented individuals may be unable to substantially benefit from using conventional hearing aids. The major flaw in conventional hearing aids is their inability to distinguish the desired stimulus (usually speech) from noise. It may not be possible for the demented person to use strategies that normal-hearing people and nondemented people use to improve signal-to-noise ratio in many situations. For instance, in a noisy environment in which a hearing aid user has difficulty understanding conversation, she or he may move closer to the speaker, or eliminate the noise source (the television, for example). Subsequently, conversation is more easily understood because the signal-to-noise ratio has been improved. A demented individual may not be able to manipulate his or her environment to gain this advantage. Further, because of central impairment, the effects of unfavorable signal-to-noise ratio may be more deleterious to understanding speech, because of the combined impairments in extrinsic and intrinsic redundancy (see Table 4.2).

Those people who are experienced hearing-aid users prior to becoming demented may have little difficulty continuing to successfully use their hearing aids. For these individuals, hearing aids are part of their routine and pose little more problem than the use of glasses or dentures. For those in whom hearing loss is diagnosed after the dementing process has begun, however, hearing-aid use may prove difficult. In such cases, a reasonable alternative to conventional hearing aids may be a personal communication device that can be used part-time. With the advent of assistive device technology for the hearing impaired and deaf, many options exist for amplifying speech other than the use of conventional, wearable hearing aids. Personal communication devices that require only that lightweight earphones be worn by the hearing-impaired individual can be used as needed to facilitate communication. Many hospitals, nursing homes, and senior centers keep such personal communication devices on hand as an alternative to shouting at hearing-impaired people (see Chapter 14 for further discussion of this topic).

Effective communication with hearing-impaired persons, including elderly and demented persons, requires not only that the acoustic speech signal is maximized, but that the visual speech signal is maximized as well. Communication arrangements that take into account the importance of visual speech information (e.g., lip movement, facial expression, body language, and environment) will increase speech understanding. The degree to which visual information can be successfully integrated with auditory information depends on a variety of factors, including visual acuity and visual-processing ability. It is possible that in the older demented person, the visual system suffers impairments similar to those seen in the auditory system. If so, this would limit the role that vision may play in speech understanding.

The rich external redundancy of speech, and the internal redundancy of the auditory pathway, allow successful understanding of speech. Any technique that increases the extrinsic redundancy present in speech information (both auditory and visual) will facilitate communication with those individuals whose internal redundancy of the central auditory pathway is compromised because of peripheral and central impairments.

## Research Needs

Much remains to be discovered about the function of the auditory system in the elderly and demented individual. At this time, particularly with the paper recently published by Uhlman, a major question is the relationship of peripheral hearing loss and dementia.[101] Does peripheral hearing loss predispose an individual to dementia, or does it simply exacerbate its effects? Or, is the relationship merely correlational, that is, that older people are likely to be both hearing impaired and demented, but do the two conditions bear no causative relationship to each other?

Of equal importance is the need to investigate ways to exploit the remaining function to maximize communication. Does visual information facilitate or confuse recognition of auditory stimuli in patients who may have both auditory and visual deficits? And finally, much remains to be learned by more detailed investigation of temporal-lobe function in patients who are demented. With the proliferation of radiologic and electrophysiologic tools to investigate structure and function of brain regions, the understanding of the nature of central impairment will certainly increase.

## Concluding Remarks

The effects of aging on the auditory system must be considered from two viewpoints. First are the effects of peripheral sensory loss, which may differ little from those of younger, peripherally impaired listeners. Second are the effects of neural changes in the CANS. In isolation, these effects may be subtle, but together, they may combine to result in performance decrements that affect the understanding of speech in everyday situations and contexts.

The effects of peripheral changes, which in a younger listener might be only a minor handicap, may be exacerbated in an elderly person. The ability to make a recognizable whole from parts, some of which are missing or distorted, may be compromised in the aged person who has peripheral hearing loss. In the person with cognitive impairment, the combined effects of peripheral hearing loss and specific temporal-lobe impairment may result in a major decrement in communication ability.

Successful rehabilitation of the auditorily impaired demented person, however one might define success, depends first on accurately defining the presence of peripheral and central components of auditory changes. Peripheral auditory impairment can be ameliorated through the appropriate use of hearing aids and assistive listening-device technology. Central impairment requires deliberate structuring of the communication environment in ways to enhance speech understanding. This can be accomplished by the reduction of noise, reverberation, and distance, and by the use of communication rules and strategies that reduce, simplify, and increase the redundancy lost through CANS impairment.

Nowhere is this more important than with the cognitively impaired, elderly individual. Methods to increase audibility and redundancy must be investigated and utilized to maximize communication with these individuals.

## References

1. Amerman J, Parnell M. The Staggered Spondaic Word Test: A normative investigation of older adults. Ear Hear 1980; 1:42–45.
2. Arnst D. Staggered Spondaic Word Test performance in a group of older adults: A preliminary report. Ear Hear 1982; 3:118–123.
3. Bergman M. Aging and the perception of speech. Baltimore: University Park Press, 1980.
4. Berlin C, McNeil M. Dichotic listening. In: Lass N, ed. Issues in experimental phonetics. New York: Academic Press, 1976:327.
5. Bocca E, Calearo C. Central hearing processes. In: Jerger J, ed. Modern developments in audiology. New York: Academic Press, 1963:337.
6. Brewer C. Electrophysiologic measures. In: Mueller H, Geoffrey V, eds. Communication disorders in aging: Assessment and management. Washington, D.C.: Gallaudet University Press. 1987:334.
7. Broadbent D. The role of auditory localization in attention and memory span. J Exp Psychol 1954; 47:191–196.
8. Brody H. Organization of the cerebral cortex. III. A study of aging in the human cerebral cortex. J Comp Neurol 1955; 102:511–556.
9. Brody H. Cell counts in cerebral cortex and brainstem. In: Katzman R, Terry R, Bick K, eds. Alzheimer's disease: Senile dementia and related disorders. Aging, Vol. 7. New York: Raven Press, 1978.
10. Brun A, Gustafson L. Distribution of cerebral degeneration in Alzheimer's disease. Arch Psychiatr Nervenkr 1976; 223:15–33.
11. Calearo C, Lazzaroni A. Speech intelligibility in relation to the speed of the message. Laryngoscope 1957; 67:410–419.
12. Committee on Hearing, Bioacoustics and Biomechanics (CHABA). Speech understanding and aging. J Acoust Soc Am 1983; 83:859–893.
13. Craik F. Age differences in dichotic listening. Q J Exp Psychol 1986; 17:227–240.
14. Creasey H, Rapoport S. The aging human brain. Ann Neurol 1985; 17:2–10.
15. Cunningham D, Cunningham C, Vise L. The effects of chronic hypoxemia on central auditory processing in patients with chronic obstructive pulmonary disease. Ear Hear 1985;6:297–303.
16. DeLeon M, Ferris J, George A, et al. Computed tomography and positron emission transaxial tomography evaluations of normal aging and Alzheimer's disease. J Cereb Blood Flow Metab 1983; 3:391–394.
17. Drachman D, Noffsinger D, Sahakian B, Kurdziel S, Fleming P. Aging, memory and the cholinergic system: A study of dichotic listening. Neurobiol Aging 1980; 1:39–43.
18. Dubno J, Dirks D, Morgan D. Effects of age and mild hearing loss on speech recognition in noise. J Acoust Soc Am 1984; 76:87–96.
19. Findlay R, Denenberg L. Effects of subtle midfrequency auditory dysfunction upon speech discrimination in noise. Audiology 1977; 16:252–259.
20. Frackowiak R, Pozzilli C, Legg N, et al. Regional cerebral oxygen supply and utilization in dementia: A clinical and physiological study with oxygen-15 and positron tomography. Brain 1981; 104:753–778.
21. Gelfand S, Hoffman S, Waltzman S, Piper N. Dichotic CV recognition at various interaural temporal onset asynchronies: Effect of age. J Acoust Soc Am 1970; 68:1258–1261.
22. Gelfand S, Silman S. Future perspectives in hearing and aging: Clinical and research needs. In: Roush J, ed. Aging and hearing impairment. Semin Hear 1985; 6:207–219.
23. Goodin D, Squires K, Starr A. Long-latency event-

23. related components of the auditory evoked potential in dementia: Brain 1978; 101:635-648.
24. Gordon-Salant S. Effects of aging on response criteria in speech-recognition tasks. J Speech Hear Res 1986; 29:155-162.
25. Gordon-Salant S. Basic hearing evaluation. In: Mueller H, Geoffrey V, eds. Communication disorders in aging: Assessment and management. Washington, D.C.: Gallaudet University Press, 1987:301.
26. Grady C, Grimes A, Patronas N, et al. Divided attention, as measured by dichotic speech performance, in dementia of the Alzheimer type. Arch Neurol 1989; 46:317.
27. Graham J, Greenwood R, Lecky B. Cortical deafness: A case report and review of the literature. J Neurol Sci 1980; 48:35-49.
28. Grimes A, Elks M, Grunberger G, Pikus A. Auditory brain-stem responses in adrenomyeloneuropathy. Arch Neurol 1983; 40:574-577.
29. Grimes A, Mueller H, Williams D. Clinical considerations in the use of time compressed speech. Ear Hear 1984; 5:114-117.
30. Grimes A, Grady C, Foster N, Sunderland T, Patronas N. Central auditory function in Alzheimer's disease. Neurology 1985; 35:352-358.
31. Grimes A, Grady C, Pikus A. Auditory evoked potentials in patients with dementia of the Alzheimer type. Ear Hear 1987; 8:157-161.
32. Grimes A. Central auditory nervous system function. In: Mueller H, Geoffrey V, eds. Communication disorders in aging: Assessment and management. Washington, D.C.: Gallaudet University Press. 1987:381-407.
33. Hannley M, Jerger J, Rivera V. Relationship among auditory brainstem responses, masking level differences and the acoustic reflex in multiple sclerosis. Audiology 1983; 22:20-33.
34. Hansen C, Reske-Nielsen E. Pathological studies in presbycusis: Cochlear and central findings in 12 aged patients. Arch Otolaryngol 1965; 82:115-132.
35. Harkins S. Effects of presenile dementia of the Alzheimer's type on brainstem transmission time. Int J Neurosci 1981; 15:165-170.
36. Harris J, Haines H, Myers C. The importance of hearing at 3 kc for understanding speeded speech. Laryngoscope 1963; 70:131-146.
37. Hart C, Cokely C, Schupbach J, Dal Canto M, Coppleson L. Neurotologic findings of a patient with acquired immune deficiency syndrome. Ear Hear 1989; 10:68-76.
38. Hawkins J, Johnsson L. Otopathological changes associated with presbycusis. In: Roush J, ed. Aging and hearing impairment. Semin Hear 1985; 6:115-134.
39. Hayes D, Jerger J. Aging and the use of hearing aids. Scand Audiol 1979; 8:33-40.
40. Hayes D. Aging and speech understanding. In: Aging and hearing impairment, Semin Hear 1985; 6:147-159.
41. Inglis J, Caird W. Age differences in successive responses to simultaneous stimulation. Can J Psychol 1963; 17:98-105.
42. Jacobson J, Deppe U, Murray T. Dichotic paradigms in multiple sclerosis. Ear Hear 1983; 4:311-317.
43. Jerger J. Diagnostic audiometry. In: Jerger J, ed. Modern developments in audiology. 2nd ed. New York: Academic Press, 1963:75-116.
44. Jerger J, Speaks C, Trammell J. A new approach to speech audiometry. J Speech Hear Disord 1968; 33:318-328.
45. Jerger J, Weikers N, Sharbrough F. Bilateral lesions to the temporal lobe: A case study. Acta Otolaryngol [Suppl] (Stockh) 1969; 258:5-51.
46. Jerger J, Jerger S. Comment on "The effects of age and the diagnostic utility of the rollover phenomenon." J Speech Hear Disord 1976; 41:556-557.
47. Jerger J, Hall J. Effects of age and sex on auditory brain-stem responses. Arch Otolaryngol 1970; 106:387-391.
48. Jerger J, Brown D, Smith S. Effect of peripheral hearing loss on the masking level difference. Arch Otolaryngol 1984; 110:290-296.
49. Jerger J, Johnson K, Jerger S. Effect of response criterion on measures of speech understanding in the elderly. Ear Hear 1988; 9:49-56.
50. Jerger J, Jerger S, Oliver T, Pirozzolo F. Speech understanding in the elderly. Ear Hear 1989; 10:79-89.
51. Jokinen K. Presbyacusis. Acta Otolaryngol 1973; 76:426-430.
52. Kaga K, Hink R, Shinoda Y, Suzuki J. Evidence for a primary cortical origin of a mid latency auditory evoked potential in cats. Electroencephalogr Clin Neurophys 1980; 50:254-266.
53. Katz J. The use of staggered spondaic words for assessing the integrity of the central auditory nervous system. J Aud Res 1962; 2:327-337.
54. Kileny P. Auditory evoked middle latency responses: Current issues. In: Jacobson J, ed. Auditory evoked potentials. Semin Hear 1983;4.
55. Kimura D. Some effects of temporal lobe damage on auditory perception. Can J Psychol 1961; 15:156-165.
56. Kimura D. Cerebral dominance and the perception of verbal stimuli. Can J Psychol 1961; 15:166-171.
57. Kirikae I, Sato T, Shitara T. A study of hearing in advanced age. Laryngoscope 1963; 73:205-220.
58. Konkle D, Beasley D, Bess F. Intelligibility of time-altered speech in relation to chronological aging. J Speech Hear Res 1977; 20:108-115.
59. Korabic E, Freeman B, Church G. Intelligibility of time-expanded speech with normally hearing and elderly subjects. Audiology 1978; 17:159-164.
60. Kraus N, Ozdamar O, Hier D, Stein L. Auditory middle latency responses (MLRs) in patients with cortical lesions. Electroencephalogr Clin Neurophys 1982; 54:275-287.
61. Kryter K. Presbycusis, sociocusis and nosoacusis. J Acoust Soc Am 1983; 73:1987-1997.
62. Lowell S, Paparella M. Presbycusis: What is it? Laryngoscope 1977; 87:1710-1717.
63. Lynn G, Gilroy J. Neuro-audiological abnormalities in patients with temporal lobe tumors. J Neurol Sci 1972; 17:167-184.
64. Marshall L. Auditory processing in aging listeners. J Speech Hear Disord 1981; 46:226-240.
65. McCoy C, Butler M, Broekhoff J. Effects of age and sex on dichotic listening: The SSW test. J Aud Res 1977; 17:263-268.
66. Mills J, Ryals B. The effects of reduced cerebrovascular circulation on the auditory brain stem response (ABR). Ear Hear 1985; 6:139-143.
67. Miltenberger G, Dawson G, Raica T. Central auditory testing with peripheral hearing loss. Arch Otolaryngol 1978; 104:11-15.
68. Moscicki E, Elkins E, Baum H, McNamara P. Hearing loss in the elderly: An epidemiologic study of the Framingham Heart Study cohort. Ear Hear 1985; 6:184-190.
69. Mueller H. Monosyllabic procedures. In: Katz J, ed. Handbook of clinical audiology. 3d ed. Baltimore: Williams & Wilkins, 1985:355-382.

70. Mueller H, Sedge R. Audiological aspects of head trauma. Semin Hear 1987; 3:191–303.
71. Musiek F, Donnelly K. Clinical applications of the (auditory) middle latency response—an overview. In: Jacobson J, ed. Auditory evoked potentials. Semin Hear 1983;4.
72. Noffsinger D, Olsen W, Carhart R, et al. Auditory and vestibular aberrations in multiple sclerosis. Acta Otolaryngol [Suppl] (Stockh) 1972; 303:4–63.
73. Novak R, Anderson C. Differentiation of types of presbycusis using the masking-level difference. J Speech Hear Res 1982; 25:504–508.
74. Olsen W, Noffsinger D, Kirdziel S. Speech discrimination in quiet and in white noise by patients with peripheral and central lesions. Acta Otolaryngol 1975; 80:375–382.
75. Otto W, McCandless G. Aging and auditory site of lesion. Ear Hear 1982; 3:110–117.
76. Ozdamar O, Kraus N, Curry F. Auditory brainstem and middle latency responses in a patient with cortical deafness. Electroencephalogr Clin Neurophys 1982; 53:224–230.
77. Palva A, Jokinen K. Presbyacusis. Acta Otolaryngol 1970; 70:232–241.
78. Parving A, Salomon G, Elberling C, Larsen B, Lassen N. Middle components of the auditory evoked response in bilateral temporal lobe lesions. Scand Audiol 1980; 9:161–170.
79. Patronas N, Deveikis J, Schellinger D. The use of computed tomography in studying the brain. In: Mueller H, Geoffrey V, eds. Communication disorders in aging: Assessment and management. Washington, D.C.: Gallaudet University Press, 1987:107.
80. Patronas N, Deveikis J, Schellinger D. The use of magnetic resonance imaging in studying the brain. In: Mueller H, Geoffrey V, eds. Communication disorders in aging: Assessment and management. Washington, D.C.: Gallaudet University Press, 1987:135.
81. Pfefferbaum A, Ford J, Wenegrat B, Tinklenberg J, Kopell B. Electrophysiological approaches to the study of aging and dementia. In: Corkin S, et al, eds. Alzheimer's disease: A report of progress, aging, vol. 19. New York: Raven Press, 1982.
82. Potash M, Jones B. Aging and decision criteria for the detection of tones in noise. J Gerontol 1977; 32:436–440.
83. Rees J, Botwinick J. Detection and decision factors in auditory behavior of the elderly. J Gerontol 1971; 26:133–136.
84. Robinson K, Rudge P. Abnormalities of the auditory evoked potentials in patients with multiple sclerosis. Brain 1977; 100:19–40.
85. Roeser R, Johns D, Price L. Dichotic listening in adults with sensorineural hearing loss. J Am Aud Soc 1976; 2:19–25.
86. Rosenhammer H, Lindstrom, Lundborg T. On the use of click-evoked brainstem responses in audiological diagnosis. II. The influence of sex and age upon the normal response. Scand Audiol 1980; 9:93–100.
87. Roush J, ed. Aging and hearing impairment. Semin Hear 1985; 6:99–219.
88. Rowe M. Normal variability of the brainstem auditory evoked response in young and old adult subjects. Electroencephalogr Clin Neurophys 1978; 44:459–470.
89. Schuknecht H. Presbycusis. Laryngoscope 1955; 65:402–419.
90. Schuknecht H. Further observations on the pathology of presbycusis. Arch Otolaryngol 1964; 80:369–382.
91. Schuknecht H. Pathology of the ear. Cambridge: Harvard University Press, 1974.
92. Smith R, Prather W. Phoneme discrimination in older persons under varying signal-to-noise conditions. J Speech Hear Res 1971; 14:630–638.
93. Sparks R, Geschwind N. Dichotic listening in man after section of neocortical commissures. Cortex 1968; 4:3–16.
94. Sparks R, Goodglass H, Nickel B. Ipsilateral versus contralateral extinction in dichotic listening resulting from hemisphere lesions. Cortex 1970; 6:249–260.
95. Speaks C, Niccum N, Van Tasell D. Effects of stimulus material on the dichotic listening performance of patients with sensorineural hearing loss. J Speech Hear Res 1985; 28:16–25.
96. Stach B, Jerger J, Fleming K. Central presbyacusis: A longitudinal case study. Ear Hear 1985; 6:304–306.
97. Stockard J, Stockard J, Sharbrough F. Detection and localization of occult lesions with brainstem auditory responses. Mayo Clinic Proceedings 1977; 52:761–769.
98. Studdert-Kennedy M, Shankweiler D. Hemispheric specialization for speech perception. J Acoust Soc Am 1969; 48:579–594.
99. Syndulko K, Hansch E, Cohen S, et al. Long-latency event related components in normal aging and dementia. In: Courjon J, Mauguierer F, Reuol M, eds. Clinical applications of evoked potentials. New York: Raven Press, 1981:279.
100. Thornton A, Raffin M. Speech discrimination scores modeled as a binomial variable. J Speech Hear Res 1978; 21:507–518.
101. Uhlmann R, Larson E, Rees T, Keopsell T, Duckert L. Relationship of hearing impairment to dementia and cognitive dysfunction in older adults. JAMA 1989; 261:1916–1919.
102. Wilson R. The effect of aging on the magnitude of the acoustic reflex. J Speech Hear Res 1981; 24:406–413.
103. Yanz J, Anderson S. Comparison of speech perception skills in young and old listeners. Ear Hear 1984; 4:64–71.
104. Yellin M, Jerger J, Fifer R. Norms for disproportionate loss in speech intelligibility. Ear Hear 1989; 10:231–235.

# CHAPTER 5

# Motor Speech Changes

IRENE CAMPBELL-TAYLOR, Ph.D.

Changes in motor speech in the early stages of a dementing illness are of diagnostic importance. This chapter will focus on these changes as they occur in many dementias. It will not address the classic dysarthrias in detail, nor is it intended to describe, in full, their perceptual and acoustic manifestations. Excellent accounts of these can be found elsewhere.[38,86] It is intended to underline the importance of the identification of motor speech changes and their relationship to underlying pathophysiology, thereby indicating the probable type of dementia.

The dysarthrias are a group of speech disorders resulting from damage to neural mechanisms that regulate speech movements.[100] They are distinct from language disorders (aphasia) and from apraxia of speech, although the latter is closely related and may be difficult to distinguish. Apraxia of speech is the result of impairment of neural mechanisms that select and sequence the position and timing of the articulators. The dysarthrias reflect pathology of the motor system and have for many years been used as indicators of neurologic dysfunction and to provide diagnostic information. Signs of weakness, slowness, and other physiologic abnormalities in gait, arm movement, eye movements, reflexes, and so on are used as indicators of underlying pathology. In the same way, speech production is a fine motor skill so that a disease that affects motor control may affect speech to some extent. For this reason, motor speech dysfunction can be utilized as a diagnostic sign.

Descriptions of motor speech in the literature on dementing illness are scarce, anecdotal, and imprecise. It is evident that, in many cases, dysphasia is confused with dysarthria, and aphonia is confused with mutism. In the first instance, as already stated, a nonfluent dysphasia can sound, to the untrained listener, very much like dysarthria, and a severe motor speech impairment that renders the patient unintelligible is often mistaken for aphasia. It is also essential to distinguish between mutism and aphonia. A patient who can whisper but who makes little or no sound when laughing or crying is aphonic, not mute. A mute patient may laugh or cry voluntarily but will make no attempt to articulate or make "phonologically relevant movements."[121]

This chapter is based on the author's clinical experience with autopsy-proven cases as well as on a review of the relevant literature.

## The Importance of Accurate Diagnosis

Why such concern about the accurate identification of incurable, relentlessly progressive conditions? There are several answers. The first is that differentiation of other dementias from senile dementia of the Alzheimer type (DAT) is critical. If a treatment for DAT is ever found, or even a potential treatment, it must be certain that the patients entered into therapy actually have the disease. It is usually true that the earlier a disease is identified, the more readily it is treated. Therefore, the early identification of dementing illness is of extreme importance. The poor results of some of the clinical trials already run may have resulted from the fact that some of the subjects were suffering from other diseases. These trials often include only small numbers of subjects, so that even one or two misdiagnoses could significantly affect the outcome. Research into the clinical, behavioral, and pathologic features of DAT also requires that subjects be accurately diagnosed. Some of the conflicting reports in the literature are no doubt attributable to misdiagnosis.

The controversy about the co-existence of Parkinson's disease and DAT is possibly a reflection of this phenomenon. It has been pointed out many times that the dementing illnesses have both cortical and subcortical pathology, but these studies involve information gleaned from postmortem results.[28,97,122] Autopsy cannot identify the structures involved at the beginning stages. It must be remembered that as the cortical dementias progress, sufferers develop movement disorders and dysarthrias as white matter as well as subcortical structures undergo neuronal loss and other pathology. At the point of diagnosis, however, dysarthria is not found in the cortical dementias.[15] It is here that identification of all signs of pathology is invaluable. In addition, continual clinical evaluation is necessary to identify the structures that become involved as these diseases progress. As far as the dysarthrias are concerned, the appearance of additional features in the motor speech can lead to inference about the progression of pathology. For example, the presence of a cognitive impairment with parkinsonian dysarthria in the very early phase would indicate a probable cortical site of lesion.

Some aspects of the subcortical dementias are potentially treatable, for example, parkinsonism. At least, one should know that an underlying extrapyramidal disorder exists and may be worsened by the administration of neuroleptic and psychotropic drugs so often used in the control of mood and behavior in the dementias.[14,32]

The labeling aspect of dementing illness must also be considered. For some reason, a diagnosis of DAT produces an often nihilistic attitude in health-care professionals. It is better to have a diagnosis that gives some ability to anticipate and prepare for changes and carries fewer connotations of hopelessness and despair. On a practical level, many nursing homes will not accept residents with a diagnosis of DAT but will accept those with Parkinson's disease, progressive supranuclear palsy, and many other dementing illnesses, although the nursing demands may be heavier for the latter cases. The difference seems to lie in the relative lack of wandering and aggressive behavior in the noncortical dementing illnesses. It is a practical consideration of extreme importance when the time comes to institutionalize a patient.

The hereditary aspects of some dementias must be considered. One form of DAT is familial, and even those cases without a strong familial component indicate an elevated risk for other family members.[11] Families of patients who are not suffering a dementia with an inheritable component need not be subject to the anguish of wondering whether they or another family member will fall victim to the disease. On the other hand, those with a strong family history of dementia should have the opportunity of making informed choices about whether to have children.

Accuracy of diagnosis is therefore vital for a variety of medical, social, ethical, academic, and practical reasons. Speech-language pathologists should be aware of the necessary role they have to play in this process.

## Dementias and the Motor System

As has been stated, patients with progressive cortical dementias do not present with dysarthria in the early stages.[4,15] Various impairments of the motor system occur in the later stages of all dementing illnesses, if the victim survives long enough.[28,53,97,122] In the major cortical dementias such as senile dementia of the Alzheimer type (DAT) and Pick's disease, the motor system is spared until the late stages. To illustrate the significance of motor signs in the differential diagnosis of the dementias, Marks et al point out that, since bowel and bladder control are spared until late in DAT, the absence of either in the beginning stages would indicate a diagnosis other than DAT.[78] Similarly, if incontinence were found early in a disease resembling Pick's and seemed to be a true motor dysfunction rather than a result of poor toilet habits, again, the diagnosis would be different. By the same token, another motor sign, namely of dysarthria, in the early stage of dementia, would indicate neither Pick's disease nor DAT but, more probably, one of the subcortical dementias.[3]

Diagnosis of probable, progressive cortical dementia such as DAT must exclude focal neurological signs.[85] Dysarthria is not, strictly speaking, a focal sign. It is a localizing sign, the nature of the motor speech impairment bearing a direct relationship to the relevant pathophysiology. It takes extensive practice as well as knowledge of the involved anatomy and physiology to identify the type of dysarthria. Although the sophisticated technology available to analyze the various components of speech should be utilized whenever possible, the trained ear remains the most frequently used instrument. With practice, it is possible to identify speech as belonging to an individual with a particular neurologic disease.[38]

Speech movements require temporal and spatial precision of a remarkable degree. For example, lip closure for the sound [$p$] can be as small as 10 mm.[63] Tongue placement for repeated [$ee$] is within 1 mm.[50,100] A subcortical dementia is one associated with a movement disorder. Unlike the "pure" movement disorders, most of these subcortical diseases do not exhibit readily identifiable types of motor speech impairment, according to accepted classifications. They tend to be mixed and difficult to identify. They also change as the disease progresses and more structures become involved. The separate components of the motor speech, respiratory, laryngeal, resonatory, and articulatory systems must be identified individually so that they can provide pointers to specific pathophysiology.

Recently, acoustic-physiologic studies have added significantly to our knowledge of the dysarthrias.[13,30,86] Most of this work has been accomplished in the relatively "pure" disorders, that is, with patients who have features of motor speech associated with Parkinson's disease, cerebellar disorders, Huntington's disease, bulbar dysfunctions, and strokes. We lack information on the "dementing dysarthrias" partly because they are seldom "pure" in nature. Further, motor speech signs have been overlooked as being important diagnostic signs.

The features of motor speech can be as important as measurements of muscle tone, weakness, and disordered movement in allowing inferences to be drawn about the nature of the disease process. Because of the pathology involved in various cortical, white matter, and subcortical sites, these dysarthrias are mixed and, often, usual. In order to be used diagnostically, it is essential that the various components be identified individually and then related to probable sites of lesion. A knowledge of the pathology of the different cortical and noncortical dementias, together with a detailed clinical history, should indicate the probable disease involved.

The reasons for developing skills in the perceptual assessment of the dysarthrias are many. Apart from the lack of instrumentation in many clinical settings, the protocol for the diagnosis of probable DAT, for example, is lengthy and expensive.[85] Identification of a treatable condition must be made as quickly as possible to allow for timely therapeutic intervention. For example, early identification of an atypical Parkinson's disease would enable the physician to instigate treatment with appropriate medication.

Language assessments are usually among the first to be performed because of the relationship between language and cognition and the need to discover the level of the patient's verbal abilities and comprehension before testing memory.[7,16,28,36,48,70,85] At the same time, motor speech should be examined closely.

At the beginning of a dementing illness, if the voice or speech sound is in any way abnormal, i.e., too soft, too loud, monotonous, or slightly indistinct, the patient should be examined by (1) an otolaryngologist, to rule out laryngeal pathology; (2) an audiologist, to rule out certain types of hearing loss that can affect speech; and (3) an experienced speech-language pathologist, to assess the possibility of a dysarthria and, if present, its type. It is often useful to ask the patient whether his or her speech has changed and if he or she is often able to speak more loudly. These can be early signs of motor speech changes. The family is also a useful source of information about changes in voice and speech.

## Causes of Motor Speech Dysfunction in the Dementias

Motor speech changes appear uniformly in the early stages of the noncortical and in many of the non-Alzheimer familial dementias. These are listed in Table 5.1.

Dysarthria early in a dementia is frequently overlooked if the articulation is still intact. Dysarthria is, in many ways, a misleading term because its root focuses on the articulatory aspects of speech. It is not generally recognized that normal speech requires the integration of many muscle groups affecting respiration, phonation, nasal resonance, articulation, and prosody. An early dysarthria in Parkinson's disease (PD) for example, does not noticeably affect articulation, but is manifest in abnormal respiration and phonation with impaired pitch and loudness control, probably because of the generalized stiffness of the whole system.[38,55] Mildly abnormal speech is usually obvious only to the trained listener; therefore, this is an area in which the contribution of the speech-language pathologist can be invaluable.

A phenomenon resembling apraxia of speech, as distinct from dysarthria, is found early in Pick's disease in patients presenting with more left than right frontotemporal pathology.[9,70,116] Literal paraphasias suggestive of verbal apraxia are common, as is the so-called "cortical stuttering."[71,96] These are not found in the beginning stages of cortical dementias such as DAT nor in the noncortical dementias because the loci of lesions are not focal nor are they confined to the left frontal cortex. Acquired dysfluency (stuttering) is found in

TABLE 5.1 **Types of Dementia Causing Dysarthria**

"Amyotrophic" Creutzfeldt-Jakob disease
Amyotrophic lateral sclerosis–Parkinson's dementia
Corticodentatonigral degeneration
Creutzfeldt-Jakob disease
Dementia and parkinsonism with non-Alzheimer amyloid plaques
Gerstmann-Sträussler-Scheincker disease
Huntington's disease
Familial olivopontocerebellar degeneration
Familial non-Alzheimer dementia
Familial myoclonic dementia
Parkinson's disease
Progressive supranuclear palsy
Thalamic dementia

dementias involving the basal ganglia. When it occurs in a cortical dementia such as Pick's, it is because of a lesion of the prefrontal cortex. When found in subcortical dementias, it is presumed also to be caused by frontal dysfunction, resulting from the intimate relationship between basal ganglia and frontal lobes. This will be discussed more fully in the section on theories of subcortical dementia.

## Loci of Lesions in the Dementing Dysarthrias

### RETICULAR, LIMBIC, AND NEOCORTICAL SYSTEMS

The reticular system ascends from lower to higher brainstem and includes the basal nuclei. Lesions can result in body parts assuming fixed postures and can impair fine muscle contractions.[62,93,99] Severe involvement can result in akinetic mutism, i.e., an inability to speak caused by the lack of ability to initiate speech movement.

Damage to the neocortex can produce an apraxia of speech, a dysarthria, or both. Internal capsule lesions affecting white matter can cause aphasia as well as dysarthria.[112] Many speakers with lesions of the cerebellum can sound apraxic and vice versa. In these cases, careful history taking is essential to identify strokes, degenerative conditions, or any other causes, and acoustic as well as perceptual evaluation may be required. Lesions of corticobulbar and corticospinal pathways may yield the so-called "pseudobulbar" or upper motor neuron dysarthria, with associated lability caused by limbic system involvement.[72,80]

### NEUROTRANSMITTERS

The role of neurotransmitters has been extensively studied in recent years.[61] Chemical neurotransmitters such as dopamine, serotonin, acetylcholine, and others mediate interneural communication.[94,97,102] Released from the nerve terminal, they diffuse across the synaptic cleft and interact with receptors on adjacent neurons. Any disruption of this process reduces the facilitative or suppressive effect of the neurotransmitter. This, in turn, affects motor activity as well as mood and cognition. It is well known that depression is endemic to Parkinson's disease (PD).[56] Motor dysfunction and, to some degree, cognitive impairment are also part of the disease. Consideration of the dysarthrias in dementing diseases must also take into account the role of neurotransmitters and their effects on distant structures.

### CRANIAL NERVES AND NUCLEI

Diseases affecting cranial nerves V, X, XI, and XII can produce speech that is perceptibly slow, hypernasal, and breathy with reduced pitch variability and loudness. Darley and others have called them the "flaccid" dysarthrias.[38] Because diseases progress at different rates, lesions of the hypoglossal nerve or its nucleus can produce either spasticity or flaccidity at a given point in time.

### CEREBELLAR LESIONS

Damage to the cerebellum or its connections via the cerebellar peduncles produces "ataxic" dysarthria.[64] The speech sounds like that of inebriation: slow, with syllables of equal duration and pitch being somewhat more variable than normal. Speakers cannot speed up and they perceive themselves as being unable to control their articulators. Because speech is involuntarily so slow, patients complain of having to think carefully about what they are saying because their intentions are running ahead of their speech. Just as speech cannot proceed faster than the formulation or intention to utter words, so the formulation must be slowed down to match the output mechanism. One often hears the complaint of slow typists that they cannot compose at the typewriter. Their thoughts run ahead of their fingers and errors result. In a similar fashion, cerebellar lesions often induce an apparent slowness of thought, ellipsis, or word substitution as a result of formulation or production mismatch. This apparent slowness and hesitation can be mistaken for word-finding difficulty.

The causes of cerebellar dysarthria are not clearly defined. There are no truly ballistic speech movements, therefore it is difficult to understand the influence of the cerebellum in speech. The function of the cerebellum in this case appears to be one of selecting appropriate muscle force.[72] Cerebellar dysfunction seems to slow the normal, precise forces, making all muscle contractions of equal duration. This leads to syllables of equal length and an inability to make unstressed syllables. The speech may sound monotonous, but the equal durations and lack of stress patterning in cerebellar speech (the so-called "scanning speech") should not be confused with the monotony of extrapyramidal parkinsonian dysarthria.

### EXTRAPYRAMIDAL LESIONS

Sufferers of Parkinson's disease (PD) show a variety of movement disorders. They tend to have a voice that is breathy, reduced in loudness, and monotonous. Logemann, Fisher, Boshes, and Blonsky have shown that laryngeal involvement is found in over 90 percent of PD patients.[77] Impairment of the articulators proceeds as the disease progresses. In the early stages, speech articulation is rarely affected, but the patient is quieter than normal with a noticeably reduced pitch variability producing the monotonous speech that is so characteristic of the disease.

Parkinsonian dysarthria is one of the most extensively studied and perhaps one of the easiest to identify.[99] Jaw and tongue muscle dysfunction in patients with idiopathic PD result from aberrations in muscle and afferent function.[1,91] Tongue muscles devoid of stretch reflexes are most impaired. Jaw-closing muscles, which have numerous spindles and a monosynaptic stretch reflex, are least impaired. Patients therefore tend to hold the jaw in a relatively fixed, closed posture because the weaker jaw-opening muscles cannot overcome the stretch of their antagonists. PD sufferers also have difficulty moving the tongue. These factors affect the configuration of the vocal tract and, in turn, intraoral air pressure and voice loudness.[18,19,98] The result is a voice reduced in intensity, with some effect on articulation. The "masked faces" of PD patients implies that the perioral musculature is affected by rigidity.[13,115] This affects articulation. Voice loudness and articulation interact because they are affected by oral cavity size, articulatory configuration, and laryngeal resistance.[18,19,63] Also, Schneider, Diamond, and Markham have shown that PD patients have complex deficits in the ability to use sensory input to organize and guide movements of the orofacial system.[114]

Caliguri and Abbs have demonstrated that rigidity and bradykinesia are two independent pathologic manifestations in PD.[21] Both may contribute to dysarthria. When rigidity is predominant, a fast and indistinct type of dysarthria is perceived, whereas when bradykinesia is predominant, the dysarthria is slow paced. A combination of the two types, accompanied by low vocal intensity, often occurs. The main markers of extrapyramidal dysarthria are initial and continuing monotony with reduced loudness levels and inappropriate phrasing.

## Neuropharmacology

The effects of medications must always be considered in the evaluation of motor speech. Neuroleptic and psychotropic drugs with anticholinergic and extrapyramidal side effects must be considered very carefully. In dementing illnesses, these medications are widely used to control behavior and mood.[105,106,111] Most importantly, extrapyramidal side effects can produce tardive dyskinesia or parkinsonian syndrome or exacerbate an underlying disease process. It must be remembered that medications have different effects in the elderly, and the window between therapeutic dosage and overdose can be vanishingly small.[40,123] The neuroleptic and antipsychotic medications are not metabolized and excreted in the same way as they are in younger adults. The half life of medications, particularly those that are lipophilic, can be many times normal.[35] An individual who is already taking such medication at the time of diagnosis may be exhibiting a motor speech impairment induced by the drug, by a combination of drugs, or by a drug-food interaction. A careful history must be taken, including the starting date of any drug, particularly the butyrophenones such as haloperidol as well as the benzodiazepines. The elderly are notoriously large consumers of over-the-counter medications as well, so that any of these drugs should be considered. A nonmedicated patient, presenting with a dysarthria, may be regarded as clearly displaying a pathologically induced motor speech disorder.

## Dementia and Dysarthria in Focal Lesions

Monrad-Krohn first identified alterations in what he called the "melody of speech" and termed this dysprosody.[92] This should not be confused with the "dysprosodias" described by Ross and Mesulam that refer to the alterations in affective speech production and comprehension found in persons with right-hemisphere lesions.[109] Kent and Rosenbeck have identified a dysarthria produced by right frontal lesions that is perceptually and acoustically indistinguishable from extrapyramidal motor speech impairment.[65] Patients with these lesions are often cognitively impaired and may have no physical sequelae of the stroke producing the lesion. They usually have no hemiplegia or hemiparesis and, if the stroke remains undetected, can be mistaken for victims of subcortical disorders. CT scans may not always identify small lesions. Scans performed many years post-insult often do not show the original damage, so a careful history is mandatory with close consideration of other clinical signs or the absence of such. These patients usually do not show the cogwheel rigidity, bradykinesia, gait disturbance, or tremor of PD.

Multi-infarct dementia may also produce a dysarthria, depending on the sites of lesions. If cortical only, a dysarthria is most often of the pseudobulbar or upper motor neuron type. If mixed cortical and subcortical, the speech impairment will correspond to the site of lesion.

Often, Binswanger's encephalopathy, lacunar infarcts of the cerebral white matter, also produces an upper motor neuron dysarthria. There is currently some debate as to whether this is a true nosologic entity. Whether or not we can call it Binswanger's, patients with such lacunar infarcts often have both a dementia and a dysarthria.

## Other Considerations in Dementia and Dysarthria

Accurate descriptions of motor speech changes in dementia are difficult to find in the literature. One must usually infer from anecdotal evidence, clinical signs such as ataxic gait, and extrapyramidal signs, to determine that a dysarthria probably exists. A knowledge of the anatomy and physiology of speech production is essential, as well as an awareness of the causes and effects of motor speech impairment.

Descriptions of word-finding difficulty in subcortical dementia must be approached with caution, partly for the reasons given above with respect to cerebellar lesions, but also because the long pauses often found in extrapyramidal syndromes can mimic word-finding difficulty.

Impairments of *voluntary* movement, including speech, are direct indications of disease severity. In extrapyramidal syndromes, the identification of such pathophysiologic signs is extremely important. *Involuntary* movement disorders usually involve a loss of sensory information from the pallidal and cerebellar pathways to the ventrolateral nucleus of the thalamus.[31] This would indicate an entirely different disease process. Voluntary movement disorders are usually the result of more diffuse cerebral dysfunction.[12] Because there is such a close relationship between voluntary and involuntary movement,[32,43] assessment of dysarthria must separate the variables relating to each as far as possible.

## Theories of Subcortical Dementia

Whitehouse has pointed out the difficulties of differentiating the cortical from the subcortical dementias.[122] The subcortical variety of dementia so often produces a frontal-lobe type cortical impairment with disinhibition, poor judgment, lack of insight, and apparent personality changes. Progressive supranuclear palsy (PSP) is an outstanding example. At autopsy, patients are found to have extensive frontal-lobe atrophy. This may be caused by deactivation of deafferentation of neocortex from subcortical structures.[2,6,27,39] Information from positron emission tomography (PET) shows extensive brainstem and cortical lesions expressed as frontal-lobe and striatal function changes.[37,49,52] There is a true frontal-lobe dysfunction, as shown by the PET traces, although the seat of pathology is in the subcortical structures. If the frontal-type cognitive impairment is given greater weight in the diagnostic process and the accompanying dysarthria ignored, the result may be a diagnosis of Pick's disease.

Dubois et al have shown that, with regard to the slowing of cognitive functioning in patients with PD or progressive supranuclear palsy (PSP), only in PSP is cognitive impairment related to frontal-lobe dysfunction.[47] They differentiate between the slowing of decision-making processes, essentially related to motor slowing in PD, and slowing of thought processes caused by frontal-lobe impairment in PSP. Both PD and PSP have a common nigrostriatal dopaminergic denervation,[57,59] but in PSP there is additional severe damage to the striatopallidal complex.[8,39,60] These structures are the main output of the basal ganglia to the frontal lobes.[2] Neuronal loss in the basal ganglia and subsequent deafferentation of the frontal lobes are possibly responsible for the cognitive impairment of the striatum, leading to disruption of its motor output but not significantly affecting its output to the prefrontal cortex. This would explain the fact that dementia is neither universal nor predominant in PD.[44,75,74,87,103]

Loss of neurotransmitters alone could account for this deactivation phenomenon. The sources of the various neurotransmitters are the very structures most often involved in the subcortical dementias: the raphe nucleus for serotonin, the locus ceruleus for noradrenaline, the mesencephalic dopamine cells for dopamine, and the nucleus basalis of Meynert for acetylcholine. The latter structure is also involved in the development of DAT, with its known reduction of acetylcholine that is essential for cognitive functioning. If it is involved in the development of subcortical dementia, it is in conjunction with the degeneration of other structures.

In early DAT, there is a focal hypometabolism in the temporal posterior-parietal cortex, as demonstrated by PET scanning.[46] Temporal and parietal cortical pathology not involving the white matter does not produce dysarthria. It is unlikely, then, that one would find a motor speech disorder early in DAT; this appears to be the case as found by Boone et al.[15]

## Types of Subcortical Dementia

### PROGRESSIVE SUPRANUCLEAR PALSY

Progressive supranuclear palsy (PSP) involves degeneration of the brainstem, basal ganglia, and cerebellum. It can be difficult to distinguish clinically from PD in the beginning stages. The characteristic opthalmoplegia, particularly paralysis of upward gaze, may not develop immediately.[41] Hallmarks of the disease include absence of tremor, a history of falls, slowly developing dementia, rigidity in the neck so that the head is held in extension, and dysfunction of extraocular movements.[27,118] Dysarthria and dysphagia are early signs, with aphonia developing quickly.[8] When frontal atrophy occurs before the onset of aphonia, one frequently finds "cortical stuttering," sometimes referred to as "palilalia." Repetition of initial phonemes and syllables may occur without the secondary behaviors usually encountered in dysfluency. The patient is unaware of this occurrence even when it involves repetitions of whole words and phrases.[71]

Presentation of the disease may be atypical, and it has been misdiagnosed frequently as DAT or other dementia in spite of the early dysarthria.[22,41] The dysarthria is mixed, falling between extrapyramidal and cerebellar with marked hypernasality. It may be described best as "pseudocerebellar." Some patients present with unusual upper-extremity movement disorders that are difficult to describe, being at times dyskinetic, dystonic, ballistic, and/or choreo-athetoid. In these patients, the extraocular signs are late developing, and there is a marked early dysarthria and dysphagia.[25] Surprisingly, articulation remains fairly well preserved in the more extrapyramidal type of PSP after the patient is aphonic, and therefore use of a voice-amplification device may be helpful. The literature often describes the dysarthria of PSP as pseudobulbar, but, given the underlying pathology, this is unlikely.[8]

## CORTICODENTATONIGRAL DEGENERATION

Rebeiz et al describe three patients with a disorder previously not identified.[104] Characterized by a severe gait disturbance, beginning with numbness and clumsiness on the left side, mild dementia developed in the later stages. Initially resembling unilateral parkinsonism, there was, however, no tremor, and the severe rigidity that developed, together with a limb apraxia, distinguished it from PD. At autopsy, in addition to cortical atrophy, there were lesions of the cortical white matter. Most severe pathology was found in the substantia nigra. The dysarthria closely resembles that of parkinsonism with cortical stuttering and early aphonia. Clinical history, limb apraxia, absence of tremor, and bradykinesia with no cerebellar features in the dysarthria distinguish corticodentatonigral degeneration from both PD and PSP.

## CREUTZFELDT-JAKOB DISEASE

Although usually described as a cortical dementia, Creutzfeldt-Jakob disease (CJD) was first called "spastic pseudosclerosis" by Jakob in 1921.[59] Lower motor neuron and pyramidal tract degeneration are commonly found.[17,33,42,76] It is usually readily identified by the dementia, rapid course, and a movement disorder including trembling and choreoathetosis with myoclonus late in the disease.[84] The visual and cerebellar systems are also involved.

## "AMYOTROPHIC" CREUTZFELDT-JAKOB DISEASE

The amyotrophic type of CJD resembles ALS-Parkinson's dementia.[42] It may be a variant of amyotrophic lateral sclerosis.[58,83] The dysarthria can be very unusual, having both lower motor neuron and cerebellar features producing a very dysprosodic output with hypernasality, lowered pitch, and "scanning" speech with even and equal stress on each syllable.[24] Salazar and others, in a review of over 2,000 cases of CJD, found that 231 had lower motor neuron disease and dementia.[110] CJD is a transmissible disease and can be passed to humans and primates by injection of tissue. Only two cases of transmission of the "amyotrophic" form have been reported; therefore, it is uncertain that it is a variant of the disease. In atypical ALS with dementia, CJD must be considered as part of the differential diagnosis, and a strong dysprosodic/cerebellar element in the dysarthria would point to the latter disorder.

## GERSTMANN-STRAÜSSLER-SCHEINCKER DISEASE

Gerstmann-Straüssler-Scheincker disease (GSSD) is a familial form of CJD with autosomal-dominant inheritance. Transmissible in the same way as CJD, its main difference lies in the involvement of the pyramidal tract. It can be mistaken for familial olivopontocerebellar degeneration. Extrapyramidal rigidity in GSSD can be mistaken for pyramidal signs, but the type of dysarthria implicates the relevant pathology. If extrapyramidal, the dysarthria is hypokinetic and similar to that found in PD. If pyramidal, it is mainly of the upper motor neuron type with a hypokinetic component. In olivopontocerebellar degeneration, the dysarthria remains almost purely cerebellar in type. In GSSD, the speech can be so severely spastic that it may resemble spastic dysphonia.[34,51]

## FAMILIAL OLIVOPONTOCEREBELLAR DEGENERATION

Olivopontocerebellar degeneration (OPCA) may be sporadic or familial (FOPCA). The familial form has an associated dementia and, when it appears early, it remains a prominent feature of the disease.[10] Dysarthria and dysphagia are significant symptoms. In its early stages, it may be confused with Friedreich's ataxia. It is actually a group of diseases, the only common factor being a loss of neurons in the ventral pons, inferior olives, and cerebellar cortex. In FOCPA, there is generalized spasticity, abnormal movements, psychomotor retardation, ophthalmoplegia, and dysarthria of the cerebellar type. In GSSD and FOCPA, the dysarthria type can be the only clinical sign that differentiates the two diseases, especially in the early stages.

## FAMILIAL MYOCLONIC DEMENTIA

Familial myoclonic dementia can also mimic CJD. It has been reported in one family with seven confirmed and two probable cases. It is autosomal dominant in inheritance and produces marked gliosis and neuronal loss in dorsomedial and midline thalamus, with hypertrophy of the medulla and superior olives.[76] The family reported above had a fulminant course of less than 1 year, with members aged 25 to 72 years affected. The disease otherwise resembled CJD, although the affected structure was the thalamus, producing both aphasia and dysarthria. The familial form of CJD comprises 5 to 15 percent of all reported cases.[82]

## AMYOTROPHIC LATERAL SCLEROSIS WITH PARKINSONISM OR DEMENTIA

In amyotrophic lateral sclerosis (ALS), atrophy and muscular weakness of the tongue contribute to the dysarthria commonly found. In addition to hypernasality and lowered pitch, the muscle bulk changes affect articulation in the early stages and exacerbate the oropharyngeal dysphagia that is a hallmark of the disease.[5,26,58]

ALS with dementia or parkinsonism can present with a dysarthria that is initially bulbar or extrapyramidal or, more often, a combination of the two with hypernasality, impaired articulation, low intensity, and inappropriate pauses. Dementia and the physical signs of the two diseases are present in varying combinations.[24] If the presentation is predominantly parkinsonian with a bulbar dysarthria or vice versa, the identification of the type of motor speech disorder can be vital to accurate diagnosis in vivo.

Mitsuyama, Kogoh, and Ata reported 20 cases in Japan.[90] The initial signs were cognitive decline, muscle wasting in the upper extremities, dysphagia, dysarthria (undescribed) leading to "muteness," no tremor, generalized rigidity, and cogwheeling with intact sensation. There was frontal and/or fronto-temporal atrophy in 11 out of 20 cases. All had significant neuronal loss in substantia nigra and anterior horn cells. It may be inferred from the pathology that the dysarthria was extrapyramidal/bulbar leading to aphonia. This type of dysarthria is found in other dementing illnesses with prominent extrapyramidal features.

## DEMENTIA AND PARKINSONISM WITH NON-ALZHEIMER AMYLOID PLAQUES

Rosenberg et al reported on a family with another inherited form of dementia.[108] Fourteen members in five generations seem to have been affected, their speech being described as monotonous and rapid, leading to unintelligibility. Major pathology found in the current and some of preceding generation consisted of non-Alzheimer amyloid plaques in the cortex, basal ganglia, thalamus, and substantia nigra. Pathology of this type would tend to produce an extrapyramidal dysarthria, and the description given supports this contention. In this family, cognitive impairment appeared before the parkinsonian signs, distinguishing it from classical PD. In DAT, extrapyramidal signs appear in the late stages whereas in this kindred, they developed in the first year of a course lasting 4 to 8 years.

Morris et al reported on a family in which dementia was characterized by initial dysphasia with literal paraphasias that quickly led to signs of PD with dysarthria and dysphagia.[96] At autopsy, signs of both DAT and PD were found. The average duration of illness was 8 years. True aphasia is not a feature of classical DAT and, in this case, was probably a result of the combination of cortical and subcortical pathology.[36,69,81]

## THALAMIC DEMENTIA

As noted above, "classic" aphasia is seldom a feature of early dementing illnesses. Progressive involvement of the thalamus is one cause of a developing aphasic syndrome and is found in the "thalamic" dementias.[88,95,117,119] These remain only partly described but do not seem to involve motor speech changes unless other structures are also affected.

## FAMILIAL NON-ALZHEIMER DEMENTIA

Diffuse dementias producing dysarthria of extrapyramidal type have been reported in some families, most notably by Kim et al[67] and Neumann and Cohn.[101] In the family reported by Kim, there was early incontinence and dysarthria, neither of which is found in early DAT or Pick's disease. Extrapyramidal signs developed early together with a frontal-type dementia. Neuropathologic examination revealed involvement of frontal cortex, cortical white matter, striatum, pallidum, thalamus, and substantia nigra.

## Case Presentations

Dementia is the presenting sign or a complication of several multisystem diseases that may be familial. Scherer was the first to propose an endogenous vulnerability in some families to dementing illness.[113] These may be initiated by exposure to viruses or environmental agents as yet undetermined. They are easily confused in the early stages with the progressive cortical dementias, and require extremely careful and detailed assessment of *all* behavioral and clinical features, including speech and language.

### CASE 1

The following case is one that was initially misdiagnosed as DAT.[75] The identification of an early dysarthria helped to indicate a noncortical dementia that was proven at autopsy.

Mr. A. was a 67-year-old man whose mother had died of a dementing illness and whose brother had a similar disease that had been classified as Pick's. At age 60 years of age, he had developed mild paranoia, apathy, poor coordination, food obsessions, and urinary incontinence. He developed bradykinesia, poor coordination of the right hand, facial masking, cogwheel rigidity, and hyperreflexia. Treated for Parkinson's disease, he developed hallucinations while on the medication with no relief of symptoms. He had slow, monotonous, and quiet speech. He had poor insight, but fair recent and remote memory. There was no disturbance of reading or writing and no constructional apraxia. He had positive palmomental, snout, and glabellar tap reflexes. Routine laboratory testing was normal. CT scan showed severe symmetric hemispheric atrophy.

When admitted for long-term care, 2 years into the course of his disease, he arrived with a diagnosis of DAT. He had imprecise, monotonous speech, impaired memory, frequent urinary incontinence, and voracious appetite. Because of the clinical signs and history, including the dysarthria and incontinence, the diagnosis was changed to subcortical dementia of unknown etiology, probably familial. He became markedly rigid, bedbound, and mute, and he died at age 67 years of bilateral aspiration pneumonia.

Autopsy findings revealed the pathology to be identical to that of the family reported by Kim.[67] There was neuronal loss and gliosis of cortex and cortical white matter. There were lesions in striatum, pallidum, thalamus, and substantia nigra. The hippocampus was not involved.

### CASE 2

Mr. B. was a 62-year-old male with a family history of a father and two brothers dying of a dementing illness with an associated movement disorder. He first developed an ataxic gait with pain in the knee joints, thought at first to be arthritis. He developed hyperreflexia, upper-extremity weakness, extrapyramidal-type dysarthria with a strong upper motor-neuron component, scanning speech, moderate cognitive impairment, and, finally, visual and hearing problems. There was a severe dysphagia. He arrived for long-term care with a diagnosis of familial olivopontocerebellar degeneration (FOPCA). The clinical history and the type of dysarthria made this diagnosis unlikely and led to the designation of probable Gerstmann-Straüssler-Scheincker disease (GSSD). This was confirmed at autopsy.

There was significant loss of cells in Clarke's nucleus and hypomyelination of posterior nerve roots, posterior columns, and dorsal spinocerebellar tracts. There was moderate loss of Purkinje cells and also cells from the substantia nigra. There were Lewy bodies as well as amyloid deposits in the cortex, cerebellum, basal ganglia, and amygdala. There was moderate loss of anterior horn cells. This represents one of the few cases of GSSD identified in vivo without a prior autopsy-proven family history.[24]

## Therapeutic Intervention

The difficulty with therapy for motor speech disorders in dementing illness is, of course, the influence of cognitive impairment. In most of the subcortical dementias that produce dysarthria, the presentation of illness or the rapid development of cognitive dysfunction is typical of a frontal-type dementia. These behavioral changes that include disinhibition and lack of insight and judgment militate against successful therapy aimed at reducing rate and varying pitch. The common clinical experience is, however, that these patients do not seem to be able to monitor their own performance.

In progressive supranuclear palsy (PSP) and some other subcortical dementias, aphonia develops early while articulation remains relatively intact; in these cases the use of a voice amplification device can help to maintain communication. In individual cases, other forms of communication augmentation can be tried, but these require highly individualized approaches because the variability of cognitive and physical involvement is so great. In all cases, working with the family to help them adjust to the changes in communication is extremely important. It may be as simple as explaining the disease process and its effects. Sometimes, the family must encourage the patient to use an amplification device or other communication prosthesis. They may be taught how to compensate in their own interactive style for the patient's particular deficits in cognition, vision, and hearing.

## Dysarthria and Dysphagia

The secondary effect of dysarthria in dementing illness is dysphagia.[20,107,114] This can develop quickly and requires timely intervention if the patient is to avoid recurrent pneumonia, malnutrition, and/or airway obstruction. The dysphagia may be mainly intraoral as in diseases with a marked cerebellar component.[25] In PD it involves reduction in laryngeal elevation and cricopharyngeal opening.[107,120] Direct intervention can sometimes help; more often treatment requires dietary adjustment and the use of special feeding techniques.[54]

In the terminal stages, feeding becomes difficult. The solution is often seen as tube-feeding, either by nasogastric tube or by gastrostomy. Unfortunately, most patients in end-stage disease are bedridden, noncommunicative, and rigid. Tube feeding these patients is hazardous because of the high risk of reflux and aspiration of stomach contents.[23] Aspiration bronchopneumonia is the immediate cause of death in the majority of patients with end-stage dementias, whether they are tube fed or not.[29] Careful spoon feeding may be more satisfactory in these cases, although it is time consuming and difficult.

## Research Needs

Although a great deal is known about the features and pathophysiology of the classic dysarthrias, the mixed motor speech disorders of the dementing illnesses remain largely unidentified. This is partly due to the fact that they change throughout the course of most of these diseases as more structures become impaired. Just as the language impairments found in dementing illnesses do not match the known aphasia profiles, so the motor speech disorders are of a different nature.

We may start by identifying, perceptually and acoustically, the speech of all patients at the inception of dementing illness and follow, at regular intervals, any changes that occur. This approach would help to answer several questions:

1. How many patients with DAT have signs of PD at the beginning of their illness?
2. What structures are becoming involved as these diseases progress?
3. What are the clinicopathologic correlations *over time*?

Answers to these questions, as well as the closer attention paid to the important behavioral sign of speech, would improve our knowledge of the dementias and reduce the incidence of misdiagnosis. Increased accuracy of diagnosis has implications for quality of life in addition to the factors outlined at the beginning of the chapter. It might go far to prevent the misplacement of elderly individuals who, though impaired, are not necessarily found in the appropriate type of institution. Several studies have shown that inaccurate diagnosis leads to misplacement, overmedication, and earlier mortality.[45,66,68] All individuals charged with the responsibility of playing a part in the diagnosis of these devastating diseases have an obligation to use whatever means possible to add to the armamentarium of diagnostic tools. One of these is the accurate and timely identification of motor speech disorders in the dementing illnesses.

### References

1. Abbs JH, Hartman DE, Vishwanat B. Orofacial motor control impairment in Parkinson's disease. Neurology 1987; 37:394–398.
2. Agid Y, Javoy-Agid F, Ruberg M, et al. Progressive supranuclear palsy: Anatomo-clinical and biochemical considerations. In: Yahr MD, Bergmann KJ, eds. Advances in neurology, vol. 45. New York: Raven Press, 1986
3. Albert ML, Feldman RG, Willis AL. The subcortical dementia of progressive supranuclear palsy. J Neurol Neurosurg Psychiatry 1979; 37:121–130.
4. Appell J, Kertesz A, Fisman M. A study of language functioning in Alzheimer patients. Brain Lang 1982; 17:73–91.
5. Aronson A, Brown JL, Willis AL. Differential diagnostic speech patterns of the dysarthrias. J Speech Hear Disord 1974; 12:246–269.
6. Baron JC, Maziere B, Lo'ch C, et al. Loss of striatal (Br-76) bromo-spiperone binding sites demonstrated by positron tomography in progressive supranuclear palsy. J Cerebral Blood Flow Metab 1986; 6:131–136.
7. Bayles KA, Tomoeda CK. Confrontation naming impairment in dementia. Brain Lang 1983; 19:98–114.

8. Behrman S, Carroll JD, Janota J, Matthews WB. Progressive supranuclear palsy: Clinico-pathological study of four cases. Brain 1969; 92:663–678.
9. Benton AL. Differential behavioral effects in frontal lobe disease. Neuropsychologia 1968; 6:53–60.
10. Berciano J. Olivopontocerebellar atrophy: A review of 117 cases. J Neurol Sci 1982; 53:253–272.
11. Bird TD, Sumi SM, Nemens EJ, et al. Phenotypic heterogeneity in familial Alzheimer's disease. A study of 24 kindreds. Ann Neurol 1989; 25:12–25.
12. Birri E, Evarts EV. Translational mechanisms between input and output. In: Schmitt FO, Adelman G, Melnechuk T, Worden FC, eds. Neurosciences research symposium summaries. Vol. 6. Control of movement. Cambridge: MIT Press, 1972.
13. Blair C, Muller E. Functional identification of the perioral neuromuscular system: A signal flow diagram. J Speech Hear Res 1987; 30:60–70.
14. Blazer DG, Federspiel CF, Ray WR, Schaffner W. The risk of anticholinergic toxicity in the elderly: A study of prescribing practices in two populations. J Gerontol 1983; 38:31–35.
15. Boone D, Boies RM, Bayles KA. Dysarthria in dementia. Paper presented at the Third Biennial Clinical Dysarthria Conference, Tucson, AZ, 1986.
16. Borod JC, Goodglass H, Kaplan E. Normative data on the Boston Diagnostic Aphasia Examination, Parietal Lobe Battery and the Boston Naming Test. J Clin Neuropsychol 1980; 2:209–215.
17. Brown P, Rodgers-Johnson P, Cathala F, et al. Creutzfeld-Jakob disease of long duration: Clinicopathological characteristics, transmissibility and differential diagnosis. Ann Neurol 1984; 16:295–304.
18. Brown WS, McGlone RE. Relation of intraoral air pressure to oral cavity size. Folia Phoniatr (Basel) 1969; 21:321–331.
19. Brown WS, McGlone RE, Tarlow A, Shipp T. Intraoral air pressure associated with specific phonetic positions. Phonetica 1970; 22:202–212.
20. Bushmann M, Dobmeyer SM, Leeker LL, Perlmutter JS. Swallowing abnormalities and their response to treatment in Parkinson's disease. Neurology 1989; 39:1309–1314.
21. Caliguri MP, Abbs JH. The influence of drug cycle on labial kinematics in dysarthria associated with Parkinson's disease. Paper presented at Clinical Dysarthria Conference, Tucson, AZ, 1986.
22. Campbell-Taylor I. Atypical presentation of progressive supranuclear palsy. Ann Neurol 1986; 20:375.
23. Campbell-Taylor I, Fisher RH. The clinical case against tube feeding in palliative care of the elderly. J Am Geriatr Soc 1987; 35:1100–1104.
24. Campbell-Taylor I, Lewis A, Black SE. Dysarthria in autopsy-proven GSSD and ALS-Parkinson's-dementia. Paper presented at American Neurological Association Meeting, New Orleans, LA, 1989. (Abstract.)
25. Campbell-Taylor I, Tamas IE. Dysarthria and dysphagia in early progressive supranuclear palsy. Paper presented at American Geriatrics Society Annual Meeting, Anaheim, CA, 1988. J Am Geriatr Soc 1987; 35:1100–1104.
26. Cha CH, Patten BM. Amyotrophic lateral sclerosis: abnormalities of the tongue on magnetic resonance imaging. Ann Neurol 1989; 25:468–472.
27. Chavany JA, van Bogaert L. Godlewski S. Sur un syndrome de rigité à prédominance axiale avec perturbation des automatismes oculo-palpébrale d'origine encephalitique. Presse Medecine 1951; 59:958–962.
28. Chui HC. Dementia: A review emphasizing clinicopathologic correlation and brain-behavior relationships. Arch Neurol 1989; 46:806–814.
29. Ciocon JO, Silverstone FA, Graver M, Foley CJ. Tube feedings in elderly patients: Indications, benefits and complications. Arch Intern Med 1988; 148:429–433.
30. Connor NP, Abbs JH, Cole KJ, Gracco VL. Parkinsonian deficits in serial multiarticulate movements for speech. Brain 1989; 112:997–1009.
31. Cooper LS. A general theory of causation and reversibility of involuntary movement disorders. Appl Neurophysiol 1981; 45:317–323.
32. Crane GE, Naranjo ER. Motor disorders induced by neuroleptics. Arch Gen Psychiatry 1971; 24:179–184.
33. Creutzfeldt HG. Uber eine eigenartige, herdformige Erkrankung des Zentralnervensystems. Zritschrift fur die Gesamte Neurol Psychiatrie 1921; 56:1.
34. Critchley M. Spastic dysphonia ("inspiratory speech"). Brain 1939; 62:96–102.
35. Crow TJ, Cross AJ, Johnstone EC. Abnormal involuntary movements in schizophrenia: Are they related to disease process or to its treatment? Are they associated with changes in dopamine receptors? J Clin Psychopharmacol 1982; 2:336–340.
36. Cummings J, Benson DF, Hill MA, Read S. Aphasia in dementia of the Alzheimer type. Neurology 1985; 35:394–397.
37. D'Antona R, Baron JC, Samson Y, et al. Subcortical dementia: Frontal cortex hypometabolism detected by positron tomography in patients with progressive supranuclear palsy. Brain 1985; 108:785–799.
38. Darley F, Aronson A, Brown J. Motor speech disorders. Philadelphia: WB Saunders, 1975.
39. David NJ, Mackey EA, Smith JL. Further investigations in progressive supranuclear palsy. Neurology 1968; 18:349–356.
40. Davidson JRT, Raft D, Lewis BF, et al. Psychotropic drugs on general medical and surgical wards of a teaching hospital. Arch Gen Psychiatry 1975; 32:507–511.
41. Davis C, McLachlan D, Bergeron C. Atypical progressive supranuclear palsy. Ann Neurol 1985; 19:113–119.
42. Davison C. Spastic pseudosclerosis (cortico-pallidospinal degeneration). Brain 1932; 55:247–264.
43. Desmedt J, Godaux E. Ballistic skilled movements: Load compensation and patterning of the motor commands. In: Desmedt J, ed. Cerebral motor control in man: Long loop mechanisms. Vol. 4. Progress in clinical neurophysiology. Basel: S. Karger, 1984.
44. Dickson DW, Davies P, Mayeux R, et al. Diffuse Lewy body disease: Neuropathological and biochemical studies of six patients. Acta Neuropathol (Berl) 1987; 75:8–15.
45. Dodd KJ, Clarke M, Palmer RL. Misplacement of the elderly in hospitals and residential homes: A survey and follow-up. Health Trends 1980; 12:74–76.
46. Duara R, Grady C, Baxby J, et al. Positron emission tomography in Alzheimer's disease. Neurology 1986; 36:879–887.
47. Dubois B, Pillon B, Legault F, Agid Y, Lhermitte F. Slowing of cognitive processing in progressive supranuclear palsy: A comparison with Parkinson's disease. Arch Neurol 1988; 45:1194–1199.
48. Forette F, Henry JF, et al. Reliability of clinical criteria for the diagnosis of dementia. Arch Neurol 1989; 46:646–648.
49. Foster NL, Gilman S, Berent S, Hichwa RD. Distinctive patterns of cerebral cortical glucose metabolism in progressive supranuclear palsy and Alzheimer's dis-

ease studied with positron emission tomography. Neurology suppl 1, 1986; (Cleveland) 36:338-341.
50. Gay T, Lindblom B, Lubker J. Production of bite block vowels: Acoustic equivalence by selective compensation. J Acoust Soc Am 1981; 69:802-810.
51. Gerstmann J, Straüssler E, Scheincker J. Uber eine einigastige hereditarz familiare Erkrankung der Zentralnervensystems. Z Neurol 1936; 154:736-762.
52. Goffinet AM, de Volder AG, Gillain C, et al. Positron tomography demonstrates frontal lobe hypometabolism in progressive supranuclear palsy. Ann Neurol 1989; 25:131-139.
53. Greiffenstein MF, Verma NP, Nichols CD, Delacruz CR. Neuropsychological validation of two dementia categories: A preliminary study. Neuropsychiatry Neuropsychol Behav Neurol 1989; 2:21-30.
54. Groher ME, ed. Dysphagia: Diagnosis and management. Boston: Butterworth, 1984.
55. Hermann K, Turner JW, Gillingham FJ, Gaze RM. The effects of destructive lesions and stimulation of the basal ganglia on speech mechanisms. Second International Symposium Stereoencephalotomy, Vienna. Continental Neurol 1965; 27:197-207.
56. Hoehn MM, Yahr Y. Parkinsonism: Onset, progression, and mortality. Neurology 1967; 17:427-442.
57. Hornykiewicz O. Dopamine (3 hydroxytyramine) and brain function. Pharmacological Revue 1966; 18:925-964.
58. Hudson AJ. Amyotrophic lateral sclerosis and its association with dementia, parkinsonism and other neurological disorders: A review. Brain 1981; 104:217-247.
59. Jakob A. Uber eigenartige Erkrankungen des Zentralnervensystems mit bemerkenswertem anatomischen Befunde Z. Gesamte Neurol Psychiatrie 1921; 64:147.
60. Jellinger K. Progressive supranuclear palsy: (Subcortical argyrophilic dystrophy.) Acta Neuropathol (Berl) 1971; 19:347-352.
61. Johnstone M, Coyle J. Development of central neurotransmitter systems in the foetus and in independent life. CIBA Foundation Symposium, London: Pitman, 1971.
62. Kent R. Brain mechanisms of speech and language with special reference to emotional interaction. In: Naremore R, ed. Language science. San Diego: College-Hill Press, 1984.
63. Kent R, Moll K. Vocal tract characteristics of the stop cognates. J Acoust Soc Am 1969; 46:1549-1555.
64. Kent R, Netsell R, Abbs J. Acoustic characteristics of dysarthria associated with cerebellar disease. J Speech Hear Res 1979; 22:627-648.
65. Kent R, Rosenbek JC. Prosodic disturbance and neurologic lesion. Brain Lang 1982; 15:259-291.
66. Kidd CB. Misplacement of the elderly in hospital: A study of patients admitted to geriatric and mental hospitals. Br Med J 1962; 2:1491-1495.
67. Kim RC, Collins GH, Parisi JE, Wright AW, Chu YB. Familial dementia of adult onset with pathological findings of a "non specific" nature. Brain 1981; 104;61-78.
68. Kirk S, Compton SA, Devaney N, Donnelly CM, McGuigan M. The elderly in long-term care: 2 An estimate of misplacement using objective criteria. Int J Geriatr Psychiatry 1989; 4:305-309.
69. Kirshner HS, Webb WG, Kelly MP. The naming disorder of dementia. Neuropsychologia 1984; 22:23-30.
70. Kirshner HS, Webb WG, Kelly MP, Wells CE. Language disturbance: An initial symptom of cortical degenerations and dementia. Arch Neurol 1984; 41:491-496.
71. Koller WC. Dysfluency (stuttering) in extrapyramidal disease. Arch Neurol 1983; 40:175-177.
72. Kornhuber H. Cerebral cortex, cerebellum and basal ganglia: An introduction to their function. In: Schmitt F, Worden F, eds. The neurosciences: Third study program. Cambridge, MA: MIT Press, 1983.
73. Lees AJ, Smith E. Cognitive deficits in the early stages of Parkinson's disease. Brain 1983; 106:257-270.
74. Leverenz J, Sumi M. Parkinson's disease in patients with Alzheimer's disease. Arch Neurol 1986; 43:662-664.
75. Lewis A, Zorzitto ML, Campbell-Taylor I. Familial non-Alzheimer dementia. Neurology; (forthcoming).
76. Little DW, Brown PW, Rodger-Johnson P, Perl DP, Gajdusek DC. Familial myoclonic dementia masquerading as Creutzfeldt-Jakob disease. Ann Neurol 1986; 20:231-239.
77. Logemann JA, Fisher H, Boshes B, Blonsky EB. Frequency and occurrence of vocal tract dysfunction in the speech of a large number of Parkinson patients. J Speech Hear Res 1978; 43:47-51.
78. Marks WA, Shuman RM, Leech RW, Brumback RA. Cerebral degenerations producing dementia: Importance of neuropathologic confirmation of clinical diagnosis. J Geriatr Psychiatry Neurol 1988; 1:187-198.
79. Marsden CD. The mysterious motor function of the basal ganglia: The Robert Wartenberg lecture. Neurology 1982; 32:514-539.
80. Marsden CD, Fahn S. Movement disorders. vol. 2. Stoneham, MA: Butterworth, 1986.
81. Martin A, Fedio P. Word production and comprehension in Alzheimer's disease: The breakdown of semantic knowledge. Brain Lang 1983; 19:124-141.
82. Masters CL, Gajdusek DC, Gibbs CJ. The familial occurrence of Creutzfeld-Jakob disease and Alzheimer disease. Brain 1981; 102:535-558.
83. Masters CL, Harris JO, Gajdusek DC, et al. Creutzfeldt Jakob disease: patterns of world-wide occurrence and significance of familial and sporadic clustering. Ann Neurol 1979; 5:177-178.
84. May WW. Creutzfeldt-Jakob disease. 1: Survey of the literature and clinical diagnosis. Acta Neurol Scand 1968; 14:1-32.
85. McKhann G, Drachman D, Folstein M, et al. Clinical diagnosis of Alzheimer's disease: Report of the NINCDS-ADRDA Work Group under the auspices of Department of Health and Human Services Task Force on Alzheimer's disease. Neurology 1984; 34:939-944.
86. McNeil MR, Rosenbek JC, Aronson AE. The dysarthrias: Physiology, acoustics, perception, management. San Diego: College-Hill Press, 1984.
87. Mesulam MM. Slowly progressive aphasia without generalized dementia. Ann Neurol 1982; 11:592-598.
88. Metter EJ, Riege WH, Hanson WP, et al. Subcortical structures in aphasia: An analysis based on (F18) fluorodeoxyglucose positron emission tomography and computed tomography. Arch Neurol 1988; 45:1229-1234.
89. Michocki RJ. What to tell patients about over-the-counter drugs. Geriatrics 1982; 37:113-119.
90. Mitsuyama HK, Kogoh H, Ata K. Progressive dementia with motor neuron disease: an additional case report and neuropathological review of 20 cases in Japan. Psychiatry Neurol Sci 1985; 235:1-8.
91. Mlcoch AC. Diagnosis and treatment of Parkinsonian dysarthria. In: Koller WC, ed. Handbook of Parkinson's disease. San Diego: College-Hill Press, 1987.
92. Monrad-Krohn GH. Dysprosody or altered "melody of language." Brain 1947; 70:405-415.
93. Moore J. Neuroanatomical considerations relating to

recovery of function following brain injury. In: Bach-y-Rita P, ed. Recovery of function: Theoretical considerations for brain injury rehabilitation. Baltimore: University Park Press, 1980.
94. Moore RY. Catecholamine neuron systems in brain. Ann Neurol 1982; 12:321–327.
95. Moosy J, Martinez J, Hann I, et al. Thalamic and subcortical gliosis with dementia. Arch Neurol 1987; 44:510–513.
96. Morris JC, Cole M. Banker BO, Wright D. Hereditary dysphasic dementia and the Pick-Alzheimer spectrum. Ann Neurol 1984; 16:455–466.
97. Morris JC, Drazner M, Fulling K, Grant EA, Goldring J. Clinical and pathological aspects of Parkinsonism in Alzheimer's disease: A role for extranigral factors? Arch Neurol 1989; 46:651–657.
98. Muller EM, Brown WS. Variations in the supraglottal waveform and their articulatory interpretation. In: Lass NJ, ed. Speech and language: Advances in basic research and practice. New York: Academic Press, 1980.
99. Mysak E. Pathologies of the speech systems. Baltimore: Williams & Wilkins, 1976:318.
100. Netsell R, Kent R, Abbs J. The organization and reorganization of speech movements. Paper presented at the Society for Neuroscience, Cincinnati, OH, 1980.
101. Neumann MA, Cohn R. Progressive subcortical gliosis: A rare form of presenile dementia. Brain 1967; 90:405–418.
102. Perry EK, Curtis M, et al. Cholinergic correlates of cognitive impairment in Parkinson's disease: Comparisons with Alzheimer's disease. J Neurol Neurosurg Psychiatry 1985; 48:413–421.
103. Rafal RD, Posner MI, Walker JA, et al. Cognition and the basal ganglia: separating mental and motor components of performance in Parkinson's disease. Brain 1984; 107:1083–1094.
104. Rebeiz JJ, Kolodny EH, Richardson EP. Corticodentatonigral degeneration with neuronal achromasia. Arch Neurol 1968; 18:20–33.
105. Rifkin A, Quitkin F, Kane JM, et al. Akinesia: A poorly recognized drug-induced extrapyramidal behavioral disorder. Arch Gen Psychiatry 1977; 34:43–47.
106. Risse S, Barnes RB. Pharmacologic treatment of agitation associated with dementia. J Am Geriatr Soc 1986; 34:368–376.
107. Robbins JA, Logemann JA, Kirschner HS, Swallowing speech production in Parkinson's disease. Ann Neurol 1986; 19:283–287.
108. Rosenberg RN, et al. Dominantly inherited dementia and parkinsonism with non-Alzheimer amyloid plaques: A new neurogenetic disorder. Ann Neurol 1989; 25:152–158.
109. Ross ED, Mesulam MM. Dominant language functions of the right hemisphere? Arch Neurol 1978; 36:144–148.
110. Salazar AM, Masters CL, Gajdusek DC, Gibbs CJ. Syndromes of amyotrophic lateral sclerosis and dementia: Relationship to transmissible Creutzfeldt-Jakob disease. Ann Neurol 1983; 14:17–26.
111. Salzman C, Van der Kolk B. Psychotropic drug prescriptions for elderly patients in a general hospital. J Am Geriatr Soc 1980; 288:188–222.
112. Sarno MT. Acquired aphasia. New York: Academic Press, 1983.
113. Scherer HJ. Zritschrift fur die Gesamte Neurol Psychiatrie 1933; 145:135.
114. Schneider LS, Diamond SG, Markham CH. Deficits in orofacial sensorimotor function in Parkinson's disease. Ann Neurol 1986; 19:275–282.
115. Schneider LS, Chui HC. Progressive supranuclear palsy manifesting with depressive features. J Am Geriatr Soc 1986; 34:633–665.
116. Scully RE, Mark EJ, McNeely BU. Case 16-1986, Massachusetts General Hospital CPC. N Engl J Med 1986; 314:1101–1111.
117. Shulman S. Bilateral symmetrical degeneration of the thalamus: A clinicopathological study. J Neuropathol Exp Neurol 1957; 17:446–470.
118. Steele JC, Richardson JC, Olszewski J. Progressive supranuclear palsy. Arch Neurol 1964; 10:333–359.
119. Stern K. Severe dementia associated with bilateral symmetrical degeneration of the thalamus. Brain 1939; 62:157–171.
120. Tamas IE, Campbell-Taylor I. Dysarthria and dysphagia in atypical PSP. Paper presented at the First International Congress, European Neurological Society, Nice, France, 1988. (Abstract.)
121. Vogel M, von Cramon D. Dysphonia after traumatic mid-brain damage. A follow-up study. Folia Phoniatr (Basel) 1982; 34:150–159.
122. Whitehouse P. The concept of subcortical and cortical dementia: Another look. Ann Neurol 1986; 19:1–6.
123. Wise TN, Mann LS, Niru Jani JD. Haloperidol prescribing practices in the general hospital. Gen Hosp Psychiatry 1989; 11:368–371.

# SECTION TWO

*Language Changes and Dementia*

# CHAPTER 6

# *Normal Aging and Language*

ELLEN BOUCHARD RYAN, Ph.D.

The purpose of this chapter is to address a variety of language issues pertaining to later life. Initially, the cognitive and psycholinguistic literature on language differences associated with healthy old age is reviewed. Then, a framework is presented that addresses the heterogeneity of language performance of older adults in terms of individual differences and environmental variations. The dependence of performance on task demands, environmental constraints, and social expectations is particularly emphasized. Finally, the clinical implications of a balanced perspective of language in normal aging are developed in terms of assessment, treatment, and communication for health professionals.

This chapter on healthy aging is intended to provide the background context within which to study the language and communication changes in dementia, the focus of this volume. Understanding changes in normal aging is prerequisite to clinical work with, as well as research of, cognitively impaired elders. Such knowledge is necessary to analytically separate the effects of disease from those of aging, individual life history, and environment. Assessment and treatment of cognitively impaired elders must take into account the fact that clients may have resources that can reduce the impact of their disease or they may have age-associated difficulties that exacerbate the functional problems associated with the disease. Moreover, assessment and treatment of cognitively impaired clients frequently involves communication with cognitively healthy, older members of the family and age peers.

Three principles underlying a balanced understanding of language in later life need to be emphasized at the outset. The first principle is that of heterogeneity among older adults in their cognitive and language performance. Individual differences based on genetic inheritance and life histories, as well as differential vulnerability to age-associated diseases and environmental changes, increase with age.[68,95] Studies comparing older and younger groups focus on group differences, but the great variability within age groups cannot be ignored. Despite averages in favor of younger adults, a considerable number of healthy elders invariably exceed the younger group's average performance. Rowe and Kahn discussed this heterogeneity as a challenge to research, in that one should examine successful aging (with little or no decline) in comparison with usual aging (with average performance declines in some domains) and ill aging (with substantial declines linked to age-associated disease), to identify modifiable factors that could move the life trajectory of the majority of individuals from one of usual aging to one of successful aging.[85]

The second principle, related to the first, is that adult age differences in language competence (knowledge of the language presumably acquired early in life) are minimal, whereas in some domains, age-associated sensory and cognitive changes lead to noticeable age-group differences in language performance.[4,60] Linguistic and pragmatic knowledge acquired in adolescence is maintained, and there are no doubt important increases based on the wealth of experiences throughout life in dealing with communication challenges.[60,70] However, performance in language tasks can be limited by age-associated changes such as hearing difficulties, decreased speed, and poor memory.[21,78,96]

The third principle is that communicative success depends not only on a person's abilities, but also on the interpersonal and environmental situation in which communication occurs. Ryan, Giles, Bartolucci, and Henwood argued that the social

---

Preparation of this chapter was partially supported by a grant from the Natural Sciences and Engineering Research Council of Canada.

context of language use has been ignored in the study of the psycholinguistic and clinical aspects of language change in aging (see also articles by Coupland et al and Light).[22,23,60,90] Whereas older adults perform best under conditions of moderate environmental challenge with appropriate support, they are frequently in environments that understimulate. In addition, they are often asked to perform tasks with little relevance to their usual environmental challenges.[58,84] Social and situational factors are addressed explicitly in the section of this chapter on variability of performance, but they are also mentioned throughout the chapter where particularly relevant to alternative interpretations of low performance scores of older adults.

## Age-Associated Language Differences

### OVERVIEW

The study of language in healthy aging persons residing within the general community has occurred primarily from cognitive, psycholinguistic, and neuropsychologic perspectives. Sociolinguistic perspectives have just recently been given consideration. Because only the highlights can be addressed in this chapter, the reader is referred to recent reviews for elaboration.[4,6,62,74,103]

A number of methodologic limitations require that generalizations based on studies of language among older adults remain tentative. First, all the major studies of language are cohort studies, except when vocabulary and other verbal measures have been administered as part of intelligence batteries. In addition to the lack of longitudinal research in this area, studies tend to involve small samples, variable representation of genders, and variable definitions of "old." Moreover, despite the large number of separate reports, only a few investigators are systematically addressing aging questions across a series of cumulative studies. Controls for educational level, socioeconomic status, English as a native rather than a second language, activity level, and health are sporadic and never simultaneous.

Given the early state of research on language among older adults, the findings of age-group difference reported here should be considered as leads for further research and as suggestions for areas to keep in mind during clinical applications.

### SPEECH AND VOICE

Anatomic, physiologic, and neurologic changes associated with normal aging result in gradual changes in specific acoustic characteristics of the human voice. Acoustic changes in aging that have been studied include reduced maximum phonation time, reduced speech rate, lowered vocal intensity, increased fundamental frequency (for men only), slight hoarseness, vocal jitter, variation, range of fundamental frequency, and nasality.[8]

Such changes can be used by trained and naive listeners to estimate speaker age, with relatively reliable accuracy within a decade.[45,79,88,100] Listeners have reported the following cues to be of use in age estimations: speech rate, pitch usage, voice quality, loudness, and fluency.[79,88] With multiple regression analysis, Ryan and Burk showed that chronologic age within an elderly group of speakers could be well predicted by laryngeal air loss, voice tremor, mean fundamental frequency, slow articulation rate, and imprecise consonants.[94] Stewart and Ryan reported that naive listeners distinguished voices of male speakers in their sixties from those in their twenties in terms of less intensity, lower pitch, increased hoarseness, greater nasality, and a marginally slower rate.[107]

Less favorable views of older adults than of younger counterparts have been observed by Ryan and others in a series of studies eliciting evaluative reactions to voices.[7,88,93,100,107] Vocal cues associated with age have been linked to stereotyped impressions of personal competence and characteristics of benevolence. Moreover, effective communication performance presented by an older voice tends not to be given the same credit as identical performance presented by a younger voice.[92,93,107] This research suggests that listeners pay less attention to the quality of speech behavior for older adults than for younger adults.

The research of Ramig highlighted the role of physical condition in producing the acoustic correlates typically associated with age.[8] Earlier work by Ramig and Ringel demonstrated that healthy elderly speakers showed the acoustic characteristics of much younger speakers, whereas speakers of the same age in poor physiologic condition sounded old.[82] Age estimations were accurate for choices in poor physiologic condition during the production of both sustained vowels and connected discourse, whereas age estimations were only good for the voices of healthy individuals for connected discourse.[81] Both Ramig and Benjamin proposed that sociolinguistic explanations could account for variation beyond the physical changes: the age-associated changes produced in connected discourse by individuals with few acoustic cues of old age and the avoidance of imprecise articulation by aging women (as compared to men, traditionally less oriented to careful pronunciation).[7,81] Benjamin concluded that because advancing age and poor physical condition are often associated, these factors interact to create the stereotypic older voice.[8]

With regard to fluency of speech production, Manning and Shirkey indicated that hesitation phenomena such as interjections and revisions increase with age.[66] It has also been suggested that some of these hesitations may result from a word-finding difficulty, but also that they could be related to social conversational dynamics, especially because interviewers are rarely age peers of the older study participants.[118]

## VOCABULARY

Vocabulary knowledge has been extensively studied, primarily as part of psychometric batteries of intellectual behavior, with the conclusion that vocabulary knowledge does not decline with age, especially when educational background is controlled.[5,98] More specific examinations of lexical performance, however, have identified aspects that are susceptible to age-group differences. The aging person's major difficulty seems to be accessing words. Hence, lexical access tasks not requiring retrieval of specific words (e.g., multiple choice vocabulary test and lexical decision tasks) are most likely to elicit good performances by older adults.[5,13] Confrontation naming tasks, and other lexical tasks requiring productive use of words, tend to show age declines from middle-aged to young-old to old-old.[11,13,56]

This difficulty with word access presumably underlies the frequent complaints of older adults about difficulty remembering names and failure to retrieve a well-known word while speaking.[112] Goodglass established that, contrary to aphasics with word-naming difficulties, healthy older adults have access to sound and orthographic features of a word on the "tip of the tongue."[40] In a diary study, older adults reported more frequent experiences of "tip of the tongue," but were likely to resolve them later.[14]

Another important type of lexical task exhibiting age differences is the verbal fluency task, which assesses the generative naming of words meeting either a structural (e.g., words beginning with a specific letter) or semantic (e.g., names of animals) criterion.[4,40] Speeded tasks have also revealed age differences in the rate of lexical access of semantic activation—a problem for elders that may contribute to a limitation of processing resources for more complex language tasks.[43]

## SYNTAX

With respect to linguistic knowledge, the lack of age differences across the adult age range (from the twenties to the seventies) when performing sentence disambiguation suggests that syntactic competence remains strong.[5] However, utilization of complex grammatic structures has been shown to be reduced among older adults in various situations, even though a number of studies report no age group differences (for an excellent review see the article by Bayles and Kaszniak).[4] It should be noted that the studies showing age associations in grammatic performance frequently place high demands on participants for sensory processing and memory.

In terms of sentence comprehension, older adults (aged 60 years and over) have been found to enact sentence meanings more poorly than younger counterparts.[32] On a variety of syntactic processing tasks, Emery observed more finely differentiated age differences in that pre–middle-aged participants (aged 30 to 42 years) performed better than elderly participants (aged 75 to 93 years), and the younger half of the elderly group performed better than the older half.[28] Similarly, age-group differences (among those in their thirties, forties, fifties, sixties, and seventies) in the accuracy of sentence comprehension were observed by Obler, Fein, Nicholas, and Albert, especially for complex syntactic constructions and semantically improbable sentences.[4]

It is generally agreed that the elderly find the loss of redundancy a bigger problem in comprehension than do younger adults, largely because of subtle hearing problems and slower processing.[21] The sentence-processing difficulties of older adults are exacerbated by noisy conditions.[46] Obler, Nicholas, Albert, and Woodward found that age differences were apparent in sentence processing through noise for low-probability sentences, but not for highly predictable sentences.[75] Although a ceiling effect prevented assessment of age differences for use of context, the fact that Hutchinson found almost one quarter of the elderly showing no advantage with predictable sentence context underscores the importance of examining individual difference factors.[46]

Stine and Wingfield have examined sentence processing under speeded conditions that would tax the presumed reduced processing resources of older adults (averaging approximately 70 years of age) as compared to university undergraduates. In the first study, they observed the predicted magnification of age differences in a sentence-repetition task under faster oral presentation rates and with less structured word strings as compared to meaningful sentences.[120] Subsequently, with long, propositionally dense sentences, they also found a particular age decrement in the speeded condition, but no age-associated difference was noted for processing sentences of varying informational load.[110] A third study replicated the differential age sensitivity to rate manipulations and supported the Cohen and Faulkner finding of greater reliance among older adults upon stress and other prosodic features.[20,109] Individual differences in sentence-repetition performance were largely accounted for by working memory and the age-associated tendency to use a meaningful reconstruction strategy.[108]

In a series of studies on sentence production, Kemper has examined the assumption that elders are most likely to experience difficulties with syntactic constructions with high attentional and memory loads. In the first study, older adults (in their seventies and eighties) experienced more difficulty than middle-aged adults (in their thirties and forties) in repeating or paraphrasing complex sentences when the sentences were long, especially when embedded clauses were in initial position.[49] Imitations in this task were made particularly challenging in that the subjects had to identify and correct any grammatic errors in the sentences. In the second study, the spontaneous speech of adults in their fifties and sixties exhibited a narrower repertoire of syntactic constructions, avoidance of constructions imposing high memory demands, and more errors in the use of simple syntactic structures.[55] The third study utilized diaries written over a lifetime to compare longitudinal and cohort differences in written use of sentences and confirmed the earlier findings of age-related decline in sentence complexity.[50] Finally, Kemper and colleagues observed age differences (between two groups aged 18 to 28 years old versus 60 to 92 years old) in grammatic complexity of oral and written statements and further identified a relationship between working memory capacity and the production of complex utterances.[51]

## DISCOURSE

### Prose Comprehension and Recall

The literature on prose comprehension and recall across the lifespan is extensive. The findings regarding age differences are highly variable and complex. Hultsch and Dixon have argued that age-related performance differences in memory for text materials are best viewed in terms of interactions between characteristics of the participants (e.g., intellectual abilities), materials (e.g., modality, genre, and concreteness), acquisition conditions (e.g., incidental versus intentional learning and time constraints), and criterial tasks (e.g., recognition and free recall).[44]

Some tentative summary statements can be made within this framework.[4,44,62] Older adults are more likely to show lower scores than are their younger counterparts in the following circumstances: when participants are poorly educated and have low intelligence, when text materials require organizational effort, when materials are youth-oriented, when working memory demands are high, when inferences or logical reasoning are required, when delayed testing is involved, or when free recall is assessed. An illustration of the interaction among these factors is the finding that age differences are likely for both main ideas and details for low-ability subjects but only for details among high-ability subjects.[44]

### Conversation Skills

Although little research has focused specifically on conversational skills, this is clearly a vital domain for the everyday life of older adults. Among community-residing elderly possessing sufficiently good communication skills to be interviewed by telephone, 18 percent of the respondents in a recent survey indicated that they had trouble in one-to-one conversations and 33 percent reported trouble with group conversations.[101]

Three laboratory studies illustrate the ways in which memory problems may influence conversational skills. Rabbitt[80] found that among adults over age 70 years, keeping track of which speaker made which statement in a multispeaker interaction was particularly difficult. Participation in the conversation also appeared to detract significantly from recall of content. Second, a study of memory in a word-retrieval task indicated that older adults showed poorer judgment about whether words had already been recalled and hence repeated words during recall.[53] This deficiency in output monitoring was interpreted as linked to the difficulty sometimes experienced by the elderly of repeating a story to the same listener. Finally, older adults were less able than younger adults to recall topics discussed in a session, even though age groups did not differ in recognition of the discussion prompts provided.[48]

Excessive loquaciousness has been identified as a problem for some older persons.[29] Gold and colleagues conducted the first empirical work on verbosity, defined as excessive off-topic talk.[39] In two studies, they examined the intellectual and personality characteristics of elderly interviewees classified as highly verbose as compared with nonverbose peers. A major hypothesis offered by clinicians, that verbose individuals were especially lonely and were more demanding in social interactions to make up for fewer interactions, was not supported. The verbose elders were older, less physically mobile, experienced more stress, were more extroverted, sought more social contacts, and expressed less concern for making favorable impressions upon others. In addition, longitudinal data indicated that verbosity was related to decline over a 40-year period in nonverbal intelligence.[39] This latter finding has led to current work by these investigators to determine whether verbosity may be associated with early dementia.

### Narrative Production

Ambiguity of reference and reduced efficiency in conveying information are the two aspects of story telling and retelling that seem to differentiate the old from the young. Obler first noted that older adults used more paraphrases and indefinite terms, presumably an indication of cognitive difficulty with the discourse.[73] The word-retrieval difficulties already discussed may be one cause of this pattern. Ulatowska and colleagues examined a variety of narrative discourse tasks in a sample of middle-aged (mean age 46 years) and older women (mean age 76 years), and observed significantly more ambiguity of reference between the middle-aged and older groups and between the younger and older halves of the elder group.[117] As the investigators suggest, research is needed to determine when linguistic variation, such as ambiguous reference, may be related to a strategy for concealing comprehension and memory problems or to an egocentric lack of sensitivity to listeners' needs for clarity.

Efficiency of conveying information also appears to be diminished among older adults. In story retelling and procedural descriptions, fewer critical units of information were included by the older adults.[71] This is supported by the norming study conducted by Shewan and Henderson.[105] Story telling by adults in their forties, based on pictures, differed from those in their sixties and seventies primarily in terms of communication efficiency. Since efficiency may not be the highest communicative goal, it is important to keep in mind variation in speaker goals and in stylistic conventions.[22,73]

The complexity of analyzing age differences in story telling is highlighted by Kemper's most recent study.[51] The same age pattern of reduced syntactic complexity is observed for oral and written discourse, but the older adults' discourse was rated more favorably in terms of interest and clarity. Such a finding underscores the hypothesis that investigators may not be asking all the appropriate questions about discourse and that research intended to find age deficits is more likely to find them than research intended to find age benefits.[22] For example, identifying story telling as an old-age appropriate domain, Mergler, Faust, and Goldstein[69] designed their study based on predictions in favor of old age. And indeed, they found that stories told orally by elders were better retained by young people than the same stories told by young or middle-aged tellers.

### Nonverbal Communication

Reception and production of nonverbal cues (e.g., facial expressions, gestures, and interpersonal distance) are an important part of overall communication. As pointed out by McGee and Barker, subtle nonverbal cues are necessary to understand and negotiate roles within conversation as well as to distinguish apparent from true communicative intention.[67] Nonverbal cues can become particularly important for elders with hearing difficulties.

Two studies have addressed the topic of age variation in nonverbal communication. Malatesta, Izard, Culver, and Nicolich asked young (aged 25 to 40 years), middle-aged (45 to 60 years), and old women (aged 65 years and older) to express various emotions under laboratory conditions and then three similar groups of women attempted to identify the emotions from facial expressions only.[65] Older women did show overall poorer decoding, but they performed significantly better for age peers and after practice. Age congruence was an even greater factor for the young women, who performed much worse in decoding emotions expressed by the elder women. Although the authors suggest that older faces may be less able to express emotions, these findings highlight the potential for intergenerational miscommunication. In a second study, older women (mean age 62 years) showed less sensitivity to auditory (content-filtered) and visual aspects of nonverbal communication.[59] In addition to the influence of fatigue on older adults making 220 judgments of novel materials, the intergenerational issues raised by the first study may be influential here.[65] Because all the affective situations were communicated by a single young woman (aged 24 years), the poorer performance of older adults may be largely attributable to the age incongruence.

Investigations of nonverbal behavior in aging have just begun, and this should be a fruitful area for new insights over the next decade. Because adults may develop a greater reliance on tactile cues as hearing and vision decline in very old age or with age-related diseases, research on the perception and production of messages through touch needs to be initiated.

### Summary

Age-associated language differences have been identified in a number of domains of speech and language performance. The key areas of age-related differences to be targeted for further, continuing research are: vocal characteristics, word retrieval, sentence processing, memory for components of conversation and for text, reference and efficiency in discourse production, and nonverbal communication. Nevertheless, disparities from youthful standards are often subtle, usually unlikely to handicap an individual in everyday communication activities, and highly linked to variables not systematically studied simultaneously.[4]

## Understanding Variability In Aged Communication

### SOCIAL-COGNITIVE MODEL OF COMMUNICATION IN LATE LIFE

In order to interpret the language performance of a given older person, it is important to consider individual life-history and environmental factors. The schematic model presented in Figure 6.1 is intended to facilitate discussion of these factors. Note that several earlier characterizations of the communication process in late life contributed importantly to the development of this model.[23,90,103,118] The model is intended to integrate the three principles introduced at the beginning of this chapter: the importance of performance-limiting factors in language usage, diversity within the elderly population, and the dependence of individual success or failure on environmental factors.

This schematic model depicts the major contributors to language performance as a function of individual differences in language competence, information-processing factors, and social strategies, as well as variations in the immediate situation. Correspondingly, the language-relevant individual differences are based on individual life histories and current abilities and predispositions. The immediate situation depends on the sociocultural environment within which individuals have lived, especially environmental variations in their current lives. In addition, the specific demands of the assessment context impose constraints on participants' opportunities to exhibit their language competence. Note that this schema is not age-dependent and can be used to compare elders to

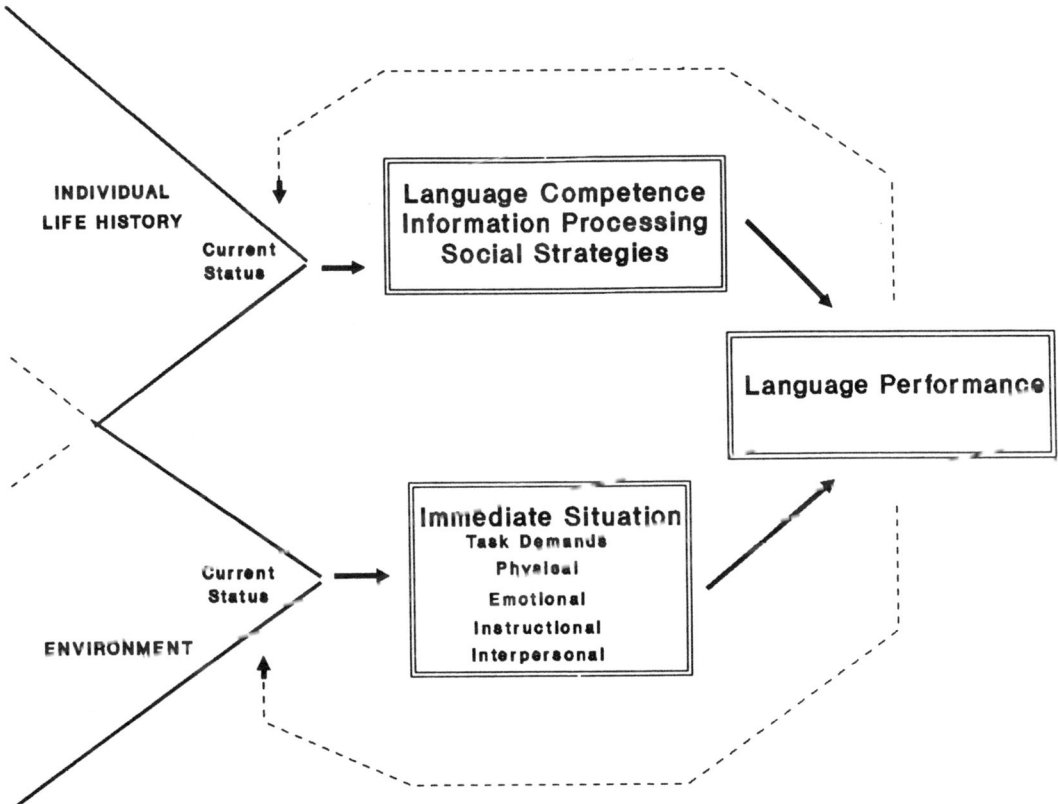

**Figure 6.1** Schematic model of individual life history and environmental contributions to language performance in a specific situation.

members of younger and older cohorts. In this section, issues relevant to individuals and environments will be addressed separately first. Then the interconnections between the components of the diagram will be discussed.

## INDIVIDUAL DIFFERENCES

### Individual Life History

Among community-residing elders with no known neurologic impairments, some persons are more likely to exhibit communication difficulties than others. Critical background variables associated with individual life history include education, socioeconomic status, bi- or multilingualism, health, gender, and personality. These can influence the level of language, information processing, and social skills that individuals bring to their old age. Moreover, several researchers have interpreted studies of reading comprehension, for example, as evidence of a threshold hypothesis according to which those with strong verbal skills appear to be less susceptible to decline with age.[44,108,114]

Thus, several groups can be identified as particularly vulnerable to language-performance difficulties in late life. Individuals of lower social class or with little education are especially likely to have difficulties with tasks requiring reading and writing. Individuals functioning in their second language may never have achieved proficiency. Even when fluent second-language functioning is achieved, there is some suggestion that a language acquired after early childhood is more susceptible to loss in late life.[17,18]

Current variations among individuals in old age can have major influences upon language competence, information-processing strategies, and social strategies. Chronologic age is obviously one key factor, in that older adults in their nineties are likely to show more language changes than those in their sixties and seventies. The link between physiologic status and vocal characteristics was discussed earlier, and the dependence of cognitive and linguistic performance upon current health cannot be overemphasized.[9] Performance difficulties can be caused or exacerbated by medical illnesses, as well as by medications.[3,37] Problems associated with nutritional status, alcohol abuse, and poor physical fitness can also reduce a person's information-processing skills.[77] Depression, the most prevalent mental-health problem among older people, limits communicative performance because it is associated with poor social relationships, social withdrawal, apathy, poor concentration, and memory complaints.[36]

### Language Competence

Language competence represents the language knowledge and optimal level of performance of which individuals are capable. As emphasized earlier, performance in specific assessment situations provides just a glimpse of the actual underlying competence. Individual variations in competence can be assumed to be relatively minor, except in cases where a person never achieved proficiency in a second language or in the education-dependent domains of reading and writing. Variations in competence play a more prominent role when neurologic impairment is involved, as in the case of dementia.

### Information Processing

The key information-processing constraints for language performance relate to sensory abilities, speed of processing, and memory. Sensory abilities are critical for processing linguistic messages as well as for processing the supporting contextual information.[76] Hearing difficulties pose the most prevalent limitations associated with aging. Despite widely varying estimates, it appears that one-third to one-half of the adults over 65 years of age experience some difficulty in hearing speech, especially in noisy or group settings (see Chapters 4 and 14).[21,119] In addition, vision changes associated with aging (e.g., lower acuity, need for greater illumination, sensitivity to glare, and diminished color discrimination) may inhibit perception of nonverbal gestures or the use of speech reading.[33] The cumulative impact of slight changes in both sensory modalities can be substantial because of the tendency to use the complementary sense to compensate for one loss and because of anxiety and social avoidance resulting from the loss of confidence.[72,77] Compensations for hearing or visual difficulties can also involve behaviors (e.g., standing too close or speaking too loud) that irritate social partners and hence negatively affect conversational opportunities.[67]

The most significant cognitive changes underlying language performance are slowed mental processing and decreased memory. The gradual slowing of perceptual, cognitive, and psychomotor processes is one of the best established findings in the psychology of aging.[96] Intensive research on memory has identified particular difficulties for elders. Of most importance here are age-group differences in memory for new information, especially when effortful processing is required, when active retrieval (versus recognition) is tested, and when the task is particularly difficult.[77,78]

These two changes have recently been combined in various formulations of the notion that the fundamental cognitive change in aging involves reduced processing resources.[19,25,60,63,97] Hence, aged individuals showing difficulties with language tasks are likely to also be experiencing reduced processing resources in terms of slowed reaction times, as well as reduced capacity for attention; on-line processing of information, storage, and retrieval. Research examining these empirical relationships is recent.[38,61,121] Yet, despite conceptual problems with the unifying notion of reduced processing resources, this perspective highlights the dependence of language performance on age-associated changes in information-processing skills.[60,62]

### Social Strategies

Social strategies contribute significantly to variation in language performance as well. Communication is a resource for coping and adapting to the stresses of life through the satisfaction of instrumental needs and the development and maintenance of social support networks.[42,102] Social rewards and a feeling of well-being are associated with good communication experiences among older adults. In addition, communication facilitates the negotiation of people's changing social identities as "older."[10,22]

Norris and Rubin reviewed the social skills of the elderly, pointing out the strengths associated with life experiences as well as potential weaknesses associated with altered environmental conditions or with declining cognition.[70] From the small number of studies in this area, it would seem that the social strategies of older adults are highly variable and specifically challenged by aging changes. Hence, some communication styles may represent strategies to compensate for declines in hearing and memory, such as avoidance of talking and conversational domination. Older adults have reported experiencing greater difficulty with a range of common social situations than have their younger counterparts, and they demonstrate a lower probability of using various appropriately assertive responses.[35] Norris and Rubin point out that possible differences in social purposes may underlie some of the performance contrasts between generations.[70] For example, efforts to form friendships in late life often have fairly short-term, limited functional objectives as compared to earlier adulthood. A sociolinguistic analysis of how elders intermingle the past and present in organized topic flow of conversations by Boden and Bielby illustrates the rich information available from studying "old" communication in itself, rather than in contrast with "young" communication.[10]

With regard to identification of aging strengths, Smith, Reinheimer, and Gabbard-Alley verified the predicted advantages of being an older adult when communicating within crowded social conditions as compared with younger adults, who seemed to depend more on personal space for optimal performance.[106] Likewise, elders have been found to exhibit more complex social perceptions and show better comprehension of social motives.[70] Investigators have only begun to explore the multiple ways in which social strategies interact with changing information processing resources as well as the increased life experiences of older adults.

## ENVIRONMENT

Individual life histories are obviously greatly affected by the sociocultural environment within which one matures. Of greatest relevance here is the influence of the current environment upon the ability of aging people to use language skillfully. According to discussions of person-environment fit, performance and growth in aging are maximized in an environment that challenges persons to perform slightly above their current levels.[58]

### Social Expectations

Stereotypes of old age and ageist bias when interpreting the behaviors of older people have been well documented, although there is a trend toward more subtle forms.[26,52,86,89] In particular, older adults are expected to show memory decline, to be slower to learn, to be less successful in achievement-oriented situations, and to show more helpfulness and friendliness than younger adults.[87,91]

Negative expectations and overprotection can pose barriers to successful communication. The self-appraisal of older adults is based to some extent on social expectations, and meeting challenges with the appropriate effort and strategies depends on a strong sense of one's capabilities.[77,84,90] Expectations that older individuals with some health limitations cannot think or speak adequately may lead to avoidance of communication, to overly constrained communication opportunities, to diminished corrective feedback about negative behaviors, to overprotection, or to patronizing behaviors such as oversimplified speech.[15,16,23,84,89,90] Ryan et al have outlined a model for understanding how age and illness stereotypes and weakened communication skills can lead to a negative spiral in which fewer and more limiting occasions for communication practice are offered to an older adult.[90] Alternatively, one could reverse this negative spiral to create a positive feedback system for assisting a communicatively at-risk individual to become more and more competent in more and more challenging situations.[54] For further discussion of this topic see Chapter 10 on learned helplessness.

### Living Arrangements and Activities

The opportunity for continued use and growth of communication skills within one's current environment can clearly influence language performance in an assessment situation.[72,90] For example, the maintenance of communication skills is hindered in environments where an older person is relegated to a position outside regular social contacts. Older adults are at a risk for loss of contact with members of their social network through retirement, illnesses, deaths, or geographic relocation. Communication in community settings, in lifelong friendships, and especially within a marriage occurs naturally and is spontaneously nurtured. If these everyday opportunities are lost, the older person is challenged to establish new friendships and intimate relationships. Reductions in the traditional social network of an older person as well as increasing dependence can also diminish the opportunities for reciprocal exchanges of support.[70,72]

As noted earlier, intergenerational communication can be more demanding and more prone to difficulty than communication with healthy age peers. However, another frequent challenge for normal elders is to communicate with language-impaired age peers, especially those with hearing loss and dementia and those recovering from strokes.[64]

The level and type of activities engaged in by older adults are reciprocally negotiated within their environment. Extroverted and experienced elders can alter the environment for themselves and for others in terms of initiating activities or encouraging others to take part. Elders participating in activities that challenge them socially, mentally, and physically are more likely to practice and extend their social and communication skills.[58,72,83] Those living and socializing within seniors-only settings can be expected to experience more difficulties in intergenerational communication than those continuing to interact frequently with individuals of all ages.

### Immediate Situation

Language performance is a function of various characteristics of the immediate situations. With regard to the specific task, time constraints and memory demands are probably the best identified factors increasing age-group differences. In addition, older adults seem to exhibit relatively greater motivation when the task is familiar and clearly relevant to everyday life and when an opportunity for practice is available.[12,78] Emotionally, test situations that are highly unusual or critical for life decisions are likely to arouse anxiety among older adults.

In terms of the testing situations, failure to consider possible information-processing factors such as sensory losses among elders can be identified in terms of small print, noisy or busy settings, glare, poor lighting, and insufficient intensity of language stimuli.[41] The increased likelihood of fatigue needs to be taken into account in terms of length of testing sessions. From an instructional perspective, the appropriateness and manner of conveying information about what is expected in an assessment situation can greatly influence participants' understanding of the task at hand as well as their comfort in participating.[115] From an interpersonal point of view, elders' performance is influenced by the typically invisible variable of experimenter age. Hence, several studies reviewed found that elders performed better with age-peers than in an intergenerational situation.[59,65]

## LANGUAGE PERFORMANCE IN A SPECIFIC SITUATION

The performance of a given individual in a given language situation can be seen from Figure 6-1 to involve contributions of the individual and environmental factors just discussed. Within this framework, chronologic age is merely one of many influences upon assessed behavior. To the extent that the situation calls for language behaviors that are a typical part of the older individual's activities, in a manner that accommodates possible limitations in information processing functions, performance is likely to be a good measure of everyday language skills. The interactive nature of the components can be illustrated by considering the apparently egotistic tendency of some older individuals to dominate a conversation. Such behavior might result from self-centeredness that is lifelong or from decline in perspective-taking ability. However, it may also arise as a social strategy for coping with hearing or memory problems.[80]

As denoted in Figure 6.1, language performance has reciprocal influences upon the individual and the environment. For example, positive experiences can enhance a person's sense of social efficacy, challenge negative social expectations, increase one's social network, and set the stage, through practice, for improved subsequent performance. Correspondingly, an unsuccessful performance can confirm negative social expectations, undermine one's sense of communication efficacy skills, lead to avoidance of similar situations, and subsequently set the stage, through failure, for even poorer performance.

## Clinical Implications

Although a considerable body of cognitive and psychometric literature attests to age-group differences in various aspects of speech and language, it is essential that clinicians keep in mind the great variability among elders, the contrast between underlying competence and observed performance, and the multitude of situational determinants of language performance.

## COMMUNICATION WITH ELDERS

Social expectations regarding old age and the elderly tend to be negative, and elders are particularly vulnerable to the expectations expressed by others in interactions.[84] Appropriately high expectations are critical to the maintenance of self-esteem among older adults, and professionals can convey these expectations in the manner in which they speak to and about older adults. The elderly themselves have become part of the effort to educate about age bias. For example, a publication by the American Association of Retired Persons skillfully addresses the unconscious biases displayed in individual conversation, group lectures, and written materials, and also illustrates good communication strategies for reducing the effects of potential difficulties with hearing, vision, and information processing.[2]

Research on conversation addressed to the elderly indicates that caregivers tend to modify their speech more in terms of stereotyped communication needs than in terms of the real, individual needs of specific older individuals.[15,16] Moreover, the tendency to overaccommodate one's utterances is exaggerated when individuals exhibit signs of disability or dependence (e.g., being wheelchair bound or blind). Although elders who are institutionalized or suffering from cognitive confusion are the most likely recipients of patronizing or infantalizing speech, healthy older adults in the community also complain of this type of behavior.[57,89,90] The affective dimensions of respect and nurturance have been highlighted as particularly relevant to communication with elders. Conveying respect and nurturance simultaneously is often a difficult challenge. Research is needed to evaluate different communication approaches and to guide the training of clinicians to meet the challenge of appropriate communication with older adults, who may or may not require modifications of speech parameters or language structures. In particular, skills for dealing with off-topic verbosity or painful self-disclosures would be useful to ease clinicians' concerns about talking to older clients.[24,39]

## ASSESSMENT

The finding of age-group differences in a number of domains for healthy community residents supports the value of developing age norms for tests used to identify neuropsychological losses resulting from pathology or injury. The work with the Boston Aphasia Test and the Shewan Spontaneous Language Analysis System is notable in this regard.[74,105] Cohort effects will inevitably be an important component of age norms, especially in domains linked to amount and type of education, such as writing style.[73] Given the variability among elders, however, the most important comparison control for an elder with suspected language or cognitive decline is earlier performance by that particular individual. Hence, periodic assessments of high-risk elders would seem to be a useful strategy.

The distinction between language competence and language performance in a specific situation is critical for the assessment of an older individual's communication potential in various situations. The social-cognitive model outlined in this chapter emphasizes the difficulty of making inferences about competence based on chronologic age and performance levels in a particular testing situation. Individuals who perform poorly because of lack of practice, social isolation, or diminished self-esteem need to be identified because their language problems may be readily remediable. Those who perform poorly because of sensory or memory difficulties need interventions that address their specific information processing problems rather than language therapy. Individuals who perform very well in low-demand situations common to daily life may still have serious language performance difficulties that would be exhibited in more demanding or more unusual settings. Sundberg, Snowden, and Reynolds argue for assessment of personal competence and incompetence in life situations, especially linked with environmental demands or constraints.[111] This approach to assessment of functional competence, with an emphasis on abilities as well as deficits, would be especially useful for older adults' communication because this type of diagnosis leads directly to remediation. Related to the notion of functional competence is the probability that older adults may have different goals for communication than younger adults, especially in terms of more emphasis upon short-term affective gain rather than informational or instrumental objectives.[22,70]

## HEALTH-PROMOTION INTERVENTIONS

Maintaining social interaction and a strong, reciprocal social-support network can be seen as an essential contribution to well-being among older adults.[30,31] For instance, those with a positive expectation about their ability to obtain needed social support are less likely to become depressed, and social support has been linked to good functional status and is buffering the effects of losses.[1,42] Moreover, Twining argues that social breakdown between caregivers and elders is an important cause of institutionalization decisions.[116]

Hence, interventions aimed at enhancing the communication skills of older adults can be viewed as health promoting. Indeed, training in communication skills has been included in health-promotion programs as well as in specific communication programs.[27,31] The only evaluative study of community elders showed that assertiveness training did yield significant increases in assertiveness and in positive self-concept, although consequent improvement of interpersonal relationships was not assessed.[34] This study also highlighted the importance of group variables, in that the effect occurred primarily for the higher-social-class participants. Given that language performance and social skills depend on memory, memory training can also be expected to promote communication performance and self-esteem in social situations.[99]

Another reason for teaching communication skills to older adults is to assist them to help others, especially their peers, with communication difficulties or with their need for counseling. Recently, Hyde taught facilitative communication skills to elderly candidates for a peer-counseling program, and demonstrated that self-esteem and social sensitivity among the trainees increased.[47] On the basis that communication difficulties are associated with very old age and with various age-associated pathologies, Shadden developed a program of precrisis intervention to prepare healthy elders to communicate effectively with others who have communication disorders.[104] Meeting the challenges to develop new skills for helping others is a growth experience that may buffer the impact of threats to the learners' own communication abilities later on. In the near future, research is needed to identify the key communication strategies for elders to learn, to develop the best methods for teaching and learning these strategies, and to evaluate the specific and generalized benefits of such training.

## Concluding Remarks and Future Research Directions

Mild age-group differences in language performance have been documented in cohort studies, with many of the performance differences probably attributable to both generational differences and age-associated changes in information processing. Better-controlled research studies, including longitudinal work, are needed now that the most likely areas for age-associated decline among healthy elders have been outlined. The most important factors for control seem to be education, gender, language history, health, and activity level.[63,77] With regard to information processing influences, hearing, vision, and memory have been identified as major individual difference variables affecting language performance.

The social-cognitive model depicted in Figure 6.1 characterizes the variety of factors affecting language performance in a specific situation. In accordance with Coupland and Coupland,[22] this chapter calls for an enriched social context within which to view the cognitive aspects of language performance. In this regard, more research on the social strategies of older adults and how these influence elder communication is needed. Although the role of compensation strategies has been recognized, clinicians need to examine the flexible and creative use of a variety of compensation strategies by elders who suffer from declines in information-processing abilities or from losses of key members of their social networks. Moreover, the less appropriate compensatory strategies, such as avoidance of social situations and overreliance on spouse, need to be highlighted so that their use can be diagnosed and addressed. Clinicians need to seek areas where the experience of long life is likely to show benefits, rather than declines, as in the perception of complex social situations.[70]

From a clinical perspective, implications for the communication of clinicians with elders have been outlined as well as for assessment and interventions. In clinical research, the principles of wide individual differences among older adults, important situational influences, and the social interdependence among older adults and others should be addressed.

In conclusion, Tamir wrote that the transition to old age challenges us to avoid loss of self-esteem, competence, and personal identity.[113] In line with Tamir and with Rodin and Langer, it would seem that a major challenge for clinicians and researchers is to understand the manner in which many older adults use social and communicative skills to meet these challenges effectively and how others might do so more successfully.[84]

### References

1. Albrecht TL, Adelman MB. Communicating social support. Newbury Park, CA: Sage Publications, 1987.
2. American Association of Retired Persons. Truth about aging—Guidelines for accurate communications. Washington, D.C.: AARP, 1984.
3. Avorn J. Biomedical and social determinants of cog-

nitive improvements in the elderly. J Am Geriatr Soc 1983; 31:137-143.
4. Bayles KA, Kaszniak A. Communication and cognition in normal aging and dementia. Boston: Little, Brown and Co, 1987.
5. Bayless KA, Tomoeda CK, Boone DR. A view of age-related changes in language function. Dev Neuropsychol 1985; 1:231-264.
6. Beasley DS, Davis GA, eds. Aging: Communication processes and disorders. New York: Grune & Stratton, 1981.
7. Benjamin BJ. Dimensions of the older female voice. Lang Commun 1986; 6:35-46.
8. Benjamin BA. Changes in speech production and linguistic behavior with aging. In: Shadden BB, ed. Communication behavior and aging: A sourcebook for clinicians. Baltimore: Williams & Wilkins, 1988:163.
9. Birren JE, Schaie KW, eds. Handbook of the psychology of aging, 2nd ed. New York: Van Nostrand Reinhold, 1985.
10. Boden D, Bielby DD. The way it was: Topical organization in elderly communication. Lang Commun 1986; 6:73-90.
11. Borod JC, Goodglass H, Kaplan E. Normative data on the Boston Diagnostic Aphasia Examination, Parietal Lobe Battery, and the Boston Naming Test. J Clin Neuropsychol 1980; 2:209-215.
12. Botwinick J. Aging and behavior, 3rd ed. New York: Springer Publishing 1984.
13. Bowles NL, Poon LW. Aging and retrieval of words in semantic memory. J Gerontol 1985; 40:71-77.
14. Burke DM, Worthley J, Martin J. I'll never forget what's-her-name: Aging and the tip of the tongue experience. In: Gruneberg MM, Morris P, Sykes RN, eds. Practical aspects of memory: Current research and issues Vol. 2. Chicester, England: John Wiley & Sons, 1988:113.
15. Caporael L. The paralanguage of caregiving: Baby talk to the institutionalized aged. J Pers Soc Psychol 1981; 40:876-884.
16. Caporael L, Lukaszewski M, Culbertson G. Secondary baby talk: Judgments by institutionalized elderly and their caregivers. Pers Soc Psychol 1983; 44:746-754.
17. Clyne M. Bilingualism of the elderly. Talanya 1977; 4:45-65.
18. Clyne M, de Bok K. Language reversion revisited. Studies in second language acquisition. (In press.)
19. Cohen G. Age differences in memory for texts: Production deficiency or processing limitations. In: Light LL, Burke DM, eds. Language, memory and aging. Cambridge, MA: Cambridge University Press, 1988:171.
20. Cohen G, Faulkner D. Does 'elderspeak' work? The effect of intonation and stress on comprehension and recall of spoken discourse in old age. Lang Commun 1986; 6:99-112.
21. Corso J. Auditory perception and communication. In: Birren JE, Schaie KW, eds. Handbook of the psychology of aging. 1st ed. New York: Van Nostrand Reinhold, 1977:535.
22. Coupland N, Coupland J. Language and later life: The diachrony and decrement predicament. In: Giles H, Robinson P, eds. Handbook of language and social psychology. Bristol: Multilingual Matters. (In press.)
23. Coupland N, Coupland J, Giles H, Henwood K. Accommodating the elderly: Invoking and extending a theory. Lang Soc 1988; 17:1-41.
24. Coupland N, Coupland J, Giles H, Henwood K, Wiemann J. Elderly self-disclosure: Interactional and intergroup issues. Lang Commun 1988; 8:109-133.
25. Craik FIM, Byrd M. Aging and cognitive deficits: The role of attentional resources. In: Craik FIM, Trehub S, eds. Aging and cognitive processes. New York: Plenum Publishing, 1982: 191-211.
26. Crockett WH, Hummert ML. Perceptions of aging and the elderly. Ann Rev Gerontol Geriatr 1987; 7:217-241.
27. Doty L. Communication and assertion skills for older persons. New York: Hemisphere Publishing, 1988.
28. Emery OB. Linguistic decrement in normal aging. Lang Commun 1986; 6:47-64.
29. Epstein LJ. Issues in communication in geropsychiatry. In: Obler LK, Albert ML, eds. Language and communication in the elderly. Lexington, MA: Lexington Books, 1980:139.
30. Evans LK. Maintaining social interaction as health promotion in the elderly. J Gerontol Nurs 1978; 5(2):19-21.
31. FallCreek S, Mettler M. A healthy old age: A sourcebook for health promotion with older adults. Seattle: University of Washington, 1984.
32. Feier C, Gerstman L. Sentence comprehension abilities throughout the adult life span. J Gerontol 1980; 35:727-728.
33. Fozard JL, Wolf E, Bell B, McFarland RA, Podolsky S. Visual perception and communication. In: Birren JE, Schaie KW, eds. Handbook of the psychology of aging. 1st ed. New York: Van Nostrand, 1977:497.
34. Franzke AW. The effects of assertiveness training on older adults. Gerontologist 1987; 27:13-16.
35. Furnham A, Pendleton D. The assessment of social skills deficits in the elderly. Int J Aging Hum Dev 1983; 17:29-38.
36. Gallagher D, Thompson L. Depression. In: Lewinson P, Teri L, eds. Clinical geropsychology: New directions and treatment. New York. Pergamon Press, 1983:7.
37. Gawel MJ. The effects of various drugs on speech. Br J Disord Commun 1981; 16:51-57.
38. Gick ML, Craik FIM, Morris RG. Task complexity and age differences in working memory. Mem Cog 1988; 16:353-361.
39. Gold D, Andres D, Arbuckle T, Schwartzman A. Measurement and correlates of verbosity in elderly people. J Gerontol Psychol Sci 1988; 47:27-33.
40. Goodglass H. Naming disorders in aphasia and aging. In: Obler LK, Albert ML, eds. Language and communication in the elderly. Lexington, MA: Lexington Books, 1980:37.
41. Gravell R. Communication problems in elderly people: Practical approaches to management. London: Croom Helm, 1988.
42. Holahan CK, Holahan CJ. Self-efficacy, social support, and depression in aging: A longitudinal analysis. J Gerontol 1987; 42:65-68.
43. Howard DV. Aging and memory activation: The priming of semantic and episodic memory. In: Light LL, Burke DM, eds. Language, memory and aging. Cambridge, MA: Cambridge University Press, 1988:77.
44. Hultsch DF, Dixon RA. Memory for text materials in adulthood. In: Baltes P, Brim OJ Jr, eds. Life-span development and behavior. Vol. 6. New York: Academic Press, 1984:77.
45. Huntley R, Hollien H, Shipp T. Influence of listener characteristics on perceived age estimations. J Voice 1987; 1:49-52.
46. Hutchinson KM. Influence of sentence context on speech perception in young and older adults. J Gerontol 1989; 44:36-44.
47. Hyde RB. Facilitative communication skills training:

Social support for elderly people. Gerontologist 1988; 28:418-420.
48. Kausler DH, Hakami MK. Memory for topics of conversation: Adult age differences and intentionality. Exp Aging Res 1983; 9:153-157.
49. Kemper S. Imitation of complex syntactic constructions by elderly adults. Appl Psycholing 1986; 7:277-288.
50. Kemper S. Life-span changes in syntactic complexity. J Gerontol 1987; 42:323-328.
51. Kemper S, Kynette D, Rash S, O'Brien K, Sprott R. Life-span changes to adults' language: Effects of memory and genre. Appl Psycholing 1989; 10:49-66.
52. Kite ME, Johnson BT. Attitudes toward older and younger adults: A meta-analysis. Psych Aging 1988; 3:233-244.
53. Koriat A, Ben-Zur H, Sheffer D. Telling the same story twice: Output monitoring and age. J Mem Lang 1988; 27:23-39.
54. Kuypers JA, Bengtson VL. Social breakdown and competence. Hum Dev 1973; 16:186-201.
55. Kynette D, Kemper S. Aging and the loss of grammatical forms: A cross-sectional study of language performance. Lang Commun 1986; 6:65-72.
56. LaBarge E, Edwards D, Knesevich JW. Performance of normal elderly on the Boston Naming Test. Brain Lang 1986; 27:380-384.
57. Lanceley A. Use of controlling language in the rehabilitation of the elderly. J Adv Nurs 1985; 10:125-135.
58. Lawton MP. Environment and aging. Monterey, CA, Brooks/Cole Publishing, 1980.
59. Lieberman DA, Rigo TG, Campain RF. Age-related differences in nonverbal decoding ability. Commun Q 1988; 36:290-297.
60. Light LL. Language and aging: Competence versus performance. In: Birren JE, Bengtson VL, eds. Emergent theories of aging. New York: Springer Publishing, 1988:177.
61. Light LL, Anderson PA. Working memory capacity, age, and memory for discourse. J Gerontol 1985; 40:737-747.
62. Light LL, Burke DM, eds. Language, memory and aging. Cambridge: Cambridge University Press, 1988.
63. Light LL, Burke DM. Patterns of language and memory in old age. In: Light LL, Burke DM, eds. Language, memory, and aging. Cambridge, MA: Cambridge University Press, 1988:244.
64. Lubinski R. A model for intervention: Communication skills, effectiveness, and opportunity. In: Shadden BB, ed. Communication behavior and aging: A sourcebook for clinicians. Baltimore: Williams & Wilkins, 1988:294-308.
65. Malatesta CZ, Izard CE, Culver C, Nicolich M. Emotion communication skills in young, middle-aged, and older women. Psychol Aging 1987; 2:193-203.
66. Manning WH, Shirley EA. Fluency and the aging process. In: Beasley DS, Davis GA, eds. Aging: Communication processes and disorders. New York: Grune & Stratton, 1981:175.
67. McGee J, Barker M. Deference and dominance in old age: An exploration in social theory. Int J Aging Hum Dev 1982; 15:247-262.
68. McPherson BD, Aging as a social process. Toronto: Butterworths, 1983.
69. Mergler NL, Faust M, Goldstein MD. Storytelling as an age-dependent skill: Oral recall of orally presented stories. Int J Aging Hum Dev 1985; 20:205-228.
70. Norris JE, Rubin K. Peer interaction and communication: A life-span perspective. In: Baltes P, Brim OG, eds. Life-Span Development and Behavior. (vol. 6). New York: Academic Press, 1984:355.
71. North AJ, Ulatowska HK, Macaluso-Haynes S, Bell H. Discourse performance in older adults. Int J Aging Hum Dev 1986; 23:267-283.
72. Nussbaum JF, Thompson T, Robinson JD. Communication and aging. New York: Harper, 1988.
73. Obler LK. Narrative discourse style in the elderly. In: Obler LK, Albert ML, eds. Language and communication in the elderly. Lexington, MA: Lexington Books, 1980:75.
74. Obler LK, Albert ML. Language skills across adulthood. In: Birren JE, Schaie KW, eds. Handbook of the psychology of aging. 2nd ed. New York: Van Nostrand Reinhold, 1985:463.
75. Obler LK, Nicholas M, Albert ML, Woodward S. On comprehension across the adult lifespan. Cortex 1985; 21:273-280.
76. Olsho LW, Harkins SW, Lenhardt ML. Aging and the auditory system. In: Birren JE, Schaie KW, eds. Handbook of the psychology of aging, 2nd ed. New York: Van Nostrand Reinhold, 1985:332.
77. Perlmutter M, Adams C, Berry J. Aging and memory. Ann Rev Gerontol Geriatr 1987; 7:57-92.
78. Poon LW. Differences in human memory with aging: Nature, cause and clinical implications. In: Birren JE, Schaie KW, eds. Handbook of the psychology of aging, 2nd ed. New York: Van Nostrand Reinhold, 1985:427.
79. Ptacek PH, Sander EK. Age recognition from voice. J Speech Hear Res 1966; 9:273-277.
80. Rabbitt P. Talking to the old. New Society 1981; 55:140-141.
81. Ramig LA. Aging speech: Physiological and sociological aspects. Lang Commun 1986; 6:25-34.
82. Ramig LA, Ringel R. Effect of physiological aging on select acoustic characteristics of voice. J Speech Hear Res 1983; 26:22-50.
83. Ratner HH, Schell DA, Crimmins A, Mittleman D, Baldinelli L. Changes in adults' prose recall: Aging or cognitive demands? Dev Psychol 1987; 23:521-525.
84. Rodin J, Langer EJ. Aging labels: The decline of control and the fall of self-esteem. J Soc Issues 1980; 36:12-29.
85. Rowe JW, Kahn RL. Human aging: Usual and successful. Science 1987; 237(July 10):143-149.
86. Rubin KH, Brown IDR. A life-span look at person perception and its relationship to communicative interaction. J Gerontol 1975; 30:461-468.
87. Ryan EB. Age-based stereotypes about memory. Paper presented to the International Congress on Gerontology, Acapulco, Mexico, 1989.
88. Ryan EB, Capadano HL. Age perceptions and evaluative reactions toward adult speakers. J Gerontol 1978; 33:98-102.
89. Ryan EB, Cole R. Evaluative perceptions of interpersonal communication with elders. In: Giles H, Coupland N, Wiemann J, eds. Communication, health, and the elderly. Manchester: University of Manchester Press. (In press.)
90. Ryan EB, Giles H, Bartolucci G, Henwood K. Psycholinguistic and social psychological components of communication by and with the elderly. Lang Commun 1986; 6:1-24.
91. Ryan EB, Heaven R. The impact of situational context on age-based attitudes. Soc Behav 1988; 3:105-117.
92. Ryan EB, Johnston DG. The influence of communicative effectiveness on evaluations of younger and older adult speakers. J Gerontol 1987; 42:163-164.

93. Ryan EB, Laurie S. Evaluations of younger and older adult speakers: The influence of communication effectiveness and noise. Paper presented to the Gerontological Society of America. San Francisco, 1988.
94. Ryan WJ, Burk KW. Perceptual and acoustic correlates of aging in the speech of males. J Commun Disord 1974; 7:181–192.
95. Salthouse TA. Adult cognition: An experimental psychology of human aging. New York: Springer Publishing, 1982.
96. Salthouse TA. Speed of behavior and its implications for cognition. In: Birren JE, Schaie KW, eds. The handbook of the psychology of aging, 2nd ed. New York: Van Nostrand Reinhold, 1985:400–426.
97. Salthouse TA. The role of processing resources in cognitive aging. In: Howe ML, Brainerd CJ, eds. Cognitive development in adulthood: Progress in cognitive development research. New York: Springer-Verlag, 1988:185.
98. Salthouse TA. Effects of aging on verbal abilities: Examination of the psychometric literature. In: Light LL, Burke DM, eds. Language, memory and aging. Cambridge: Cambridge University Press, 1988:17–35.
99. Scogin F, Storandt M, Lott L. Memory skills training memory complaints, and depression in older adults. J Gerontol 1985; 40:562–568.
100. Sebastian RJ, Ryan EB. Speech cues and social evaluation: Markers of ethnicity, social class, and age. In: Giles H, St. Clair RN, eds. Recent advances in language, communication and social psychology. London: Erlbaum, 1985:112–143.
101. Services for seniors study—Mapping the way to the future for the elderly: Report of findings and recommendations. Regional Municipality of Hamilton-Wentworth (Ontario) and Hamilton-Wentworth District Health Council, 1988.
102. Shadden BB. Interpersonal communication patterns and strategies in the elderly. In: Shadden BB, ed. Communication behavior and aging: A sourcebook for clinicians. Baltimore: Williams & Wilkins, 1988:182.
103. Shadden BB, ed. Communication behavior and aging: A sourcebook for clinicians. Baltimore: Williams & Wilkins, 1988.
104. Shadden BB. Pre-crisis intervention: A tool for reducing the impact of stroke-related personal family crisis. J Gerontol Soc Work 1983; 6:61–74.
105. Shewan CM, Henderson VL. Analysis of spontaneous language in the older normal population. J Commun Disord 1988; 21:139–154.
106. Smith MJ, Reinheimer RE, Gabbard-Alley A. Crowding, task performance, and communicative interaction in youth and old age. Hum Commun Res 1981; 7:259–272.
107. Stewart MA, Ryan EB. Attitudes toward younger and older adult speakers: Effects of varying speech rates. J Lang Soc Psychol 1982; 1:91–109.
108. Stine EL, Wingfield A. Levels upon levels: Predicting age differences in text recall. Exp Aging Res 1987; 13:179–183.
109. Stine EL, Wingfield A. Process and strategy in memory for speech among younger and old adults. Psychol Aging 1987; 2:272–279.
110. Stine EL, Wingfield A, Poon IW. How much and how fast: Rapid processing of spoken language in later adulthood. Psychol Aging 1986; 1:303–311.
111. Sundberg ND, Snowden LR, Reynolds WM. Toward assessment of personal competence and incompetence in life situations. Ann Rev Psychol 1978; 29:179–221.
112. Sunderland A, Watts K, Baddeley AD, Harris JE. Subjective memory assessment and test performance in the elderly. J Gerontol 1986; 41:376–384.
113. Tamir L. Communication and the aging process. New York: Pergamon Press, 1979.
114. Taub HA. Comprehension and memory of prose materials by young and old adults. J Gerontol 1979: 33:725–730.
115. Taub HA, Baker MT, Sturr JF. Informed consent for research: Effects of readability, patient age, and education. J Am Geriatr Soc 1986; 34:601–606.
116. Twining TC. Social skill, psychological disorder, and aging. Int J Aging Hum Dev 1983; 17:7–13.
117. Ulatowska HK, Cannito MP, Hayashi MM, Fleming SG. Language abilities in the elderly. In: Ulatowska HK, ed. The aging brain: Communication in the elderly. San Diego: College-Hill Press, 1985:125–139.
118. Walker VG, Hardiman CJ, Hedrick DL, Holbrook DL. Speech and language characteristics of an aging population. In: Lass NJ, ed. Speech and language: Advances in basic research and practice. Vol. 6. New York: Academic Press, 1981:143–202.
119. White JD, Regan MMS. Otologic considerations. In: Mueller HG, Geoffrey VC, eds. Communication disorders in aging: Assessment and management. Washington, D.C.: Gallaudet University Press, 1987:36.
120. Wingfield A, Poon IW, Lombardi L, Lowe D. Speed of processing in normal aging: Effects of speech rate, linguistic structure, and processing time. J Gerontol 1985; 40:579–585.
121. Wingfield A, Stine EAL, Lahar CJ, Aberdeen JS. Does the capacity of working memory change with age? Exp Aging Res 1988; 14:103–107.

# CHAPTER 7

# *Language Changes in Dementia of the Alzheimer Type*

DANIEL KEMPLER, Ph.D.

In 1907 Alzheimer described a demented woman who "frequently used perplexing phrases...some paraphrastic expressions" (*milk-pourer* instead of *cup*) and suffered from a significant language comprehension deficit.[4] Language disorders continue to be one of the most obvious and well-studied symptoms of dementia and are particularly pronounced in dementia of the Alzheimer type (DAT). The incidence of language impairment in dementia is estimated to be between 88 and 95 percent, and is close to 100 percent in DAT.[30,127] This chapter will (1) describe the language disorder associated with various stages of DAT; (2) review several prominent research questions about the origin and interpretation of these language disorders; (3) discuss clinical implications of this research for diagnosis and treatment of language disorders in DAT; and (4) sketch out important areas of future research.

## Overview of Language in DAT

The many descriptions of language in dementia that have appeared over the past decade confirm and expand Alzheimer's original observation of word-finding deficits, paraphasias, and comprehension impairment.[3,9,30,64,91,106,108] It should be noted that Alzheimer patients have little or no peripheral weakness or incoordination, and have no obvious motor speech deficits: control of phonation, articulation, and resonance remains intact until the latest stages. In addition, the ability to arrange words into grammatical sentences appears to be relatively spared throughout the course of the disease. The communication problems of this population are largely confined to the two aspects of language: lexicon (word knowledge) and pragmatics, the use of contextually appropriate language. As might be expected with a degenerative process, the deficits change over time, and each phase of the disease is characterized by a distinct profile of language deficits.*

## EARLY-STAGE DEFICITS

The earliest language deficit observed in DAT is anomia. DAT patients have difficulty coming up with words in structured tasks such as word-list generation (e.g., name as many animals as you can) as well as in elicited narratives and spontaneous conversation.[72,104,105] Semantically empty words (e.g., *thing, stuff, do*) are scattered throughout the DAT patient's utterances in place of content words, thereby maintaining fluency and sacrificing informational content. Language comprehension for simple, structured, concrete material appears intact during these early stages. However, comprehension of abstract language that does not rely on meaning of single words in syntactic structures, but rather requires inference (e.g., Rome wasn't built in a day; She took a sudden turn for the worse), is poor even in the earliest stages of DAT.[25,74] Also, early on, patients have a difficult time generating spontaneous language via writing, although the mechanics of writing and

---

*Throughout this chapter, the terms "early/mild," "moderate," and "severe/late" will be used to describe the nondiscrete stages associated with the 5 to 15 year course of DAT, which begins with mild cognitive symptoms and ends in a persistent vegetative state.

reading remain intact.[30,58,113] At this point, DAT patients can communicate sufficiently for most social situations, although they may not be able to follow complex conversations and may tend to digress or repeat themselves. Although the DAT patient is often initially aware of his or her own language deficits, this awareness appears to wane by the end of the early phase.

A sample of a narrative description (from Kempler) of the cookie theft picture from The Boston Diagnostic Aphasia Examination (Fig. 7.1) illustrates some of these points.[69] Note particularly the repetition of ideas (Momma's washing dishes), empty words (somebody's doing), paraphasias (single pencil), difficulty with appropriate use of pronouns (My teacher...they...), and a hint of awareness of the difficulty (My teacher should be here...). Despite these difficulties, this patient is able to describe the major events and participants in the picture.

**Examiner**

I want you just to tell me what's going on in this picture.

**Alzheimer patient**

Momma's washing dishes and children are taking jam or jelly or something from the jar, and the little fella's about ready to fall on the floor. And Momma's washing dishes.

**Examiner**

Good. Anything else?

**Alzheimer patient**

Well, the overflow of the water.

**Examiner**

That's right. What about that?

**Alzheimer patient**

That's the overrun of, I said, of the dishwater on the floor.

**Examiner**

Why do you think that's happening?

**Alzheimer patient**

You can see her mouth is open and she is talking, and not paying any attention. That's about all I can think of. Or somebody's going, one of the children are about to climb, or something like these one, these ones. My teacher should be here and they'd throw me out the door.

**Examiner**

Oh, you're doing a good job. What about here (point to girl taking cookie)?

**Alzheimer patient**

The little one? She's asking her mother for a cookie. It's very easy. They're very, uh, well done, you know, by a single, uh, jar, no, I mean single pencil, whatever they're using.

**Examiner**

Great.

## MODERATE-STAGE DEFICITS

By the moderate stages of DAT, patients begin to have more difficulty with both production and comprehension of language. In production, anomia worsens and word-finding deficits are made more obvious by copious substitutions of empty words and circumlocutions for information-bearing nouns and verbs. The utterances of moderate DAT patients are often difficult to follow because of pragmatic deficits, including poor topic maintenance and poor use of pronouns.[12,55,104,114,128] It is somewhat surprising that in the context of these pronounced discourse deficits, certain other discourse skills, such as turn-taking in conversation, remain undisturbed. Comprehension for complex material (e.g., sequential instructions) is often impaired by this stage.[3] Although the mechanics of reading aloud and writing remain unimpaired, deficits in producing well-formed coherent writing and reading for comprehension parallel problems observed in auditory-spoken language.[3,30,31] In the moderate stages, DAT patients'

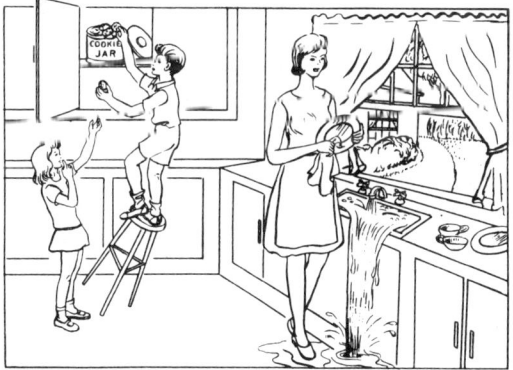

Figure 7.1 Cookie theft picture. Reprinted from Goodglass H, Kaplan E. The assessment of aphasia and related disorders. Philadelphia: Lea & Febiger, 1972.

conversations become difficult to follow, and the patients may withdraw slightly from social situations in which communication demands may occur. They often appear unaware of their communicative deficits at this point.

The more severe language deficits associated with this stage are illustrated by another narrative description of the cookie theft picture.[69] At this point, the empty words and paraphasias render the narrative largely uninterpretable. The patient's use of descriptive phrases that have no direct relationship to the picture (canned goods, politically well known) elicit several requests for clarification from the examiner. However, the patient appears unable to clarify the narrative. Notice the preservation of sentence structure, including some syntactic complexities (e.g., "apparently because he has a tendency to be falling").

#### Examiner

I just want you to describe what's going on in this picture. Tell me what's going on here.

#### Alzheimer patient

This picture incorporates a certain amount of coming and going, and cheating, and doing the things in the world...[pause]...planning some for uh money on the floor, not worrying about it. Falling over onto the ground.

#### Examiner

Speak a little louder.

#### Alzheimer patient

Oh that he has the ability to—she has the ability to change the timing and then and then the wind is blowing in the wind, blowing in the floor. Wind is blowing on the canned goods.

#### Examiner

The wind is blowing on the canned goods?

#### Alzheimer patient

Yeah, splattering.

#### Examiner

What's she doing (point to woman at sink)?

#### Alzheimer patient

She is not only losing, doings, washing her payplate there, but also being careful of the child, apparently because he has a tendency to be falling this, slipping. And then there's a child slipping again, or more normally.

#### Examiner

More normally?

#### Alzheimer patient

Yeah, politically well known.

#### Examiner

Politically well known. What's going on over here (point to stool)?

#### Alzheimer patient

Well, it seems to be that they're trying to, filling up and ideal of it inside there...(pause)...things that we eat...play with and maybe get hurt. Candy or something.

## LATE-STAGE DEFICITS

By the later stages of the disease, verbal production becomes uninterpretable because of paraphasias (word and sound substitutions) and lack of coherence. Late in the course of the disease, dysarthria may impair speech intelligibility. Eventually, the patients manifest echolalia (repetition of others), palilalia (repetition of self), and muteness. At this point, comprehension is impaired in all modalities, even for single words, and the patients are no longer successfully participating in social interaction through language or any other communicative modalities.

## INTERPRETING LANGUAGE DEFICITS IN DAT

A few important observations about language in DAT must be mentioned before proceeding. First, there are language impairments that do *not* occur in DAT. For instance, there are no reports of agrammatism of the type associated with Broca's aphasia in DAT. There are also no reports of disproportionate difficulty with repetition: in fact, unbidden repetition in the form of echolalia and palilalia is one of the characteristics of late-stage DAT. And finally, there are no descriptions of phonologic disturbance; that is, DAT patients apparently do not violate the phonotactic constraints of their native language (using nonnative sounds or sound combinations) or make errors in prosodic aspects of language.[3,104,127] We emerge with a picture of language breakdown in DAT that is quite specific: Semantic and pragmatic deficits are marked; morphosyntactic deficits are rare, and phonologic deficits are rarer still.

Second, many authors have attempted to describe the language disturbance of DAT by comparison with focal aphasia, arriving at the conclusion, for example, that transcortical sensory and Wernicke's aphasias are frequent in DAT.[3,30] I have avoided classifying the language disturbance of DAT as an "aphasia" for two reasons. First, although the term aphasia can be used to describe any language disorder, it has become associated with syndromes where language disorder is primary, or significantly worse than any other symptom. This is not true for the DAT population. Although the language of DAT does manifest some typical aphasic symptoms (anomia, semantic paraphasias, and comprehension deficits), the language disorder of DAT is not primary or isolated but rather persists among other intellectual impairments. I concur with Holland et al that "aphasia...is a difficult, if not glib, diagnosis to apply in such cases. In the context of general deterioration of intellectual function, language disorder typically becomes intertwined with so many concomitant neurobehavioral changes as to render the term aphasia almost useless."[57] Second, identifying the language disorder of DAT as an aphasia may imply (by association with focal aphasias) that there is a static quality to the disorder and that there is the possibility of recovery. However, because DAT is unrelentingly progressive and degenerative, so are the language disorders associated with it. The language deficits are continually changing and recovery has never been observed. The language patterns of focal aphasias may be similar to the language disorder of DAT in some ways, but also differ in many important respects (see also Ulatowska et al for discussion).[128] This must be remembered when planning research, considering diagnoses, or contemplating treatment.

## Research: Dissociations and Associations

Four areas of current research on language functions in DAT will be reviewed here: semantic impairment, syntactic preservation, pragmatic deficits, and brain-behavior relationships.

### SEMANTIC IMPAIRMENT IN DAT

Anomia (word-finding difficulty) is the earliest and most common language symptom of DAT. As such, accurate description of the symptoms and origins of anomia in DAT has been the subject of much research.

The earliest explanation for anomia in DAT was a visual perceptual deficit. Several pieces of evidence support this claim: naming by DAT patients is improved if the patients are allowed additional sensory cues (e.g., touching the object).[7] DAT patients often use the name of an object that is visually similar to the stimulus in tasks of confrontation naming (e.g., calling an anchor a "hammer");[115] these patients are better able to name objects that are very familiar and thus require less visual recognition (e.g., body parts) than less familiar objects.[15] Kirshner, Webb, and Kelly systematically investigated the effect of visual perception on naming by comparing object naming of actual objects, photographs, line drawings, and visually degraded drawings.[79] Their results indicated that perceptual difficulty did play a significant role in anomia of DAT patients. However, problems with this theory are obvious: First, it does not explain why DAT patients are anomic in spontaneous conversation where no visual perceptual skills come into play,[72] and, second, the theory is not consistent with the finding that most verbal paraphasias in DAT are substitutions of semantically (not visually) related object names.[11,60,70] Further evidence against the visual perceptual argument comes from recent studies that demonstrate that DAT patients with significant anomia perform relatively well on independent measures of visual form discrimination.[20,61]

The search for clues into the origin of anomia in DAT has continued beyond the visual perceptual theory and has focused on specifically semantic deficits, that is, problems in (1) impaired lexical access and (2) deterioration of lexical representations. There is some evidence that underlying lexical representations are intact and that naming difficulties arise from a problem in lexical access or retrieval for verbal production. Evidence supporting this view includes the findings that:

1. In tasks of confrontation naming, DAT patients can often give a related name or circumlocution, suggesting that they know much about the meaning of the word but cannot find the exact name (e.g., "cutter" for saw; "this is for your eyes" for glasses).[11,70]
2. Comprehension of words is generally superior to production of the same words, indicating that the underlying representation can often be accessed in a passive comprehension task when the name cannot be generated or retrieved on demand.[70]
3. DAT patients can utilize phonemic cues to help retrieve words, indicating again that the information is there but cannot be easily retrieved.[52,103]
4. There have been several reports of DAT patients using gesture to indicate the function of an object that they could not name, suggesting that the deficit is limited to

lexical retrieval and may not affect basic symbolic representations presumed to underlie both gestural and language productions.[52,70,119]

Another source of support for this view comes from semantic priming data that indicate that subconscious semantic associations may be intact in DAT.[98,100,101] The findings of semantic priming in DAT are perhaps the most curious of all and require some explication. Several researchers have demonstrated that, like normal subjects, DAT patients react faster in lexical decision formats (i.e., is it a word?) if the target word (e.g., nurse) is preceded by a related word (e.g., doctor) than if it is preceded by an unrelated word (e.g., shoe).[101] Initially, this was taken to indicate that underlying semantic associations were intact and that the anomia was not the result of permanent underlying semantic problems but must be an effect of impaired lexical access. However, findings from other studies have not always confirmed intact semantic priming in DAT. For instance, Smith et al found that DAT patients did not exhibit any effect of priming,[126] and Albert and Milberg found semantic priming only in a subset of DAT patients.[2] Several other studies have found that DAT patients actually show *greater* priming effects than control subjects.[20,99] In addition, Chertkow et al found that hyperpriming in DAT was associated specifically with words that were shown to be semantically degraded on a variety of other tasks (e.g., responses to probe questions).[20]

In summary, the positive results of the early priming studies suggested intact semantic representations in DAT, but follow-up studies have demonstrated abnormal responses to semantic priming including (1) lack of priming effects; (2) subgroup differences; and (3) hyperpriming. Perhaps most interesting, the finding of hyperpriming appears to coincide with *degraded* semantic representations for particular words and has been used to support the theory that DAT patients suffer from disrupted semantic representations.[20] It is to this possibility that we now turn.

Perhaps the first convincing evidence for the proposal that anomia in DAT is a reflection of impaired semantic representations was presented in a case study.[119] Through a variety of methodologies to examine lexical knowledge (e.g., naming, verbal, and nonverbal match to sample), Schwartz et al were able to attribute the naming errors (e.g., calling a dog a "cat") to an erosion of referential boundaries. This finding has been supported by observations that many DAT naming errors are within-category errors (e.g., "truck" for car), a finding consistent with a deficit in the underlying conceptual and semantic representations.[70] Additional evidence that representations within semantic categories may be degraded in DAT comes from studies that have demonstrated correspondence between naming and word comprehension errors and consistency of response across several testing sessions.[20,54,71,89] These findings are consonant with the notion of central degeneration of lexical representation, which would be expected to permanently affect both comprehension and production of specific items. Although there is a growing consensus that DAT patients do exhibit evidence of impaired lexical representations, there are only general proposals about the type of disruption that occurs within the lexical representation. For instance, Schwartz et al discussed the problem as a "breakdown in the structure of the underlying categories,"[119] while Chertkow et al referred to the "degraded" semantic representations,[20] and Grober et al proposed that the representations are disorganized.[50] Specific models of the exact nature of the representational deficit will undoubtedly be the subject of future research.

In summary, word-finding problems are among the earliest and most obvious symptoms of DAT, but the underlying cause(s) of anomia remain disputed.[9,11,30] Although most researchers concur that the origins are primarily cognitive, there is still considerable disagreement about whether the deficit is best characterized as a processing limitation that interferes with lexical access or as a deficit in the underlying lexical representations. Further, because DAT patients have significant problems in attention and memory, correlations between performance on tests of attention and tests of naming have led other researchers to attribute anomia in DAT to problems in attention and concentration.[105,120] This review of recent research suggests that the anomia of DAT is heterogeneous and that no single explanation can account for the naming performance of any group of DAT patients. Visual perception, attention, lexical access, and deterioration of lexical representations all play a role in anomia of DAT. It is likely that individual patients may be more or less affected by one particular deficit and that groups of DAT patients fall into distinct subgroups demonstrating anomia for different reasons.[71]

## SYNTACTIC ABILITIES IN DAT

Although most descriptions of language in DAT have observed that syntactic ability appears intact, few experimental investigations have addressed this question. The earliest detailed investigation of this phenomenon was Whitaker's description of a severely demented patient who spontaneously corrected agrammatic but not semantically anomalous sentences in repetition (e.g., "There are two book on the table" was repeated as "There are few books on the table" while "The book is very happy" was repeated verbatim).[131] This finding was taken to indicate that grammatical competence was selectively preserved and, therefore, must be somehow autonomous from the rest of cognition. Schwartz, Marin, and Saffran also examined a single subject in detail and found that their patient, despite severely deteriorated semantic ability, was able to manipulate syntactic structures (e.g., turn an active in a passive), again supporting the notion that the syntactic processor may in fact be special and neuropsychologically insulated from cognitive and cortical degeneration seen in DAT.[119] Subsequent attempts to address this issue have found DAT patients to produce syntactically complex and well-formed sentences in spontaneous speech as well.[55,72]

Kempler et al evaluated the spontaneous speech of 10 DAT patients and 10 normal controls, and demonstrated that the spontaneous speech of DAT patients contained few syntactic errors and many lexical semantic errors.[72] More important, the range and frequency of sentence types (e.g., relative clauses, questions, and adverbial clauses) were almost identical to the normal controls (rank order correlation, $p = .9833$; $p < .0000$), and there was no difference between the DAT patients and the control population on a measure of structural complexity. A second study reported by Kempler et al further confirmed the relative preservation of syntactic competence through a dictation task adapted from Schwartz et al.[72,119] Twenty DAT patients and 20 normal controls were asked to write short phrases containing a homophone, a word that has one pronunciation (si) but two spellings (sea/see) and two meanings (body of water/visual perception). In each case, the words can be disambiguated by semantic cues (a word with a similar meaning such as "*lake*-sea," "*look*-see") or a syntactic cue (a word with little semantic content but definite syntactic restrictions on what can follow such as "*the* sea, "*I* see"). The DAT patients made significantly more errors than did the control subjects with both types of cues, and significantly more errors with the semantic cues than with the syntactic cues, suggesting that the disease does seem to spare the ability to use syntactic (more than semantic) knowledge in a writing task of this sort.

Comprehension of syntax has not proven to be as consistently intact as production of syntax. Schwartz, Marin, and Saffran[119] demonstrated intact comprehension of four syntactic forms (active, passive, preposition, and comparative adjectives) by a single demented patient. However, Emery, using the Test of Syntactic Complexity[34] and the Chomsky Test of Syntax,[21] has documented syntactic comprehension deficits in a larger sample of 20 DAT subjects.[35] These tests evaluate the patient's comprehension of syntax by eliciting verbal responses to grammatically complex stimuli (e.g., "The dog was bitten by the cat; which animal bit the other and which was bitten?") or gestural responses to similarly complex auditory stimuli (e.g., "Mickey tells Donald to hop up and down; make him hop."). In contrast to Schwartz et al's findings of preserved comprehension of grammatically complex structures, Emery found significant impairment in DAT patients' ability to process syntactically complex grammatical constructions.

It is not simple to evaluate the intactness of grammatical knowledge with conflicting data: intact production versus impaired comprehension. Uneven profiles of grammatical abilities across tasks have been observed in other forms of brain damage, and explanations for these dissociations fall into two broad categories:[83] those that postulate modality specific blockage (e.g., a motor output problem in the case of preserved comprehension and impaired production in Broca's aphasia) and those that postulate selectively impaired independent processors for different grammatical tasks.[134] The dissociation between intact syntactic production and impaired comprehension in DAT may have another explanation: Overall memory and processing demands may have affected performance on comprehension tasks more than production tasks. Emery argued against this explanation, citing the finding that DAT patients were able to *repeat* all of the stimuli accurately even though they could not comprehend them, suggesting that the problem is not necessarily one of memory but more likely the result of deterioration of complex syntactic processing.[35] A recent study by Smith investigated the relative contribution of syntactic knowledge and general processing demands to performance on tests of syntactic comprehension.[125] Smith presented a group of 22 DAT patients with a picture-pointing task to assess comprehension of reciprocals and reflexives, systematically varying elements that contribute to processing difficulty and syntactic complexity (e.g., two- versus four-choice response arrays and different position of the reflexive in the sentence). The results demonstrated that both DAT patients and controls showed performance decrements as task difficulty increased, and both groups showed a similar pattern of errors. These results were interpreted to indicate that comprehension deficits in DAT may be attributed to general processing limitations and not to a specifically syntactic deficit.

We are left with the finding that despite severe lexical semantic deficits, DAT patients retain grammatical ability in (1) spontaneous utterance production; (2) tasks of sentence comprehension; and (3) writing to dictation. This dissociation between syntactic and semantic abilities has been explained by recourse to the notion of automaticity.[66,72,122] Syntactic structure has the characteristics of a domain that could be run by an automatic processor: The number of syntactic structures is limited, and each instance is frequent. Syntactic ability appears to fit the characteristics of automaticity insofar as syntactic processes "operate independently of the subject's control...do not require attention...and they do not use up short-term capacity."[118] Lexical selection, on the other hand, can be characterized as a system operated by a controlled processor: There is a large range of alternatives for each occurrence, and each word is relatively infrequent when compared with each syntactic structure. On the basis of this dichotomy, it has been suggested that automatic functions may be preserved in DAT,[66] and that grammatical ability may be just one instance of an automatic cognitive operation being preserved in the context of general cognitive decline.[72]

The research on syntactic abilities in DAT has more general implications for theories of mental functions. Dissociations between mental functions reveal the cognitive and neurologic independence of these abilities and have led scientists to many of the important discoveries of hemispheric specialization and localization of function.[16,44,130] Age-old arguments about the relative interdependence of cognitive functions continue today under the terms modularity[38,39] and connectionism.[117] Although the research in these areas increasingly relies on mathematic models and computational solutions, data from abnormal populations still provide supporting evidence for the relative interdependence of various cognitive abilities. As such, syntactic sparing in DAT demonstrates that syntactic ability can function in the adult without support from semantic and other cognitive or conceptual operations.

## PRAGMATICS: UNEXPLAINED DEFICITS

Pragmatics, the study of language use in context, includes a large variety of language skills from turn-taking to appropriate topic introduction and overall discourse structure, all generally considered within the context of interpersonal interaction. In its broadest sense, pragmatics covers everything relevant to communication beyond sentence structure and linguistic semantics, often including extralinguistic features of facial expression and body language. In comparison with other language functions, we know least about pragmatic disturbance in DAT. Because very little research has been reported on the pragmatic abilities of DAT patients, much of what can be said about this area is anecdotal and in need of confirmation (see Chapter 8 for more detail on discourse and dementia).

Some aspects of discourse are clearly preserved in DAT through the mild and moderate stages: DAT patients take conversational turns when appropriate and often produce socially ritualized parts of the conversations (e.g., greetings and leave takings) with appropriate timing, affect, and linguistic structure. These observations indicate that DAT patients are able to adhere to basic structures and obey pragmatic rules of some verbal interactions. However, there are also subtle pragmatic problems early on, such as a tendency to repeat things unnecessarily and to lose the topic of the conversation. At this stage the deficits are often attributed to failing attention and memory.

By the moderate stages of the disease, the discourse of DAT patients often becomes irrelevant, lacking in topical cohesion, and grossly insensitive to the needs of the listener.[12,55,104,114,128] Hutchinson and Jensen analyzed conversations of 10 dementia patients (and 5 healthy controls) and found several pragmatic abnormalities including: (1) patients produced fewer utterances and more turns, resulting in fewer utterances per turn; (2) patients produced more directives (utterances aimed at getting the listener to do something, such as explain or clarify); (3) patients produced more utterances for which no intent could be determined; and (4) patients initiated more new topics, often inappropriately.[63] Further investigations of discourse in DAT have confirmed and expanded Hutchinson and Jensen's original findings.[114,128] Particular attention has focused on the production of decreased information content and lack of coherence. Ripich and Terrell suggested that the perception of conversational incoherence on the part of DAT patients might be attributed to "absent pieces of discourse that should provide relationships between preceding texts and that which follows."[114] Ulatowska et al found that decreased informativeness could be traced back, at least in part, to problems in reference such as the overuse of demonstratives (e.g., here, there) and exophoric reference (e.g., *this* without a clear antecedent).[128]

Still unaddressed are the underlying causes of the discourse problems in DAT. These deficits could be secondary to existing and documented problems such as anomia, decreased attention, and poor memory. On the other hand, they may result from more general pragmatic deficits that impair the ability of the DAT patient to take the perspective of the listener and to judge what information is important in the particular discourse. Further, DAT may selectively affect specific discourse knowledge. For instance, certain discourses are structured largely on the basis of internalized scripts—rules about what type of information is mentioned first, second, and so on. This knowledge of narrative superstructure, much like internal representation of lexical items, could deteriorate and cause discourse breakdown. Any of these deficits could create incoherent conversations.

One investigation specifically looked for associations between discourse impairments and other language deficits for a clue to the underlying cause of the discourse problems. Nicholas et al compared DAT patients' performance on the Boston Naming Test (BNT)[46] with elements of empty speech in narrative descriptions of the cookie theft picture,[47] in an attempt to evaluate the claim that discourse incoherence could be attributed to anomia.[104] The authors reported a significant negative correlation between the score of DAT patients on the Boston Naming Test and the use of indefinite terms (e.g., "thing" and "stuff") and a significant positive correlation between the BNT and the production of "content elements" (i.e., references to characters and activities, in cookie theft stories). They concluded that the naming deficit did not underlie the emptiness of discourse, presumably because many other measures of discourse emptiness (e.g., paraphasias, pronouns with antecedents, and deictic terms) did not correlate with the BNT scores. The data, however, also suggest that at least some of the referential problems that make discourse difficult to follow might be a result of anomia. That is, to the degree to which patients are anomic and substitute or omit content elements, their discourse will be difficult to interpret. Nicholas et al are undoubtedly correct in their general conclusion that the anomia *does not underlie* the discourse deficits, but it is unarguable that the anomia *does contribute* to the observed discourse deficits.

Further description of the discourse problems in DAT can be used to delineate which aspects of pragmatics are related to which aspects of linguistic and nonlinguistic cognition. For instance, it can be hypothesized that some aspects of discourse (e.g., topic maintenance) depend on recent memory but may be independent of lexical and morphosyntactic function. Therefore, we could predict that these features would correlate with decreased memory and be deficient early on in the disease. Conversely, some aspects of discourse are more structural (e.g., the use of definite and indefinite articles to signal new versus old topics) and may be retained with morphosyntactic abilities. Other aspects of pragmatics may be unrelated to either memory or morphosyntax (e.g., politeness and use of speech registers) and therefore should not correlate with either. At this time, these are only conjectures to be investigated in the future. In summary, although little research has been reported to date, DAT is a likely place to start identifying the cognitive bases of pragmatic knowledge.

## BRAIN-BEHAVIOR RELATIONSHIPS

Any neurogenic language disorder provides the opportunity to learn more about the language, the brain, and the relationship between the two. By correlating language disturbance with various types and locations of brain lesions, we have learned a great deal about the neural representation (lateralization and localization) of language.[18,76] Although the language and neuropathologic changes associated with DAT are not as focal and specific as in cases of cerebral vascular accident (CVA), neither are they global or diffuse. For instance, we have seen that language changes affect semantics and pragmatics preferentially but leave grammatical and phonologic abilities relatively spared. Likewise, the neurologic picture is multifocal: Excessive numbers of neurofibrillary tangles, plaques, neuronal loss, gliosis, and amyloid angiopathy are found in association cortex and in the limbic system, but the primary motor and sensory areas are characteristically spared.[23,29]

There are both direct and indirect methods of investigating the neurologic bases of language deficits in DAT. Direct observation of neuropathology is possible only through brain biopsy or autopsy. Because of the time course of the disease, direct histologically derived clinicopathologic correlations are difficult to specify in DAT; the distribution of plaques and tangles at postmortem can tell you little about the relationship between the brain and language performance at the point of interest some years earlier. Nonetheless, grossly spared versus grossly pathologic areas of the brain correlate with what is known about behavior in DAT and contribute to our theories of brain function. Chui reviewed clinicopathologic correlations in DAT and associated the fluent speech production of DAT with sparing of the primary motor and sensory cortex, while the impaired semantics was associated with deteriorated temporal-parietal association cortex.[23] Clinicopathologic correlations, then, suggest that expressive fluency and syntactic ability may be subserved by primary motor and sensory areas in the anterior portions of the cerebral hemispheres, while semantic abilities depend on temporal and parietal association cortex. By inference, this strong association between fundamental linguistic and basic sensorimotor abilities lends support to theories of brain function that have stressed the functional and even evolutionary connections between neural control of motor and sequencing skills and the specialized linguistic capacity of man's left hemisphere.[77]

Noninvasive, indirect measurements of brain structure and function have the distinct advantage of allowing comparison of brain structure and function at or near the time of language evaluation. In vivo measures can be divided into two general categories: those showing brain structure—computed tomography (CT) and magnetic resonance imaging (MRI)—and those showing brain function—electroencephalogram (EEG), positron emission tomography (PET), and single photon scanning (SPECT). Studies of structural abnormality in DAT have been relatively unrevealing. DAT patients tend to have enlarged ventricles and widened cortical sulci on CT and MRI, and these changes generally do not correlate with the presence or severity of dementia.[42,68,85] Although this is essentially a negative result, it highlights the interesting fact that structural abnormality on CT and MRI scans is in no way prerequisite to serious, permanent language disturbance.

Studies of brain function in DAT have shown that the structural damage that may be minimal or invisible on CT or MRI has significant consequences for brain function as measured by blood flow or glucose utilization. Decrease in cerebral blood flow is a consistent finding in DAT;[135] it appears to correlate with severity and to be most pronounced in the parietal regions.[65] The particular patterns of brain dysfunction in comparison with language deficits are of interest here. Recent research has demonstrated that there are subgroups of DAT patients that present with primarily language or constructional deficits, and these subgroups display different patterns of cortical hypometabolism in the expected directions: Patients with marked anomia demonstrated lower metabolic rates in the left temporal regions; patients with focal visuo-constructive impairment showed relatively more hypofunction in the right temporal and parietal regions.[19,41,88] These studies extend our notions of brain-behavior relations to include measures of glucose utilization. To date, most studies appear to coincide with the familiar division of function between the hemispheres and between the lobes that we have come to accept from years of clinicopathologic correlations.

The next step toward deciphering the neurofunctional code is to perform detailed case studies in which we can correlate specific language and cognitive deficits with specific patterns of brain dysfunction. One case study with serial PET scans of a DAT patient has attempted to do this.[32] In this case, although the patient showed significant memory deficits early on, the initial PET scan showed no abnormality. In addition, although no additional neuropsychologic deficits appeared during the course of the study, the patient showed decreased parietal metabolism in the two later scans. This case highlights the lack of correlation between observed behavior and measurable brain function when DAT patients are examined individually.

In summary, the investigations into brain-behavior relationships with DAT tend to uphold traditional models of cerebral function of language, but force us to expand those models in certain ways. It is clear that gross left-hemisphere structural change is not prerequisite for a lasting language disorder and that measures of brain function (e.g., blood flow) are not yet sensitive enough to correlate with language dysfunction on an individual case basis. It is also clear that the type of structural and functional damage seen in DAT spares primary motor and sensory regions as well as areas thought to subserve syntactic function. Further research into brain function in DAT will undoubtedly add to our knowledge of the neural representation and neuropathology of language.

## Clinical Issues

Any clinical consideration of dementia or DAT must include a discussion of evaluation, differential diagnosis, and potential treatment. Each of these issues will be taken up in turn. For further discussion of diagnostic and treatment issues, see Chapters 13 and 15.

### EVALUATION

The goal of the language evaluation is to reach or confirm a diagnosis and, ultimately, to develop a treatment plan. Language evaluation of dementia patients combines two elements not usually relevant to other populations: age and multiple cognitive deficits. The special considerations that need to be addressed because of the relatively old age of these patients are well described in a recent chapter by Groher, and include admonishments for the clinician to: (1) allow ample time for all aspects of the evaluation to compensate for the inevitable slowing that accompanies age; and (2) compensate to the degree possible for peripheral disturbance (e.g., decreased vision and hearing) within the test environment to prevent these factors from contaminating the evaluation of central language abilities.[51]

The second important point to remember in evaluation of a demented patient is the likelihood of multiple cognitive deficits in addition to language disturbance. It is essential to establish the relative severity of nonlanguage deficits in memory, attention, nonverbal problem solving, daily living skills, and spatial orientation. These factors will be important for reaching a diagnosis as well as for implementing a treatment program. For instance, severely impaired episodic memory (memory for personal experiences) will preclude direct teaching of any compensatory techniques (e.g., self-cueing); the self-care level will tell you what the patient's daily interactions are like and what type of language production and comprehension skills the patient needs in his particular social environment.

Both formal and informal tests should be used. Standardized aphasia batteries are valuable for their inclusion of many aspects of language functioning (naming, comprehension, reading, writing, spontaneous speech, repetition),[47,75,112] and the Communication Abilities in Daily Living (CADL) provides additional information about functional skills.[36] However, with the exception of The Arizona Battery for Communication Disorders of Dementia, standardized tests have little or no normative data for the demented population.[10] Other specific tests (e.g., Token Test, Reading Comprehension Battery for Aphasia, and Boston Naming Test) are valuable for in-depth analysis of particular aspects of language. Analysis of language samples taken from conversation is also important because they provide a gauge of an individual's communicative abilities in a relatively unstructured situation.

## DIFFERENTIAL DIAGNOSIS

Differential diagnosis refers to the characteristics that distinguish one disease from another. It is an important step in reaching a probable diagnosis and crucial in arriving at a useful treatment plan. With most dementias and with DAT in particular, definite diagnosis can only be made on the basis of histopathology and is therefore limited to patients who agree to a brain biopsy or have come to postmortem. Therefore, there is a great need to improve our ability to diagnose DAT on the basis of clinical evaluation. The issue of the differential clinical diagnosis of DAT has been taken up by a special composite panel of NINCDS-ADRDA personnel that produced published guidelines for diagnosis of probable DAT.[90] The criteria include documented dementia with deficits in two or more areas of cognition (including language), progressive worsening of cognitive deficits, no disturbance of consciousness, and the absence of other disorders or diseases that could account for the progressive deficit in memory and cognition. Some researchers have proposed somewhat more stringent criteria for the clinical diagnosis of DAT, requiring deficits in three areas of cognition and even suggesting that language disturbance be required for the diagnosis.[30] From the perspective of the speech-language pathologist, it is hoped that an adequate description of language in DAT will help to distinguish this from other forms of dementia, including multi-infarct dementia, normal pressure hydrocephalus, and dementia associated with extrapyramidal disorders. An adequate history of language symptoms and a thorough language evaluation should go a long way toward differentiating DAT from other forms of dementia. Language features that help to distinguish DAT from other dementia syndromes include: presence or absence of specific language symptoms, onset and course of language disorder, and order of appearance of language disorder vis-a-vis other problems such as motor disturbance. The remainder of this section will highlight the use of language disorders for discriminating between various dementia syndromes.

### Reversible Dementias

There are many causes of potentially reversible dementia, including intracranial conditions (e.g., tumors and hydrocephalus), vitamin-deficiency states, endocrine disorders, drug intoxication, exposure to toxins or infections, and dementia resulting from affective disorders.[29] Some studies estimate that up to 30 percent of the demented population may be suffering from a potentially reversible dementia. A thorough history and medical work-up are the best ways to differentially diagnose reversible dementias. A few of the more common reversible dementias, however, do distinguish themselves from DAT on the basis of language symptoms, or more specifically, their lack of language symptoms. For instance, the dementia associated with normal pressure hydrocephalus, resulting from impairment in the circulation of cerebrospinal fluid through the ventricles, is perhaps the most common potentially treatable cause of dementia.[87] Hydrocephalic dementias generally present with a triad of dementia, ataxia of gait, and urinary incontinence. Although language deficits are generally not present, these patients may *appear* to have a sentence-formulation problem or anomia caused by the substantial psychomotor retardation (mental slowing) that typically accompanies the syndrome. Unlike those with DAT, hydrocephalic patients can eventually generate the appropriate word or sentence without cues and have no language comprehension deficits. The absence of true language disturbance and the presence of a motoric (gait) disturbance early on in the course of the disease should alert the clinician to a clinical presentation *inconsistent* with DAT.

Another potentially reversible form of dementia is the "pseudodementia" associated with affective disorders such as depression. The dementia syndrome accompanying depression typically presents with psychomotor slowing, forgetfulness, disorientation, impaired attention, and disturbed ability to abstract and grasp the meaning of situations.[29] Signs of cortical impairment such as language disturbance are not present. This dementia, if recognized and treated appropriately, has the same cure rate as any depressive illness.

## Subcortical Dementia

Dementia is a common and debilitating symptom associated with extrapyramidal disorders such as Huntington's disease, Parkinson's disease, and progressive supranuclear palsy.[27,28] Although motor disturbance is generally the earliest and most pervasive symptom in subcortical diseases, cognitive deficits occur in a large percentage of these patients. The standard symptoms of subcortical dementias include disorders of motivation, mood, attention, memory, personality, slowness of thought processes, and impaired ability to manipulate acquired knowledge (see Chapter 2).[1,27,29] These patients generally do not present with agnosia or apraxia. It has also been assumed that, although communication is severely impaired by dysarthria and cognitive deficits, patients with subcortical dementia are not aphasic. However, recent research calls into question the status of preserved language in subcortical dementia: Demented patients with Huntington's disease are anomic and demonstrate a range of other language deficits including reduced syntactic complexity;[17,48] demented patients with progressive supranuclear palsy (PSP) have been noted to have deficits in word selection;[107] and demented Parkinson's patients have been shown to have severely impaired syntactic comprehension.[82] The data demonstrating impaired comprehension in Parkinson's disease are particularly important because they demonstrate a language deficit beyond language production, one that cannot be easily attributed to motoric or memory impairment. These studies that have found evidence of language deficits in subcortical dementia are consistent with data suggesting the presence of aphasia in patients with subcortical strokes and with an integrated view of brain systems in which damage to certain subcortical regions strongly influences the functioning of cortical areas traditionally tied to language ability.[93,97]

## Cortical Dementias

Alzheimer's and Pick's diseases are the two most common cortical dementias, but DAT is by far the most common, accounting for approximately 50 percent of dementias, and being 10 to 15 times more common than Pick's disease.[29] They differ pathologically in that Pick's disease affects primarily the anterior temporal and frontal areas of the brain, while the pathology of DAT is concentrated more posteriorly, including parietal and temporal lobes and the hippocampi. Neuropsychologically, the two dementias are similar in preserved motor functions, impaired language, and altered personality through the early and moderate stages. They differ primarily in the areas of memory and visuo-spatial abilities that are spared in Pick's until later stages and impaired in DAT from the beginning. Descriptions of the language impairments in these two syndromes look grossly similar: anomia in the early stages, progressing to more marked language disturbance with comprehension deficits in the moderate stages, progressing ultimately to echolalia and terminal muteness. A case study by Holland et al, in one of the few detailed descriptions of language dissolution in Pick's disease, documented a pattern uncharacteristic of language deficits in DAT.[57] This patient presented with spoken language marked by literal paraphasias and some omissions of grammatical words, and eventually progressed to muteness. Auditory comprehension deficits were also observed. However, other language skills, including reading and writing, were relatively preserved and few other signs of dementia appeared through much of the 12½-year course. This case description is unlike DAT in several respects: The Pick's patient had preservation of memory and the "creative" aspects of language (semantics), while DAT patients typically present with significant memory deficits and semantic impairment. In addition, the Pick's patient appeared mute before the severe stages of the disease, but muteness is a late-appearing symptom in DAT.

Occasionally, DAT, Pick's, or Creutzfeldt-Jakob patients present with an isolated and progressive language disorder and only subsequently go on to develop other symptoms and an identifiable dementia syndrome.[86,123,129] Another group of patients also present with progressive language deficits but do not develop a dementia syndrome.[73,91,92,96] There has been lively discussion about whether or not these patients, if followed and tested carefully, will develop a range of neuropsychological deficits consistent with DAT or other dementia syndromes.[78,91,96,102,110,111] So far, there has been little agreement about the appropriate diagnosis for these patients, and it has become clear that distinguishing the slowly progressive aphasia from dementia is not always easy. Serial evaluations documenting isolated and progressive language impairments can lead to a provisional diagnosis of slowly progressive aphasia. However, follow-up testing and thorough neuropsychological evaluations are essential in order to distinguish this syndrome from more widely recognized forms of dementia such as DAT and Pick's disease.

## Mixed Dementias

The second most common cause of dementia is vascular or multi-infarct dementia (MID), which results from multiple cerebral infarctions and often presents with a combination of cortical and subcortical signs and symptoms. The symptoms are varied and are therefore sometimes difficult to distinguish from the symptoms of DAT. A thorough history can document abrupt onset, stepwise deterioration, and a fluctuating course that contrasts with the insidious onset and gradual course typical of DAT.[116] Moreover, interim recovery of lost function is often observed in MID but not in DAT. A history of hypertension or strokes, with focal neurologic signs, also suggests vascular dementia.

One vascular dementia, the angular gyrus syndrome (AGS), resulting from posterior middle cerebral-artery lesions, has been particularly easy to confuse with DAT.[15] The lesions in AGS are often too small to be visible on CT scans, and focal motor-sensory signs may be absent, leaving diagnosis largely dependent on neuropsychological findings, which appear similar to DAT, particularly in the area of language. AGS presents with fluent aphasia, alexia with agraphia, acalculia, left-right disorientation, finger agnosia, and constructional disturbances. The differences between AGS and DAT lie mainly in the preserved nonverbal memory and preserved awareness of language disorders in AGS.

Two important caveats must be made regarding the differential diagnosis of DAT. First, although up to 84 percent of dementia patients are clinically diagnosed with a primary degenerative dementia consistent with DAT, the diagnosis is complicated by factors of accuracy and specificity: 20 percent or more of cases with the clinical diagnosis of Alzheimer's disease are found at autopsy to have other conditions and not Alzheimer's disease, and dementia patients, like most older patients, tend to have multiple disease processes at work.[90] For instance, in the case of DAT, 15 to 20 percent of the patients have been shown to have pathologic features consistent with both DAT and multi-infarct dementia.[29] These facts force us to temper any generalizations we make about the behavior of clinically diagnosed DAT patients without histologic confirmation.

The second problem for differential diagnosis is variability of language symptoms within the DAT population. Alzheimer patients differ from one another. Some of the differences may be because of premorbid dispositions, and some may be because of stage of the disease. However, there remains a good likelihood that differences observed in language functions will be traced to subgroups of DAT patients with different etiologies.[22] The most frequently mentioned subgroup of patients are those with genetic or familial DAT.[95] The association between familial DAT and language disorders has been difficult to ascertain because researchers have found correlations between language deficits and positive family history of DAT,[40] negative family histories,[80] as well as no relationship between language disturbance and family history.[24] Other subgroups based on language differences have been proposed, citing correlations between language disorders and age at onset[36,37] and rate of progression,[80,121] but these too have not been replicated.[13,30,88,120] Therefore, it is clear that some DAT patients show more or less language disturbance than others, but the extent of these differences and the source of the variation are yet to be determined.

## Treatment Implications

Once a diagnosis has been reached, a treatment strategy is designed. Although there is currently no cure for DAT, it is possible to compensate for some of the language problems described in this chapter. Candidacy for treatment will depend on the stage of the disease, the patient's social environment, the patient's awareness of his or her deficits, the nature and degree of other (e.g., cognitive) impairments, and, finally, the clinical judgment of whether treatment can help (see Chapter 15 for perspectives on treatment alternatives).[45,84]

Traditional direct language therapy, as used to treat focal aphasias,[59] may not be appropriate with DAT patients for several reasons. It is important to remember that DAT patients have a language disorder that differs in crucial ways from typical aphasias. For instance, unlike patients with focal aphasia, DAT patients present with intact grammatical and phonologic abilities, and the bulk of treatment must focus on semantic and pragmatic deficits. Because there has been a substantial body of research in the area of lexical semantics in DAT, there is now information that can be used to structure treatment. Unlike focal aphasia, where the anomia can be largely attributed to impaired lexical access,[82] the anomia in DAT is probably polygenic (having multiple causes).[14,71,132] Therefore, treatment and compensation will have to be multidimensional and tailored to individual patients. To the extent that visual perceptual impairment and lexical access deficits underlie the anomia, environmental support (e.g., good lighting) and lexical probing (Is it an X?) may alleviate the problem. However, because at least some of the anomia appears to stem from degraded lexical representations, probes, cues, and environmental support are less likely to be of any help. In these instances, because research has demonstrated that superordinate category information remains relatively intact in DAT, communication might benefit from use of superordinate category names (e.g., furniture and tools) rather than basic level names (e.g., footstool and socket wrench).[20]

It is also crucial to bear in mind that the language disorders of DAT are embedded in a dementia syndrome and therefore occur among other, often more severe, cognitive deficits. These other aspects of the dementia preclude the use of traditional therapeutic techniques that rely largely on self-monitoring and on the acquisition of strategies to aid performance. Therefore, therapeutic intervention must emphasize compensation for lost function with little emphasis on learning. This includes indirect therapy such as counseling for the patient's caregivers and investigation of methods to enhance the patient's communicative abilities. A few compensation strategies that might prove useful with DAT patients are discussed below. Remember, however, that there is still very little research demonstrating positive effects of these approaches on communicaton.

Gestural communication has been used to compensate for language deficits in aphasia and might be considered as an augmentative strategy with DAT patients.[53,124] In fact, the literature on naming impairment in DAT includes several observations that DAT patients spontaneously pantomime the use of objects that they are unable to name.[52,119] Although this indicates that DAT patients might be able to use gesture to compensate for anomia, several studies have also documented a decline in DAT patients' ability to produce and understand pantomime, which parallels deficits in spoken language and indicates that compensation through gesture may be difficult for this group.[70,81] It should be noted, however, that the research has *not* found a one-to-one correspondence between word loss and gesture loss. Therefore, even if the patient cannot produce or understand a specific word, he may still be able to make use of a related gesture and vice versa. No research has systematically explored the efficacy of gestural compensation in the treatment of DAT patients.

Because DAT impairs multiple aspects of cognition, and many of these nonlanguage deficits will impair communication, language therapy need not be limited to treating only the language deficits. For instance, deficits in memory and orientation may result in language comprehension problems and pragmatic deficits of poor topic maintenance and discourse incoherence. Improving these nonlinguistic cognitive abilities would likely have beneficial effects on communication. Perhaps the oldest and most common cognitive intervention for dementia is "reality orientation therapy." This consists of providing orienting information to the patient with the goal of improving all aspects of functioning that rely on orientation (including daily communication and participation in therapies). Studies on the effectiveness of reality orientation therapy suggest that although this type of therapy may have a positive overall effect, the benefits are difficult to document objectively.[8]

Other cognitive intervention strategies for DAT patients are drawn from the literature on methods to improve and compensate for memory deficits in normal aging.[5,26] One technique for improving recall involves structuring the input to aid memory. If language addressed to DAT patients could be structured so that it is encoded more completely and remembered more thoroughly, language comprehension and discourse abilities that depend on memory might improve. In one series of experiments, DAT patients were asked to remember a series of objects that were presented in different conditions (e.g., objects, objects with an instruction to tell the function of each one, and objects with a motoric instruction) and asked to recall the list of items in various conditions.[6] One important finding is that the input condition appears to have different effects at different stages of the disease. For example, for mild DAT patients, the conditions with multiple input modalities (e.g., object and action) did not appear to affect performance significantly, suggesting that multiple modality input does not enhance memory at this stage of the disease. However, for moderate and severe DAT patients, verbal input alone was the optimal condition for free recall, sparking speculation that a "pure verbal presentation enables these patients to use verbal repetition to a greater extent than in the other conditions."[6] These initial findings suggest that multimodality input may be of little help to memory in the initial stages and may be a hindrance later on. Other memory-enhancing strategies such as "subject performed tasks" during encoding (e.g., lift the cup, put on the glove) appear to enhance memory at all stages of DAT,[67] indicating that some interventions, particularly those that rely on motor acts, may be more effective for the population as a whole. Although many investigations have demonstrated effects of encoding manipulations on memory performance, the effects of such manipulations on language performance are unclear.

One research project has tested the effect of altered input directly on language comprehension. Young and Kennedy presented two patients with severe DAT with pragmatic or linguistic orienting cues prior to a simple picture-pointing comprehension task.[136] The pragmatic cue consisted of an "alerting strategy," in which the examiner called the subject's name, made eye contact, and then gave the instruction (e.g., "Point to snow plow").

The linguistic cue consisted of a semantic context as in "Show me something that clears the road in winter. Point to snow plow." One subject profited from both cue conditions, but more so from the simple pragmatic alerting cue. The other subject's performance did not improve with either cue. This study highlights both the potential effectiveness for improving language comprehension by a simple alerting cue prior to stimuli presentation and the importance of considering individual differences in any treatment program: What works for one DAT patient may not work for another.

There are many other techniques that may be effective in enhancing communication with DAT patients, although there is very little research to prove their efficacy. For instance, a reduced rate of speech has been shown to improve auditory comprehension in normal elderly, and may be effective with DAT patients as well.[133] Ostuni and Santo-Pietro[109] and Bayles and Kaszniak[10] recommend many simple and potentially helpful alterations in caregiver's speech that might enhance communication with DAT patients. These include: using short sentences; paraphrasing a sentence when repeating it; avoiding open-ended questions; being redundant; avoiding analogies; establishing eye-contact before addressing the patient; using pictures, objects, and gestures to enhance the message; and allowing time for processing.

Finally, it must be emphasized that, because there is no cure for DAT, and direct treatment is of unproven value with this population, caregivers are crucial participants in any treatment for DAT patients. The caregivers must be educated about the disease itself (etiology, course, and complications) and counseled about the patient's impairments and abilities. There are now many good, comprehensive books that can help to educate caregivers.[33,43,49,109] Thorough language evaluations will help the caregivers understand the communicative strengths and limitations of the patient, and repeat evaluations can be a valuable method of monitoring the progress of the disease. It is the caregivers who will be primarily in charge of implementing the therapeutic strategy on a daily basis, and it is they who will ultimately benefit most from improved communication.[84]

## Future Research

There are many places where our research needs to be expanded, and I will make only a few suggestions here. There is ample evidence that there are individual differences in language abilities and deficits within the DAT population and that these differences are not random. It is crucial that variability of language impairments be documented, and if reliable subgroups exist, they must be adequately described. Much of the inconsistency in current research findings will ultimately be attributed to variability within the population rather than variability in experimental paradigms. Considering the extent of behavioral variability within the DAT population, it is essential that future treatment for this population be empirically derived and tailored to individual patients.

Over the past decade, there has been an almost blind devotion to studying the lexical deficits in DAT to the exclusion of other aspects of language. This makes sense in that anomia is one of earliest and most apparent deficits in the disease. However, we have produced little basic research on pragmatic and discourse deficits that are also early and apparent in DAT, and we have produced even less clinical research to document how and when intervention is most effective. Both of these areas deserve more attention in the next decade.

Collaboration across disciplines must also be increased. This may come in the form of collaboration with psychopharmacologists who are testing new drugs and need behavioral measures to test the effect of their medicines on cognitive deficits. It may come in the form of collaboration with epidemiologists attempting to sort out the behavioral markers of familial versus sporadic subtypes of DAT. It should certainly come in collaboration with caregivers and other clinical specialists (e.g., primary care physicians, nurses, and occupational therapists) who communicate daily with DAT patients.

## References

1. Albert ML, Feldman RG, Willis AL. The subcortical dementia' of progressive supranuclear palsy. J Neurol Neurosurg Psychiatry 1974; 37:121–130.
2. Albert M, Milberg W. Semantic processing in patients with Alzheimer's disease. Brain Lang 1989; 37:163–171.
3. Appell J, Kertesz A, Fisman M. A study of language functioning in Alzheimer patients. Brain Lang 1982; 17:73–91
4. Alzheimer A. Of a particular disease of the cerebral cortex. Zentralblatt vur Nervenheilkunde und Psychiatrie 1907; 30:177–179. Translation and commentary by Wilkins RH, Brody IA. Alzheimer's disease. Arch Neurol 1969; 21:109–110.
5. Backman L. Compensation and recoding: A framework for aging and memory research. Scand J Psychol 1985; 26:193–207.
6. Backman L, Herlitz A. Memory functions in normal aging and Alzheimer's disease: The issue of utilization of environmental support. Paper presented at 10th Biennial Meeting of the International Society for the Study of Behavioral Development. Finland, July, 1989.
7. Barker MG, Lawson JS. Nominal aphasia in dementia. Br J Psychiatry 1968; 114:1351–1356.

8. Barnes JA. Effects of reality orientation classroom on memory loss, confusion, and disorientation in geriatric patients. Gerontologist 1974; 14:138–142.
9. Bayles KA. Language function in senile dementia. Brain Lang 1982; 16:265–280.
10. Bayles KA, Kaszniak AW. Communication and cognition in normal aging and dementia. Boston: Little, Brown and Co, 1987.
11. Bayles KA, Tomoeda CK. Confrontation naming impairment in dementia. Brain Lang 1983; 19:98–114.
12. Bayles KA, Tomoeda CK, Kaszniak AW. Verbal perseveration of dementia patients. Brain Lang 1985; 2:102–116.
13. Becker JT, Huff FJ, Nebes RD, Holland A, Boller F. Neuropsychological function in Alzheimer's disease. Arch Neurol 1988; 45:263–268.
14. Benson DF. Neurologic correlates of anomia. In: Whitaker H, Whitaker H, eds. Studies in neurolinguistics. Vol. 4. New York: Academic Press, 1979:293–328.
15. Benson DF, Cummings JL, Tsai SY. Angular gyrus syndrome simulating Alzheimer disease. Arch Neurol 1982; 39:616–620.
16. Broca P. Localization of speech in the third left frontal convolution. Translated by Berker EA, Berker AH, Smith A. Arch Neurol 1986; 43:1065–1072.
17. Butters N, Sax D, Montgomery K, Tarlow S. Comparison of the neuropsychological deficits associated with early and advanced Huntington's disease. Arch Neurol 1978; 35:585–589.
18. Caplan D. Neurolinguistics and linguistic aphasiology. Cambridge: Cambridge University Press, 1987.
19. Chase TN, Foster NL, Fedio P. Regional cortical dysfunction in Alzheimer's disease as determined by positron emission tomography. Ann Neurol 1984; 15:170–174.
20. Chertkow H, Bub D, Seidenberg M. Priming and semantic memory loss in Alzheimer's disease. Brain Lang 1989; 36:420–446.
21. Chomsky C. The acquisition of syntax in children from 5 to 10. Cambridge: The MIT Press, 1979.
22. Chui HC. The significance of clinically defined subgroups of Alzheimer's disease. J Neural Transmission, [suppl.] 24:57–68.
23. Chui HC. Dementia: A review emphasizing clinicopathologic correlation and brain-behavior relationships. Arch Neurol 1989; 46:806–814.
24. Chui HC, Teng EL, Henderson VW, Moy AC. Clinical subtypes of dementia of the Alzheimer type. Neurology 1985; 35:1544–1550.
25. Code C, Lodge B. Language in dementia of recent referral. Age Ageing 1987; 16:366–372.
26. Craik FIM, Byrd M, Swanson JM. Patterns of memory loss in three elderly samples. Psychol Aging 1987; 2:79–86.
27. Cummings J. Subcortical dementia. Br J Psychiatry 1986; 149:682–697.
28. Cummings JL. The dementias of Parkinson's disease: Prevalence, characteristics, neurobiology and comparison with dementia of the Alzheimer type. Eur Neurol 1988; 28:15–23.
29. Cummings JL, Benson DF. Dementia: A clinical approach. Boston: Butterworth, 1983.
30. Cummings JL, Benson DF, Hill MA, Read S. Aphasia in dementia of the Alzheimer type. Neurology 1985; 29:315–323.
31. Cummings JL, Houlihan JP, Hill MA. The pattern of reading deterioration in dementia of the Alzheimer type: Observations and implications. Brain Lang 1986; 29:315–323.
32. Cutler NR, Haxby JV, Duara R. Brain metabolism as measured with positron emission tomography: Serial assessment in a patient with familial Alzheimer's disease. Neurology 1985; 35:1556–1561.
33. Dippel RL, Hutton JT. Caring for the Alzheimer patient: A practical guide. Buffalo, NY: Prometheus Books, 1988.
34. Emery OB. Test for syntactic complexity. Lang Commun 1986; 6:63–64.
35. Emery OB. Language and memory processing in senile dementia Alzheimer's type. In: Light LL, Burke DM, eds. Language, memory and aging. New York: Cambridge University Press, 1988:221–243.
36. Faber-Langendoen K, Morris JC, Knesevich JW. Aphasia in senile dementia of the Alzheimer type. Ann Neurol 1988; 23:365–370.
37. Filley CM, Kelly J, Heaton RK. Neuropsychologic features of early- and late-onset Alzheimer's disease. Arch Neurol 1986; 43:574–576.
38. Fodor J. The modularity of mind, an essay on faculty psychology. Cambridge: The MIT Press, 1983
39. Fodor J. Precis of the modularity of mind. Behav Brain Sci 1985; 8:1–42.
40. Folstein MF, Breitner JCS. Language disorder predicts familial Alzheimer's disease. In: Corkin S, ed. Alzheimer's disease: A report of progress. New York: Raven Press, 1982:197.
41. Foster NL, Chase TN, Fedio P. Alzheimer's disease: Focal cortical changes shown by positron emission tomography. Neurology 1983; 33:961–965.
42. Fox JH, Topel JL, Huckman MS. Use of computerized tomography in senile dementia. J Neurol Neurosurg Psychiatry 1975; 38:948–953.
43. Glickstein JK. Therapeutic interventions in Alzheimer's disease: A program of functional communication skills for activities of daily living. Rockville, MD: Aspen Publishers: 1988.
44. Goldstein K. Language and language disturbances. New York: Grune & Stratton, 1948.
45. Golper L. Communication and dementia: A clinical perspective. In: Shadden B, ed. Communication behavior and aging: A sourcebook for clinicians. Baltimore: Williams & Wilkins, 1988:279.
46. Goodglass H, Kaplan E. The assessment of aphasia and related disorders. Philadelphia: Lea & Febiger, 1983.
47. Goodglass H, Kaplan E. The Boston Naming Test. Philadelphia: Lea & Febiger, 1983.
48. Gordon WP, Illes J. Neurolinguistic characteristics of language production in Huntington's disease: A preliminary report. Brain Lang 1987; 31:1–10.
49. Gruetzner H. Alzheimer's: A caregivers guide and sourcebook. New York: John Wiley, 1988.
50. Grober H, Buschke H, Kawas C, Fuld P. Impaired ranking of semantic attributes in dementia. Brain Lang 26:276–286.
51. Groher M. Modifications in speech-language assessment procedures for the older adult. In: Shadden B, ed. Communication behavior and aging: A sourcebook for clinicians. Baltimore: Williams & Wilkins, 1988:248.
52. Harrold RM. Object naming in Alzheimer's disease: What is the cognitive deficit? Unpublished Ph.D. dissertation, Claremont Graduate School, 1987.
53. Helm-Estabrooks NA, Fitzpatrick PM, Barresi B. Visual action therapy for global aphasia. J Speech Hear Disord 1981; 47:385–389.

54. Henderson V, Mack W, Freed D, Kempler D, Andersen E. Naming consistency in Alzheimer's disease: Evidence for lexical semantic loss. Unpublished manuscript, 1989.
55. Hier D, Hagenlocker K, Shindler A. Language disintegration in dementia on a picture description task. Brain Lang 1985; 25:117-133.
56. Holland A. Communication abilities in daily living. Baltimore: University Park Press, 1980.
57. Holland AL, McBurney DH, Moossy J, Reinmuth OM. The dissolution of language in Pick's disease with neurofibrillary tangles: A case study. Brain Lang 1985; 24:36-58.
58. Horner J, Heyman A, Dawson D, Rogers H. The relationship of agraphia to the severity of dementia in Alzheimer's disease. Arch Neurol 1988; 45:760-763.
59. Howard D, Hatfield FM. Aphasia therapy: Historical and contemporary issues. Hillsdale, NJ: Erlbaum, 1987.
60. Huff FJ. The disorder of naming in Alzheimer's disease. in: Light LL, Burke DM, eds. Language, memory and aging. New York: Cambridge University Press, 1988:209.
61. Huff FJ, Corkin S, Growdon HJ. Semantic impairment and anomia in Alzheimer's disease. Brain Lang 1986; 28:235-249.
62. Huff FJ, Mack L, Mahlmann J, Greenberg S. A comparison of lexical-semantic impairments in left hemisphere stroke and Alzheimer's disease. Brain Lang 1988; 34:262-278.
63. Hutchinson JM, Jensen M. A pragmatic evaluation of discourse communication in normal and senile elderly in a nursing home. In: Obler L, Albert M, eds. Language and communication in the elderly. Lexington, MA: D.C. Heath and Company, 1980:59-74.
64. Irigaray L. Le Langage des dements. The Hague: Mouton, 1973.
65. Johnson KA, Holman BL, Mueller SP. Single photon emission computed tomography in Alzheimer's disease: Abnormal iofetamine I 123 uptake reflects dementia severity. Arch Neurol 1988; 45:392-396.
66. Jorm AF. Controlled and automatic information processing in senile dementia: A review. Psychol Med 1986; 16:77-88.
67. Karlsson T, Backman L, Nilsson LG, Winblad B, Osterlind PO. Memory improvement at different stages of Alzheimer's disease. Neuropsychologia 1989; 27:737-742.
68. Kaszniak AW, Fox J, Gandell DL. Predictors of mortality in presenile and senile dementia. Ann Neurol 1978; 3:246-252.
69. Kempler D. Syntactic and symbolic abilities in Alzheimer's disease. Ph.D. dissertation, UCLA, 1984.
70. Kempler D. Lexical and pantomime abilities in Alzheimer's disease. Aphasiology 1988; 2:147-159.
71. Kempler D, Andersen E, Hunt M. Language subgroups in Alzheimer's disease. Paper presented at the Gerontological Society of America. Minneapolis, MN, November, 1989.
72. Kempler D, Curtiss S, Jackson C. Syntactic preservation in Alzheimer's disease. J Speech Hear Res 1987; 30:343-350.
73. Kempler D, Jackson CA, Metter EJ. Slowly progressive aphasia. In: Prescott T, ed. Clinical aphasiology (vol. 18). San Diego: College-Hill Press, 1989:257-270.
74. Kempler D, Van Lancker D, Read S. Proverb and idiom interpretation in Alzheimer disease. Alzheimer disease and associated disorders 1988; 2:38-49.
75. Kertesz A. Western Aphasia Battery. London, Ontario: University of Western Ontario, 1980.
76. Kertesz A. Aphasia and associated disorders: Taxonomy, localization and recovery. New York: Grune & Stratton, 1979.
77. Kimura D, Archibald Y. Motor functions of the left hemisphere. Brain 1974; 97:337-350.
78. Kirshner HS, Tanridag O, Thurman L, Whetsell WO. Progressive aphasia without dementia: Two cases with focal spongiform degeneration. Ann Neurol 1987; 22:527-532.
79. Kirshner HS, Webb WG, Kelly MP. The naming disorder of dementia. Neuropsychologia 1984; 22:23-30.
80. Knesevich JW, Toro FR, Morris JC, LaBarge E. Aphasia, family history, and the longitudinal course of senile dementia of the Alzheimer type. Psychiatry Res 1985; 14:255-263.
81. Langhans JJ. Pantomime recognition and expression in persons with Alzheimer's disease. Unpublished doctoral dissertation. University of Arizona, AZ, 1985.
82. Lieberman P, Friedman J, Feldman LS. Syntax comprehension in Parkinson's disease. J Nervous Ment Disease (In press.)
83. Linebarger M, Schwartz M, Saffran E. Sensitivity to grammatical structure in so-called agrammatic aphasics, Cognition 1983; 13:361-392.
84. Lubinski R. A model for intervention: Communication skills, effectiveness and opportunity. In: Shadden B, ed. Communication behavior and aging: A sourcebook for clinicians. Baltimore: Williams & Wilkins, 1988:294.
85. Luxenberg JS, Haxby JV, Creasey H, Sundaram M, Rapoport SI. Rate of ventricular enlargement in dementia of the Alzheimer type correlates with rate of neuropsychological deterioration. Neurology 1987; 37:1135-1140.
86. Mandell AM, Alexander MP, Carpenter S. Creutzfeldt-Jakob disease presenting as isolated aphasia. Neurology 1989; 39:55-58.
87. Marsden CD, Harrison MJG. Outcome of investigation of patients with presenile dementia. Br Med J 1972; 2:245-252.
88. Martin A, Brouwers P, Lalonde F. Towards a behavioral typology of Alzheimer's patients. J Clin Exp Neuropsychol 1986; 8:594-610.
89. Martin A, Fedio P. Word production and comprehension in Alzheimer's disease: The breakdown of semantic knowledge. Brain Lang 1983; 19:124-141.
90. McKhann G, Drachman D, Folstein M. Clinical diagnosis of Alzheimer's disease: Report of the NINCDS-ADRDA work group under the auspices of Health and Human Services Task Force on Alzheimer's disease. Neurology 1984; 34:939-944.
91. Mesulam M. Slowly progressive aphasia without generalized dementia. Ann Neurol 1982; 11:592-598.
92. Mesulam M. Primary progressive aphasia—Differentiation from Alzheimer's disease. Ann Neurol 1987; 22:533-534.
93. Metter EJ, Riege WH, Hanson WR. Subcortical structures in aphasia: An analysis based on (F-18)-fluorodeoxyglucose, positron emission tomography, and computed tomography. Arch Neurol 1988; 45:1229-1234.
94. Miller E. Language impairment in Alzheimer type dementia. Clin Psychol Rev 1989; 9:181-195.
95. Miner GD, Richter RW, Blass JP, Valentine JL, Winters-Miner LA. Familial Alzheimer's disease: Molecular

genetics and clinical perspectives. New York: Marcel Dekker, 1989.
96. Morris JC, Cole M, Banker BQ, Wright D. Hereditary dysphasic dementia and the Pick-Alzheimer spectrum. Ann Neurol 1984; 16:455–566.
97. Naesser M, Alexander JP, Helm-Estabrooks H. Aphasia with predominantly subcortical lesion sites: Description of three capsular/putaminal aphasia syndromes. Arch Neurol 1982; 39:2–14.
98. Nebes RD. Semantic memory in Alzheimer's disease. Psychol Bull 1989; 106:377–394.
99. Nebes RD, Brady CG, Huff FJ. Automatic and attentional mechanisms of semantic priming in Alzheimer's disease. J Clin Exp Neuropsychol 1989; 11:219–230.
100. Nebes RD, Boller F, Holland A. Use of semantic context by patients with Alzheimer's disease. Psychol Aging 1986; 1:261–169.
101. Nebes RD, Martin DC, Horn LC. Sparing of semantic memory in Alzheimer's disease. J Abnorm Psychol 1984; 93:321–330.
102. Neils J, Barrett E. The evolution of slowly progressive aphasia. Paper presented at the annual meeting of the American-Speech-Language-Hearing Association. New Orleans, November, 1987.
103. Neils J, Brennan MM, Cole M, et al. The use of phonemic cueing with Alzheimer's disease patients. Neuropsychologia 1988; 26:351–354.
104. Nicholas M, Obler L, Albert M, Helm-Estabrooks N. Empty speech in Alzheimer's disease and fluent aphasia. J Speech Hear Res 1985; 28:405–410.
105. Ober BA, Dronkers NF, Koss E, Delis DC, Friedland RP. Retrieval from semantic memory in Alzheimer-type dementia. J Clin Exp Neuropsychol 1986; 8:75–92.
106. Obler LK. Language and brain dysfunction in dementia. In: Segalowitz S, ed. Language functions and brain organization. New York: Academic Press, 1983.
107. Obler LK, Cummings JL, Albert ML. Subcortical dementia: Speech and language functions. Washington, D.C.: American Geriatric Society, 1979.
108. Obler LK, Albert MC. Language in the elderly aphasic and in the dementing patient. In: Sarno MT, ed. Acquired aphasia. New York: Academic Press, 1981:385.
109. Ostuni MJ, Santo-Pietro E. Getting through: Communicating when someone you know has Alzheimer's disease. Princeton: The Speech Bin, 1986.
110. Poeck K, Luzzatti C. Slowly progressive aphasia in three patients: The problem of accompanying neuropsychological deficit. Brain 1988; 111:151–168.
111. Pogacar S, Williams RS. Alzheimer's disease presenting as slowly progressive aphasia. R I Med J 1984; 67:181–185.
112. Porch B. Porch Index of Communicative Abilities. Palo Alto, CA: Consulting Psychologists Press, 1981.
113. Rapcsak SZ, Arthur SA, Bliklen DA, Rubens AB. Lexical agraphia in Alzheimer's disease. Arch Neurol 1989; 46:65–68.
114. Ripich DN, Terrell BY. Cohesion and coherence in Alzheimer's disease. J Speech Hear Disord 1988; 53:8–14.
115. Rochford G. A study of naming errors in dysphasic and in demented patients. Neuropsychologia 1971; 9:437–443.
116. Rosen WG, Terry RD, Fuld PA, Katzman R, Peck A. Pathological verification of ischemic score in differentiation of dementias. Ann Neurol 1980; 7:486–488.
117. Rumelhart D, McClelland J, PDP Research Group. Parallel distributed processing: Explorations in the microstructure of cognition. Cambridge, MA: The MIT Press, 1986.
118. Schneider W, Shiffrin R. Controlled and automatic human information processing: I. Detection, search and attention. Psychol Rev 1977; 84:1–66.
119. Schwartz M, Marin O, Saffran E. Dissociations of language function in dementia: A case study. Brain Lang 1979; 7:277–306.
120. Selnes OA, Carson K, Rovner B, Gordon B. Language dysfunction in early- and late-onset possible Alzheimer's disease. Neurology 1988; 38:1053–1056.
121. Seltzer B, Sherwin I. A comparison of clinical features in early- and late-onset primary degenerative dementia. Arch Neurol 1983; 40:143–146.
122. Shiffren RM, Schneider W. Controlled and automatic human information processing: II. Perceptual learning, automatic attending and a general theory. Psychol Rev 1977; 84(2):127–190.
123. Shuttleworth EC. Atypical presentations of dementia of the Alzheimer type. J Am Geriatr Soc 1984; 32:485–490.
124. Skelly M. Amerind gestural code based on universal American Indian handtalk. New York: Elsevier North Holland, 1979.
125. Smith S. Syntactic comprehension in Alzheimer's disease. Paper presented at the Academy of Aphasia. Santa Fe, NM, October, 1989.
126. Smith S, Butters N, Granholm E. Activation of semantic relations in Alzheimer's and Huntington's disease. In: Whitaker H, ed. Neuropsychological studies of nonfocal brain damage. New York: Springer-Verlag, 1988:265–285.
127. Thompson IM. Language in dementia. Int J Geriatr Psychiatry 1987; 2:145–161.
128. Ulatowska H, Allard L, Donnell A. Discourse performance in subjects with dementia of the Alzheimer type. In: Whitaker H, ed. Neuropsychological studies in nonfocal brain damage. New York: Springer-Verlag, 1988:108–131.
129. Wechsler A. Presenile dementia presenting as aphasia. J Neurol Neurosurg Psychiatry 1977; 40:303–305.
130. Wernicke C. Der aphasiçhe symtomenkomplex. Breslau, Germany: Rohn & Weigert, 1874.
131. Whitaker H. A case of the isolation of the language function. In: Whitaker H, Whitaker H, eds. Studies in neurolinguistics. Vol. 4. New York: Academic Press, 1976:1–58.
132. White-Williams BW, Mack W, Henderson VW. Multiple factors contribute to the naming disorder of Alzheimer's disease (abstract). Paper presented at the International Neuropsychological Society. Washington, D.C., November, 1986.
133. Wingfield A, Poon LW, Lombardi L, Lowe D. Speed of processing in normal aging: Effects of speech rate, linguistic structure and processing time. J Gerontol 1985; 40(5):579–585.
134. Wulfeck BB. Grammaticality judgments in sentence comprehension in agrammatic aphasia. J Speech Hear Res 1988; 31:72–80.
135. Yamaguchi F, Meyer JS, Yamamoto M, Sakai S, Shaw T. Noninvasive regional cerebral blood flow measurements in dementia. Arch Neurol 1980; 37:410–418.
136. Young EC, Kennedy J. An investigation of language facilitation in two patients with Alzheimer's disease. Paper presented at American Speech-Language-Hearing Association. Boston, MA, 1988.

# CHAPTER 8

# *Discourse Studies*

HANNA K. ULATOWSKA, Ph.D.
SANDRA BOND CHAPMAN, Ph.D.

This chapter describes a methodologic approach to the study of communicative function in dementia. First, pertinent literature concerning communication breakdown in dementia is reviewed, focusing primarily on discourse studies, although studies of other linguistic functions essential to communicative competence are also mentioned. The highlighted findings delineate deficits and preserved abilities pertinent to communicative function in dementia. Interpretations offered to explain communicative decline in dementia are summarized. As the literature review shows, considerable groundwork has been laid in isolating deficits in dementia. There is still need, however, for an increased understanding of the mechanisms underlying deterioration of communication.

The second portion of this chapter describes a specific methodologic approach used by our research group in Dallas for investigating communicative function in dementia. Our methodology builds on the work of other investigators. The experimental paradigm described herein explores relationships across seemingly isolated deficits. The results of a pilot study comparing patients with senile dementia of the Alzheimer's type (DAT) to other clinical populations including old-elderly (>85 years), aphasic, and normal aged-matched control subjects are summarized.

In the final section, the clinical applications and implications of the described methodology are presented. Implications for clinical management and further research needs are also discussed.

## Discourse Studies

Current interest in discourse performance is motivated by the explanatory power provided by discourse. Although discourse may be composed of a single word, a phrase, a sentence, or a combination of all the above, discourse typically consists of a sequence of connected sentences. The coherence of discourse is determined by how well this sequence of sentences is related. Discourse provides a promising avenue for investigating behavioral changes in dementia because discourse can be manipulated to explore how cognitive impairment impinges on linguistic functioning and communicative competence. This approach is possible because of the inherent nature of discourse, which entails a complex interaction among *linguistic*, *communicative*, and *cognitive* processes. Precisely, discourse is expressed linguistically (i.e., via words and sentences) and is defined communicatively (i.e., a unit of language that conveys a message). Moreover, complex cognitive processes (e.g., memory, attention, perception, and retrieval) underlie discourse comprehension and production. Communicative competence presupposes both linguistic and cognitive abilities. Both abilities are utilized in the process of effectively communicating a message within a given context. Knowledge of discourse performance in different neurologic populations such as dementia increases our understanding of brain-behavior relationships. Recent evidence in aphasia has shown a dissociation between communicative and linguistic abilities.

## DISCOURSE DEFICITS

For almost a decade, communicative deficits have been described or at least alluded to in dementia. Numerous studies have delineated facts describing deficits and preserved language abilities in dementia. To date, the identified verbal deficits include reduction of information, incoherent discourse, verbosity, tangentiality, and perseveration of ideas. Relatively preserved abilities include phonologic and syntactic processes. These facts have provided the necessary empirical groundwork to foster further research of communicative function in dementia.

## Reduction of Information

A number of studies have documented reduced information in dementia. Informativity relates to the most essential or core information on a given task. That is, the reduction of information does not correspond to the total amount of language produced. Informativity is reduced when a speaker fails to adequately express the essential components of a message. The studies below demonstrate that informativity cannot be assessed merely by quantifying the amount of language produced.

Information reduction in dementia has been reported on a variety of discourse tasks, including picture description, narrative recall, self-generated narratives, and other procedures. Hier, Hagenlocker, and Shindler[8] found that demented patients produced fewer relevant observations than did normal, age-matched, control subjects when describing the "cookie theft" picture from the Boston Diagnostic Aphasia Examination.[6]

Reduced information was described in a study by Bayles, Boone, Tomoeda, Slauson, and Kaszniak.[3] They evaluated patients with dementia of the Alzheimer's type (DAT) on fourteen tasks proposed as being sensitive to differential diagnosis of dementia. Four of the fourteen tasks were directly relevant to discourse performance. These included two orally presented narratives for retelling (an immediate and a delayed condition) and two picture descriptions, one oral and the other written. The picture stimuli for the latter two measures were Norman Rockwell prints. The DAT subjects produced fewer "ideas" than did normal control and aphasic subjects on retelling the brief narratives, in both immediate and delayed conditions. Specific "idea units" were identified and divided into main and supplemental ideas for the retelling tasks. The single most discriminating measure for DAT versus normal subjects was the delayed story retelling task. This finding indicates that informativity in dementia suffers greater reduction when memory is involved. For mild versus moderate DAT subjects, the story-retelling measure immediately discriminated between the two populations. This pattern suggests that informativity decreases as dementia progresses. On the oral and written picture description tasks (Norman Rockwell), the performance of demented patients as compared to normal controls was also reduced in terms of information units.

Further evidence for reduction of information in dementia was found in both narrative and procedural discourse genres.[16] Narrative tasks used by Ulatowska and colleagues included four narratives: two verbally self-generated, one auditory retelling, and one written. In addition, a summary and a moral were elicited for one story. Generating summaries and morals is a more complex cognitive task in terms of information manipulation than simply producing a narrative. The DAT subjects produced fewer a priori propositions for both genre types, i.e., narratives and procedures, as compared to normals. The gap in performance between the two populations increased on the summary and moral formulation tasks. These findings suggest that as cognitive demands increase, greater impairment of discourse occurs. In contrast, only minimal difference was found between the DAT and normal control subjects on total amount of language. Thus, the DAT subjects produced less information than normals, despite the fact that they produced as much language.

## Disrupted Coherence and Cohesion

Impairment of coherence and cohesion has also been documented in the discourse of demented subjects. Coherence of discourse operates at a cognitive level and represents conceptual organization of information. Conceptually, discourse is coherent if the ideas relate to a global theme and seem to follow a logical sequence determined by one's world or script knowledge. That is, coherent discourse has unity. Discourse is perceived as incoherent when the flow of ideas seems to be disjointed. Ripich and Terrell reported impaired coherence in DAT subjects' topic-directed discourse, as judged by listeners.[14] The specific foci where listeners perceived incoherence coincided with occurrences of missing information units in DAT subjects' utterances. Ulatowska et al described intrusions in the flow of information in DAT discourse that interrupted coherence. The intrusions consisted of irrelevant and incorrect propositions.[16]

Whereas *coherence* of language is primarily cognitive in nature, *cohesion* operates primarily at a linguistic level. Certain linguistic devices such as reference, connectors, and verb tense contribute to cohesion. Disturbances of cohesion in dementia have been documented for the use of reference. Ripich and Terrell identified referential errors as the most frequent coherence error in DAT patients' discourse.[14] The presence of referential errors in the discourse of demented subjects has been described in other studies as well. Ulatowska et al found referential errors in dementia evidenced by greater pronoun-to-referent ratios.[16] Hier, Hagenlocker, and Shindler found greater use of pronouns and empty words in patients with dementia.[8] DAT subjects use more vague terms such as "thing, that, or somebody" than do normal controls.[12]

The relationship between coherence and cohesion is poorly understood and complex. There is no doubt that coherence and cohesion are interrelated and interdependent; however, the parameters important to this relation are not well understood. Ripich and Terrell noted that perceived incoherence could not be equated with distribution of specific cohesive devices or grammaticality of sentences.[14] The DAT subjects used similar proportions of cohesive devices as did normal control subjects, and yet their discourse was evaluated as incoherent. Despite subjects' facility with syntax, they were unable to produce coherent discourse.

### Verbosity and Taciturnity

Although verbosity and taciturnity are at opposite ends of the verbal output continuum, both phenomena are described in dementia. Verbosity tends to be present more at early stages of the disease, while taciturnity is described more often at the later stages.[5,13] Ripich and Terrell reported that DAT subjects produced greater amounts of language when compared to normal controls.[14] The increased amount of language, however, occurred in a greater number of turns in an interview dialogue. The increased output did not occur as an extended monologue but rather resulted from probing and facilitation by the interviewer. Other researchers have described different patterns according to dementia type. Verbosity was more characteristic of DAT discourse, whereas laconic speech was more characteristic of subjects with stroke-related dementia.[8]

### Tangentiality

Obler described tangentiality in the discourse of demented subjects, characterized by digressions from the topic.[12] In early-stage dementia, the demented subjects sometimes returned to the topic, whereas late-stage subjects typically failed to do so. Digressions (tangential comments) were also reported in narrative and procedural discourse of demented subjects.[16]

### Perseverations

Repetition of ideas in dementia has been identified by a number of researchers. Hier et al found perseverations in both DAT and stroke-related demented subjects.[8] A significant amount of information redundancy was found in DAT subjects' formulation of a memorable experience.[16] The redundancies were attributed either to failure to self-monitor or to memory deficits that caused the patient to lose the "trace" of previously produced information.

## PRESERVED ABILITIES

The presence of linguistic deficits in dementia has received less attention than cognitive and communicative processes, primarily because demented patients seem to talk with relative ease. On the surface, demented subjects have little difficulty producing sounds or using grammatically correct sentences. For the most part, studies of phonology and syntax have shown relative preservation of these processes. Demented subjects recognize and correct phonologic errors even at severe stages of the disease.[2,19] Kempler, Curtiss and Jackson described preserved syntactic abilities in DAT subjects.[10] The DAT subjects produced a similar range and frequency of syntactic constructions as well as a similar level of syntactic complexity as compared to normals. Schwartz, Marin, and Saffran described relative preservation of syntax in dementia as manifested by use of syntactic cues to disambiguate homophones.[11] The same subjects had significant difficulty using semantic cues for disambiguation purposes. Although most studies report intact syntactic abilities, the intactness of this system may be relative. Other studies indicate that, although syntax is grammatically correct in DAT subjects, syntactic simplification occurs.[8,16] This disparity may be because of the difference in tasks, as syntactic complexity varies according to the type of discourse. (See Chapter 7 for more detail on language abilities.)

## SUMMARY

Important empirical facts relevant to communication deficits in dementia have been identified. Evidence indicates that communication is disrupted by reduction of essential information, despite increased verbal output, and by impaired coherence and tangential and perseverative language. Considerable groundwork has now been laid in identifying deficits in dementia. Currently there is need to focus attention on explanations for patterns of losses and preserved abilities. The next section discusses interpretations offered for the findings in dementia research.

## Explanations of Findings

Clinically, differential diagnosis is only the first step in the management and treatment of disease. Once a diagnosis is made, the next step is to offer explanations for the behavioral disruptions. Specifically, it is necessary to consider the underlying mechanisms contributing to the difficulties. For example, how can one account for the presence of verbosity at one stage and taciturnity at a later stage? Is the verbosity seen in various clinical populations, e.g., demented patients, Wernicke's aphasic patients, and healthy old-elderly persons, caused by the same or similar mechanisms? Understanding what underlies the problem leads to development of appropriate treatment alternatives. Differential diagnosis needs to be closely tied to treatment for clinical advancement.

Several explanations for the behavioral losses and preservations have been suggested or implied in the literature. The most commonly proposed interpretations for performance patterns in dementia revolve around observed *dissociations*: dissociations between cognition and language, dissociations between language components and within language components, and dissociations between automatic versus volitional language function. Other interpretations relate to brain-behavior relations. Finally, some believe that deficits result from an interaction between cognitive and linguistic functions.

## DISSOCIATIONS

Dissociations between cognition and language have evolved from evidence that verbal performance in dementia is more resistant to deterioration than other intellectual functions. In fact, language is claimed to be compromised only in the later stages of the disease.[5,7] This perspective holds that communicative deficits in dementia occur secondary to cognitive rather than linguistic deficits. Bayles, however, contends that this disparity between cognitive and linguistic performances is because of the differential ways in which the two are assessed.[1] The cognitive tasks upon which such conclusions were drawn are more complex than the linguistic tasks. Hence, researchers have now begun to look more closely at linguistic function in dementia.

Linguistic studies have demonstrated dissociations between syntactic and semantic language systems. Several explanations for these findings are provided. One is that syntax represents a more automatic process whereas semantic performance is more volitional.[10,19] These researchers acknowledge that certain semantic tasks, e.g., counting, naming days and months, can be more automatic and that certain syntactic abilities can be more volitional. They suggested that automatic tasks (syntactic or semantic) are relatively spared, whereas volitional tasks are more likely to be impaired. Different neural organizations for automatic versus volitional functions are proposed. For example, Schwartz et al suggested that the semantic system may be more diffusely organized, whereas syntax is more locally organized in the brain.[15] Such an explanation would account for why syntax may be more impaired following a focal lesion such as that seen in aphasia than in diffuse organic brain involvement seen in dementia.

Other evidence suggests that syntax of DAT subjects may not be "intact" after all. Syntax in DAT subjects appears to be simplified when compared to normals on self-generated discourse.[8] As the disease progresses, syntactic simplification increases and paragrammatic errors occur.[8,11] Further evidence for impaired syntax is reported by Whitaker, whose subject had more difficulty on a self-correction task as the syntactic complexity increased.[19] DeAjuriaguerra and Tissot found that severely demented subjects failed to correct complex sentences containing causal and temporal clauses but did correct relatively simple morphosyntactic errors such as errors in noun-verb agreement.[4] Schwartz and colleagues agree that cognitive decline may affect the syntactic as well as semantic system in DAT subjects, but the underlying mechanisms are probably quite different than those that produce the syntactic disturbances seen in agrammatic aphasic patients.[15] Another explanation given is that the syntactic disturbances seen in dementia may occur in patients with an associated focal pathology. Hier et al reported abbreviated responses in stroke-related dementia.[8] It is unclear whether these abbreviated responses were in any way agrammatical.

Others have offered explanations that relate linguistic and cognitive function. Ulatowska et al suggested that comprehension difficulties may be caused by attentional deficits.[16] Specifically, DAT subjects may have failed a comprehension task because of inadequate encoding rather than because of inability to access the information. In addition, these researchers offer several interpretations for reduction of information. One possible explanation is memory deficits underlying reduction of essential information. Another is difficulties in organizing thought, resulting in simplification of information. An alternative explanation is impaired understanding of the task demands. Although not explicitly stated, the schemata underlying the various tasks in the Bayles et al study suggest that memory may underlie some deficits.[3] These explanations indicate that language and cognitive abilities are intricately related processes that do not function autonomously. According to this view, generalized cognitive impairments are seen to affect both language and communication.

## SUMMARY

Thus far, empirical facts have been summarized regarding deficits and preserved abilities in dementia and provided possible explanations for such findings. Although some explanations have been offered, continued efforts are needed in this direction to unravel the complex interaction of cognition, linguistic function, and communication. The next section describes one approach to investigating communicative decline in dementia. This represents only one of the many possible ways to study the relation between cognition and language in dementia.

## Methodology

The major purpose of this pilot study is to present a methodologic approach for exploring the interrelationship among cognitive, linguistic, and communicative processes in dementia. The approach uses the same experimental paradigm to assess these three processes, as opposed to evaluating cognitive performance on certain measures and communicative and linguistic performance on different measures. The methodology is used to evaluate various geriatric populations that are relevant to understanding discourse in dementia. After describing the population and methodology, the important trends relevant to discourse performance in dementia are presented. Because this is a pilot study, the data are not subjected to statistical analysis; rather, comparisons are descriptive and based on raw data. This methodology is an initial attempt to explore the mechanisms underlying impaired communicative competence in dementia.

### POPULATIONS

Four groups of subjects were used in this study. Each group consisted of five subjects and included patients with dementia of the Alzheimer's type, age- and education-matched normal controls, old-elderly persons (>85 years of age), and aphasic patients. Four of the DAT subjects were in their early to mid-sixties, and one was in his seventies. The aphasic subjects were somewhat younger. The Alzheimer's and aphasic groups included patients with mild and moderate levels of impairment. Severity for the DAT subjects was assessed by their performance on the Mini-Mental Status Exam (MMSE), and severity for aphasic subjects was assessed by the Boston Diagnostic Aphasia Examination (BDAE). All subjects were screened for adequate hearing and vision. These four groups of subjects were selected because of their relevance to dementia.

Studies of contrasting clinical populations provide insight into the nature of a disease process as well as the underlying mechanisms of the disease. Characteristic features of a disease become more apparent when compared to diagnostic features of other populations. For example, patients with Alzheimer's disease were compared to aphasic patients because both represent neurologically impaired populations and because similar verbal behaviors are reported for DAT and Wernicke's aphasic patients. Alzheimer's and aphasic patients differ in cortical focus and the progressive aspect of the disease. Nonetheless, linguistic features of Alzheimer's discourse, e.g., emptiness and relative verbosity, are often said to be similar to that observed in the language of Wernicke's aphasic patients.[11] Comparisons between these two neurologically impaired populations provide insight into whether different mechanisms are producing similar surface manifestations. Also, comparisons between these two populations are of interest because of the converse relation between language and cognition. It is believed that in Alzheimer's disease, language is preserved relative to cognitive abilities, whereas in aphasia, cognition is preserved relative to language performance. Exploring the contrast between these two populations can provide valuable insight into the complex interaction between cognitive and linguistic processing.

The comparison between Alzheimer's subjects and old-elderly persons addresses the issue of whether the dementing disease represents an early aging process. Old-elderly persons are often compared with Alzheimer's subjects because of similar behavioral manifestations, e.g., memory impairment and verbosity. Furthermore, diffuse brain involvement may be present in both populations. The rate and degree of deterioration, however, are not similar. A slower rate of deterioration may allow old-elderly persons to develop compensatory strategies over time.

### EXPERIMENTAL PARADIGM

The design for the experimental tasks described herein was derived from theoretic and clinical perspectives. Theoretically, the empiric facts regarding deficits in dementia served as a guide in determining what behaviors to tap. Behavioral deficits across cognitive, linguistic, and communicative domains were of interest. The methodologic approach utilized tasks with various components so that the same experimental paradigm could be used to tap all three domains. From a clinical perspective, measures of behaviors identified as important to differential diagnosis were incorporated into the tasks.

The primary purpose of this pilot study of dementia was to identify linguistic, communicative, and cognitive deficits underlying discourse production and to consider the interrelationships across these deficits. Our particular bias is that deficits in the three domains (i.e., linguistic, communicative, and cognitive) do *not* occur independently but, rather, arise from related underlying processes. Therefore, it is important to evaluate these three domains on the same experimental paradigm, as opposed to separate measures. Two issues were addressed. The first issue was the relation between performance at various levels of language (i.e., lexical-semantic, syntactic, and discourse). The premise was that there would be a dissociation between the different levels of language, namely discourse being impaired and syntax being relatively spared in dementia. The second issue focused on the ability to manipulate information necessary for discourse production. To address this second issue, information contained in the discourse tasks was elicited using paradigms that place different cognitive demands on information processing. Our hypothesis was that DAT subjects may have difficulty formulating discourse because of underlying cognitive impairments, e.g., impairments in selecting, isolating, or sorting information, to mention a few.

## RATIONALE FOR NARRATIVE DISCOURSE

Narratives are actually stories that relate a sequence of events where one or more characters are involved. Narratives represent the most basic discourse genre from which other discourse genres such as jokes and procedures are derived. Narrative discourse was chosen for several reasons. The most important reason is that the interrelationship between language and cognition can be best studied at a discourse level.[17] Sentential level aspects of language do not reflect this relationship as readily. The nature of discourse is optimally suited for building tasks to tap different types of knowledge. Second, this is the area of our relative expertise, as we have studied discourse and the relation between language and cognition in a variety of adult populations. For example, discourse studies in aphasia have provided insight into a dissociation between cognitive and linguistic abilities. Specifically, aphasic patients had preserved information structure despite severe disruption in linguistic abilities.[18] Third, deficits at a discourse level in dementia have been well documented in the literature reviewed above.

In addition, narrative discourse is a familiar form of connected language, making it ecologically salient. Narratives are a natural part of daily interactions as current and past life experiences are shared with others. We chose Norman Rockwell prints to elicit narratives because they belong to the salient era of our subjects' lives. Task salience is a critical factor in research with DAT subjects because failure to perform may result from a lack of motivation or a fear of failure and not necessarily from reduced abilities. In addition, not only are narratives familiar to all speakers, they also represent a clear organization of information. Story structure and chronologic sequence of events are intuitive to all speakers because this information is derived from world-knowledge schemas developed early in life.

Finally, narrative discourse was chosen because it is optimally suited for experimental purposes. Patterns of narrative production are more predictable, thus more interpretable, than other forms of discourse, e.g., conversation where response predictability is much lower. From a cognitive point of view, well-organized narratives are more resistant to memory decay because they may be supported by world knowledge. This interaction between memory and language is not as readily apparent in conversational discourse. In addition, complexity level of narratives can be easily manipulated to assess subjects at various severity levels. Complexity of both content and depicted organizational schema may be controlled. As described subsequently, narrative complexity was manipulated by using both single-frame pictures (Norman Rockwell) and sequenced pictures to elicit narratives.

## STIMULI

The primary stimuli for this experiment were pictorial. By using pictorial stimuli, some control over the input is provided without controlling the structure of subjects' responses. Thus, the subject is allowed to create his or her own story using a personally driven internal schema. Such is not the case for auditory retelling tasks where information is already structured. A creative aspect is an important factor in tapping differences at mild stages of dementia. Pictures, as opposed to auditory stories, can be processed by patients with a wider range of deficits, e.g., auditory comprehension impairments, memory, or attention deficits.

Two types of visual stimuli were used to elicit narratives. The first type was a single-frame picture where a single event was frozen in time. For this picture-type, the events leading up to the single-frame, as well as those following the depicted event, were implicit and had to be interpreted by the subject. This first type was more open-ended and allowed more originality or creativity of the story line. The second type of stimuli, sequence pictures, depicted the events from beginning to end. In this type, the narrative content was explicitly stated.

The *single-frame pictures* included five Norman Rockwell prints. The pictures differed according to the relationship between the depicted characters. In three of the stories, all the depicted characters (two or three) were central to the story. An example of this story type was the picture of a father, his son, and the boy's dog, waiting for a train to take the boy to college. In the other two stories, there were many characters (10 or more) focused on one participant. These characters did not play a central role in the story. Their role was that of observer. This type was exemplified by the homecoming picture where a soldier was returning home from war and was greeted by his girlfriend, family members, and neighbors. These two types of pictures could be used to determine whether the number of depicted characters affects performance.

The *picture sequences* included five different sequences ranging from four to seven frames. The story themes revolved around simple, everyday events, e.g., caring for a pet and losing one's possession. The subjects were asked to order the pictures before verbally generating a story. By having the subjects sequence the pictures, a patient's ability to logically organize pictured information could be assessed. This ability to sequence pictures could then be compared with ability to sequence information verbally.

## PROTOCOL

The experimental paradigm included a number of components designed to address the two central issues of this research that were outlined previously. The components are described below according to the two issues and are summarized in Table 8-1.

### Relation Between Levels of Language

In order to address the issue of the relation between performance at various levels of language, 15 narratives were elicited from each of the subjects. The narratives provided a means of assessing both the subjects' ability to structure large amounts of information in narrative form as well as the subjects' syntactic ability on individual sentences comprising the narrative. Facility with information structure relates to communicative ability. The lexical-semantic level of language was evaluated at both a single word and discourse level. The subjects were asked to name the people and items in the picture so that their naming ability on a confrontation task could then be compared to their ability to use specific reference terms during ongoing story formulation.

### Ability to Manipulate Information

In order to address the issue of the possible sources of discourse problems, the paradigm included subtasks that manipulated (1) memory; (2) isolation of information; (3) sorting information

TABLE 8.1 Experimental Tasks*

| STIMULI | NORMAL ROCKWELL PICTURES (5) | SEQUENCE PICTURES (4 to 7 FRAMES) |
|---|---|---|
| Sequencing pictures | | X |
| Reducing story by removing pictures | | X |
| Telling story (pictures present) | X | X |
| Telling story (pictures withdrawn) | X | |
| Eliciting titles for the story (pictures present) | X | X |
| Probe questions (pictures withdrawn) | | |
| 1. Setting | | |
|   a. place of story | X | |
|   b. time of story | X | |
| 2. Yes/No questions | X | |
|   a. Presence of items in story | X | |
|   b. Importance of items in story | X | X |
| Naming | X | |

*The tasks included for each pictorial stimulus are indicated by an "X"

according to importance; (4) reduction of information; and (5) sequence of information. *Memory* was tapped at both a discourse and word level. Subjects were asked to retell the story and to name the people and items that they remembered from the the picture after the stimulus was withdrawn. By adding a memory component to the experimental paradigm, subjects' language performance with and without supporting visual cues could be compared.

Probe questions soliciting specific information were incorporated in the task to evaluate ability to *isolate information*. The specific information consisted of temporal and locative information and questions requiring yes or no responses. Temporal questions probed *when* the story took place and locative questions probed *where* the story took place. Temporal and locative information is considered to be the most essential information to narratives. If temporal and locative information is not spontaneously produced in a narrative, then it is diagnostically important to determine if the subject can identify the information in response to individual probe questions. Cognitively, a person may have difficulty organizing important information in ongoing discourse but still may process isolated "chunks" of information. Additionally, yes or no questions were asked regarding whether certain props or characters were present in the pictorial stimulus, after the stimulus was withdrawn. The probe questions included foil items of thematically related and unrelated items. These probe questions involved both memory and ability to isolate information.

Ability to *sort information* according to importance was measured by asking subjects if certain items were important to the story. It was explained that unimportant items could be removed without changing the story, whereas important items would alter the story if they were removed. Examples were given for further clarification. For the picture-sequence stories, subjects were asked to identify any pictures that could be removed without changing the story. For the single pictorial stimulus, subjects were asked to identify the most important actors and items to the story. Ability to *reduce information* was measured by asking the subjects to formulate titles for their narratives. Producing story titles requires abstracting the gist of a story and expressing the global meaning in a few words. These latter two components tap higher level cognitive and linguistic processes and entail certain perceptual or cognitive evaluations. Structuring the tasks in such a manner provided a way to evaluate subjects' abilities to organize information hierarchically and express it verbally. Thus, both cognitive and linguistic function could be tapped simultaneously.

## DATA ANALYSES

The experimental language tasks were audiorecorded and transcribed verbatim. For cases of ambiguous text, transcripts were verified for accuracy by a second listener and consensus for interpretation was reached. The texts were then separated into propositions, an informational unit consisting of a predicate with one or more associated arguments. To address issue one (i.e., the relation between levels of language), all narratives were analyzed at multiple levels, i.e., sentential, content, and discourse levels, in order to fully understand communicative performance. Looking at any level in isolation will provide an incomplete picture. Although isolated deficits may be identifiable by assessing individual language levels, explanations will be incomplete. For example, sentential analysis may be the most tedious and least revealing, in light of the fact that syntactic abilities are relatively preserved in dementia. Nonetheless, some measure of intactness of basic syntactic units is important because syntax represents the form of language and represents units of thought. Some researchers have suggested that syntax in dementia is simplified. First, the issue of whether syntax is indeed simplified needs to be addressed. If it is, then the aspects that are simplified need to be identified. Finally, explanations need to be offered to account for why the simplification may occur. Perhaps reduction of syntax is a compensatory mechanism to monitor the train of thought during ongoing speech. Alternately, certain linguistic devices necessary for complex syntactic formulations may no longer be available, resulting in syntactic reduction.

**Sentential Analysis.** The basic unit for segmenting the data was a sentential unit, specifically a T-unit. A T-unit is defined as one independent clause plus any dependent modifiers of that clause.[9] Sentential analyses included the components of (1) number of T-units; (2) length of T-units measured by number of words; and (3) a complexity measure as determined by clauses per T-unit and type of clauses.

**Content Analysis.** The basic unit for evaluating content is the proposition defined above. Content analyses included three components. First, amount of language was measured by number of propositions. Second, amount of information produced was measured against a set of a priori propositions. The set of a priori propositions was derived by analysis of the stimulus material and agreed upon by five judges. All judges were speech-language pathologists with extensive experience with adult neurogenic populations. Finally, number of incomplete propositions was measured.

**Discourse Analysis.** The 15 narratives (5 with

Rockwell prints present, 5 with Rockwell prints removed, 5 with picture sequences) were evaluated using both genre-type and story-grammar characteristics. The different genre types included narratives, descriptions, or combinations of narrative and description. According to story grammar, the following components are considered necessary for a narrative: setting, complicating action, and resolution. Optional elements include abstract, code, and evaluation. In addition, the use of reference in narratives was investigated according to pronoun-to-referent ratio. Errors of reference were also tabulated. An error of reference occurred if (1) no clear referent for a pronoun could be found, or (2) more than one referent could be assigned to a pronoun.

## Results and Discussion

ISSUE ONE: *Relation between levels of language.*

### Word Level

Word level abilities were measured by having the subjects name pictured items. Difficulties in naming were present for both the DAT and old-elderly groups but were minimal for the normal controls and aphasic subjects. Evidence of reduced naming abilities supports previous evidence of difficulties in dementia on generative naming tasks. The naming difficulties may reflect attentional deficits manifested by poor scanning strategies. Subjects may superficially scan the picture in a rather disorganized fashion.

It is interesting to note that the DAT and old-elderly subjects tended to use sentences to identify items rather than to produce labels. The subjects responded as if they were retelling the story again, even when specifically instructed to just name the items. This may have been a type of contextual cuing strategy they adopted to aid their naming ability.

### Sentential Level

The raw data for sentential measures are represented in Table 8-2 to illustrate the trends across the four populations. These trends may be supported by additional studies on larger sample sizes. Quantity of language was measured by total number of words and number of T-units. As can be seen from Table 8-2, the old-elderly group produced more language on both the single-picture and picture-sequence narratives than the other groups. Comparing the two story tasks, the old-elderly group was the only group that exhibited more verbal output on the picture-sequence narratives than on the single-picture narratives. Interestingly, the DAT subjects were the second most

TABLE 8.2 Comparison of DAT, Old-Elderly, Aphasic, and Control Subjects on Selected Linguistics Measures. Numerical Values Represent Raw Figures per Task

| MEASURE | DAT | OLD ELDERLY | APHASIC | CONTROLS |
|---|---|---|---|---|
| **Mean Number of Words** | | | | |
| Rockwell | 185 | 230 | 152 | 166 |
| Sequence | 104 | 276 | 118 | 120 |
| **Mean Number of T-units** | | | | |
| Rockwell | 16 | 22 | 17 | 12 |
| Sequence | 9 | 26 | 14 | 8 |
| **Mean Number of Words per T-unit** | | | | |
| Rockwell | 11.6 | 10.7 | 11.6 | 9.1 |
| Sequence | 11.5 | 10.5 | 11.5 | 8.6 |
| **Mean Number of Clauses per T-unit** | | | | |
| Rockwell | 1.8 | 1.8 | 1.6 | 1.9 |
| Sequence | 2.1 | 1.7 | 1.5 | 2.4 |

verbal on the single-picture narrative but the least verbal on the picture-sequence narratives. Little difference in verbal output was found for either the aphasic or normal control subgroups between the two tasks.

In terms of sentential length, the aphasic group showed the greatest reduction, followed by old-elderly and DAT subjects. Normal subjects had the longest sentences in terms of both words and clauses per T-unit (see Table 8–2). The relative distribution of clause-types was evaluated across populations. The results showed a similar distribution of clause-types, with noun clauses and relative clauses being the most frequent types for all groups. Low-frequency clauses were virtually absent from the language of aphasic subjects. The finding of similar clausal distribution supports the notion of a continuum of language change across populations. The continuum of language change occurs because the inherent structure of language allows only a limited number of ways for language to be expressed.

For the most part, the above findings were consistent with those anticipated. Reduction in sentential length and clausal types in aphasia is a well-established fact. The finding of increased verbal output in the old-elderly has been reported previously.[12] The trend observed in DAT subjects of increased amount of language on single-picture as compared to output on picture-sequence narratives suggests that the nature of the task affects performance. We can only speculate on the reasons for the differences in the DAT subjects between the two tasks. Perhaps the structure and explicit information offered in the picture-sequence task helped the demented patients to organize information and to reduce extraneous detail and redundancies of information. Another alternative explanation is that the DAT subjects found the picture-sequence task simplistic, reducing motivation on the task. Possibly the difficulty described later in sequencing the picture-sequence narratives may have been reflected in reduced language.

One question raised was whether verbosity is characteristic of DAT subjects. The DAT subjects ranked second in amount of output as measured by total number of words, on the single-picture narrative only. When individual demented subjects were reviewed, however, a considerable range in performance between DAT subjects was observed. For example, one moderately impaired DAT subject displayed more language as measured by number of words, longer sentences, and more embedding than any other DAT or old-elderly subject. In contrast, a mildly impaired DAT subject produced less language with shorter sentences than old-elderly or normal subjects. Sample stories of these two DAT subjects are presented in Appendix A. For this small study, verbosity was not associated with mild disease stage of dementia. Verbosity probably reflects premorbid tendencies as well as disease progression. The disparity of performances between the two DAT subjects described above may be indicative of the lack of homogeneity among DAT subjects in general.

The failure to find any conspicuous differences in sentential complexity between DAT and normal subjects may have resulted from the nature of the tasks. Methodologically, the task simplicity may have obscured any real differences. Narrative discourse does not require higher ranges of sentential complexity, because the information can be expressed with relatively simple syntax. This is particularly true of narratives elicited from picture-sequence stories. Expository discourse, on the other hand, entails more diverse syntax with complex clausal embedding. Thus, complex discourses such as expositions may be more sensitive to changes in sentential structure.

## CONTENT ANALYSIS

The most important finding regarding content was marked reduction of information in DAT subjects as compared to normal control subjects. Normal subjects produced approximately 88 percent of the core information determined by a priori propositions, whereas DAT subjects produced only 58 percent. DAT subjects produced less information than the other three groups. Aphasic subjects produced 82 percent of the a priori propositions. The aphasic subjects performed at a similar level to the normal subjects on this measure of essential content information. Old-elderly subjects performed poorer than normal and aphasic subjects (74 percent), but better than DAT subjects.

Content analysis revealed parallel performances between certain populations. Performances by DAT and old-elderly subjects appeared similar, whereas aphasic and normal control subjects exhibited similar performances. DAT subjects did however, exhibit more incomplete propositions than old-elderly or any other population.

## DISCOURSE ANALYSIS

### Genre Type

Differences in discourse genre types (narrative versus descriptive) were found across the four populations, although the populations clustered in a similar way as reported for content measures. Both DAT (48 percent) and old-elderly (48 percent) subjects produced more descriptive genre types than did aphasic (24 percent) and normals (28 percent). The latter two populations produced more *narra-*

*tive* genre-type discourses. Thus, changes in discourse structure were observed in DAT and old-elderly as compared to normals. A possible explanation for the differences in genre type is discussed later.

### Story Grammar Analysis

Differences in distribution of information were found across populations. Distribution of information was evaluated by the story components of setting, complicating action, and resolution. Although all four populations produced setting information, this component represented the greatest amount of information in DAT narratives. That is, amount of setting information was increased in the DAT subjects as compared to other populations. In addition, action sequences were poorly developed in the moderately impaired DAT subjects. Finally, resolutions were rarely produced in narratives of DAT subjects.

The co-occurrence of descriptive genre type and inclusion of setting information is consistent in two ways. Settings and descriptive discourse genres are simpler to express both linguistically and cognitively. Linguistically, descriptive discourse and setting information are expressed with stative verbs (e.g., forms of *to be*) and require limited diversity in verb forms. Cognitively, both descriptive discourse and setting have a simpler set of underlying relations because information consists of components that are not closely related.

### Coherence

Impairment of coherence was measured by the number of reference errors, i.e., instances of referent without an antecedent or ambiguous referents. These disruptions were especially evident in old-elderly subjects and in some DAT subjects. Few reference errors were found in the aphasic subjects. Disruptions of reference were more evident in Norman Rockwell stories for all four groups. In addition to errors of reference, other variables such as number of incomplete propositions, false starts, and poorly developed story line seemed to have an impact on coherence, especially for the DAT subjects.

ISSUE TWO: *Ability to Manipulate Information*

### Memory

Memory was tapped at three levels: (1) telling a story from memory; (2) naming objects from memory; and (3) answering yes/no probes as to whether certain items appeared in a picture. On the story task, productions of narrative, as opposed to merely descriptive discourse, increased on the second telling for the mildly impaired DAT and old-elderly subjects. In contrast, moderately impaired DAT subjects' performance did not improve. In some instances, subjects at the moderate severity level completely lost the pictured story from memory. It is of clinical interest to note that production of narrative as opposed to descriptive genre types increased from the first to second telling for all populations except the moderately impaired DAT subjects. This pattern occurred even though the second telling was from memory. The fact that the aphasic, old-elderly, and mild DAT subjects did better on the second story in terms of appropriate genre type suggests that they were helped in some way by the probe questions between the two tellings. The probe questions may have helped the subjects structure pieces of information necessary for building discourse.

Although most of the subjects produced more narrative-type discourse on the second telling (from memory), they did not necessarily produce as much of the core information on the second telling (from memory) as they produced in the first telling (picture present). The effects of memory loss were seen for both the DAT and old-elderly subjects on the story from memory condition. These two groups produced fewer "core" propositions when telling the story from memory as compared to telling the story with the picture in front of them. This reduction of core information in the memory condition was not observed in the aphasic and normal control subjects.

Reduction of information in the memory condition may occur because of memory decay or pragmatic factors involved in telling the same story for a second time. The normal and aphasic subjects in this study exhibited relatively good memory. Narrative information content was not adversely affected when they told the story from memory. For old-elderly and DAT subjects, both memory and pragmatic factors may have contributed to the significant deterioration in performance. Memory decay seems to be the strongest factor for two reasons. First, all subjects made some effort to respond. Second, some DAT subjects remarked that the story was "gone from their head" or they told parts of stories from previously seen pictures.

Naming performance from memory deteriorated for both DAT and old-elderly subjects, as compared to aphasic and normal subjects. DAT subjects showed the greatest decrement in performance. The DAT and old-elderly subjects did not appear to be aided by a general context provided by a pictured story. Context seems to facilitate labeling in normal subjects by providing an organizing framework. If an organizational schema is not in force, elements may become more difficult to retrieve from memory. This may explain why naming performance by DAT and old-elderly subjects deteriorated in the memory condition.

## Isolation of Information

The specific information solicited included yes/no probes in regard to the presence of specified items depicted in the pictures (picture withdrawn) as well as locative and temporal information. The probe questions were included to compare naming from memory to answering yes/no questions. Both were related to identifying pictured items. Failure to recall an item may be attributable to either a naming deficit or memory impairment. Yes/no questions were included to measure identification of pictured items without having the subjects label the items. The DAT subjects made almost twice as many errors (mean number of errors per patient) as old-elderly subjects and almost three times the number of errors per subject compared with aphasic and normal subjects on the yes/no probes.

## Sorting Information According to Importance

Two tasks were used to measure ability to organize information according to perception of importance, one on the single-frame stories and one on the picture-sequence stories. As described earlier, subjects were asked probe questions as to whether certain items were important to the single-frame stories (Norman Rockwell prints). In addition, reasons for how the items were important to the story were solicited. DAT subjects showed a response bias toward an affirmative response to the yes/no probes. Perhaps they felt an item must be important simply because the examiner asked if it was. This response bias was not seen in the other three populations. In supplying a reason, DAT subjects tended to respond with the same words as in the question. That is, a common rationale was that the item could not be removed without changing the story because it was important to the story.

On the picture-sequence stories, subjects were asked to remove any picture that could be taken out without changing the story. This task involved reducing information to include only the most essential information and proved to be difficult for the DAT and old-elderly subjects. Conversely, the aphasic and normal control subjects had no difficulty on this task. The DAT and old-elderly subjects were either unable to reduce the information or were reluctant to do so. This reluctance may have been because of rigidity of thinking.

## Reduction of Information

Title creation requires abstracting the main point or gist of a story and expressing it in a few words. Title formulation results in a wide range of responses even for normal individuals, making response analysis difficult. The titles generated by all subjects were assessed at two levels, first at a global level and then at a more descriptive level. Globally, titles were classified as either relevant or irrelevant to the story content. The results at this level revealed no interesting differences. Even moderately impaired DAT subjects produced relevant topics. DAT subjects appeared to be able to glean a global impression of the content, even though they had difficulty organizing the information.

At a more specific level of analysis, classifications of titles included metaphoric titles at one end of the spectrum and shortened stories or descriptions at the other end. Metaphoric titles represent the most abstract level, whereas shortened stories or descriptions reflect a more concrete level of response. Metaphoric titles were produced predominately by the normal control subjects, with some being produced by old-elderly subjects. No DAT subject produced a title at this abstract level. Metaphoric titles included "Injured Pride" and "The Price of Carelessness." There was considerable overlap in performance between DAT and old-elderly subjects at the more concrete level where subjects tended to recount the story again, although in a shortened version. Other title descriptions included evaluative comments and identification of main props. An example of an evaluative title is "Smashed Window is not Good." This type of title is higher level than retelling the story. Evaluative titles were observed in aphasic subjects. Their titles seemed to focus on the main props or actors, for example, "The Bird and the Little Girl," "The Thief and the Satchel." DAT subjects produced titles classified as perseverative, personalized, or empty. Examples of perseverative titles included: "A Lost Bird," "The Lost Dog," and "The Lost Cap." Personalized titles included: "Feeding *My* Birds," "*My* New Dog," and "Training *My* Dog." An example of an empty title was "Little Man and Big Man and a Little Thing."

The results showed considerable overlap in performance across the four populations. Aphasic subjects had difficulty because of linguistic impairments. Counter to the hypothesis that DAT subjects would not be able to produce titles, some DAT subjects were able to produce abbreviated titles, demonstrating an ability to organize information hierarchically. A method that may be more sensitive to differential diagnosis is to request one statement that best represents the story. This task may be more effective than a title formulation task in tapping ability to focus on the single most important aspect of a story.

## Sequence of Information

Finally, subjects' ability to sequence information without verbal expression was evaluated by having the subjects sequence the picture-sequence stories. The most notable finding was the inability of the moderately impaired DAT subjects to correctly sequence any of the five stories. Their performance was completely random. The aphasic and normal control subjects correctly sequenced all of the stories, while the mildly impaired DAT and old-elderly subjects sequenced only 60 percent and 75 percent of the stories, respectively. Greater difficulties for the latter two populations were also manifested by increased time to complete each task.

## HESITATION PHENOMENA IN INFORMATION PROCESSING

In addition, certain indicators of information-processing difficulties were present in the flow of speech of mildly impaired DAT subjects. These indicators included: (1) "hedges," or terms of uncertainty, e.g., presumably, I assume, possibly; (2) hesitations, defined as unfilled pauses of duration of 5 seconds or more; and (3) false starts. The use of "hedges" seemed to differentiate DAT from old-elderly subjects. "Hedges" occurred in language of old-elderly, aphasic, and normal subjects only one-third as frequently as in the language of DAT subjects. Hedging terms may be used for different reasons in DAT and normal subjects. Normal subjects may not want to commit themselves to a particular interpretation, whereas DAT subjects simply may not have the information. The second indicator of processing difficulties was hesitations. A similar incidence of hesitations occurred in both DAT and old-elderly. Hesitations were more frequent in the speech of aphasic subjects as compared to normals, but almost half as frequent as in DAT subjects. Hesitations are reflective of different underlying mechanisms. In aphasia, the hesitations may be more of a motor control or language problem, whereas in dementia the problem may be cognitive or linguistic. False starts, the third indicator of processing difficulties, were more characteristic of old-elderly subjects. They were also characteristic of aphasic subjects, but to a lesser degree than old-elderly subjects. DAT subjects produced approximately one-half the number of false starts as did the old-elderly subjects.

## RATINGS

Although the primary data analyses described above involved objective measures, subjective rating measures were also included. Ratings were conducted by four speech-language pathologists with extensive experience with adult neurogenic communication disorders. We felt it important to verify the objective measures against some subjective evaluation. Objective measures may suggest differences not apparent to listeners and, vice versa, listeners may perceive problems to which objective measures are insensitive. Thus, we wanted to see if unbiased listeners rated the groups differently on five communicative aspects: (1) genre type; (2) story content; (3) story clarity; (4) perceived communicative difficulties; and (5) quality of story with visual stimuli compared to story from memory. In addition, the raters, blinded to subjects' diagnosis, were asked to classify each subject according to which of the four populations (DAT, aphasic, old-elderly, and normal control) they felt the subject belonged. In general, the subjective measures paralleled the objective measures. DAT and old-elderly subjects were rated lower on content and clarity measures than aphasic or normal subjects. Aphasic subjects were rated lowest of all groups on perceived difficulties in communicating. This lowered rating may relate to impairment of aphasics' language at a sentential level that is readily apparent to listeners.

The attempted diagnosis of the subject groups added support to the evidence of overlap between DAT and old-elderly subjects. Old-elderly subjects were misdiagnosed more frequently than any other subgroup. The misclassifications were that of DAT. Furthermore, misclassifications for DAT tended to be old-elderly. Aphasic and normal subjects were rarely misclassified.

## Concluding Remarks

This section integrates the findings from the multilevel analyses and offers global interpretations. We will then discuss the implications from both a clinical and research perspective.

The evidence from this study suggests that DAT subjects suffer from impairment of communication and not language. Documentation of communicative decline in DAT subjects was supported by the described deficits in information content and structure. Impairment of information content was manifested by (1) reduction of information and (2) reduction of specificity of information. The former impairment of content was characterized by reduction of essential information when responses were matched against a particular stimulus. The latter impairment was characterized by disruption of reference. Problems with reference produced vagueness of expression. This vagueness could not be attributed to language deficits, as is the case in aphasia. Impairment of information structure was manifested by (1) difficulties sequencing information in a logical order and (2) rigidity in restructuring information. The rigidity in restructuring information was observed in (1) tasks requiring removal of relatively unimportant information; (2) reduction of information, as in title creation; and (3) isolation of an information item, as in naming. DAT subjects tended to name items within the context of retelling the story rather than simply labeling the objects. Labeling was characteristic of aphasic and normal subjects. Perhaps the failure to isolate labels may reflect a perseveration problem in that the subjects have difficulty shifting tasks. Indeed, perseveration may be one manifestation of rigidity of thought. Alternately, the retelling instead of labeling may reflect a compensatory strategy adopted to aid them in identifying a target item.

Although the primary deficits were in information content and structure, these deficits were reflected in other levels of analysis, i.e., discourse, sentential, and word levels. At a discourse level, DAT subjects exhibited impaired narrative superstructure. The distribution of information was skewed toward excessive setting, with action poorly developed and resolution typically absent. In addition, DAT subjects produced discourse that lacked coherence. They had difficulty connecting language components, as evidenced by disruption of reference and presence of incomplete propositions.

At a sentential level, no obvious impairment was found except for reduced length. Failure to find differences at this level may be because of the sample sizes or the simplistic nature of the tasks. More complex discourse types, e.g., expository discourse, may be more illuminating in terms of sentential level differences, although increased complexity may be appropriate for only mildly impaired subjects. At some level, incomplete propositions may affect sentential measures. For example, DAT subjects may produce what appears on the surface to be paragrammatic errors. Without more in-depth analysis, it cannot be ascertained whether paragrammatic errors reflect impaired use of functors or whether the errors reflect difficulties organizing thought.

Perhaps the most important implication from this study is the clustering of the clinical populations. DAT subjects more closely resembled the old-elderly subjects than any other population in terms of information content and structure. In contrast, aphasic subjects, the other neurologically impaired population, were more similar to normal control subjects on measures of information content and structure. This finding once again raises the issue of whether deficits identified in DAT subjects are a result of pathologic early aging. Perhaps this question can best be addressed by a multidisciplinary approach to the study of dementia in which behaviors are carefully characterized and neuroanatomic and neurophysiologic parameters are compared.

## Clinical and Research Implications

From a clinical perspective, implications for the present findings are discussed. First, a multidisciplinary approach to the study of dementia will provide an in-depth understanding of the mechanisms underlying the deficits. A speech-language pathologist should play a key role in a team approach, because a primary deficit is decline in communicative function. In performing this role, however, the speech-language pathologist is handicapped by the lack of appropriate standardized tests. Although a number of aphasia batteries are available, these tests are designed to tap the linguistic deficits central to communicative impairments in aphasia and are not appropriate for dementia. Unfortunately, measures of communicative function secondary to cognitive decline are not presently available. Major efforts are needed to design test batteries to tap the communicative deficits in dementia.

We believe a promising conceptual schema for a test battery would include measures to tap language processing at multiple levels. This is based on the present evidence that DAT subjects have difficulty isolating and restructuring linguistic information. Tasks that may be particularly sensitive to dementia are discourse tasks requiring creativity of responses, inferencing, and generalizing ideas. Information content at the various levels needs to be thematically related so that the interrelationship of performance across levels (sentential, content, and discourse) and processes (cognitive, linguistic, and communicative) can be tapped. Identification of isolated deficits may provide important information regarding differential diagnosis. However, identifying isolated deficits does not offer explanations for the difficulties or directions for management. An integrated approach ties communicative breakdown to cognitive and linguistic performance and can provide guidance for therapeutic intervention. Tests that tap a wide range of abilities are necessary so that the batteries can measure decline in performance as the disease progresses.

At the current level of knowledge, it is not clear to what extent comprehension measures need to be included in batteries for dementia. Although a number of researchers have noted deficits in the latter stages of the disease, no systematic study has documented comprehension in dementia in early stages. DAT patients are frequently said to make irrelevant comments in response to questions. This may be because of deterioration of comprehension and attention as well as deterioration of hearing acuity (see Chapter 4). More documentation is needed in this modality.

Additionally, the evidence presented herein suggests that comparisons of DAT subjects to old-elderly may provide insight into the disease process unavailable through comparisons to normal aged-matched control subjects. Comparisons to old-elderly populations address the question of whether DAT is premature aging of the brain or another pathologic disease process. Studies of language and communicative function alone will probably not enable us to answer this question. Behavioral studies need to be done in conjunction with neuropathologic studies. Observation of one old-elderly subject classified (incorrectly) by three raters as DAT makes us suspect that some differences exist despite similar behavioral manifestations. On a less structured, more creative task, this old-elderly subject held the floor for 1½ hours, providing a sociolinguistic perspective of society and aging to a graduate-level class. Although some difficulties in fielding questions were noted, this subject produced elaborate and well-developed stories of real-life experiences. Thus, communicative impairment in old-elderly may be more pronounced on artificial tasks, as has been reported in the literature.

The gap in performances between DAT and aphasic subjects in this study suggests that use of the term aphasia to describe language deficits in dementia may be inappropriate. Little overlap in performance occurred between these two populations. Any similarities in performance appear to be because of different reasons. Thus, collapsing the classification of aphasia to describe language behavior in dementia my be misleading.

There is also need for more studies directed toward differential diagnosis of other types of dementia. Comparing and contrasting DAT subjects with other forms of dementia will provide valuable insight into differential disease processes and the impact of these processes on cognitive, linguistic, and communicative function.

In closing this chapter we would like to emphasize the need for naturalistic studies in dementia to complement methodologies as described in our experiment. Observation of patients in a variety of real-life situations provides a more complete picture of dementia, not only the deficits but also preserved abilities. For example, we are presently involved in assessment of communicative abilities of demented patients in a group setting in a geriatric day-care center. Communicative behavior of the patients is observed in a number of different activities such as playing games, talking about daily events, reminiscing about past events, and singing. On the basis of this evaluation, a communication profile for each patient is established in the form of a five-point scale. Communication behaviors include, among others, initiating appropriate spontaneous comments, requesting clarification, following simple directions, and using nonverbal language. Single-case studies of demented patients in their home environments are another way of in-depth investigation of patients who may have clearly delineated areas of preservations with severe disruptions of other competences. Functional tasks routinely performed by the patient, such as writing checks, can be used to tap preserved competences. The longitudinal nature of such studies may illuminate the nature of slow versus fast deterioration of specific functions in the course of a dementing illness.

As clinicians working with demented patients, we are made keenly aware of the progressive deterioration and devastation that these patients exhibit. Consequently, we frequently overlook and discount behavioral evidence of past talents, wit, and good spirit that they display on rare occasions. On such occasions, we get a glimpse of the dissociations described in this chapter and hence come closer to understanding the disease. From a human point of view, we come to terms with our own passage through time and the indestructible trace we leave behind.

### References

1. Bayles KA. Communication in dementia. In: Ulatowska HK, ed. The aging brain. San Diego: College-Hill Press, 1985:157.
2. Bayles KA, Boone DR. The potential of language tasks for identifying senile dementia. J Speech Hear Disord 1982; 47:210–217.
3. Bayles KA, Boone DR, Tomoeda CK, Slauson TJ, Kaszniak A. Differentiating Alzheimer's patients from the normal elderly and stroke patients with aphasia. J Speech Hear Disord 1989; 54:74–87.
4. DeAjuriaguerra J, Tissot R. Some aspects of language in various forms of senile dementia. In: Lenneberg E, Lenneberg E, eds. Foundations of language development: A multidisciplinary approach. New York: Academic Press, 1975:323.
5. Gustafson L, Hagberg B, Ingvar D. Speech disturbances in presenile dementia related to local cerebral blood flow abnormalities in the dominant hemisphere. Brain Lang 1978; 5:103–118.
6. Goodglass H, Kaplan E. The assessment of aphasia and related disorders. 2nd ed. Philadelphia: Lea & Febiger, 1983.
7. Hagberg B, Ingvar DH. Cognitive reduction in presenile dementia related to regional abnormalities in the cerebral blood flow. Br J Psychiatry 1976; 128:209–222.
8. Hier DB, Hagenlocker D, Shindler AG. Language disintegration in dementia: Effects of etiology and severity. Brain Lang 1985; 25:117–133.
9. Hunt KW. Grammatical structures written at three grade levels. Research report no. 3. Champaign, IL: National Council of Teachers of English, 1965.
10. Kempler D, Curtiss S, Jackson C. Syntactic preservation in Alzheimer's disease. J Speech Hear Res 1987; 30:343–350.
11. Obler L. Review of Le langage des dements. Brain Lang 1981; 12:375–386.

12. Obler LK. Language and brain dysfunction in dementia. In: Segalowitz S, ed. Language functions and brain organization. New York: Academic Press, 1983:267-282.
13. Obler LK, Albert ML. Language in the elderly aphasic and in the dementing patient. In: Sarno M, ed. Acquired aphasia. New York: Academic Press, 1981: 385-398.
14. Ripich DN, Terrell BY. Patterns of discourse cohesion and coherence in Alzheimer's disease. J Speech Hear Disord 1988; 53:8-19.
15. Schwartz M, Marin O, Saffran E. Dissociations of language function in dementia: A case study. Brain Lang 1979; 7:277-306.
16. Ulatowska HK, Allard L, Donnell A, et al. Discourse performance in subjects with dementia of the Alzheimer type. In: Whitaker H, ed. Neuropsychological studies of nonfocal brain damage. New York: Springer-Verlag, 1988:108-131.
17. Ulatowska HK, Cannito M, Hayashi M, Fleming S. Language abilities in the elderly. In: Ulatowska H, ed. The aging brain. San Diego: College-Hill Press, 1985: 125-139.
18. Ulatowska HK, Freedman-Stern R, Weiss–Doyel A, Macaluso-Haynes S. Production of narrative discourse in aphasia. Brain Lang 1983; 19:317-334.
19. Whitaker H. A case of the isolation of the language function. In: Whitaker H, Whitaker HA, eds. Studies in neurolinguistics. New York: Academic Press, 1976: 1-58.

# APPENDIX

# Samples of DAT Subjects' Language

## DAT Subject 1

**Age:** 61
**Education:** 17 Years
**Occupation:** Mechanical & Electrical Engineer
**Diagnosis:** Probable senile dementia of Alzheimer's type based on physical examination, neurologic examination, neuropsychological evaluation, laboratory evaluations, and neural imaging at the Alzheimer's Unit at Southwestern Medical School
**Onset:** 7 Years
**MMS:** 22
**Global Deterioration Scale:** 4
**Stage:** Early
**Neural Imaging:**
    Magnetic resonance imaging (MRI): Mild prominence of ventricles and sulci, consistent with age
    Single photon scanning (SPECT): Normal
**EEG:** Reduced alpha, abnormal delta. Results consistent with encephalopathic disorder such as DAT
**Other diagnoses ruled out:** Cerebral infarct, head trauma, infectious process, drug or alcohol abuse
**Example:** First telling of single Rockwell picture
**Discourse type:** Description, not narrative

| Subject 1 | Observations |
|---|---|
| OK, I'm going to start talking out loud for a moment. | Comment to examiner |
| Uh...there's a young boy in this picture and a more elderly man. | Identification of participants |
| And there seems to be uh...truck that they're sitting on the running board. | Location |
| There's a lantern over here sitting on some kind of box or something. | |
| And there's a collie dog there. | |
| And *apparently* this kid is going off to school. | Hedging |
| There's, he's got his...uh...luggage...uh | |
| *You don't know, don't know where the boy is* | |
| But I rather ex...expect that that he is uh...the grandson...or...uh... | |
| Those are the elements I see. | Closing |

**Example:** Second telling
**Discourse type:** Narrative

| | |
|---|---|
| OK we *don't know really*, with uh...with the starting of this story, to know just exactly where they are. | Hedging |
| But it *seems to be* that the uh...boy has come out either on the farm *maybe*. | Participant and location<br>Event |
| *Maybe* the others live in the uh...in the city, But he's out there to see his granddad and uh...get some advice, so forth. | |
| Uh...I'm sure that the grandfather was giving him some sage advice. | |
| Uh...he...the grandfather is *probably* not a uh...college graduate. | Event |

But he's trying to give good advice.
Uh...and I'm sure the boy was uh...happy to have it.
So uh...as soon as they got through with their little chat uh...the boy uh...left and went off to school. — Event / Event resolution

## DAT Subject 2:

**Age:** 58
**Education:** 17 Years
**Occupation:** Accountant
**Diagnosis:** Probable DAT
**Onset:** 55 Years
**Stage:** Mild
**EEG:** Unremarkable
**Example:** First telling of a single Rockwell picture
**Discourse type:** Description, not narrative

| Subject 2 | Observations |
|---|---|
| This picture of a uh... *apparently* at a uh... pardon me and uh... | Hedging |
| It has a uh...uh...old time...uh...radio sitting on uh...on the back of this | |
| And uh...there's a uh...uh...box here where pies and so forth were kept primarily and until they sell 'em and so forth. | |
| And there's a uh...uh...special today listing of uh...what they're, of what you could buy there for that day. | |
| And sitting that, the person that uh...runs this place is talking to a policeman. | |
| And they are | |
| And the policeman and a small boy is sitting there at the counter. | Identification of participants |
| And they are talking to each other | |
| Uh...the uh...there's a uh...uh... | |
| They have three stools shown here | |
| And uh...it shows uh...uh...that there's somebody *probably* had had some coffee because there's a cup and and and uh...so forth there with it. | Hedging |
| And uh...the uh...uh...*apparently* uh...that the person that runs this store uh...cafe...uh...*apparently* it's his son there. | Hedging / Hedging |
| And uh...he, the son was talking to the policeman. | |
| And uh...it doesn't uh...show whether exactly what they're talking about | |
| But they are talking to each other | |
| And and the boy has and | |
| The policeman are are looking to both together are looking for to each other | |
| And uh...the boy his his uh...uh...coat laying over his lap while he's sitting there | |
| And his | |
| And the policeman is sitting on a stool | |
| And he's got his uh...boots on the place there where they could put their feet | |
| And the boy couldn't reach that. | |

# CHAPTER 9

# *Bilingual Dementia: Pragmatic Breakdown*

LORAINE K. OBLER, Ph.D.
SUSAN de SANTI, M.S.
JOAN GOLDBERGER, M.A.

Bilingualism, for the purposes of this paper, can be defined as the ability to use two or more languages in proficient conversation with native speakers of each language. Not only are bilingual speakers able to use the linguistic structures of their two languages, they also master pragmatic and sociolinguistic norms of the culture surrounding each language. For example, the healthy bilingual is extremely sensitive to when it is appropriate to use which language. Moreover, the healthy bilingual has mastered code-switching—the ability to mix the two languages in linguistically, pragmatically, and sociolinguistically appropriate ways—by an early age. As a rule, bilingual aphasics make language choice and code-switching decisions appropriately, yet there is some indication that in the demented patient these abilities break down. This breakdown contributes to the impairment of communication between demented patients and caregivers who may often be frustrated and unaware of what exactly is occurring. Many elderly and demented patients in the Americas are bilingual because of immigration patterns at the end of the last century and at the beginning of the present one. Their numbers are particularly great in urban centers. Thus, it behooves professionals working with them to learn more about the communicative consequences of bilingualism.

This chapter reviews existing literature on breakdowns in code-switching and discusses a study reported more fully in de Santi et al,[1] documenting differences among individuals in ability to maintain appropriate language choice. The chapter concludes with suggestions for diagnostic and rehabilitive practice as well as ideas for further research.

## Review of the Literature

There have been anecdotal reports of grandparents speaking to their grandchildren in the grandparent's native tongue despite the fact that the grandparent had previously known that the grandchild did not speak the language. We were unable, however, to document this breakdown in a patient with dementia of the Alzheimer's type (DAT), studied at the Gerontological Neurolinguistic Laboratory of the Boston VA Medical Center and in the Boston Aphasia Research Center. The subject was a 73-year-old speaker of German origin who had immigrated to the United States in his early twenties. He was tested in both English and German at our laboratory. Despite moderate to severe DAT, he exhibited no problems in choosing the appropriate language to use either with German speakers or English speakers, nor was there any mixing of one language into the other in the hour-long test sessions or during conversations. This is particularly surprising as the patient was in the stage where his language resembled that of a Wernicke's aphasic, that is, it was fluent and empty, with poor comprehension, neologisms, and paraphasias. It is well known that the monitoring of speech errors is absent in both groups of patients, especially in the middle and late stages of DAT. One might have expected the apparent lack of ability to monitor one's own speech in this stage of Alzheimer's dementia to result in inappropriate switching or language choice.

Several papers have been presented or published, however, that report apparent difficulties in either language choice or code-switching in patients with DAT. Hyltenstam and Stroud reported on two patients with DAT (one a speaker of

Swedish and Finnish, the other a speaker of Swedish and German).[6] These patients both had two kinds of difficulties with language choice: (1) They would choose the inappropriate language as a base language when speaking to a monolingual interlocutor, and (2) they would code-switch with a monolingual interlocutor. Although these patients made many pragmatic errors in each of their languages (for example, in turn-taking and lexical search), Hyltenstam and Stroud saw that there was differential ability for these patients in their two languages.[6] One patient showed a substantial advantage in the first-learned language and the other patient showed a smaller advantage in the first-learned language.

If all demented patients experienced advantages in the first-learned language, it would be particularly striking because this is not the rule in polyglot aphasics. In some instances where differential recovery is reported in bilingual or polyglot aphasics, it is the first-learned language that is better spared. The rule that accounts significantly for differentially spared abilities in bilingual aphasics, however, is that the language that the aphasic has been using at the time of onset is the one that is spared, according to Obler and Albert.[9] Thus, it is simply by chance whether it is the first-learned language that is spared for bilingual aphasics. In the case of immigrants to a country where the use of a second language is necessary, the first-learned language is not generally the one that is being primarily used at the time of the onset of the disease.

Another interesting finding in the Hyltenstam and Stroud paper relates to the linguistic appropriateness of code-switching.[6] Although code-switching is used in many bilingual linguistic communities for a number of purposes including emphasis, speech play, and more sociolinguistic variables like group solidarity, it is not at all linguistically random, as it may appear to the monolingual listener; rather it conforms to a number of rules. Poplack abstracted two of importance: (1) the free-morpheme constraint and (2) the equivalence constraint.[12] The free-morpheme constraint is that code-switching cannot take place within a free morpheme, but only between two free morphemes. This would rule out saying "garcons scouts" for *boy scouts*, as the morphemes are bound in that word but would permit "Boys chantent" (sing) because the noun and the verb are independent morphemes. Thus, excepting young children, a healthy individual will not mix languages within a single word, even across bound morphemes.

The equivalence constraint is somewhat more complex. Poplack developed it on the basis of her study of code-switching in Spanish-English speakers.[12] According to this constraint, code-switching can only take place at a point before and after which there is structural equivalence between the two languages. The example cited above, "Boys chantent" conforms to this rule as well, because both French and English permit noun-verb sequences. Nishimura has modified Poplack's equivalence constraint as it applied to Spanish and English, to apply to languages without many shared structures.[8] She observed that in Japanese-English speakers code-switching can occur at points where constituents on either side of the code-switch do not share word order. She attributes the differences between her findings and those of Poplack to the fact that Japanese and English share many fewer structures than Spanish and English.

Given these relatively sophisticated constraints, it is somewhat surprising that Hyltenstam and Stroud found virtually no linguistically inappropriate code-switching either for their Swedish-German speaker (Swedish and German being structurally closely related languages) or for their Swedish-Finnish speaker (Swedish and Finnish being significantly less closely related to each other).[6]

Dronkers and her colleagues (1986)[3] and de Vreese and his colleagues[2] each report a single case of a multilingual demented patient. In the case of Dronkers et al, the subject, aged 76 years, was a native speaker of Dutch who had lived in England and then in the United States, and who had been speaking English for 45 years when her dementia was evaluated. The authors reported her to have equal language abilities in both English and Dutch. However, with dementia, this patient inappropriately spoke Dutch to non-Dutch speakers and would mix languages within sentences to monolingual speakers.

de Vreese and colleagues reported a case of a 65-year-old Italian-born businessman who had learned a number of languages in school and early adulthood that he used regularly in his business.[2] When he became demented he would mix languages inappropriately and translate spontaneously even in front of individuals who did not know the language(s) into which he was translating. Curiously, on days when he could not produce utterances in French he could nevertheless translate into French from Italian.

## Methodology

In order to determine the kinds of code-switching and language choice errors that may occur in bilingual patients, four Yiddish-English speakers were tested and interviewed. Two patients were born in Russia, one in Poland, and one in the United States. All spoke Yiddish at home from an early age. (The ones born outside the United States also spoke Russian and/or Polish, but our testing was only for Yiddish and English.) The mean age of the subjects was 92 (ranging from 87 to 96 years). The subjects were not highly educated: three of them had completed elementary school and one secretarial school. All had worked outside their home for a period of time and had used English at their work. All continued to use some Yiddish throughout their lives. Those who had immigrated to the U.S. had done so by their midteens.

Two different testers evaluated the patients, one a monolingual English speaker and one a bilingual Yiddish-English speaker. The monolingual English speaker could convincingly say she did not understand when she was spoken to in Yiddish. The bilingual examiner would repeat in Yiddish what a patient said when the patient switched to English, because the bilingual examiner could not honestly feign ignorance of English.

Patients were tested in four to six sessions, on different days, in Yiddish and English. Testing sessions were audio recorded and transcribed, then scored for the parameters of the study. Any segments that did not sound English were reviewed by the bilingual examiner and, in difficult cases, other speakers of Yiddish, in order to determine whether code-switching had occurred or whether neologisms had been produced.

Formal testing was done with the patients in order to determine their level of language breakdown. Data from formal testing that included inappropriate language use were studied as well as data from the informal interviews. Subtests of the Boston Diagnostic Aphasia Exam,[5] the Boston Naming Test,[7] and the Action Naming Test[11] were used to determine that patient B was at stage two (mild-moderate by the Obler and Albert staging),[10] patient D was at stage three (moderate), patient C was at stage four (mid-late stage, similar to Wernicke's aphasia), and patient E was between stages three and four.

## Results

As can be seen in Table 9.1, the four patients presented a diversity of problems common to the language and communication breakdown of dementia of the Alzheimer's type. These include naming problems, paraphasic errors, neologisms, circumlocutions, perseverations, illogical responses, and topic loss. Note that only one patient, patient C, evidenced apparently equal problems in the two languages, although, in the case of patient C, this dichotomous scale masks the actual differences that occurred in degree of deterioration in the two languages. In the other cases, it should be noted that the dementia appeared to cause differential breakdown in the two languages of the patients. However, it is hard to rule out the possibility that differential breakdown reflected differences in language use, early language proficiency, or recent language use before the onset of the dementia. Note that patient D, who learned English earliest of all four patients, nevertheless had problems in every listed aspect in English and fewer in Yiddish. This suggests that we cannot make a general rule that for multilingual patients with dementia of the Alzheimer's type, early-learned languages are spared.

The question of language choice can be divided into two components: (1) simply choosing English or Yiddish appropriately and (2) choosing to code-switch. In speaking to the monolingual examiner, the true test case, it would be inappropriate either to code-switch or to choose extended discourse in Yiddish. Two of the four patients, patient B and patient D, always chose the appropri-

TABLE 9.1 **General Language Behavior of Four Bilingual Demented Subjects**

| LANGUAGE BEHAVIOR | PATIENT B | | PATIENT C | | PATIENT D | | PATIENT E | |
|---|---|---|---|---|---|---|---|---|
| | E | Y | E | Y | E | Y | E | Y |
| Naming problems | + | n/a | + | + | + | − | + | + |
| Paraphasic errors | + | − | + | + | + | − | + | + |
| Neologisms | − | − | + | + | + | − | + | + |
| Circumlocutions | − | − | + | + | + | − | + | + |
| Perseveration | + | − | + | + | + | + | + | + |
| Illogical responses | − | − | + | + | + | + | + | + |
| Topic loss | − | − | + | + | + | − | + | − |

From de Santi S, Obler L, Sabo-Abramson H, Goldberger J. Discourse abilities and deficits in multilingual dementia. In: Joanette Y, Brownell H, eds. Discourse ability and brain damage. New York: Springer-Verlag, 1990:224.

Key: E = English, Y = Yiddish, n/a = not available
  + = The problem listed was evidenced in our sessions
  − = The problem listed was not evidenced in our sessions

ate language when speaking with the monolingual examiner. Two patients, D and E, were able to choose the appropriate language, that is, the one the examiner indicated, when speaking to the bilingual examiner (Table 9.2).

This was a tougher test of the patients' language choice abilities because it was in fact not fully inappropriate to code-switch or switch to English with the bilingual examiner. It should be noted that patient C, who chose the "wrong language" with both examiners, was the most severely demented of all the patients. Patient D, who appropriately performed language choice with both examiners, was the only patient who had been born in the United States and simultaneously learned English and Yiddish. Presumably she also learned rules of appropriate language choice and code-switching from the earliest age. It is possible, then, that the ability to perform language choice correctly deteriorates in later stages of demented language decline.

Only two of our patients chose to do extensive code-switching, patients C and E, although all four patients did some code-switching. Interestingly, the equivalence constraint was followed in a high percentage of instances, ranging from 83 percent in patient C to 100 percent in patient B (who also had the fewest code-switches altogether). Violation of the equivalence constraint occurred in 17 percent of patient C's code-switches and 11 percent of patient E's (Table 9.3).

However, these violations of Poplack's equivalence constraint appeared not to be violations in the light of Nishimura's modification, which appears to be appropriate because Yiddish and English do not share as many word order patterns as Spanish and English do.

Moreover, only one instance of breaking the free-morpheme constraint obtained. In reciting the days of the week in Yiddish, patient D composed the word *Thurshtik*, of the morpheme *Thurs* in English and *tik* for *day* in Yiddish. Otherwise, although there were numerous opportunities, these patients did not violate any linguistic constraints. Recall, however, that they violated pragmatic constraints in code-switching inappropriately when speaking with the monolingual examiner (see Table 9.2).

One further phenomenon that was stressed in the de Vreese et al case was the patients' curiously *spared* and *impaired* abilities to translate.[2] It is worth noting that one of our subjects translated from Yiddish into English either spontaneously (which is only appropriate when one is addressing a monolingual examiner to clarify an inappropriate code-switch) or when she was asked for clarification. While talking about life in Russia, patient C spontaneously translated "If /zain tada/, if your father wants to do something he can." This subject, however, did not translate when speaking to the bilingual examiner, which was also pragmatically inappropriate given that the bilingual examiner presumably understood words in either language. Patient E was likewise able to translate when requested to, in this case by the bilingual examiner who did not know a particular word that the patient had used. Most surprisingly, patient E actually took it upon herself to correct the bilingual examiner's use of an incorrect word. The bilingual examiner said "Hant, aieh hob a pur bilders tse kiken (today I have a few pictures to see)." Patient E made a correction "tse zein" (to look at). Although this is not a form of translation, it is a pragmatic ability that suggests a certain metalinguistic sophistication on the part of the patient.

One final fine point must be made with regard to the neologisms in the corpora discussed here. The data on neologisms were analyzed for their phonologic components in order to discover whether there were phonemes appropriate only to Yiddish or only to English. Neologisms, like code-switching, were produced only by patients C and E. In the case of the 29 neologisms produced by patient C, half (15) had phonemes peculiar to Yiddish, whereas the other half (14) could have occurred in either language. For patient E, by contrast, 6 of the 7 neologisms had distinctive Yiddish phonology, whereas only one could have occurred from either language. This suggests that if a "random language generator" is responsible for neologisms, it can weight its "random" phoneme choice toward one or the other language.

TABLE 9.2 **Language Choice of Four Bilingual Demented Subjects**

| INTERACTION | ENGLISH | YIDDISH |
| --- | --- | --- |
| Appropriate | Patient B, Patient D | Patient D, Patient E |
| Inappropriate | Patient C, Patient E | Patient B, Patient C |

From de Santi S, Obler L, Sabo-Abramson H, Goldberger J. Discourse abilities and deficits in multilingual dementia. In: Joanette Y, Brownell H, eds. Discourse ability and brain damage. New York: Springer Verlag, 1990:224.

TABLE 9.3 Code-Switching with Bilingual and Monolingual Interlocutors

**WITH BILINGUAL INTERLOCUTOR**

| Subject | # C-S | + EQ | − EQ | − FM |
|---|---|---|---|---|
| Patient B | 4 | 4 (100%) | 0 | 0 |
| Patient C | 87 | 72 (83%) | 15 (17%) | 3 (03%) |
| Patient D | 24 | 23 (96%) | 1 (04%) | |
| Patient E | 57 | 50 (88%) | 6 (11%) | 1 (02%) |

**WITH MONOLINGUAL INTERLOCUTOR**

| Subject | # C-S | # Utter | + EQ | − FM |
|---|---|---|---|---|
| Patient B | 0 | 350 | 0 | 0 |
| Patient C | 68 | 888 | 68 (100%) | 0 |
| Patient D | 0 | 944 | 0 | 0 |
| Patient E | 23 | 1664 | 21 (91%) | 0 |

Key: # C-S = Number of code-switches
# utter = number of utterances
+ EQ = number of code-switches that follow the equivalence constraint
− EQ = number of code-switches that do not follow the equivalence constraint
− FM = number of code-switches that do not follow the free morpheme constraint

From de Santi S, Obler L, Sabo-Abramson H, Goldberger J. Discourse abilities and deficits in multilingual dementia. In: Joanette Y, Brownell H, eds. Discourse ability and brain damage. New York: Springer-Verlag, 1990:224.

## Discussion

Dronkers and colleagues attribute the difficulty that their patient had in choosing the appropriate language for English interlocutors as being the result of a memory deficit typical to Alzheimer's type dementia.[3] The results of our study suggest, rather, that it is a pragmatic monitoring ability that fails when language-choice is impaired. Healthy speakers must monitor the match between their utterances and those of their interlocutor. The healthy bilingual is able to choose appropriately to use language A or B or code-switch between A and B. The demented bilingual no longer makes these distinctions.

It is particularly of interest to consider this phenomenon in the light of Paradis's argument (personal communication) that the healthy bilingual's monitoring of which language to speak or whether to code-switch is simply an extension of the monolingual's ability to choose *speech* register. Choosing speech register involves deciding whether to use language features appropriately addressed to a child, for example, or those appropriate for an adult, and among adults whether to use the language features appropriate when speaking to one's colleagues as compared to those used with people who do not know one's field. If Paradis is correct, we would expect to have breakdown in a register among monolinguals and bilingual patients with dementia as well, because we have breakdown in language choice and code-switching in some bilingual demented patients. Because the authors know of no reports nor have ourselves observed such breakdown in monolingual or bilingual DAT patients, it would appear that the ability of healthy bilingual adults to monitor pragmatically the language they use to be appropriate for their interlocutors is organized independently from their monitoring of register within a language.

Code-switching is sometimes thought to be a default phenomenon, that is, to arise when a subject—even a healthy one—cannot say something in language A and therefore needs to switch to language B. In the authors' experience this is rarely the case, and is more likely to account for the borrowing of one lexical item from another language instead of switching for more than a single word to the other code. Rather, we regard code-switching as a relatively sophisticated device when it is used appropriately. The fact that it is inappropriately used by the bilingual demented patient may be explained by disinhibition as de Vreese and colleagues did in referring back to Green.[2,4] In the particular case of bilingual demented patients, the argument should be, we maintain, that code-switching is a natural speech style, indeed a "language" like language A or language B. The healthy individual, however, must choose only one of the three languages (language A, language B, or code-mixing between the two). The demented patient does not make this language choice appropriately and therefore does not inhibit the other two of the three languages.

## Clinical and Research Implications

When evaluating the speech and language abilities of a demented patient, important information is gathered about the patient. Before administration of the traditional speech and language assessments, one must ask the patient or the family to complete a language history questionnaire. A complete language history inventory includes information such as the languages the patient can speak, read, write, and comprehend; the age at which each language was acquired; and the language use and proficiency prior to the patient's illness. A language history for each parent of the patient and the spouse of the patient should also be obtained when possible. In this way, the clinician will know the languages the patient has been exposed to and the premorbid proficiency of the patient in each of these languages. By gathering a complete language history, the clinician is prepared to evaluate the variety of language phenomena that may be exhibited during testing such as accents, apparent paraphasias, and code-switching. Without this knowledge, the clinician might classify a code-switch as jargon, or a subtle accent as a motor-speech problem.

Ideally, a speech and language evaluation in each of the languages the patient knows would provide important details about the present language abilities. The patient's languages can be compared within the semantic, syntactic, phonologic and pragmatic domains, and code-switching and language-choice abilities determined. The effect of dementia on each of the languages could then be determined as well as how proficiency within each language changes as the disease progresses.

The patient's family is important when obtaining information on spontaneous language. Specifically, they can report on the way the patient communicates in each of their languages with someone who is a familiar communication partner. Some family members may visit patients and participate in discourse with the patient. This enables the clinician to compare code-switching when the partner is familiar and when the partner is a relative stranger, the examiner. Because much of the therapy we discuss below involves the family, this interaction provides important information regarding how the family communicates with the patient and how they handle the patient's language difficulties overall, inducing language choice errors.

As with much work in patients with dementia of the Alzheimer's type, there are no immediately obvious plans to recommend for rehabilitation, because the patient's ability to learn is impaired. Education of family and caregivers then becomes the primary responsibility of the practitioner. In the case of health-care workers and family members who must deal with bilingual demented patients, it is important to educate them to the fact that language choice and code-switching errors may occur. After describing the nature of these errors through concrete examples, it is important to stress that they do not occur in all patients, as our data indicate. When errors do occur, moreover, it is sometimes possible to get the patients to translate, or to redirect them into the appropriate language by stressing that the interlocutor does not understand. One may combine techniques, e.g., looking puzzled and saying "What? Is that English? I only speak English!"

It may also be useful to stress that code-switching per se is not a language breakdown but rather a breakdown in the ability to monitor what information is available to the interlocutor. The practitioner should emphasize that the interlocutor must not be impatient when asking the patient to translate or when attempting to redirect the patient. Repeating the input using a supportive tone of voice while telling the patients that you do not understand them is important, as a nonsupportive tone of voice may negatively affect the patient's performance.

It has been the experience of these authors that extended code-switching occurred when the bilingual patients were upset or in distress. At these times, translation or language choice redirection may be unsuccessful. A picture board or a communication board may solve the immediate problem as the patient can point to pictures or vocabulary items to help the caretaker better understand the problem. The caretaker can also point to selected pictures or words to verify the patient's intended meaning. In this manner there may be less frustration for the caretaker and the patient as well as more successful communication.

## Future Research

Further research in this area should relate the difficulties in language choice of bilingual demented patients to the other pragmatic difficulties they exhibit. Attempts to correlate difficulties in language choice with other behavioral phenomena generally associated with frontal damage could be used to test whether disinhibition indeed accounts for breakdown of language choice for those patients in whom it is evidenced. Further work to determine why language choice abilities are *spared* in some patients even in the middle and later stages of dementia should contribute to our understanding of individual differences in demented performance and the cognitive, neuroanatomic, and neurophysiologic factors involved in communication breakdown in demented patients.

## References

1. de Santi S, Obler LK, Sabo-Abramson H, Goldberger J. Discourse abilities and deficits in multilingual dementia. In: Joanette Y, Brownell H, eds. Discourse abilities and brain damage: Theoretical and empirical perspectives. New York: Springer-Verlag, 1990:224.
2. de Vreese LP, Motta A, Toschi A. Compulsive and paradoxical translation behaviour in a case of presenile dementia of the Alzheimer type. J Neuroling 1988; 3:233–259.
3. Dronkers N, Koss E, Friedland R, Wertz R. "Differential" language impairment and language mixing in a polyglot with probable Alzheimer's disease. Paper presented at European International Neuropsychological Society Meeting. 1986.
4. Green D. Control activation and resource: A framework and a model of the control of the speech in bilinguals. Brain Lang 1986; 27:210–223.
5. Goodglass H, Kaplan E. The assessment of aphasia and related disorders. Philadelphia: Lea & Febiger, 1972.
6. Hyltenstam K, Stroud C. Bilingualism in Alzheimer's disease: Two case studies. In: Hyltenstam K, Obler LK, eds. Bilingualism across the lifespan: Aspects of acquisition, maturity and loss. Cambridge, MA: Cambridge University Press, 1989.
7. Kaplan E, Goodglass H, Weintraub S. Boston Naming Test. Philadelphia: Lea & Febiger, 1983.
8. Nishimura M. Intrasentential code-switching: The case of language assignment. In: Vaid J, ed. Language processing in bilinguals: Psycholinguistic and neuropsychological perspectives. Hillsdale, NJ: Erlbaum, 1986.
9. Obler LK, Albert ML. Influence of aging on recovery from aphasia in polyglots. Brain Lang 1977; 4:460–463.
10. Obler LK, Albert ML. Language in aging. In: Albert ML, ed. Clinical neurology of aging. New York: Oxford University Press, 1984.
11. Obler LK, Albert ML. Action Naming Test. Experimental Version. Boston: Boston VA Medical Center, 1986.
12. Poplack S. "Sometimes I'll start a sentence in Spanish Y TERMINO EN ESPAÑOL": Toward a typology of code-switching. Centro de Estudios Puertorriqueños Working Papers 1979; 4:1–79.

# SECTION THREE

*Social Impact of Dementia*

# CHAPTER 10

# *Learned Helplessness: Application to Communication of the Elderly*

ROSEMARY LUBINSKI, Ed.D.

Elderly individuals with dementia are among the most devalued members of our society, regardless of their lifelong characteristics and contributions. Gradually, difficulties in remembering, performing routine activities, acting responsibly, and communicating clearly and meaningfully multiply into a negative image that family and caregivers identify and respond to as sickness and deviance. Individuals who once fit into the mainstream of society, demonstrating competence and productivity over their life span, now become marginal members within their immediate families and even more so within the larger social framework.[8]

Family and friends generally have limited experience in interacting with handicapped individuals and even less with those with dementia. Social proscriptions and prejudicial behavior toward the handicapped, including stereotyping, aversion, fear of contamination, and avoidance, are transferred automatically toward those with dementia. The elderly demented individual bears the double stigma of age and mental handicap.

The perception of incompetence associated with dementia determines the social and communication opportunities the individual will have and eventually the care that the individual will receive. This perception involves not only the identification of real behaviors but covertly combines the perceiver's own reactions and difficulties in coping with the actual behaviors exhibited by the demented person. The caregivers, be they family or health-care workers, segregate the individual in his or her "best interest."[61] This can be done by limiting or withdrawing the person from activities outside the home, locking doors, restricting access to particular areas, restraining the individual, or discouraging others from coming into the home.

The ultimate segregation is institutionalization, where the setting is usually physically and psychologically designed to keep the individual closely monitored and restricted to a confined area.[26] Segregation protects the demented individual from potential dangers, curtails interaction with those outside the immediate environment, and reduces any opportunities for demonstrating intact skills. Posner states that nursing homes are actually oriented toward the most incompetent, and there are few advantages to being competent in this setting.[53] Similarly, Berger and Rose hypothesize that "social withdrawal behaviors such as reduced verbalizations and interactions may be shaped by nursing home staff," who manage quiet patients more easily.[7] Thus, reduced communication may be a result of the environmental expectations as well as inherent diminishing skills of the dementia patient.

This chapter discusses the social process of an elderly individual with dementia. The chapter is based on the premise that dementia is not only a real change in cognitive, emotional, and communicative behavior but is also a learned behavior emanating from the perceptions of those in the environment. Specifically, the chapter addresses the concepts of learned helplessness and the social breakdown syndrome as they apply to elderly demented individuals, particularly those in institutional settings. This chapter focuses on (1) the problem of diagnosing dementia; (2) the cycle of incompetence and learned helplessness; (3) the application of learned helplessness theory to communication of the elderly demented; and finally (4) some suggestions for breaking the cycle of incompetence and thus minimizing learned helplessness among these individuals.

## Diagnosis of Dementia

When an elderly individual exhibits differences in behavior, such as memory difficulties, disorientation, and inappropriate behaviors, the response from others in the environment is often to ignore the behaviors as long as possible and cope with them until some crisis occurs. During the early stages of dementia, the family may ascribe memory problems to the "forgetfulness of old age" and the individual him- or herself may deny any problems such as memory difficulties. As the dementia progresses, the family may react more actively toward behavior problems and may adjust their life-style and home environment. Families are likely to discuss concerns with other family and friends prior to seeking professional guidance.[29] At some point, tolerance and adaptability cannot keep pace with the enormity of the need, and professional help is sought. Usually, the person is taken to the family physician, who listens to the complaints of the caregivers.[68] The elderly individual rarely initiates the medical visit and may even resent going to the physician.

Because dementia can only be confirmed by autopsy or brain biopsy, its diagnosis is limited to the evaluation of observational data and the patient's interaction with the physician or others in the environment.[17] The diagnosis of dementia in many elderly persons is not always accompanied by a thorough medical, neurologic, and psychiatric evaluation to rule out possible reversible etiologies or look-alike disorders. The usual scenario for diagnosis is a process whereby a family member or caregiver lists symptoms and the patient is given a routine physical examination and interview. The interview consists of asking the patient several "orientation" questions such as "Who's the President of the United States?" and "What day of the week is it?" Undoubtedly, the patient often fails to answer correctly these or similar isolated, unrelated, and acontextual questions. Considering the person's age, the complaints of the family member, and the apparent disorientation of the individual, the diagnosis becomes dementia or some other term such as organic brain syndrome. Rathbone-McCuan and Hashimi hypothesize that some physicians may have a limited knowledge base regarding dementia.[57] Consequently, physicians may make recommendations that "promote dependence and rob clients of the opportunity to gain experience in problem solving and the confidence that it builds."

## PROBLEMS IN DIAGNOSIS

Several problems emerge from this process. First, a wrong diagnosis may be made. For example, a person who has a series of transient ischemic attacks (TIAs) may exhibit aphasic symptoms that may be interpreted as dementia, particularly when the patient is elderly. TIAs may result in intermittent difficulties in communication, perception, cognition, and physical abilities. Right-hemisphere strokes may also demonstrate symptomatology similar to dementia. For example, the individual with damage to the right hemisphere may exhibit subtle difficulties in auditory comprehension, show flat affect, and have major problems in visuospatial processing.[45] Depression may also mimic dementia, particularly when the person shows little response to interaction. Nott and Fleminger estimate that close to 15 percent of demented patients actually have a primary diagnosis of affective disorders such as depression.[48] Visual impairments may contribute to dementia-like symptoms. Snyder, Pyrek, and Smith found that older persons with visual deficiencies were more likely to score poorly on the Mental Status Questionnaire (MSQ).[64]

Further, hearing loss and central auditory disorders may also be complicating factors in accurate diagnosis of dementia. Presbycusis, the hearing loss associated with aging, is characterized by difficulty hearing high-frequency sounds such as [s] and [z]. These sounds are common in English and mark important aspects of language such as tense, possession, and plurals. Individuals with presbycusis may not respond appropriately to conversation if they do not hear or process the words. This may be misdiagnosed as confusion. See Chapters 4 and 14 on hearing disorders and dementia.

To compound the problem of accurate diagnosis, those elderly individuals who have limited proficiency in English may not be able to describe their own symptomatology and therefore rely on a family member for description and will not be able to answer questions posed during the orientation part of the evaluation by the physician. Similarly, age and cultural differences between patients and staff may create subtle barriers that influence testing results. Elderly patients may feel foolish answering "childlike questions" for a young examiner and refrain from exposing their abilities and difficulties. Patients and families may not be comfortable expressing their needs and problems to ethnically or racially different staff.

A second diagnostic problem emerges in that the process itself may be too superficial. At present there are no widely accepted standardized tests that diagnose dementia although a wide variety of batteries are available, including the CAPE,[50] FROMJE,[40] Mental Status Questionnaire,[35] Mini-

Mental State Examination,[24] Global Deterioration Scale,[59] and Brief Cognitive Rating Scale.[59] For reviews of psychological assessment of the elderly, see references by Birrin and Sloan, Butler and Lewis, Cummings and Benson, Eisdorfer and Freidel, Raskin and Jarvik, and Wattis and Hendmarch.[9,12,17,21,56,71]

The primary physician, family, and even the individual him- or herself may be reluctant to refer for series of physical and psychometric tests that will only identify the "obvious." Regardless, as complete an evaluation as possible should be attempted. Cummings and Benson suggest that although detailed evaluation may not be possible on all patients, "an assessment of intellectual competence is necessary in addition to general physical, neurologic, and laboratory tests."[17] Some studies warn that at least 20 percent of those diagnosed as demented have a potentially reversible form that a complete evaluation might reveal. (See Cummings and Benson[17] and Libow[40] for discussion of reversible dementias.)

The labeling of dementia begins a potentially irreversible chain of events, attitudes, and outcomes. The elderly individual is now a "senile" patient, one with chronic brain syndrome or organic brain syndrome or, perhaps more specifically, "Alzheimer's." Once the label is given it is permanent. The physician's labeling of dementia is perpetuated by other health-care givers including nurses and rehabilitation specialists who copy verbatim on their reports the diagnosis of dementia. Rarely is the diagnosis of dementia questioned or supporting evidence required. It is impossible to tell how the initial labeling of dementia influences future tests, observations, and results obtained by professionals.

Campbell-Taylor, in a recent review of the literature concerning the diagnosis of dementia, summarized various international studies by stating that 50 percent of those individuals given the diagnosis of dementia who entered into a long-term care institution are likely to die within 1 year "whether the diagnosis is accurate" or not.[13] This clearly illustrates the importance of accurate identification of dementia and the judicious use of its label. It is hypothesized that, accurate or not, this diagnosis will create a cycle of incompetence and learned helplessness.

## Learned Helplessness and the Cycle of Incompetence

Learned helplessness occurs when individuals perceive that events and outcomes are independent of their responses and that any further action is fruitless.[18] When demented persons perceive that their responses are futile, they stop responding.

The demented individual receives *outcome cues* that include responses from others in the environment concerning the inadequacy of performance. (See Miller and Norman for a discussion of the attribution-theory model of learned helplessness.[43]) The source of the difficulty is perceived as an internal, general, and stable attribute within the individual, namely the dementia. Significant others in the environment do not expect the individual to perform capably and provide direct feedback concerning both actual and potential failure. For example, caregivers may verbally or nonverbally tell a person that they cannot perform a task, may repeatedly correct communication that is in error, or limit communication opportunities.

Similarly, the structure of the environment sends *situational cues* to the individual that he or she is no longer expected to act responsibly or competently. The physical environment may be highly restricted, or potentially dangerous objects may be placed out of reach or removed. The fact that demented individuals are monitored or watched so closely to prevent potential harm, embarrassment, or difficult situations is yet another clear indication that the demented individual cannot be expected to act responsibly.

Miller and Norman state that outcome and situational cues are inextricably intertwined.[43] Together they help set up expectancies by both the demented individual and significant others as to what can be expected from the demented individual. The social environment sends clear signals that no one expects the demented individual to participate competently or meaningfully, usually by reducing opportunities for such interaction. Caregivers may unconsciously create opportunities for dependency to develop.[65] Dependent patients are easier to manage because the caregivers assume the responsibility for the person's well-being.

Gradually, demented individuals have fewer opportunities to demonstrate any skills, motivation to participate declines, and individuals realize at some level that they are no longer in control of their own behavior or any part of their environment. The natural response is to "give up." Martin and Seligman, in their study of learned helplessness, state that fear, frustration, and depression naturally ensue.[42]

Eventually, institutionalization may occur where the range of expected abilities, movement, and social opportunity is optimally reduced. Rathbone-McCuan and Hashimi state that "many nursing homes approach these patients from a perspective of 'overcare.'"[57] Solomon states that health-care workers in institutional settings stereotype the aged patient and respond primarily to their custodial and maintenance needs rather than to their behavior.[65] The institutional environment, by its all-encompassing nature coupled with dependency-making by staff, magnifies the actual problems the individual exhibits to the point where the individual has little reason or motivation to try to act competently.

This discussion does not negate the apparent fact that demented persons are truly helpless. Fuller states that aging itself contributes to being vulnerable to helplessness because of erosion of psychological reserves.[25] Factors such as retirement, role changes and loss, financial problems, death of a spouse, and health, personality, or cognitive changes all contribute to this vulnerability. Bengston adds that with aging there is an increasing dependency on "external sources of self labeling, many of which communicate a stereotypic portrayal of the elderly as useless and obsolete."[6] Kalish further suggests that some older persons hold ageist attitudes themselves.[36] Thus, at least some elderly live up to the societal and perhaps their own expectation of dependency and helplessness.

Indeed, with aging and dementia, older persons cannot behave in their previously competent manner, and they do demonstrate a certain amount of innate helplessness. Innate helplessness is defined as the actual reduction in abilities related to the variety of cognitive, emotional, and communicative changes within the individual and the reduction of self-initiated compensatory strategies. Although there is a certain amount of innate helplessness, and, in fact, this may progress significantly, this does not imply that meaningful, competent performance cannot be expected, particularly with regard to communication. The stereotyping of perceived and innate helplessness leads to overgeneralization of incompetency and hence to reduction in opportunities to demonstrate intact skills. Edwards proposes that skills cannot be maintained in the face of reduction of opportunity to perform them.[19] Furthermore, stereotyping consequently results in an imposed helplessness far greater than the innate helplessness of the individual. Gradually the cycle of incompetence is bred, reinforced, and maintained.

Zussman describes this process as the social breakdown syndrome, whereby others' perception of an individual combines with his or her self-concept to produce a "vicious spiral of negative psychological functioning."[75] He portrays this process as an increasing susceptibility to breakdown as a person is labeled as incompetent and inducted into the sick or patient role with its ensuing dependency and atrophy of remaining skills, so that finally, the individual accepts his or her incompetence (see Fig. 10.1).

This concept can be applied easily to elderly demented patients. They are susceptible to being perceived as being incompetent by virtue of being old as well as by their actual disabilities (innate helplessness). Their problem behaviors are now diagnosed as "dementia"; there is a clear reduction of options and expectations, and, consequently, the person is institutionalized, the ultimate dependent context. The individual begins to realize that others perceive him as different and incompetent, and because the physical and social environment reinforce the incompetency, the diagnosis must be true. Thus, rather than demonstrate any possible competent behaviors and adopt coping strategies, it is easier to conform to the expectations of the caregivers, for indeed, she or he is dependent on them for basic life needs (see Fig. 10.2).

Wolfensberger and Tullman, in discussing the principle of normalization, summarize this concept in the following statement:

> How a person is perceived and treated by others will in turn strongly determine how that person subsequently behaves. The more consistently a person is perceived as deviant, therefore, the more likely it will be that he or she will conform to that expectation and emit the kinds of behavior that are socially expected, often behaviors which are not valued by society.[73]

The philosophy of the social breakdown syndrome can be applied directly to the demented individual's communication skills and opportunities. Elderly demented individuals do communicate differently and thus are more susceptible to the social breakdown that occurs. The results of numerous research studies in the past 15 years indicate that there are changes in the semantic and pragmatic aspects of discourse.[2,4,37,46,49,60,70] As individuals progress through the syndrome of

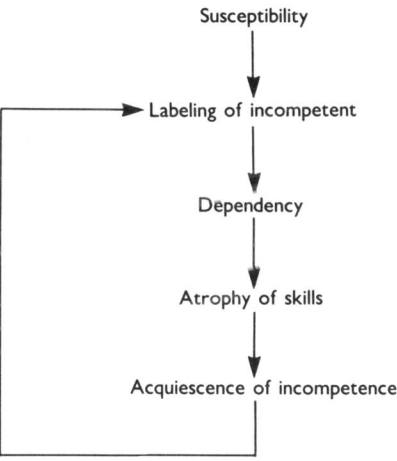

Figure 10.1 Schematic of social breakdown syndrome. Adapted from Zussman J. Some explanations of the changing appearance of psychotic patients: Antecedents of the social breakdown syndrome concept. Millbank Q 1966; 44:363–396.

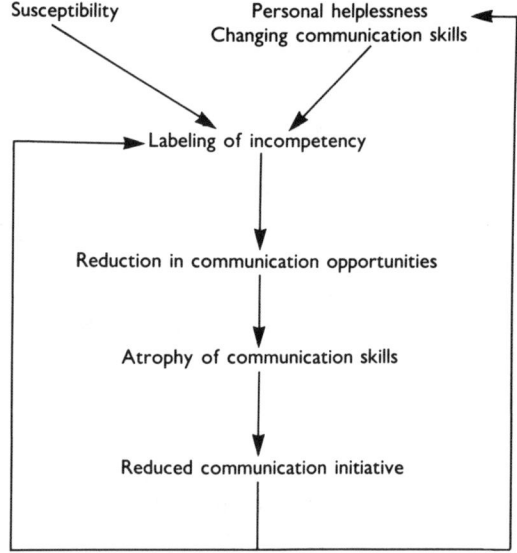

**Figure 10.2** Social breakdown syndrome as applied to communication.

dementia, their communication is likely to reflect difficulty with comprehension, word retrieval, appropriate word use, and adherence to the rules of conversation. By the late stages, patients may not appear to comprehend at all, they make few attempts to communicate, and their spontaneous speech may be filled with repetitions and meaningless jargon. Thus, the progressive deterioration in their communication abilities will reinforce the caregivers' perceptions of the individual's incompetence. See Chapters 7 and 8 for discussion of language and pragmatic changes in dementia.

Communication is a primary tool through which the demented individual's cognitive skills and competencies are evaluated. Communication becomes a critical determiner in the availability and style of communication occurring with demented patients. For example, Browne found that there was a significant difference in the amount of time nurses interacted with "oriented versus disoriented patients."[11] Oriented patients received interaction from nurses 15 percent of the time as compared with the 5.6 percent received by disoriented patients.

Basky, in a study of patient-aide communication, investigated how aides change their communication dependent on the patients' mental diagnosis.[3] She found that when patients had a "severe mental diagnosis" such as dementia, aides tended to (1) talk less; (2) use longer pauses; (3) talk even less when patients failed to respond; (4) speak only about the here and now; and (5) call patients by first or nicknames as contrasted with those without such a diagnosis. She concluded that aides' utterances to severely mentally impaired patients were in many ways similar to the "motherese" of mothers to language-learning children.

In another study of communication between institutionalized elderly and caregivers, it was found that "baby talk" constituted 22 percent of the communication to all patients, regardless of their characteristics such as presence of dementia. Caporael also found that communication categorized as "non-baby talk" with patients was not regular adult speech but consisted of "help offer" statements that promoted dependency.[14] Caporael cautions that we do not know whether baby talk is interpreted by patients as nurturing or as condescending; it may actually be the non-baby talk in an "institutional" register that promotes helplessness among the elderly demented.

Sigman, who studied the social patterning of conversational topics in a nursing home, found that there are patterns of topics between resident and staff that are based on the status identity of the staff members.[63] Sigman found that staff members check a patient's mental status by determining if a topic matches the staff member to whom it was addressed. Patients who might confuse staff members and inappropriately address communication to them would thereby be labeled "confused."

The danger here is the overgeneralizations that are likely to occur. A patient may legitimately make an error in addressing a topic to a staff member for a variety of reasons: (1) visual and/or hearing difficulties may limit clear identification of and response to staff; (2) a patient unfamiliar with nursing-home protocol may communicate with anyone available; (3) staff change so frequently that the patient may be unsure of staff identities; (4) the patient may have difficulty communicating with staff because of other types of communication disorders including aphasia, apraxia, and dysarthria; and (5) patients may have an immediate need to communicate, particularly with regard to their physical needs and therefore may address communication to anyone who can provide that help quickly.

For example, the patient who says "bedpan" to the maintenance person cleaning a bathroom will be perceived as confused, because physical care is not the job of this staff member. This "error" is referred to the nurse who may interpret the behavior as confusion. The patient's request may be disregarded and his resulting incontinence is one more confirming piece of evidence of his incompetence. In actuality, the patient may not have distinguished the color of the staff member's clothes, not clearly heard the staff member's contradiction, and have addressed his immediate need to the closest person perceived as capable of helping.

## Minimizing Helplessness

Although there are undoubtedly many suggestions that could be offered to help minimize helplessness of the demented, this chapter will focus on six aspects of care that need improvement: (1) accurate diagnosis; (2) enhanced social role; (3) improved communication skills and opportunities; (4) normalization of self and physical environment; (5) improved sense of control; and (6) in-service training for staff and support for family. These concepts are not necessarily mutually exclusive but, in fact, relate closely to each other in practice.

First, accurate diagnosis is prerequisite. The label of dementia must be eliminated where it is inaccurate or not substantiated. This involves a team approach by physicians, therapists, psychologists, nurses, family, and the affected individual. The diagnosis should be made only by a team when the evidence is compelling. Complete vision and hearing evaluations as well as other laboratory and psychological or psychiatric tests should be mandatory to rule out possible reversible etiologies or compounding factors before the label of dementia is given.

The diagnostic evaluation should not be performed when the person has just been hospitalized or immediately following a severe illness, surgery, anesthesia, or personal trauma such as loss of a spouse, relocation to a new living facility, or change in financial status. Each of these life events and others may precipitate symptoms of confusion in many elderly.[20,72] Given time to recover from illness or adjust to personal crises the individual may no longer exhibit these symptoms. Similarly, diagnosticians need to carefully document the individual's use of prescribed and over-the-counter medications and to determine their possible effects on cognitive and communicative performance.[15]

This diagnostic process should take place over time and should stress not only the disabilities of the person with dementia but also skills that are still preserved. Successful living with the dementia patient either in the home or institutional setting can be maximized when caregivers know what abilities are productive and what strategies maintain these positive abilities. Rathbone-McCuan and Hashimi state that caregivers need strategies that are "supportive, not negative of performance ability while at the same time assuring that they are not introducing more stress into the life of an individual who is struggling to cope with losses."[57]

Further, the label of dementia should not be written on a patient's record unless there are data to support the diagnosis. Physicians, nursing-home personnel, and governmental and accrediting agencies of nursing homes should not be in a hurry to label individuals as demented and then set about proving the diagnosis.

Second, the elderly individual with dementia should have some social role other than that of a demented patient. Both labels of demented and patient lead to diminished role opportunities within the family and community. Every effort should be made to provide individuals with dementia with decision-making opportunities and a sense of internal locus of control over both the physical and social aspects of their environment. Wolfensberger and Tullman suggest that if caregivers expect behaviors to occur, they will create opportunities for them to happen.[73] They state that role expectations are conveyed through (1) the structure of the physical environment; (2) the activities available; (3) the communication concerning role behaviors; (4) the opportunities for interaction; and (5) other images and symbols. Thus, the more we expect of those with dementia, the more opportunities we provide for positive behaviors to occur. Communication plays a vital role in conveying the expectations of those in the environment.

Third, attempts must be made to identify the characteristics of the demented individual's *communicative behavior* that contribute to helplessness and role loss. The fields of communication disorders, linguistics, and neuropsychology have just begun to explore the cognitive and communicative difficulties associated with dementia. Little research exists on what strategies facilitate communicative competence in this population. Specific research is needed to determine what communication partners can do to maintain conversations, what techniques are most productive, and how long communication competence at some level can be maintained. Further, communication-disorders specialists and others interested in improving the communication effectiveness of the elderly demented need to become aware of existing research on improving communicative effectiveness.[1,7,10,22,23,27,28,31–34,41,44,47,51,55]

It has been too easy for communication-disorders specialists to say that demented persons are untestable or untreatable. More emphasis at the graduate training level and in postgraduate education in both speech-language pathology and audiology is needed to develop more sophisticated attitudes and skills for working with the elderly demented.

Fourth, because it is difficult to break the cycle of incompetence once it has begun, our efforts must be directed toward preventing it or at least forstalling it. One possible way of achieving this is through "normalization principles." Gunzberg and Gunzberg define normalization as "making available...conditions of everyday life which are as close as possible to the norms and patterns of our society."[30] Safilios-Rothschild cautions that "normal" does not mean the "absolute state of health or ability but rather the lack of a societal label of deviance."[61] Thus, normalization involves providing opportunities for individuals to live as much within the mainstream of society as possible. It involves helping the demented individual to dress appropriately in clothes that reflect personal style, to live in settings that are home-like and personal, and to participate in activities that are age-appropriate and complement previous life experiences and interests. Demented individuals should also have ample opportunity to engage in activities outside the institutional setting with life-long family and friends. Wolfensberger and Tullman caution that physical integration is insufficient without "personal social integration and valued social participation."[73]

Perhaps most important of all, normalization means having a sense of control over one's daily life and activities. Schultz defines personal control as the "ability to manipulate some aspect of the environment."[62] Several studies have investigated the effect of variables related to control among the healthy elderly and the institutionalized elderly. Thomas and Hooper, in a study of healthy elderly, suggest that adequate social bonds and an internal locus of control are closely related to good health.[69] Langer and Rodin, in a study of personal responsibility and choice among the institutionalized elderly, found that 93 percent of the patients who were encouraged to participate in decision making and were given responsibilities within the setting increased their interpersonal activities and showed overall improvement on a variety of variables.[38] These two studies clearly indicate that elderly individuals, including those whose status requires long-term care, benefit from making their own choices. Langer and Rodin sum up this theory by stating that the "notion of competence (control) is indeed central to much of human behavior."[38] Lefcourt adds that the sense of control is a critical factor in sustaining life.[39] There is little reason to believe that this human need is any less for those with dementia.

The question then becomes, how can elderly demented individuals demonstrate a sense of control, particularly in an institutional environment that by its very nature tends to withdraw opportunities for such expressions? The first goal in this setting is to change or enhance caregivers' attitudes about what the elderly demented can do or might be expected to do. The second goal is to provide staff with strategies that enhance their ability to work and communicate with these patients. Staff themselves may be the best source of these strategies.

Normalization of demented patients will not occur simply because they look better or attend social functions. It basically emanates from the personal regard of their caregivers. Many of these caregivers come to the institutional setting with the same misconceptions, prejudices, and fears about old demented persons. Benedict and Ganikos state that three types of age bias, including age restrictiveness, age distortion, and ageism, may be held by medical and rehabilitation professionals.[5] The cycle of incompetence is reinforced daily by staff members who lack understanding of the nature and effects of dementia and institutionalization. Improved personal regard emanates from better understanding and is reflected in increased opportunities for the elderly demented to demonstrate their competencies. Bengston suggests that patients may actually develop a better sense of control if "those who envision themselves as serving the elderly divest some of their own power and control."[6]

Improved attitudes toward institutionalized, demented elderly patients and enhanced strategies could be fostered through continuing in-service education for care givers, particularly for nursing assistants who provide so much of the intimate daily care for the elderly demented. Nursing assistants frequently have the least education and preparation for their positions and little opportunity to provide input into the decision making and management of the institutional setting. In-service training should focus on encouraging understanding of the cognitive and emotional effects of dementia on the individual and family as well as the progression of the disorder, identifying strengths and abilities of patients rather than deficits, and learning strategies for communicating more effectively. Staff need to understand that the behavior of patients is related to caregivers' attitudes and behavior as well as the physical and psychological characteristics of an institutional setting. Role playing of difficult communicative situations with demented patients can be used to help staff generate their own ideas and critique their own as well as other staff members' actions in dealing with problem communications. (See Chapter 17 on in-service training methods and strategies.)

Such in-service training must not be a "one-time" affair, but should be extended over time. This would provide staff with opportunities to learn to observe more closely, to focus on abilities as well as disabilities, and to identify options for expressions of control and normalization by patients. Staff members need time to try strategies, evaluate them, and restructure them to meet individual needs. To make these in-service sessions more than perfunctory, staff need reinforcement for their improving insights and suggestions. Although some reinforcement will come from seeing patients who respond more competently, reinforcement is also needed from institutional leaders, possibly through financial incentives or other "perks" for attending in-service training and implementing suggestions in everyday care. Performance evaluations by supervisors should also focus on carryover of in-service concepts. In addition, time should be built into the work week for discussion of perceptions, frustrations, and insights.

Similarly, family members also need to learn about the nature and progression of dementia, support in everyday coping, strategies for maintaining and facilitating independent activities of daily living, and specific training in strategies for communicating more effectively with their loved ones. This may result in improved ability of family to comfortably retain the individual in the community, preservation of lifelong social roles, and reduction of the cost to family and society for long-term care. Further, special attention should be paid to the families of those dementia patients who are institutionalized. These families need help in adjusting to institutionalization and strategies to use in communicating during visits. Family are frequently overwhelmed by the need for institutionalization, the nature of the setting, the rules for interacting with caregiving staff, and the deterioration of their loved one. Their visits to the nursing home may become painful and decrease in frequency, thus depriving the dementia patient of needed interaction. The gradual loss of one's lifelong and primary communication partner may be one of the greatest devastations and burdens associated with dementia.

Orange, in Chapter 12, discusses the perceptions of family members about the nature of the communicative problems their demented family member exhibits and the strategies they find effective for continued interaction. Rau, in Chapter 11, also presents a detailed discussion of the impact of dementia on family systems.

## Research Needs

The effects of helplessness on dementia and the communication of those with dementia have received no attention. Research efforts might be directed toward identifying what aspects of the symptom complex of dementia are most vulnerable to helplessness. Other research questions might focus on premorbid personality of dementia patients, caregiver characteristics that promote helplessness, and physical and psychosocial aspects of the environment that promulgate helplessness. In addition, how the communication of dementia patients contributes to the feelings of helplessness of communication partners warrants investigation.

## Concluding Remarks

Dementia, by its nature, results in progressive and deteriorating changes and decreases in well-established cognitive, communicative, and social skills. The problem becomes magnified, however, by caregivers' withdrawal of opportunities for demonstrating any intact abilities. Individuals with dementia must cope with the real changes in ability plus those consciously and unconsciously imposed by persons in their home or institutional environment.

Perhaps professionals and family members need to reflect on Norman Cousin's comments on helplessness. He says in his book *Human Options*, "Humans are not helpless. They have never been helpless. They have only been deflected, or deceived, or dispirited."[16] Dementia is truly a deflection of the human mind and ability. Must we also deceive and dispirit these individuals by withdrawing all opportunity for demonstrating any competence? The answer begins in our own recognition of the problem, our acceptance of our own fears and helplessness, and our own willingness to work with the demented individual despite frustrations and failures.

### References

1. Abrahams JP, Wallach H, Divens S. Behavioral improvement in long-term geriatric patients during an age-integrated psychosocial rehabilitation program. J Am Geriatr Soc 1979; 27:218–221.
2. Appel J, Kertesz A, Fisman M. A study of language functioning in Alzheimer patients. Brain Lang 1982; 17:73–91.
3. Basky P. Aides' communication to the elderly patients in a nursing home. Unpublished masters thesis. Pennsylvania State University, 1982.
4. Bayles KA, Kazniak AW, Tomoeda C. Communication and cognition in normal aging and dementia. Boston, MA: College-Hill Press, 1987.
5. Bendict R, Ganikos M. Coming to terms with ageism in rehabilitation. J Rehabil 1981; 47:10–18.
6. Bengston V. Social psychology of aging. Columbus, OH: Bobbs-Merrill, 1973.
7. Berger R, Rose S. Interpersonal skill training with institutionalized elderly patients. J Gerontol 1977; 32:346–353.
8. Biber B. The evaluation of the developmental-interaction point of view. In: Shapiro E, Weber E, eds. Cognitive and affective growth: Developmental interaction. Hillsdale, NJ: Erlbaum, 1981:9.
9. Birrin J, Sloan R. Handbook of mental health and aging. Englewood Cliffs, NJ: Prentice-Hall, 1980.
10. Blackman D, Howe M, Pinkstone E. Increasing participation in social interaction of the institutionalized elderly. Gerontologist 1976; 16:69–76.
11. Browne K. Confusion in the elderly. Nursing 1984; 2:698–705.
12. Butler R, Lewis M. Aging and mental health. St. Louis: C.V. Mosby, 1982.
13. Campbell-Taylor I. Dimensions of clinical judgement in diagnosis of Alzheimer's disease. Unpublished doctoral dissertation. State University of New York at Buffalo, 1984.
14. Caporael L. The paralanguage of caregiving: Baby talk to the institutionalized elderly. J Pers Soc Psychol 1981; 40:876–884.

15. Chaperon D, Besdini RW. Drugs as an obstacle to rehabilitation of the elderly: A primer for therapists. Top Geriatr Rehabil 1987; 2:63–81.
16. Cousins N. Human options. New York: W.W. Worton, 1981.
17. Cummings J, Benson DF. Dementia: A clinical approach. Boston: Butterworth, 1983.
18. Decker SD, Kinzel S. Learned helplessness and decreased social interaction in elderly disabled persons. Rehabil Nurs 1985; 10:31–32.
19. Edwards A. Restoring functional behavior of senile elderly. In: Ferguson J, Taylor C, eds. The comprehensive handbook of behavioral medicine. (Vol. 3) New York: Medical and Scientific Books, 1980:45.
20. Eisdorfer C. Stress, disease and cognitive change in the aged. In: Eisdorfer C, Friedel RO, eds. Cognitive and emotional disturbances in the elderly. Chicago: Year Book Medical Publishers, 1977:27.
21. Eisdorfer C, Friedel RO. Cognitive and emotional disturbances in the elderly. Chicago: Year Book Medical Publishers, 1977.
22. Ernst P, Beran B, Safford F, Kleenhauz M. Isolation and the symptoms of chronic brain syndrome. Gerontologist 1978; 18:468–474.
23. Feier CD, Leight G. A communication-cognition program for elderly nursing home residents. Gerontologist 1981; 21:408–416.
24. Folstein MF, Folstein SE, McHugh PR. "Mini-mental state": A practical method for grading the mental state of patients for the clinician. J Psychiatr Res 1975; 12:189–198.
25. Fuller SS. Inhibiting helplessness in elderly people. Gerontol Nurs 1978; 4:18–21.
26. Goffman E. Asylums. New York: Anchor Books, 1961.
27. Gray P, Stevenson J. Changes in verbal interaction among members of resocialization groups. J Gerontol Nurs 1980; 6:86–90.
28. Green G, Linsk N, Pinkstone E. Modification of verbal behavior of the mentally impaired elderly by their spouses. J Appl Behav Anal 1986; 19:329–336.
29. Gruetzner H. Alzheimer's: A caregiver's guide and source book. New York: John Wiley and Sons, 1988.
30. Gunzberg H, Gunzberg A. Mental handicap and physical environment. London: Baillière Tindall, 1973.
31. Hoyer W, Kafer RA, Simpson SS, Hoyer FW. A reinstatement of verbal behavior in elderly mental patients using operant procedures. Gerontologist 1974; 14:149–152.
33. Hussian R, Davis R. Responsive care: Behavioral interventions with elderly persons. Champaign, IL: Research Press, 1985.
34. Jeffers FC, Nichols CR. The relationship of activities and attitudes to physical well-being in older people. J Gerontol 1961; 16:67–70.
35. Kahn RL, Goldfarb AI, Pollack M, Peck A. Brief measures for the determination of mental states of the aged. Am J Psychiatry 1960; 117:326.
36. Kalish RA, ed. The later years. California: Brooks/Cole Publishing, 1977.
37. Kempler P, Curtis S, Jackson C. Syntactic preservation in Alzheimer's disease. J Speech Hear Res 1987; 30:343–350.
38. Langer EJ, Rodin J. The effects of choice and enhanced personal responsibility for the aged: A field experiment in an institutional setting. J Pers Soc Psychiatry 1976; 34:191–198.
39. Lefcourt H. The function of the illusion of control and freedom. Am Psychol 1973; 18:417–425.
40. Libow LS. Senile dementia and "pseudosenility": Clinical diagnoses. In: Eisdorfer C, Friedel R, eds. Cognitive and emotional disturbances in the elderly. Chicago: Year Book Medical Publishers, 1977:75–88.
41. MacDonald M. Environmental programming for the socially isolated aging. Gerontologist 1978; 18:350–354.
42. Martin E, Seligman W. Helplessness: On depression, development and death. San Francisco: WH Freeman and Co., 1975.
43. Miller IW, Norman WH. Learned helplessness in humans: A review and attribution theory model. Psychol Bull 1979; 86:93–118.
44. Mueller DJ, Atlas L. Resocialization of regressed elderly residents: A behavioral management approach. J Gerontol 1972; 27:390–392.
45. Myers P. Right hemisphere communication impairment. In: Chapey R, ed. Language intervention strategies in adult aphasia. Baltimore: Williams & Wilkins, 1986:444.
46. Nicholas M, Obler LK, Albert ML, Helm-Estabrooks N. Empty speech in Alzheimer's disease and fluent aphasia. J Speech Hear Res 1985; 28:405–410.
47. Nigl AJ, Jackson B. A behavioral management program to increase social responses in psychogeriatric patients. J Am Geriatr Soc 1981; 29:92–95.
48. Nott R, Fleminger J. Presenile dementia: The difficulties of early diagnosis. Acta Psychiatr Scand 1975; 51:210–217.
49. Obler L. Language and brain dysfunction in dementia. In: Segalowitz SJ, ed. Language functions and brain organization. New York: Academic Press, 1983:267–282.
50. Pattie AH, Gilleard CJ. Manual of the Clifton assessment procedures for the elderly (CAPE). Sevenoaks, England: Hodder and Staughton, 1979.
51. Peterson RG, Knapp TJ, Rosen JO, Pither BF. The effects of furniture arrangement. Behav Ther 1977; 8:464–467.
52. Poon L. Handbook for clinical memory assessment of older adults. Washington, D.C.: American Psychological Association, 1986.
53. Posner J. Notes on the negative implications of being competent in a home for the aged. Int J Aging Hum Dev 1974; 5:357–364.
54. Post F. Diagnosis of depression in geriatric patients and treatment modalities appropriate for the population. In: Gallant PM, Simpson GM, eds. Depression: Behavioral, biochemical, diagnostic and treatment concepts. New York: Spectrum Publications, 1976:205–234.
55. Quilitch HR. Purposeful activity increased on a geriatric ward through programmed recreation. J Am Geriatr Soc 1974; 22:226–229.
56. Raskin A, Jarvik LF. Psychiatric symptoms and cognitive loss in the elderly: Evaluation and assessment techniques. Washington, D.C.: Hemisphere Publishing, 1979.
57. Rathbone-McCuan E, Hashimi J. Isolated elders. Rockville, MD: Aspen Systems, 1982.
58. Reisberg B, Ferris SH, de Leon MJ, Crook T. The Global Deterioration Scale for the assessment of primary degenerative dementia. Am J Psychiatry 1982; 139:1136–1139.
59. Reisberg B, Schenck MK, Ferris SH, Schwartz GE, de Leon MJ. The Brief Cognitive Rating Scale (BCRS): Findings in primary degenerative dementia (PDD). Psychopharmacol Bull 1983; 19:47–50.
60. Ripich DN, Tervell BY. Patterns of discourse cohesion and coherence in Alzheimer's disease. J Speech Hear Res 1988; 53:8–15.

61. Safilios-Rothschild C. The sociology and social psychology of disability and rehabilitation. New York: Random House, 1970.
62. Schultz R. Effects of the control and predictability on the physical and psychological well-being of the institutionalized aged. J Pers Soc Psychol 1976; 33:563–573.
63. Sigman S. Who pushed the button to drop the A-Bomb? Contexts and conversations in a nursing home. Paper presented at the International Communications Association. Philadelphia, 1979.
64. Snyder LH, Pyrek J, Smith KC. Vision and mental function of the elderly. Gerontologist 1976; 16:491–495.
65. Solomon K. Social antecedents of learned helplessness in the health care setting. Gerontologist 1982; 22:282–287.
66. Stewart RB. Drug use and adverse drug reactions in the elderly: An epidemiological perspective. Topics Geriatr Rehab 1987; 2:1–10.
67. Teeter R, Garetz F, Miller W, Heiland W. Am J Psychiatry 1976; 133:1430–1434.
68. Thal L. Diagnosing and treating dementia. Drug Ther 1982; 12:53–68.
69. Thomas PD, Hooper EM. Healthy elderly: Social bonds and locus of control. Res Nurs Health 1983; 6:11–16.
70. Ulatowska HK, Allard C, Donnell A, et al. Discourse performance in subjects with dementia of the Alzheimer's type. In: Whitaker H, ed. Neuropsychological studies of nonfocal brain damage: Dementia and trauma. ASHA. New York: Springer-Verlag, 1986:108–131.
71. Wattis JP, Hendmarch I. Psychological assessment of the elderly. New York: Churchill Livingstone, 1988.
72. Wolanin MO, Halloway J. Relocation confusion: Intervention for prevention. In: Burnside I, ed. Psychological nursing care of the elderly. New York: McGraw-Hill, 1980.
73. Wolfensberger W, Tullman S. A brief outline of the principle of normalization. Rehabil Psychol 1982; 27:131–145.
74. York J, Calsyn R. Family involvement in nursing homes. Gerontologist 1977; 17:500–505.
75. Zussman J. Some explanations of the changing appearance of psychotic patients: Antecedents of the social breakdown syndrome concept. Milbank Q 1966; 44:363–396.

# CHAPTER 11

# Impact on Families

MARIE T. RAU, Ph.D.

Within the last decade, a rapidly growing body of literature has focused on family caregivers of dependent elderly adults. These family caregivers have been called the "hidden patients" and the "hidden victims" of Alzheimer's disease.[36,107] They have been described as putting in a "36-hour day."[70] Dr. Lewis Thomas of the Sloan-Kettering Institute, in a 1983 New York Times interview, stated "Alzheimer's causes more damage to the family than any other disease I can think of."[98] Research studies have now clearly documented the devastating physical, psychosocial, and financial costs of such long-term caregiving.[2,14,19,24,37,42,85,108]

Why has there been this burgeoning interest in the family as a caregiving resource and in the impact of caregiving responsibilities? This has occurred for a number of related reasons. It is estimated that family members provide 80 to 90 percent of the ongoing, long-term care of frail elderly adults who live in the community, many of whom are dementia victims.[27,53,93] Projections that populations in Western society will continue to age, and that the numbers and proportions of very elderly persons will increase, have resulted in predictions that there will be increasing numbers of persons with dementia and with other chronic illnesses and disabilities who will need ongoing care. (See Chapter 1 for information on the incidence and prevalence of dementia.) The evidence for strong family involvement in caregiving and projected increases in the number of dementia victims cause concern about the prohibitive and continually escalating costs of prolonged institutional care. This has led health-care policy makers to view family caregivers as a significant financial resource to society, with resulting increased support for research on the impacts of long-term caregiving. Finally, within the past few years, caregivers themselves have begun to speak out through a variety of self-help and support groups such as the Alzheimer's Association (formerly the Alzheimer's Disease and Related Disorders Association, ADRDA). This has focused attention on the plight of caregivers.

There are a number of reasons why the impacts of dementia on family caregivers should be of particular interest to speech-language pathologists and audiologists. The roles of these professionals in providing services to dementia patients and their families have been expanding, as articles in professional journals, recent conference program content, and other chapters in this text document. In the future, referrals of patients with communicative disorders who are demented will increase as the population ages. Speech-language pathologists and audiologists need to be aware of the impact of dementing illness on families because they must work closely with caregivers to implement management strategies that will facilitate communication with impaired family members. Clinicians must be knowledgeable concerning the stresses these families face every day in order to counsel them appropriately regarding ways to cope with the gradual deterioration of communicative functions in dementing illness. Familiarity with particular family situations and with the amount of caregiving support available to the primary caregiver will assist the clinician in making realistic and practical suggestions for communication management. Awareness of the impact of dementia on the family will alert the speech-language pathologist or audiologist to signs of caregiver stress and to the need for referral to other professionals when appropriate. Finally, clinicians who have a holistic view of the impact of dementia on both the patient and the family can function more effectively as members of interdisciplinary dementia teams.

The purposes of this chapter are to summarize the current state of knowledge regarding the impact of dementia on families and to glean implications for clinical practice and future research from this information. The chapter will first provide a background for considering the impact of caregiving by defining informal caregiving and its dimensions and by reviewing some of the demographics of caregiving, largely from United States data. Next, the chapter will explore the impacts of dementia on families within the broader context of what is known about the effects of caring for the frail elderly in general, and what is known about the caregivers of other patient groups with chronic, disabling illnesses such as stroke. The specific notion of "caregiver burden" will be discussed in some detail.

The following section of the chapter will review what is known about caregiver interventions. Next, the clinical implications of the information in this chapter will be discussed. The last section of the chapter examines future research directions and questions that need to be answered regarding the impact of dementia on the family and on the patient as part of a family context.

## Formal Versus Informal Caregiving

In this chapter, the focus will be on "informal" caregivers of the demented elderly, in contrast to the care provided to this population through formal structures: government agencies, private organizations, institutions, and paid, professional in-home care providers. Examples of formal caregiving to dementia victims would be those services provided in nursing homes, adult day-care programs, foster care, and formal respite-care programs. In contrast, the terms "informal caregiving" and "informal caregivers" are commonly used interchangeably with the terms "family caregiving" and "family caregivers" to refer to the many types of unpaid assistance provided by family and close friends. Chapter 16 on the care environment and Chapter 17 on staff in-service training focus on aspects of formal caregiving.

### WHO ARE THE INFORMAL CAREGIVERS?

National data present us with a picture of families very involved in the provision of ongoing care to their elderly relatives, including those with dementing illness.[96] It has been estimated that 60 percent to 80 percent of the care to the dependent elderly is provided by the informal care system, that is, family and friends.[77] Seventy-five percent of community-dwelling elderly persons rely solely on the informal care system, while only 5 percent receive care only from paid sources.[66] Ongoing, long-term care to this population is provided almost exclusively by family members.[27,53,57,93] Furthermore, research suggests that any use of the formal care system typically occurs after care needs become more than the family can handle alone and that when supportive services are offered, family requests from the formal care system are modest.[15,73,95]

For both cultural and demographic reasons, family caregiving is largely, although not exclusively, a women's issue. The demographics of our elderly population reflect the fact that most spouse caregivers are female because women tend to outlive their husbands. Furthermore, studies have consistently shown that adult daughters and daughters-in-law are the major source of support when a spouse is not present or when the level of spouse-provided support is insufficient.[17,93,96]

Data from the 1982 Long-Term Care Survey (LTCS) and Informal Caregivers Survey (ICS) help us to describe these family-member caregivers.[96,97] Their average age is 57 years, although one-fourth are age 65 to 74 and another 10 percent are 75 years of age or older. Thus, one-third of informal caregivers to the elderly are elderly themselves. These caregivers are more likely to be female (72 percent) and to live in the same household as the care recipient (75 percent). They are less likely to be employed than their counterparts in the general population and more likely to be poor or near-poor (33 percent). They are more likely to report their health to be only fair or poor (33 percent) than similar-aged persons in the general population. Seventy percent of these caregivers describe themselves as the primary care provider, and one-third report that they are the only provider of care to a frail elderly person.

Although there are no national data available from a representative sample of caregivers of exclusively dementia patients, one study[63] compared the demographic characteristics of a large sample (N = 632) of dementia caregivers with the caregiver samples in both the LTC/IC Survey[96] and the National Long Term Care Channeling Demonstration.[61] Lawton and his colleagues found that their nonrepresentative sample of caregivers of dementia victims was very similar to the two national comparison samples on most demographic characteristics.[63] Some differences were noted, however. The comparison samples, which included both physically and mentally impaired elderly, had a greater proportion of care receivers living alone. They also had a lower proportion of spouse-caregivers than did the dementia sample.[63] The caregivers in the dementia sample rated their own health more negatively than did the respondents in the national surveys. Finally, the dementia caregivers were somewhat higher in socioeconomic status than caregivers in the national surveys.

There is additional evidence that the caregiving networks of persons with dementia may have different structural and compositional characteristics than do the support systems of dependent elderly persons who are not demented. Birkel and Jones compared the support networks of 20 elderly, physically disabled but lucid individuals with those of 20 equally physically impaired but also significantly demented elderly persons.[12] All of these elderly care receivers lived with an adult child. Birkel and Jones found that the demented subjects were cared for primarily by a core group of members of the immediate household, whereas the caregiving networks of those who were not demented included a greater number and proportion of non-household family, friends, and paid helpers. Although Birkel and Jones suggest that these different patterns of caregiving networks may in some ways reflect an adaptive phenomenon (that is, it may be easier to care for a person with cognitive and behavioral impairments within a family/household structure of a few familiar persons), they also point out the potential depletion over time of the emotional, physical, and financial resources of the family and suggest that this "adaptation" may lead to family isolation and "burnout." The authors conclude by recommending that in cases of dementia attention to family concerns and specific aspects of household functioning may be especially critical.[12]

In summary, these statistics imply a number of stresses on family-member caregivers of the elderly and on the caregivers of persons with dementing illness in particular. Many caregivers are dealing with health problems and other difficulties of aging themselves. As a group, they are experiencing financial strains. These family members are typically providing care 7 days a week, with perhaps a small amount of help from other caregivers. If the care receiver has a dementing illness, the available data suggest that he or she is more likely to be living with the primary caregiver and that the individual providing care is more likely to be a spouse or a small group of immediate household members who are utilizing few outside resources.

## WHO ARE THE RECEIVERS OF INFORMAL CARE?

In the United States there are between 4.6 and 5.1 million elderly who are functionally impaired and living in the community.[66,71] It is estimated that as many as 1 million of these impaired, community-dwelling elderly are dementia victims being cared for by their families.[88] The majority of older persons with dementia of the Alzheimer's type (DAT) and related dementias, in fact, remain at home under the care of at least one family member.[85]

It is not necessarily the case that impaired elderly persons who live in the community are less severely disabled than those living in nursing homes. Shanas estimated that for every older person residing in a nursing home, there are two elderly individuals with a similar level of impairment living in the community.[93] Liu and colleagues stated that only one in five elderly persons with long-term care needs lives in a nursing home.[66] Demented persons residing in nursing homes are not necessarily more impaired in functional abilities than those with dementia living in the community.[38] It has also been found that elderly persons with family supports enter nursing homes with much higher levels of impairment than those without such supports, providing further evidence that families tend to care for their impaired relatives at home until they can no longer manage physically, emotionally, or financially.[6,32]

There are limited demographic data about the demented population available at the present time, other than prevalence and incidence statistics. (See Chapter 1 for detailed prevalence and incidence information.) These prevalence and incidence statistics suggest that the "typical" person with progressive dementia who lives in the community will be a very elderly female whose primary caregiver is a daughter who is likely to be middle aged or elderly herself. On the other hand, studies of nursing-home residents and other institutionalized populations would suggest that those persons with progressive dementia who are married have a much greater chance of remaining in the community to be cared for by a spouse and other family members.[16,17] Recently published figures suggest that dementia is common in old age and that previous reports have probably underestimated the number of elderly persons and their family-member caregivers who experience the impact of these devastating illnesses.[35]

## Dimensions of Caregiving

Because family members provide the bulk of caregiving, they must perform a great variety of tasks and assume a number of different and sometimes unfamiliar caregiving roles. Clark and Rakowski, in a comprehensive review of the caregiving literature, categorized the types of tasks that caregivers need to accomplish into three broad areas.[22] Table 11.1 outlines Clark and Rakowski's summary of caregiving roles and provides some examples of tasks under each role. It is clear that caregivers not only accomplish tasks directly related to providing assistance to the impaired older person but also must look after themselves while living up to the expectations of other family members and of society. In all, Clark and Rakowski identi-

TABLE 11.1 **The Spectrum of Caregiving Roles and Examples of Caregiving Tasks**

**TASKS INVOLVING PROVISION OF DIRECT ASSISTANCE**

Be available when needed
Supervise prescribed treatment and general recommendations
Evaluate options for treatment and services
Cope with upsetting behavior of the care receiver
Maintain adequate communication with the care receiver

**PERSONAL TASKS**

Compensate for emotional drain from constant responsibility
Compensate for or recover personal time
Readjust personal routines
Compensate for disruption of sleep
Emotionally accept the likelihood of a progressive downward course

**FAMILIAL TASKS**

Designate other "responsible caregiver(s)"
Cope with loss/restriction of family future planning
Maintain family communication and exchange of information
Balance the giving of assistance with responsibilities to other family members
Manage feelings toward other family members who do not regularly help

**SOCIETAL TASKS**

Interact with medical, health, and social service professionals
Maintain knowledge of the service system and options
Act as advocate or third-party negotiator for the care receiver
Maintain knowledge of reimbursement mechanisms

Adapted from Clark NM, Rakowski W. Family caregivers of older adults: Improving helping skills. Gerontologist 1983; 23:637–642.

fied from the literature 14 tasks facing family caregivers, 8 tasks related to other family members, and 4 tasks involving interaction with various societal structures. Although Clark and Rakowski's taxonomy represents only one way of classifying caregiving tasks, it does provide a broad perspective on the many roles that caregivers need to assume when a family member has dementia.

Cicirelli has described some of the roles assumed by caregivers of dementia victims in particular, delineating seven tasks that family members fulfill[21]:

1. Seeking an early diagnosis when the family member's behavior seems different from normal
2. Assessing the demented person's need for care and assistance over time and as the disease progresses
3. Providing direct care or arranging for care related to survival and basic needs
4. Providing for the dementia's victim's safety
5. Managing home medical care and behavior problems
6. Providing social stimulation and activity within the dementing person's capabilities
7. Providing an atmosphere that will make the demented individual as comfortable as possible and encourage positive moods, a sense of belonging, and participation in family activities

The progressive nature of dementia requires that family caregivers assume additional roles as the patient's cognitive and physical functions deteriorate. Furthermore, in progressive dementia there is never the prospect that some of these caregiving roles can be relinquished because the patient will improve or "get better." These circumstances, taken together with the strong preference of families to care for their dementing relatives at home, make it inevitable that caregivers will experience many dementia-related stresses and that these stresses will have substantial impacts on both the primary caregiver and on the family as a whole.[94] The next section discusses some of these stresses and their impacts.

## The Stresses of Caregiving

Studies on the impacts of caregiving were first published in the 1950s in the United States and in the 1960s in Great Britain.[23,47–49] These early reports dealt with the families of psychiatric patients, some of whom were elderly, with organically based dementias. Since this early work, many reports have described the multiple stresses experienced by caregivers of dependent adults.[3,17,19,20,36,44,85] These documented stresses have included: restrictions on the caregiver's personal and social life; competing demands of intergenerational family obligations, those of the workplace, and caregiving responsibilities; family conflicts over issues of caregiving; and the need to deal with the requirements, demands, and sometimes difficult behaviors of the care recipient. Cantor, in describing caregiving in the United States, wrote of caregiver "strain"—a term that she defined as including the following: worry about several aspects of the care receiver's situation; the emotional, physical, and financial stresses that caregiving itself entails; and the impacts of caregiving that involve for the caregiver a sense of deprivation in the areas of other family obligations, personal needs, and socialization.[19]

## THE STRESSES OF CARING FOR SOMEONE WITH DEMENTIA

The studies referred to above have looked at caregiving for dependent elderly family members in general, including those with only physical incapacities. The question must be asked: Are the caregiving stresses different or more severe when the one being cared for is cognitively and behaviorally impaired, as is the case in dementing illness?

Several studies have documented that caring for someone with cognitive and behavioral impairments is more stressful than caring for someone who is physically frail.[4,29,43,47,48,59,74,90] Deimling and Bass reported that the disruptive and socially inappropriate behaviors of impaired elderly care recipients were particularly distressing to the family members with whom they lived, whereas cognitive deficits themselves were less directly stress producing.[29] Gilleard examined the psychological well-being of family caregivers of patients attending either geriatric or psychogeriatric day-care programs in Great Britain, using the General Health Questionnaire (GHQ) as the dependent measure.[43] He found that when neither communication nor behavior disturbances were present in the dependent family member, just over one-third (37 percent) of the primary support persons reported symptoms of psychiatric disorder, whereas in the presence of both communication and behavior disturbance, 39 of 56 (70 percent) of caregivers showed symptoms of psychiatric disorder. When either a communication disorder or behavior disturbance was present in the patient, 50 percent of family caregivers reported symptoms of psychiatric disorder.

In a study that found somewhat different results, Eagles and colleagues reported no greater levels of psychiatric morbidity in coresident supporters of elderly demented persons compared with the caregivers of a nondemented elderly control group.[34] These researchers did find, however, significantly higher levels of "stress" among the caregivers of the demented elderly. They also found that relatives' stress scale scores correlated highly with measures of the dependent elders' cognitive impairment and level of behavioral disturbance. In another recently published study, no relationship was found between rates of caregiver depression and whether or not the care receiver was cognitively impaired.[41]

It has been suggested that families of dementia victims experience different types of stresses during different phases of the illness.[20] Strains on primary support persons in the early phases of the illness may include anxiety and concern about changes noted in their loved one, bearing the brunt of the demented individual's anger and resentment when help is offered or problems pointed out, frustration at not being able to convince health-care personnel that something is wrong, and denial of problems by other family members. After a diagnosis has been made, stresses may involve dealing with feelings of disbelief, anger, confusion, and helplessness. As the illness progresses and the dementia victim further deteriorates, becoming more behaviorally difficult and physically dependent, stresses will be related to the need for constant care and supervision and to the caregiver's feelings of anticipatory grief.[11] Financial stresses will also be likely to increase for many families with the duration of the illness.

What are the stresses that the primary support persons of frail elderly persons find most difficult to tolerate? This is an important question and is often related to the decision to institutionalize a family member.[76] In a study by Sanford, caregivers living with impaired older adults cited their own sleep disruption (related to the care receiver's night wandering, shouting, or inability to get to the bathroom unaided), and the care receiver's fecal incontinence and general immobility as poorly tolerated behaviors.[90] In a study involving family caregivers of dementia patients, Chenoweth and Spencer found that behavioral problems and incontinence were each cited by about 20 percent of caregivers as the reason for institutionalization.[20] Caregivers interviewed by Rabins and colleagues reported violent resistance to care, memory disturbance, incontinence, catastrophic patient reactions, hitting, and suspicious and accusatory behavior as the most serious problems with which they had to deal.[85] Although few families reported communication difficulties to be among the most serious problems, 74 percent endorsed communication difficulties as a problem causing frustration and catastrophic patient reactions.

Evidence suggesting that communication-related difficulties are among the most distressing patient behaviors with which family caregivers must cope is provided by Greene, Smith, Gardiner, and Timbury, who interviewed 38 relatives of community-dwelling dementia patients.[50] Eight out of 10 items labeled "apathetic/withdrawn" behaviors on a Behavior and Mood Disturbance Scale (BMD) developed by these authors related directly to communication (see Table 11.2). Caregivers' levels of personal distress and overall stress, as measured by a Relatives' Stress Scale, were significantly related to care receivers' scores on the "apathetic/withdrawn" subscale.

To summarize this section on the stresses of caregiving, numerous studies have provided evidence that the caregiver role imposes many physical, psychological, and financial stresses on those most directly involved. Yet the caregiving literature strongly suggests that the presence of the same objective stressors does not mean that all caregivers will feel equally stressed. The impacts of caregiving and the degree of burden experienced depend on many interacting variables. The next sections of the chapter will explore some of these factors.

## Impacts of Caregiving

Given the multiple stresses of caregiving, it is not surprising that research reports have rather consistently described a variety of negative impacts of long-term caregiving on family members. Negative effects on the physical health and financial well-being of family caregivers have been noted; however, the literature suggests that the most pervasive negative impacts of providing care are related to caregivers' mental health and psychological well-being. The evidence that caregiving adversely affects physical health of caregivers will be briefly reviewed before discussing more fully what is known about the psychological and psychosocial impacts of providing long-term care.

## THE PHYSICAL HEALTH EFFECTS OF CAREGIVING

There is conflicting evidence that caregiving per se has measurable negative effects on the physical health of caregivers. These conflicting results may be due in part to the fact that heterogeneous patient samples have been used in many caregiver impact studies. Montgomery and Borgatta found that 85 percent of a large sample of family caregivers (N = 514) of a mixed group of impaired elderly persons reported their physical health to be "good, very good, or perfect" on initial interview.[73] On re-interview 12 months later, these caregivers' self-reported health status remained the same. Despite the fact that few of these caregivers used any of the available support services offered to them in this intervention study, it appears that they did not view their physical health as having suffered. In a Canadian study, Marcus and Jaeger found that 57 percent of a sample of 54 elderly caregivers rated their own health as "good," while only 15 percent rated their health as "poor."[72] Furthermore, neither sex, age, nor burden score was related to health rating. George and Gwyther, in comparing dimensions of self-reported health and well-being in a large sample of caregivers of de-

---

TABLE 11.2 **Items Related to Aspects of Communication on The Apathetic/Withdrawn Subscale of The Behavior and Mood Disturbance Scale**

Does not take part in family conversations

Does not read newspapers, magazines, etc

Does not show an interest in news about friends and relatives

Does not start and maintain a sensible conversation

Does not respond sensibly when spoken to

Does not understand what is said to him/her

Does not watch and follow television

Adapted from Greene JG, Smith R, Gardiner M, Timbury GC. Measuring behavioural disturbance of elderly demented patients in the community and its effects on relatives: A factor analytic study. Age Ageing 1982; 11:121–126.

mented adults (N = 510) to several large community samples, found that the dementia caregivers neither used more medical services nor rated their physical health worse than did respondents in the random community samples.[42] Pruchno and Resch reported that two-thirds of their sample of 315 spouse caregivers of dementia patients rated their physical health as good or excellent and only 8 percent rated their health as poor.[83]

However, some evidence to support negative physical health effects for dementia caregivers has been reported. Haley and co-workers compared a group of 44 family caregivers of dementia patients and 44 matched controls on a variety of measures including several physical health indicators.[55] The dementia caregivers reported poorer health, more prescription medication use, and higher utilization of health-care services than did the control group. Lawton et al found that a large sample of dementia caregivers had poorer self-reported physical health status than did two national representative samples of caregivers of the frail elderly.[63] In an interesting study that obtained physiologic measurements (blood samples and nutritional analyses) and psychological data from 34 family caregivers of DAT victims and 34 matched controls, evidence for negative health effects of caregiving was found.[62] The DAT caregivers had significantly lower percentages of total T lymphocytes and helper T lymphocytes than did comparison subjects, as well as significantly lower helper-suppressor cell ratios and higher antibody titers to the Epstein-Barr virus. The dementia caregivers were also more distressed than the control group on the psychological measures. The authors concluded that these results suggest that chronically stressed family caregivers of DAT patients show neither immunologic nor psychological adaptation to the level of non-care-providing age peers.

There is some evidence that caregiving takes a toll on the physical health of spouse caregivers in particular. Chenoweth and Spencer, in a study of 289 family members of dementia patients, found that of 32 family caregivers who reported serious illnesses and injuries that they related to caregiving, 31 were spouses.[20] In the George and Gwyther study, spouse caregivers reported significantly more doctor visits and poorer self-rated health than did other caregivers, even after statistically controlling for age effects.[42] Interestingly, physical health indicators were not related to patient living arrangements, even though a substantial percentage of the dementia patients in this study (34 percent) lived in nursing homes.

To summarize the evidence for possible negative physical health effects of caregiving, the data are somewhat equivocal; however, it appears that dementia caregivers, in particular, may experience negative impacts on their physical well-being and may be more vulnerable to physical illness because of chronic stress.

## MENTAL HEALTH EFFECTS OF CAREGIVING

Most studies that have examined the impacts of caregiving have focused on psychological health and well-being. Results of such studies consistently point to the negative mental health effects of this stress-producing situation, including feelings of low morale, anger, and guilt, as well as increased levels of depression and anxiety. Investigations have found, for example, rates of depressive symptoms three to seven times higher in caregiver samples than in comparable community samples of the elderly.[13,24,28,31,41,74,87,91] Not all of these studies have focused exclusively on caregivers of dementia victims, but it is informative to examine the impacts of caregiving on the caregivers of other chronically ill or disabled elderly populations in order to compare caregiver outcomes.

## DEPRESSIVE SYMPTOMS IN OTHER CAREGIVER GROUPS

A number of researchers have measured depressive symptomatology in the primary support persons of frail elderly patients, usually employing well-standardized self-report scales. Rau, for example, found that almost half (45 percent) of 50 spouse caregivers of persons who had suffered an initial stroke 6 to 8 months previously scored above the cutoff level on the Center for Epidemiologic Studies Depression Scale,[86] indicating that they were at high risk for depression.[82] Gallagher and colleagues studied two groups of caregivers, a group of 158 help-seekers caring for a heterogeneous frail elderly population, and a group of 58 volunteers participating in a longitudinal study of DAT.[41] The latter group was made up of the spouses of recently diagnosed or early DAT victims. Using strict criteria for the diagnosis of depression, these researchers found that 46 percent of the help-seeking group had a depressive disorder, and an additional 22 percent exhibited some depressive symptoms. Although no gender differences were found overall, caregiving wives were significantly more depressed than caregiving husbands. In the spouses of the early DAT patients, only 18 percent were clinically depressed, while two-thirds showed no evidence of depressive symptoms. The discrepancy in the prevalence of depression in the two caregiver groups might be explained by the fact that the dementia patients were still in the early phase of the disease and that their caregivers had been providing support for a significantly shorter period of time. Another interesting finding of this study was that for the help-seeking sample there was no relationship found between the presence or absence of significant cognitive impairment in the care receiver and depression in the caregiver.

## MENTAL HEALTH SYMPTOMS IN DEMENTIA CAREGIVERS

Although the literature on the effects of caregiving is difficult to sort through because many studies have used heterogeneous samples in terms of the care receiver's diagnosis (using such terms as "dependent elderly" or "frail elderly"), a number of recent studies have limited their samples to caregivers of dementia victims, or to support persons of individuals with probable DAT. Most are characterized by heterogeneity in terms of the caregiver's relationship to the dependent person. These studies have looked at depression and other symptomatology in the care providers and are in general agreement concerning negative impacts of the caregiving situation. A few have compared caregivers of dementia patients with representative normative samples or age-matched control groups. Some illustrative studies are cited below.

Anthony-Bergstone, Zarit, and Gatz compared the responses of 184 family caregivers of dementia patients on nine subscales of the Brief Symptom Inventory (BSI)[30] with published age-matched community norms.[2] They found that all of the caregivers (subdivided by age and gender into older and younger male and female groups) had significantly higher scores on the Hostility subscale, and that female caregivers also scored significantly higher on the Anxiety subscale. Only the older women, three-fourths of whom were spouses, scored significantly higher than the norms on the Depression, Obsessive-Compulsive, and Psychoticism subscales as well.

Cohen and Eisdorfer investigated the relationship of attributional style and living arrangements to depression in 46 primary caregivers of 27 dementia patients.[24] They found that 55 percent of family member caregivers (80 percent of whom were spouses) who were living with the patient had a clinical depression, whereas none of those not living with the patient were diagnosed as depressed. Depression was measured by the Beck Self-Report Depression Scale.[10] In terms of attributions, depressed caregivers were more likely to perceive themselves as lacking control over their situation and to feel that they should have more control over events related to caregiving than were those who were not depressed. Another interesting finding of this study was that no patient status characteristics (duration or severity of dementia) were predictive of depression in the caregiver.

George and Gwyther found that family-member caregivers of dementia victims were doing less well on several measures of mental health compared to community samples from several large-scale studies.[42] Caregivers reported almost three times as many stress symptoms as did the comparison samples and had considerably lower levels of well-being and life satisfaction. A higher proportion (28 percent) of the care providers reported using psychotropic medications. They also reported considerably lower levels of social participation than did the comparison samples and were generally dissatisfied with the amount of social interaction they had. In a community sample of elderly, community-dwelling couples in Scotland, a significant relationship between depression in husbands and cognitive impairment in their wives was found, but the reverse was not found to be true.[33] Although this review of the literature would suggest that the negative impacts of caregiving are universal, some caregivers report levels of psychological well-being and physical health status that are as high as those reported by non-caregivers. The concept of "caregiver burden" and its correlates may help to explain some of these differences among caregivers.

### Caregiver Burden

Although it is generally agreed that the chronic care of a patient with dementia produces a number of stresses that may have significant negative impacts on the caregiver, important questions remain. Why do some caregivers appear to cope better with this demanding situation? Why are some families able to continue caring for a demented relative while others make institutional placement decisions relatively soon? In seeking answers to these questions, researchers have explored the concept of "caregiver burden," or the perceptions and cognitions of the caregiver that their caregiving situation or particular aspects of it are stressful or burdensome. The notion of "caregiver burden," then, is predicted in some conceptual frameworks to depend more on the caregiver's subjective view of the situation than on more objective factors such as the care receiver's cognitive status, limitations in ADL functioning, or severity of behavior problems.

Some researchers have viewed caregiver burden as a global, unidimensional construct.[108,109] Zarit and colleagues, for example, have defined caregiver burden as "the extent to which caregivers perceive their emotional or physical health, social life, and financial status as suffering as a result of caring for their relative."[109] A Caregiver Burden Scale constructed by Zarit and colleagues and used frequently by other researchers reflects this view of burden as a unitary concept.[108] Other investigators have viewed caregiver burden as a complex, multidimensional concept that is differentially related to aspects of patient functioning, caregiver characteristics, and environmental factors.[75,82]

Morycz proposed four factors related to what he called "family burden": (1) patient behaviors and characteristics; (2) caregiver limitations and characteristics; (3) environmental factors; and (4) interactive factors.[75] Table 11.3 presents examples of the first three factors. Interactive factors are those that involve the interaction of two or more of these factors. For example, the caregiver's less-than-robust health, along with the care receiver's need for high levels of care, could together contribute to a sense of isolation and "burnout" in the caregiver.

Poulshock and Deimling present both a conceptual framework and empirical evidence to support their contention that caregiver burden should be viewed as a multidimensional construct.[82] They suggest that burden plays a central role as a mediating variable, a "subjective filter" between the care receiver's impairments and the relatively objective impacts of caregiving on the family. In an analysis of data from a study of 614 families living with an impaired older person, Poulshock and Deimling predicted that burden would be differentially related to aspects of the dependent elder's impairments (physical dependence and cognitive, social, and behavioral incapacities) and to impacts on the caregiver and family. They constructed burden measures to correspond to each aspect of elder impairment examined. Results confirmed Poulshock and Deimling's predictions. Care receivers' mental incapacities were more strongly related to impacts on family relationships, while elders' ADL needs were more strongly related to ADL burden measures and to caregiver activity restrictions. Burden measures associated with physical dependence and with mental impairment were relatively independent, suggesting that they are different aspects of subjective burden.

Other researchers have proposed that the caregiving experience cannot be characterized adequately in terms of subjective burden and negative impacts alone.[64,78] Lawton and his co-workers offer evidence from a factor analytic study that the subjective experience of caregiving is best described by the term "caregiving appraisal," which is multifaceted and includes the factors of caregiving satisfaction, subjective burden, and caregiving impact. Other authors have pointed out the tendency of researchers in this area to overlook the positive aspects of caregiving as they are perceived by the person providing care.[52,56,69] The positive feelings that a caregiver may receive from coping effectively, repaying past kindnesses, and providing quality care to a loved one may serve to buffer the stresses of caregiving.

TABLE 11.3 **Factors Related to Caregiver Burden**

**PATIENT BEHAVIORS AND CHARACTERISTICS**

Sleep disturbances
Wandering
Inability to perform ADLs
Aggressive outbursts
Other behavior problems

**CAREGIVER LIMITATIONS AND CHARACTERISTICS**

Anxiety
Depression
Negative attitudes/expectations toward aged
Insufficient physical strength
Health problems
Feelings of embarrassment related to patient's behavior
Sensitivity to criticism
Low tolerance for deviant behavior

**ENVIRONMENTAL FACTORS**

Physical barriers
Space limitations
Financial burdens

Adapted from Morycz RK. An exploration of senile dementia and family burden. Clin Soc Work J 1980; 8:16–27.

## CORRELATES OF PERCEIVED BURDEN

What are the factors that might assist in identifying those caregivers who are at risk for experiencing high levels of burden and stress in the caregiving role? This is a central question in terms of planning appropriate interventions and preventing early and inappropriate institutionalization of the person with dementia. Researchers have examined characteristics of the care receiver, characteristics and perceptions of the caregiver, and aspects of the patient/caregiver relationship in seeking answers to this question. The available data concerning some of these factors will be examined next.

### Severity and Duration of Patient Impairment and Other Care Receiver Behaviors

Contrary to what might be expected, severity of care receiver impairment and duration of symptoms have not been found to be strongly predictive of the degree of perceived caregiver burden when homogeneous dementia patient samples have been studied.[24,42,68,79,103,108] Zarit, for example, found that the caregiver's expressed tolerance for the patient's memory and behavior problems was significantly related to level of subjective burden, whereas the reported frequency and severity of these problems were not.[103] Zarit, Todd, and Zarit later confirmed these findings in a follow-up study.[109] Colerick and George found that caregiver characteristics and well-being, rather than characteristics of the patient, were more important predictors of institutional placement decisions.[26]

Conversely, certain behaviors of the care receiver have been found to be related to caregiver burden. Pruchno and Resch examined relationships between the self-reported mental health of 262 spouse caregivers of community-dwelling persons with DAT and care receivers' forgetful, disoriented, and asocial behaviors.[83] They found that asocial and disoriented behaviors of the impaired spouse were linearly related to level of reported caregiver burden, specific mental health problems associated with caregiving, and the extent to which caregivers gave up aspects of their social lives. That is, as reported levels of these behaviors increased, so did levels of burden and other consequences of caregiving. Asocial behaviors were also related to global measures of caregiver depression. Interestingly, forgetful behaviors were not related to burden or other outcome measures in a linear fashion. As forgetful behaviors increased from occurring not at all to occurring sometimes or often, levels of burden, negative mental health effects of caregiving, and social life changes increased. On the other hand, caregivers whose spouses had high levels of forgetful behaviors expressed degrees of stress similar to those of caregivers whose spouses exhibited mild memory impairments. These findings offer support for a multidimensional notion of caregiver burden. Behaviors that are less predictable (e.g., asocial and disoriented behaviors) become increasingly stressful as they increase in frequency. Forgetful behaviors, however, tend to increase linearly and predictably as the course of the disease progresses. They gradually become less stressful, suggesting adaptation on the part of the caregiver to increasing memory impairment in the care receiver.

Pearson, Verma, and Nellett examined several aspects of patient functioning and caregiver perceptions in terms of their contributions to caregiver burden.[80] Their mixed patient sample consisted of 46 elderly psychiatric patients referred to a geriatric assessment unit and their caregivers, 16 of whom shared a household with the patient. About one-quarter of the patients were described as having "possible dementia," while slightly more than half were referred for evaluation of depression. Significant predictors of caregiver burden that were measured with the Relatives' Stress Scale (RSS) were disruptive patient behavior; caregiver distress, which the authors stated was related to, but a separate construct from, caregiver burden; and patient limitations in performing activities of daily living (ADLs).[50] These results, as the authors point out, contradict those obtained in studies of caregiver burden in which homogeneous samples of dementia patients and their caregivers were used.[108]

### Age, Gender, and Relationship Factors

What are the impacts of caregiver age, gender, and relationship to the care receiver on the degree of reported caregiver burden? Currently available data suggest that these factors may interact in determining the level of burden experienced. Some studies have indicated that caregiving wives experience more negative mental health impacts than do caregiving husbands.[37,41,44,84,103] In one study that looked at both caregiver burden and several aspects of psychological well-being, husbands and wives of dementia patients were found to experience similar levels of subjective burden, but wives reported more depressive symptoms. Interaction effects of age and gender were also found.[37] Younger spouses were more resentful of their circumstances and lonelier. Younger wives and older husbands appeared to be the most at-risk groups. Pruchno and Resch found caregiving wives to be more depressed and to feel more burden than caregiving husbands.[84] Ill health and less emotional investment in the relationship were both predictive of depression in the wives, while only ill health was predictive of depression in the husbands. Higher levels of burden in the wives were associated with poorer health, less emotional investment, greater spouse impairment, and the provision of more assistance with tasks. No significant predictors of burden were found in this study for the husbands.

Other studies have not found gender differences in degree of burden experienced when relationship to the patient was controlled. Zarit, Todd, and Zarit, for example, in a longitudinal study that looked at perceived burden in spouse caregivers, found that husbands and wives experienced similar levels of burden over time, although wives had initially reported higher burden scores.[109] In another study that explored gender effects in relationship to caregiver burden, no gender effects were found for degree of perceived burden in spouse caregivers when degree of patient memory or behavior problems, age of the caregiver, and number of negative social contacts were controlled.[8]

When both gender of the caregiver and relationship to the care recipient are considered together, somewhat different burden outcomes have been found. Some researchers have suggested that caregiving daughters, particularly if they are employed, may experience higher levels of burden than other caregivers.[17,102] Spouses may view caring for a partner, whether physically frail or mentally impaired, as a normative role expectation, and thus experience less burden.

### Perceptions of the Caregiving Role

How do the caregiver's perceptions of the caregiving situation and of the care receiver influence the amount of caregiving help provided and the degree of stress that is experienced? There is evidence that family members will continue to provide basic care to a frail relative regardless of the quality of the previous relationship and despite the absence of feelings of affection, probably because feelings of family obligation are strong.[1,18,58,81] Nevertheless, Horowitz and Shindelman point out that caregiving takes place in a historical context of past relationships and interactions.[58] In their research, these authors found that expressed affection for the frail elderly care receiver was positively related to feelings of commitment and negatively related to the extent of caregiving impact; that is, positive feelings toward the care receiver did mediate potential strains of caregiving. Furthermore, Horowitz and Shindelman found that positive feelings toward the care receiver were related to the level of caregiving commitment, that is, the stronger the emotional bond, the more assistance provided to the frail elderly relative.[58] Pruchno and Resch also found perceptions of the quality of the previous relationship and degree of emotional investment to be predictive of level of burden for wives who were caregivers.[84] This has important implications for clinicians intervening with families of dementia patients. Obtaining information about the degree of closeness between caregiver and care receiver would help to identify those caregiving situations in which obligation rather than feelings of affection is the primary motivating factor for continued patient support. This would allow for the planning of specifically targeted interventions that might avoid or delay institutional placement of the dementia patient, such as counseling and concrete support services.

### SUMMARY: CORRELATES OF CAREGIVER BURDEN

When considering all of the factors that may contribute to a sense of caregiver burden and that may have negative impacts on the individual with dementia, those variables related to the characteristics, perceptions, and attitudes of the caregiver appear to be the most important. Caregiver age, physical health, gender, and relationship to the patient need to be considered in assessing the potential for negative impacts. The caregiver's perceptions of both the satisfactions and frustrations of caregiving, and his or her satisfaction with the amount and quality of social support available, will likewise influence decisions regarding care options.[92,108]

## Caregiver Interventions

### TYPES OF CAREGIVER INTERVENTIONS

As the negative impacts of long-term caregiving have come to be recognized, considerable interest has been generated in strategies to alleviate the stresses on family caregivers. Subsequently, a number of intervention approaches have been described.[40,51,54,65,101,105,106] A variety of strategies can be identified in this literature. Some interventions have adopted a support-group model, in which sharing of information, venting of feelings, and psychosocial support are primary goals.[5,46] Another intervention model employs an educational focus and stresses providing information and teaching behaviorally based strategies to help caregivers cope more effectively. Gallagher has described a psychoeducational approach, employed in Classes for Coping with Caregiving at the Palo

Alto VA Medical Center, in which cognitive and behavioral skills are taught in small groups.[39] The aims of these groups are to improve participants' sense of self-efficacy and their overall ability to cope successfully. Most support groups use a combined support and education approach.[100]

Zarit and Zarit describe a comprehensive model in which individual counseling with the caregiver, family meetings, and support groups are employed.[105] The aims of the family meeting are to bring the family's level of information (about dementia) up to that of the caregiver, to answer questions about dementing illness and its likely course over time, to identify the caregiver's most pressing needs, and to solve problems with the family. The ultimate goal of such an approach is to strengthen the caregiver's support system.

Another way in which support groups may differ in structure has to do with whether they are professionally led or peer-led. Although there are advantages and disadvantages to each type of model, recent evidence suggests that professionally led groups may show greater benefits in terms of caregiver psychological well-being while peer-led groups may be more effective in increasing the informal support networks of participants.[101]

## EFFECTIVENESS OF CAREGIVER INTERVENTIONS

Caregivers almost universally express satisfaction with support-group interventions when such measures are obtained. Likewise, the clinical impressions of authors who have reported on such groups are that many positive outcomes are observed. Nevertheless, the caregiver intervention literature lacks clear evidence that support-group participation is related to important outcomes such as improved caregiver well-being and more effective coping skills. Excellent reviews of this literature are listed in the references for this chapter.[22,40,100] In the few studies that have utilized control groups, mixed results as to the support intervention's effectiveness have been found.

Zarit and his colleagues compared two intervention approaches, individual family counseling and support groups, and measured their effectiveness in relieving family stress and subjective burden.[106] Although subjects in both groups made significant gains compared to baseline and maintained these gains over a 1-year follow-up period, they did not differ in gains made from a waiting-list control group or from each other. Haley et al also compared two types of support-group interventions (support group and support-plus-skills group) in a design that included random assignment to groups and a waiting-list control condition.[54] These researchers found that group participation did not result in improvement on measures of depression, life satisfaction, social support, or coping effectiveness, although participants rated the groups as helpful. Some forms of adaptive coping did increase in caregivers who attended either of the support groups compared to the waiting-list subjects.

Some intervention researchers have found that support groups were effective. Kahan et al reported that support-group subjects showed a significant decrease in total family burden and significant improvement on a measure of knowledge of dementia compared to a waiting-list control group.[60] Subjects were not randomly assigned to groups, however. In a study with a very small number of subjects, Lazarus and his colleagues found that support-group participants reported a greater sense of control over their lives and less dissatisfaction with changes in the family unit compared to a control group, although no group differences were found on self-reported measures of anxiety, depression, trust, or self-esteem.[65] In a carefully designed efficacy study that utilized random assignment to groups, Lovett and Gallagher found that caregivers who participated in either of two psychoeducational intervention groups demonstrated decreases in depression and increases in morale compared to caregivers on a waiting list.[67] The degree of perceived stress reported by caregivers was not affected by group participation, however. The two interventions, one designed to increase caregivers' life satisfaction and one designed to increase problem-solving skills, appeared to be equally facilitative.

Individualized caregiver intervention approaches are also effective and may even be more appropriate for some caregivers (e.g., those who are identified as suffering from a clinical depression) and in the late stages of caregiving.[39] It has also been suggested that some of the stresses of caregiving might be more effectively dealt with within a more individualized treatment framework.[46] These individual interventions, provided by someone trained in counseling skills, include cognitive or behavioral therapy, brief psychodynamic therapy, and supportive counseling.

## SUMMARY: CAREGIVER INTERVENTIONS

Helpful interventions in the early stage of caregiving, which Gallagher describes as focused on the "coping process," may include caregiver workshops, educationally oriented support groups, and structured psychoeducational programs such as life satisfaction and problem-solving classes.[39] These interventions should focus on the caregiver's need for mastery over a relatively new situation, education about the process, and on the mobilization of resources to assist adaptation. In the late stages of caregiving, which Gallagher describes as characterized by the "grief process," facilitating interventions might include individual psychotherapy focusing on the grief process, family meetings to help ease caregiver "burn-out," and psychotherapeutically oriented support groups.[39] Such supportive therapy should be planned to deal with the caregiver's more intense emotions, including depression, anxiety, guilt, fear of the future, emotional fatigue, and need to prepare in both emotional and practical terms for a future alone.

## Clinical Implications

One obvious clinical implication of the research cited in this chapter is that clinicians dealing with persons with dementia-related communication disorders will need to obtain information in some detail about the primary caregivers of these clients if they are to plan effective interventions. Questions concerning the type and quality of the patient-caregiver prior relationship, the family environment, and caregiver perceptions of and reactions to the caregiving situation need to be asked. Demographic characteristics of the caregiver, such as age, gender, health status, work status, financial situation, and other roles and responsibilities need to be noted. Self-administration of a relatively short subjective burden scale by the caregiver will allow the clinician to informally assess current levels of caregiver stress. Examples of burden scales are contained in references at the end of the chapter.[50,89,108] A caregiver assessment checklist such as that presented by Given, Collins, and Given can be useful in obtaining information from caregivers in a systematic way.[45] Hasselkus suggests the use of descriptive questions at the beginning of assessments and caregiver interviews (e.g., "Would you start by telling me what your day is like?") as a means of communicating to the caregiver that his or her perspectives are important.[56] This also provides an opportunity for the clinician to listen and learn from the family member.

Secondly, specific clinical implications can be drawn from the evidence cited that communication difficulties are a major source of frustration for caregivers of persons with dementia. Clinicians need to plan specific interventions to assist caregivers in (1) understanding the reasons for communication breakdowns in dementing illness; and (2) developing strategies for optimizing communication with their impaired relative (see article by Bayles and Kaszniak[9] and Chapters 10, 12, 15, and 16). Collaboration with the caregiver in planning practical interventions that will not contribute additional burden will likely be the most effective strategy. Interventions may be informational or behavioral in focus, depending on particular needs. Each caregiver–dementia patient dyad will need to be assessed individually in terms of their communication patterns and needs, for the caregiver intervention literature clearly suggests that no single approach will be effective with all or even the majority of caregivers.[40,54,100,104,105]

Some descriptive information obtained from caregivers suggests that spouses providing care have a strong preference for employing coping strategies that involve actions taken alone to solve problems.[7] Spouse caregivers in this study were most satisfied with this coping strategy and rated actions taken alone to solve problems as most successful. This has implications for those planning caregiver interventions, in that programs designed solely to increase caregivers' use of services and social support may be less than successful. Barusch suggests a two-pronged approach that might be most appropriate for dementia caregivers.[7] Initially, interventions designed to enhance the care provider's sense of personal control and ability to cope should be employed. Later interventions should focus on providing information about community resources and material that deals with feelings about accepting help.

## Research Issues and Questions

There are a number of research questions regarding the impact of caregiving on families that are relevant to speech-language pathologists and audiologists and to communication issues.

First, there needs to be systematic investigation into whether there are identifiable interpersonal stages of caregiving and what specific communication problems and issues might be associated with such stages. Questions such as the following need to be addressed: As caregiving demands increase, what changes in caregiver–care receiver interactions occur? Is there an observable pattern here? As communication abilities and capacities of the dementia patient to interact with his or her caregiver diminish, how does this impact the caregiver and the interaction between the two individuals? Are communication declines that are assumed to be part of the dementing process in part related to how the care providers interact with the care receiver? Can communication strategies be related to the stages of caregiving, if such "stages" exist?[20,22,25]

A second group of research questions relates to caregiver interventions. Who are the persons most likely to benefit from our interventions at different points in time? What tools would help clinicians identify those caregivers most "at risk" for negative impacts at different points in time?[99] What tools would help us identify those caregivers most likely to benefit from interventions? Which types of interventions will be most effective with which caregivers, and what should the timing of these interventions be?

Third, if one adopts a "family-systems" perspective, research questions that need to be asked include: How is the individual with dementia affected by our interventions with the caregiver? How could we measure any positive changes in the behavior, affect, and/or well-being of the person with dementia, as a result of our caregiver interventions? Especially in the mild, early period of dementing illness, are there direct interventions with the dementia victim that could alleviate family strain and caregiver burden? What strategies might be employed? How can we systematically identify what those strategies are and which dementia victims are most likely to benefit from them?

We need much more information about how the person who carries a diagnosis of early or mild dementia feels about himself or herself and how they perceive others' reactions to them and behavior toward them. This information, in turn, could be extremely helpful to use in caregiver education and information-providing sessions.

Fourth, research is needed to answer questions about the "core content" of an education and information support package focused on communication for dementia caregivers and dementia victims. What specific information needs to be presented, and when should such information be presented? What specific communication strategies and skills need to be taught to caregivers? To date, the few published reports that have dealt with this topic have contained common-sense suggestions that do have some face validity. Some have also obtained subjective evaluations of the interventions from caregiver participants that suggest at least short-term benefits of such informational and supportive interventions. Still lacking, however, are objective data supporting the effectiveness of communication-focused interventions with dementia caregivers and the relative effectiveness of specific approaches. In other areas of clinical practice, such data have been gathered over the past several years. The area of interventions with caregivers of dementia patients is new territory for speech-language pathologists and audiologists, and there is much to be done.

## References

1. Adams BN. Kinship in an urban setting. Chicago: Markham Publishing, 1968.
2. Anthony-Bergstone C, Zarit SH, Gatz M. Symptoms of psychological distress among caregivers of dementia patients. Psychol Aging 1988; 3:245–248.
3. Aronson MK, Lipkowitz R. Senile dementia, Alzheimer's type: The family and the health care delivery system. J Am Geriatr Soc 1981; 29:568–571.
4. Baillie V, Norbeck JS, Barnes LE. Stress, social support, and psychological distress of family caregivers of the elderly. Nurs Res 1988; 37:217–222.
5. Barnes RF, Raskind MA, Scott M, Murphy C. Problems of families caring for Alzheimer patients: Use of a support group. J Am Geriatr Soc 1981; 29:80–85.
6. Barney JL. The prerogative of choice in long-term care. Gerontologist 1977; 17:309–314.
7. Barusch AS. Problems and coping strategies of elderly spouse caregivers. Gerontologist 1988; 28:677–685.
8. Barusch AS, Spaid WM. Gender differences in caregiving: Why do wives report greater burden? Gerontologist 1989; 29:667–676.
9. Bayles KA, Kaszniak AW. Communication and cognition in normal aging and dementia. Boston: Little, Brown and Co., 1987.
10. Beck AT, Beamesdorfer A. Assessment of depression: The depression inventory. In: Pichot P, Oliver-Martin R, eds. Psychological measurements in psychopharmacology: Modern problems of pharmacopsychiatry. Basel, Switzerland: Karger, 1974.
11. Berezin MA. The psychiatrist and the geriatric patient: Partial grief in family members and others who care for the elderly. J Geriatr Psychiatry 1970; 4:53–64.
12. Birkel RC, Jones CJ. A comparison of the caregiving networks of dependent elderly individuals who are lucid and those who are demented. Gerontologist 1989; 29:114–119.
13. Blazer D, Williams CD. Epidemiology of dysphoria and depression in an elderly population. Am J Psychiatry 1980; 137:439–444.
14. Brocklehurst JC. Brain failure in old age—social implications. Age Ageing 1977; 6(Suppl):30–41.
15. Brody EM. The long haul: A family odyssey. In: Jarvik LF, Winograd CH, eds. Treatments for the Alzheimer patient. New York: Springer Publishing, 1988:107–122.
16. Brody EM. The role of the family in nursing homes: Implications for research and public policy. In: Harper MS, Lebowitz B, eds. Mental illness in nursing homes: Agenda for research. Washington, D.C.: NIMH, U. S. Government Printing Office, 1985:234.
17. Brody EM. Women in the middle and family help to older people. Gerontologist 1981; 21:471–480.
18. Brown AS. Satisfying relationships for the elderly and their patterns of disengagement. Gerontologist 1974; 14:258–262.
19. Cantor MH. Strain among caregivers: A study of experience in the United States. Gerontologist 1983; 23:597–604.
20. Chenoweth B, Spencer B. The experience of family caregivers. Gerontologist 1986; 26:267–272.
21. Cicirelli VG. Family relationships and care/management of the dementing elderly. In: Gilhooly MLM, Zarit SH, Birren JE, eds. The dementias: Policy and management. Englewood Cliffs, NJ: Prentice-Hall, 1986:93–110.
22. Clark NM, Rakowski W. Family caregivers of older adults: Improving helping skills. Gerontologist 1983; 23:637–642.
23. Clausen JA, Yarrow MR. The impact of mental illness on the family. J Soc Issues 1955; 11:3–64.
24. Cohen D, Eisdorfer C. Depression in family members caring for a relative with Alzheimer's disease. J Am Geriatr Soc 1988; 36:885–889.
25. Cohen D, Kennedy G, Eisdorfer C. Phases of change

25. in the patient with Alzheimer's dementia: A conceptual dimension for defining health care management. J Am Geriatr Soc 1984; 32:11–15.
26. Colerick EJ, George LK. Predictors of institutionalization among caregivers of patients with Alzheimer's disease. J Am Geriatr Soc 1986; 34:493–498.
27. Comptroller General of the United States. Home health: The need for a national policy to better provide for the elderly. (HRD-78-19). Washington, D.C.: U. S. General Accounting Office, 1977.
28. Coppel DB, Burton C, Becker J, Fiore J. Relationships of cognitions associated with coping reactions to depression in spousal caregivers of Alzheimer's disease patients. Cognitive Ther Res 1985; 9:253–266.
29. Deimling GT, Bass DM. Symptoms of mental impairment among elderly adults and their effects on family caregivers. J Gerontol 1986; 41:778–784.
30. Derogatis LR, Spencer PM. The Brief Symptom Inventory (BSI): Administration and procedures Manual-1. Baltimore, MD: Johns Hopkins University School of Medicine, Clinical Psychometric Research Unit, 1982.
31. Drinka TJK, Smith JC, Drinka PJ. Correlates of depression and burden for informal caregivers of patients in a geriatrics referral clinic. J Am Geriatr Soc 1987; 35:522–525.
32. Dunlop BD. Expanded home-based care for the impaired elderly: Solution or pipe dreams. Am J Public Health 1980; 70:514–519.
33. Eagles JM, Beattie JAG, Blackwood GW, Restall DB, Ashcroft GW. The mental health of elderly couples. I. The effects of a cognitively impaired spouse. Br J Psychiatry 1987; 150:299–303.
34. Eagles JM, Craig A, Rawlinson F, et al. The psychological well-being of supporters of the demented elderly. Br J Psychiatry 1987; 150:293–298.
35. Evans DA, Funkenstein HH, Albert MS, et al. Prevalence of Alzheimer's disease in a community population of older persons. JAMA 1989; 262(18):2551–2556.
36. Fengler AP, Goodrich N. Wives of elderly disabled men: The hidden patients. Gerontologist 1979; 19:175–183.
37. Fitting M, Rabins P, Lucas MJ, Eastham J. Caregivers for dementia patients: A comparison of husbands and wives. Gerontologist 1986; 26:248–252.
38. Fumich J, Poulshock SW. Stress provoking tasks in family caregiving situations. Paper presented at the meeting of the Gerontological Society of America. Toronto, November, 1981.
39. Gallagher DE. Individual and group therapies for family caregivers. Presented at the workshop, Creative coping with caregiving: Clinical and policy making areas. Foster City, CA: February 2–3, 1989.
40. Gallagher DE. Intervention strategies to assist caregivers of frail elders: Current research status and future research directions. Ann Rev Gerontol Geriatr 1985; 5:249–282.
41. Gallagher D, Rose J, Rivera P, Lovett S, Thompson LW. Prevalence of depression in family caregivers. Gerontologist 1989; 29:449–456.
42. George LK, Gwyther LP. Caregiver well-being: A multidimensional examination of family caregivers of demented adults. Gerontologist 1986; 26:253–259.
43. Gilleard CJ. Problems posed for supporting relatives of geriatric and psychogeriatric day patients. Acta Psychiatr Scand 1984; 70:198–208.
44. Gilhooly MLM. The impact of care-giving on caregivers: Factors associated with the psychological well-being of people supporting a dementing relative in the community. Br J Med Psychol 1984; 57:35–44.
45. Given CW, Collins CE, Given BA. Sources of distress among families caring for relatives with Alzheimer's disease. Nurs Clinics North Am 1988; 23:69–82.
46. Glosser G, Wexler D. Participants' evaluation of educational/support groups for families of patients with Alzheimer's disease and other dementias. Gerontologist 1985; 25:232–236.
47. Grad J, Sainsbury P. An evaluation of the effects of caring for the aged at home. In: World Psychiatric Associations Symposium, Psychiatric disorders in the aged. Manchester: Geigy, 1965.
48. Grad J, Sainsbury P. Mental illness and the family. Lancet 1963; 1:544–547.
49. Grad J, Sainsbury P. The effects that patients have on their families in a community care and a central psychiatric service—a two-year follow-up. Br J Psychiatry 1968; 114:265–278.
50. Greene JG, Smith R, Gardiner M, Timbury GC. Measuring behavioural disturbance of elderly demented patients in the community and its effects on relatives: A factor analytic study. Age Ageing 1982; 11:121–126.
51. Greene VL, Monahan DJ. The effect of a support and education program on stress and burden among family caregivers to frail elderly persons. Gerontologist 1989; 29:472–477.
52. Gubrium JF, Lynott RJ. Measurement and the interpretation of burden in the Alzheimer's disease experience. J Aging Studies 1987; 1:265–285.
53. Gurland B, Dean L, Gurland R, Cook D. The dependent elderly in New York City. Dependency in the elderly of New York City. New York: Community Council of Greater New York, 1978.
54. Haley WE, Brown L, Levine EG. Experimental evaluation of the effectiveness of group intervention for dementia caregivers. Gerontologist 1987; 27:376–382.
55. Haley WE, Levine EG, Brown SL, Berry JW, Hughes GH. Psychological, social, and health consequences of caring for a relative with senile dementia. J Am Geriatr Soc 1987; 35:405–411.
56. Hasselkus BR. Meaning in family caregiving: Perspectives on caregiver/professional relationships. Gerontologist 1988; 28:686–691.
57. Horowitz A. Family caregiving to the frail elderly. In: Lawton MP, Maddox GL, eds. Ann Rev Gerontol Geriatr 1985:194–246.
58. Horowitz A, Shindelman LW. Reciprocity and affection: Past influences on current caregiving. J Gerontol Soc Work 1983; 5(3):5–20.
59. Isaacs B, Livingstone M, Neville Y. Survival of the unfittest. London: Routledge & Kegan Paul, 1972.
60. Kahan J, Kemp B, Staples FR, Brummel-Smith K. Decreasing the burden in families caring for a relative with a dementing illness. J Am Geriatr Soc 1985; 33:664–670.
61. Kemper P, et al. The evaluation of the national long term care demonstration: Final report. Princeton, NJ: Mathematica Policy Research, 1986.
62. Kiecolt-Glaser JK, Glaser R, Shuttleworth EC, et al. Chronic stress and immunity in family caregivers of Alzheimer's disease victims. Psychosom Med 1987; 49:523–535.
63. Lawton MP, Brody EM, Saperstein AR. A controlled study of respite service for caregivers of Alzheimer's patients. Gerontologist 1989; 29:8–16.
64. Lawton MP, Kleban MH, Moss M, Rovine M, Glicksman A. Measuring caregiving appraisal. J Gerontol Psychol Sci 1989; 44:61–71.
65. Lazarus SW, Stafford B, Cooper K, Cohler B, Dysken M. A pilot study of an Alzheimer patients' relatives

discussion group. Gerontologist 1981; 21:353-358.
66. Liu K, Manton K, Liu BM. Home care expenses for the disabled. Health Care Financing Rev 1986; 7:51-58.
67. Lovett S, Gallagher D. Psychoeducational interventions for family caregivers: Preliminary efficacy data. Behav Ther 1988; 19:321-330.
68. Lowenthal MF, Berkman P, et al. Aging and mental disorders in San Francisco. San Francisco: Jossey-Bass, 1967.
69. Lyman KA. Bringing the social back in: A critique of the biomedicalization of dementia. Gerontologist 1989; 29:597-605.
70. Mace NL, Rabins PV. The 36-hour day. Baltimore: The Johns Hopkins University Press, 1981.
71. Macken CL. A profile of functionally impaired elderly persons living in the community. Health Care Financing Rev 1986; 7(4):33-49.
72. Marcus L, Jaeger V. The elderly as family caregivers. Can J Aging 1984; 3:33-42.
73. Montgomery RJV, Borgatta EF. The effects of alternative support strategies on family caregiving. Gerontologist 1989; 29:457-464.
74. Moritz DJ, Kasl SV, Berkman LF. The health impact of living with a cognitively impaired elderly spouse: Depressive symptoms and social functioning. J Gerontol Soc Sci 1989; 44:S17-27.
75. Morycz RK. An exploration of senile dementia and family burden. Clin Soc Work J 1980; 8:16-27.
76. Morycz RK. Caregiving strain and the desire to institutionalize family members with Alzheimer's disease. Res Aging 1985; 7:329-361.
77. National Center for Health Statistics. Current estimates from the health interview survey. 1978. Vital and health statistics, series 13. No. 130. Washington, D.C.: U.S. Government Printing Office, 1979.
78. Niederehe G, Fruge E. Dementia and family dynamics: Clinical research issues. J Geriatr Psychiatr 1984; 17:21-56.
79. Novak M, Guest C. Caregiver response to Alzheimer's disease. Int J Aging Hum Devel 1989; 28:67-69.
80. Pearson J, Verma S, Nellett C. Elderly psychiatric patient status and caregiver perceptions as predictors of caregiver burden. Gerontologist 1988; 28:79-83.
81. Peterson JA. Therapeutic intervention in marital and family problems of aging persons. In: Schwartz AN, Mensh IN, eds. Professional obligations and approaches to the aged. Springfield, IL: Charles C Thomas, 1974.
82. Poulshock SW, Deimling GT. Families caring for elders in residence: Issues in the measurement of burden. J Gerontol 1984; 39:230-239.
83. Pruchno RA, Resch NL. Aberrant behaviors and Alzheimer's disease: Mental health effects on spouse caregivers. J Gerontol Soc Sci 189; 44:S177-182.
84. Pruchno RA, Resch NL. Husbands and wives as caregivers: Antecedents of depression and burden. Gerontologist 1989; 29:159-165.
85. Rabins P, Mace N, Lucas M. The impact of dementia on the family. JAMA 1982; 248:333-335.
86. Radloff LS. The CES-D scale: A self-report depression scale for research in the general population. Appl Psychol Meas 1977; 1:385-401.
87. Rau MT. Elderly stroke patients and their partners: A longitudinal study of social support and well-being changes associated with a disabling stroke. (Doctoral dissertation, Portland State University, 1986). Diss Abstr Int 47:2274.
88. Report of the Secretary's Task Force on Alzheimer's Disease, U. S. Dept. of Health and Human Services. Alzheimer's disease. DHHS Publication No. (ADM) 84-1323. Washington, D.C.: U.S. Government Printing Office, September, 1984.
89. Robinson BC. Validation of a caregiver strain index. J Gerontol 1983; 38:344-348.
90. Sanford JRA. Tolerance of debility in elderly dependents by supporters at home: Its significance for hospital practice. Br Med J 1975; 3:471-473.
91. Schulz R, Tompkins CA, Rau MT. A longitudinal study of the psychosocial impact of stroke on primary support persons. Psychol Aging 1988; 3:131-141.
92. Scott JP, Roberto KA, Hutton JT. Families of Alzheimer's victims: Family support to the caregivers. J Am Geriatr Soc 1986; 34:348-354.
93. Shanas E. The family as a social support system in old age. Gerontologist 1979; 19:169-174.
94. Shanas E, Maddox GL. Aging, health, and the organization of health resources. In: Binstock R, Shanas E, eds. Handbook of aging and the social sciences. New York: Van Nostrand Reinhold, 1976.
95. Soldo BJ, Manton KG. Health status and service needs of the oldest old: Current patterns and future trends. Milbank Q 1985; 63:286-319.
96. Stone R, Cafferata GL, Sangl J. Caregivers of the frail elderly: A national profile. Gerontologist 1987; 17:616-626.
97. Subcommittee on Human Services, Select Committee on Aging, U. S. House of Representatives. Exploding the myths: caregiving in America. Committee Publication No. 99-611. Washington, D.C.: U.S. Government Printing Office, January, 1987.
98. Thomas L. Interview. New York Times Magazine 1983; January 16.
99. Tompkins CA, Schulz R, Rau MT. Post-stroke depression in primary support persons: Predicting those at risk. J Consult Clin Psychol 1988; 56:502-508.
100. Toseland RW, Rossiter CM. Group interventions to support family caregivers: A review and analysis. Gerontologist 1989; 29:438-448.
101. Toseland RW, Rossiter CM, Labrecque MS. The effectiveness of peer-led and professionally led groups to support family caregivers. Gerontologist 1989; 29:465-471.
102. Young RF, Kahana E. Specifying caregiver outcomes: Gender and relationship aspects of caregiving strain. Gerontologist 1989; 29:660-666.
103. Zarit JM. Predictors of burden and distress for caregivers of senile dementia patients. Unpublished doctoral dissertation, University of Southern California, Los Angeles, 1982.
104. Zarit SH, Anthony CR. Interventions with dementia patients and their families. In: Gilhooly MLM, Zarit SH, Birren JE, eds. The dementias: Policy and management. Englewood Cliffs, NJ: Prentice-Hall, 1986:66.
105. Zarit SH, Zarit JM. Families under stress: Interventions for caregivers of senile dementia patients. Psychother Theory Res Pract 1982; 19:461-471.
106. Zarit SH, Anthony CR, Boutselis M. Interventions with care givers of dementia patients: A comparison of two approaches. Psychol Aging 1987; 2:225-232.
107. Zarit SH, Orr NK, Zarit J. The hidden victims of Alzheimer's disease: Families under stress. New York: New York University Press, 1985.
108. Zarit SH, Reever KE, Bach-Peterson T. Relatives of the impaired elderly: correlates of feelings of burden. Gerontologist 1980; 20:649-655.
109. Zarit SH, Todd P, Zarit JM. Subjective burden of husbands and wives as caregivers: A longitudinal study. Gerontologist 1986; 26:260-266.

# CHAPTER 12

# *Perspectives of Family Members Regarding Communication Changes*

JOSEPH B. ORANGE, M.H.Sc.

*I often miss someone. Is it my weakness or is it perhaps a natural human condition? Yet, when someone is regularly around me and close, my noticing him becomes habitual and thus progressively less meaningful. But when that person is absent, at once my awareness of him is awakened. Although this moment is often dark and worrying, the projected image of him is subtly sweet and, as it were, transcends reality. Then I start to miss him almost resentfully because of an intense feeling of incompleteness which is painful.*[12]

Jaroslav Havelka's quote is poignant, especially as relates to this chapter. Family members of individuals suffering from dementia often describe the loneliness, isolation, and emptiness they agonizingly bear while caring for their demented relative. This chapter will address some of these feelings as recorded during a study that examined family members' perceptions of the communication skills of community-dwelling individuals with dementia of the Alzheimer's type (DAT). The initial section of the chapter will emphasize the importance of using family caregivers as sources of insightful information on communicative changes in older adults, especially those with dementia. Then relevant studies on perceptions of communicative functions of the healthy and brain-injured elderly will be briefly reviewed. The remaining portion of the chapter will discuss the results of a study, including perspectives of communication in normal, older adults gathered from a sample of healthy, elderly controls. Clinical and research implications of the results will be highlighted in the final two sections.

## Importance of the Perspectives of Family Members

Over the past 2 decades, researchers representing a number of well-established disciplines have directly examined and sought to explain the communicative behavior of older adults and individuals diagnosed with dementia. Contrasting profiles have emerged. Documented contrasts between the two groups include: (1) the organization and manipulation of concepts in semantic knowledge; (2) the use and comprehension of selective discourse features and pragmatic functions; and (3) the disproportionate retention of skills in the domains of syntax, morphology, and phonology. Despite numerous studies, little is known about the communicative and linguistic skills of the elderly as observed in natural contexts by their most frequent conversational partners, family caregivers. Furthermore, few studies have employed family members as sources of information on the communicative behaviors of the elderly.

With approximately 5 percent of the elderly in the United States institutionalized at any one time, family caregivers provide the majority of care for older cohorts in the community.[30] Families contribute over 80 percent of the health, emotional, physical, and social care of the elderly in the United States.[30] It is evident that family members are the most likely candidates to have regular, ongoing communication with older adults.

As a group, family caregivers have unique opportunities to observe, in natural contexts, real communicative changes associated with normal and abnormal aging processes. Their perceptions provide investigators with distinctive views of the communicative behaviors of the elderly. Family caregivers are exposed to opportunities wherein they may be able to describe subtle features of communicative change that researchers find difficult to record through traditional data collection methods. The ecological validity of investigations analyzing the communicative skills of the elderly is strengthened when family members' observations are included. That is, the representativeness of the communicative features may be more accurately reflected when careful consideration is given to family caregivers' descriptions.

Family members are influenced, however, by a number of factors that may prejudice their perceptions of real communicative change. These factors work collectively to constrain perceptions. They include, but are not limited to: (1) the many years of intimate contact that may limit objectivity; (2) the caregiver's understanding of what constitutes real change in functional communication skills; and (3) the subtle adjustments caregivers may make in their interactive style that anticipates and minimizes the expression of communicative disturbances.

## PERSPECTIVES OF BEHAVIOR IN DEMENTIA

Recent studies investigating various types of behavior in individuals with dementia have employed family members as sources and recorders of valuable information.[4,6,7,11,25,35] Written accounts of relatives' personal experiences appearing in texts and popular magazines (*Life, Time,* and *Newsweek*) have given insight into caregivers' emotions and perceptions of behavior in dementia.[27] Family members' observations clearly show that the devastating features of dementia affect not only the individual with the syndrome but the family as a whole.[29] Family members suffer isolation, anxiety, frustration, and loneliness along with their demented relative.[27,29] Chapter 11 provides an excellent summary of the impact of dementia on the family unit.

## PERSPECTIVES OF COMMUNICATIVE BEHAVIORS

Although there have been a limited number of studies describing family members' perspectives of the communicative behaviors of healthy older adults and of aphasic relatives,[13,16,18,31,32] relatively little attention has been directed to family members' views of communication changes in dementia. An interview-style format adopted by Shadden posed yes/no and open-ended probe questions to older healthy adults, children of older parents, and a select group of professionals who work with the elderly.[31] Shadden's interviews gathered data on the perceptions of how older healthy adults communicate in general, how they communicate with other older persons, their common topics of conversation, with whom they communicate, and the frequency of their communicative contacts. She found that slightly over 60 percent of the older respondents acknowledged that people change the way they communicate as they grow older, but only 22 percent believed these changes constituted a worsening of communicative skills. The older participants acknowledged the heterogeneity of communicative skills in the elderly and the diversity of their conversational topics. The majority of the older respondents agreed that the elderly communicated more often with other older adults, that elders had a restricted range of communicative partners, and that older adults had less frequent communicative interactions than younger adults.

In a related study, Lubinski, Morrison, and Rigrodsky examined the perceptions of institutionalized healthy elderly and chronically ill older adults regarding communication in a long-term care setting.[16] They reviewed respondents' perceptions of the quantitative and qualitative features of communication in the older population. The study showed that there was a strong desire for the elderly to communicate but that opportunities for productive and meaningful interaction were limited in quantity and scope. Communication was limited by the administrative and physical structures of the facility, the quantity and variety of accessible partners, and the effective modes of communication available to residents.

In the aphasic population, Shewan and Cameron studied how well family members were aware of their aphasic relative's communication-related problems.[32] They found that family caregivers "had some appreciation of how bothersome these problems were." Further, Helmick, Watamori, and Palmer determined that spouses rated aphasic's communication to be less impaired than did clinicians.[13] This distinction between the perceptions held by the two groups underscores the importance of including family members' perceptions and observations in studies of functional communication in older adults.

With respect to demented individuals, Rabins and colleagues found that family caregivers of a relative with senile dementia cope with the majority of problems associated with their care but that some caregivers perceive certain behaviors more burdensome than others.[25] Almost 70 percent (34/50) of the responding families reported communication disorders in relatives with dementia. Of those noting the occurrence, nearly 75 percent (25/34) stated that communication difficulties were a caregiving problem. Morycz examined caregiver and care receiver characteristics contributing to caregiving strain and the desire to institutionalize family members with Alzheimer's disease.[20] Communication disturbances were included as global measures on a vigilance-disruptiveness scale for caregivers. Morycz found that communication difficulties contributed to caregiving strain but were less important than factors such as: (1) being widowed; (2) physical labor involved in care; and (3) whether the caregiver lived alone with the demented person. Unfortunately, individual contributions of specific communicative problems to the degree of caregiving strain and burden were not identified in the scale.

Indirect measurements of communicative disturbances have been identified in other studies exploring family members' caregiving burden and strain. Family caregivers have reported general communicative problems in their demented relative through factors reflecting difficulty with social interaction and social functioning.[5,8,10,24] Although studies have examined the perceptions of communicative change associated with normal aging processes, issues of perceived communicative disturbances in dementia and their impact on family dynamics remain unaddressed.

## The Study

The purpose of this study was to examine family caregivers' perceptions of communicative changes in community-dwelling relatives with DAT. Family caregivers' perceptions and observations were gathered in participants' homes through a series of selective, open-ended questions in a structured interview that focused on the primary domains of communicative function.

### RESEARCH QUESTIONS

If family caregivers of individuals with dementia perceive general disturbances in communication as obstacles in the caring process as Rabins et al and others suggest, then a number of interesting questions are raised. First, are family caregivers able to perceive and describe in relative detail the nature of the communication skills of relatives with DAT? If they are, when did they first perceive changes and what were those changes? These questions have both theoretical and clinical significance in that they may address early indications of decline in communicative, linguistic, and cognitive functions.

Second, what aspects within the domains of communication undergo change as Alzheimer's disease progresses? What is the perceived nature of the deteriorations over time? The longitudinal changes viewed by family members may assist researchers monitoring the subtle progression of communicative and linguistic disturbances in dementia. (See Chapter 7 on communicative disturbances in DAT and Chapter 8 on discourse features in DAT.)

Third, and of clinical relevance, what do family members perceive to be their most effective management strategies for communicative distress in DAT? What interventions do family caregivers commonly employ to circumvent or anticipate problems in communication? Further, what environmental conditions are perceived to influence communicative effectiveness between individuals with DAT and their family caregivers?

Fourth, what is the perceived impact of the changes in communication on the relationship between the caregiver and the care receiver? Finally, how do family members' judgments of communication changes in individuals with DAT compare with the perceptions held by family members of normal, healthy older adults? These research questions guided the interview study.

### INTERVIEW

Data on perceived communicative behavior of individuals with DAT and healthy, elderly normals were obtained through a structured interview in participants' homes. The protocol was developed and modified after pilot use with family members of normal elderly and persons with dementia. A family member of each DAT individual and each normal elderly control was interviewed. The interview with the DAT family member consisted of a series of over 40 open-ended questions. Nearly 30 open-ended questions were presented to family respondents of the normal elderly. All responses were audio-recorded, orthographically transcribed, and categorized according to related answers among family members of both subject groups. The entire screening, history, and interview sessions for the family member of the DAT individuals lasted approximately 1½ hours, while the sessions for each normal adult lasted approximately 45 minutes.

### PARTICIPANTS

#### DAT Individuals

Fifteen individuals with probable DAT were nonrandomly recruited from the practices of two physicians: a neurologist and a geriatrician. All 12 males and 3 females met the diagnostic criteria as established by the NINCDS-ADRDA task force on research in DAT.[19] The consulting physicians used the Global Deterioration Scale (GDS) to determine severity; 3 to 4 early stage, 5 to 6 middle stage, and above 6 the late stage.[26] Eight individuals were classified as early stage, five as middle, and two as late stage.

### Normal Older Adults

To provide baseline data for perceived changes in communication related to normal aging processes, 13 healthy elderly individuals were used as controls, including 8 females and 5 males. Student's t-tests (p = ≤ .05) showed no significant difference between the normal and DAT groups for age or for years of education. Tables 12.1 and 12.2 summarize the profiles of the two groups.

### Family Members

The spouses of the DAT individuals and the normal elderly were solicited to act as respondents to the survey questions. In lieu of a spouse, a daughter, son, niece, or nephew who had daily communication with their family member for at least the past 2 years was eligible to be a respondent.

## HISTORIES

All DAT and healthy older individuals and all family members were unilingual, literate, native speakers of English, with a minimum of an eighth-grade education. None were taking medications to alter mental status. None had an associative history of neurologic disease (e.g., Parkinson's disease, Huntington's disease, or multiple sclerosis), psychiatric disease (e.g., depression, manic depressive illness, or schizophrenia), metabolic, toxic, alcoholic, or vascular disorders. All of the normal elderly and all individuals with DAT, with the exception of two, and all family members underwent pure-tone hearing testing at 500, 1000, 2000, and 4000 Hz. All participants achieved a minimum of 40 dB or lower scores in their better ear. Of the two DAT subjects unable to be tested, family members reported no associative history of hearing impairment. A vision screening test consisting of oral reading of size and boldness controlled phrases and a form-orientation task ("Which direction does the letter 'E' face?") was administered to all participants. All achieved 90 percent or better scores on the accuracy of oral reading and the form arrangement task. All of the normal elderly and all but one recent exception of the DAT individuals were community-dwelling in their own residences.

## RESULTS

In the initial part of this section, results will be presented of a comparison between family members' perceptions of the older normal adults' communicative skills and the DAT individuals' skills before the onset of dementia. This matching will demonstrate the similarities in perceived communicative performance between the two groups and establish a base from which to make further comparisons. Next, the perceived changes in the communicative skills of normal controls will be presented. These results will help to distinguish perceived changes associated with normal aging processes and those occurring as a result of dementia. The major portion of the results section will address family members' descriptions of communicative features in relatives with DAT. Family caregivers' comments of communicative changes will be presented so as to correspond to the temporal progression of dementia, i.e., initial changes, progressive changes, and present skills. The results of a comparison between communicative problems and other troublesome behaviors in DAT will be briefly reviewed. In addition, family members' perceptions of features in the psychosocial and physical environments that influence communication for the normal controls and DAT individuals will be discussed. Further, the strategies DAT family members stated they used to manage communication problems will be described. In the final segment of this section, results will be given of family members' descriptions of the impact of communication problems on their relationship with their relative.

### Communication Skills for Normal Controls at Present and DAT Subjects Before Onset of Illness

The perceptions held by normal control family members concerning their relative's communication skills *at the present time* were similar to the perceptions held by the DAT family members concerning their relative's skills *before* the onset of dementia. That is, a comparison of the perceptions of all family members revealed that all subjects: (1) were alike in amount of talking; (2) experienced little difficulty verbally expressing themselves; (3) were able to understand what was said to them; (4) talked about and listened to similar topics that included items of personal interest (e.g., their jobs, church activities, hobbies, news, politics and current events, sports, vacations, family, movies, music, and past life experiences); and (5) had comparable communication partners (e.g., friends, family, and people with parallel interests).

TABLE 12.1 **Summary Profile of Dementia of the Alzheimer's Type (DAT) Dyads**

| DYAD | SEX | AGE | EDO | S | ED | OCCUPATION |
|---|---|---|---|---|---|---|
| 1 D | F | 54.7 | 3–4 | M | 12 | Housewife |
| 1 R/H | M | 52.8 | — | — | 8 | Mechanic |
| 2 D | M | 56.6 | 6 | M | 12 | Health insurance rep. |
| 2 R/W | F | 50.7 | — | — | 12 | Sales clerk |
| 3 D | M | 72.1 | 4–5 | E | 17 | Mechanical engineer |
| 3 R/W | F | 71.8 | — | — | 13 | Housewife |
| 4 D | M | 74.4 | 4 | M | 8 | Inventory controller |
| 4 R/W | F | 72.0 | — | — | 10 | Sales representative |
| 5 D | M | 79.5 | 12 | E | 11 | Aircraft mechanic |
| 5 R/D | F | 36.11 | — | — | 14 | Office manager |
| 6 D | M | 65.5 | 5.5 | E | 12 | Real-estate agent |
| 6 R/W | F | 61.10 | — | — | 10 | Housewife |
| 7 D | F | 60.7 | 3.5 | L | 12 | Legal secretary |
| 7 R/H | M | 63.11 | — | — | 8 | Machinist |
| 8 D | F | 71.6 | 6 | L | 11 | Housewife |
| 8 R/H | M | 73.9 | — | — | 11 | Tool and dye maker |
| 9 D | M | 71.3 | 5 | M | 8 | Auto-body repairman |
| 9 R/W | F | 79.10 | — | — | 8 | Housewife |
| 10 D | M | 69.2 | 5–6 | E | 10 | Painter |
| 10 R/W | F | 61.11 | — | — | 10 | Legal secretary |
| 11 D | M | 80.11 | 3.5 | M | 11 | Machinist |
| 11 R/W | F | 74.6 | — | — | 9 | Housewife |
| 12 D | M | 66.6 | 5 | E | 19 | Dentist |
| 12 R/W | F | 64.10 | — | — | 16 | Bookkeeper |
| 13 D | M | 71.7 | 6 | E | 16 | Civil servant |
| 13 R/W | F | 65.10 | — | — | 10 | Housewife |
| 14 D | M | 68.0 | 6 | E | 12 | Bank manager |
| 14 R/W | F | 61.2 | — | — | 12 | Housewife |
| 15 D | M | 67.7 | 12 | E | 12 | Carpenter and mechanic |
| 15 R/W | F | 63.1 | — | — | 9 | Housewife |

| Age (years) | DAT | Family Members |
|---|---|---|
| M: | 68.6 | 63.3 |
| SD: | 7.3 | 10.9 |
| Range: | 54.7–80.11 | 36.11–79.10 |
| Education (years) | DAT | Family Members |
| M: | 12.2 | 10.7 |
| SD: | 3.0 | 2.4 |
| Range: | 8–19 | 8–16 |

EDO = Estimated date of onset by family member (years ago)
S   = Stage: E = early, M = middle, L = late
Ed  = Years of education
D   = DAT individual
R   = Relative: D = daughter, H = husband, W = wife
M   = Mean
SD  = Standard deviation

These results compare favorably with those obtained by Shadden in her study of communication patterns in the normal healthy elderly.[31] Overall, it appeared that normal controls and individuals prior to developing DAT were similar in many communicative respects.

## Communication Changes for Normal Controls Over Past Year

More than 70 percent of respondents for the normal controls perceived that their relative's communicative abilities had not changed over the past

TABLE 12.2 **Summary Profile of Normal Elderly Control Dyads**

| DYAD | SEX | AGE | ED | OCCUPATION |
|---|---|---|---|---|
| 1 C | M | 67.1 | 18 | Professor |
| 1 R/W | F | 66.0 | 15 | High school teacher |
| 2 C | F | 66.0 | 15 | High school teacher |
| 2 R/H | M | 67.1 | 18 | Professor |
| 3 C | M | 65.7 | 16 | Sales representative |
| 3 R/W | F | 62.3 | 19 | Professor |
| 4 C | F | 62.3 | 19 | Professor |
| 4 R/H | M | 65.7 | 16 | Sales representative |
| 5 C | F | 60.1 | 12 | Secretary |
| 5 R/H | M | 63.6 | 18 | Manufacturing consultant |
| 6 C | M | 63.6 | 18 | Manufacturing consultant |
| 6 R/W | F | 60.1 | 12 | Secretary |
| 7 C | F | 70.9 | 8 | Housewife |
| 7 R/D | F | 49.9 | 10 | Nurses aide |
| 8 C | F | 65.6 | 9 | Sales clerk |
| 8 R/D | F | 37.11 | 12 | Sales clerk |
| 9 C | F | 63.2 | 8 | Telephone operator |
| 9 R/N | F | 37.11 | 12 | Sales clerk |
| 10 C | F | 73.5 | 14 | Secretary |
| 10 R/H | M | 75.9 | 12 | Sales representative |
| 11 C | M | 75.9 | 12 | Sales representative |
| 11 R/W | F | 73.5 | 14 | Secretary |
| 12 C | M | 72.3 | 8 | Train engineer |
| 12 R/W | F | 64.4 | 13 | Secretary |
| 13 C | F | 64.4 | 13 | Secretary |
| 13 R/H | M | 72.3 | 8 | Train engineer |

| Age (years) | Controls | Family Members |
|---|---|---|
| M: | 66.9 | 61.2 |
| SD: | 4.8 | 12.5 |
| Range: | 60.1–75.9 | 37.11–75.9 |
| **Education (years)** | **Controls** | **Family Members** |
| M: | 13.1 | 13.8 |
| SD: | 4.0 | 3.3 |
| Range: | 8–19 | 8–19 |

Ed = Years of education
C = Normal control
R = Relative: D = daughter, H = husband, N = niece, W = wife
M = Mean
SD = Standard deviation

year. Those infrequent changes that were noted reflected adjustments in life-style (retirement), modest alterations in auditory attending, and age-related modifications in word-finding abilities. (For a summary of changes in communication, language, speech, and voice skills associated with normal aging processes, refer to Chapter 6.)

The age-related adjustments in expressive and receptive skills for this sample of older normals were perceived by most families as having minimal impact on their relative, the family unit, and their friends. One spouse, however, stated that her husband had a restricted range of conversational topics and that communication was no longer important to him because of his recent retirement. Members of that family, especially the spouse, found coping with these restrictions particularly difficult. As a consequence to alterations in communicative content and style, the spouse was forced to become more active in planning a variety of social engagements with relatives and friends. Below are some of her comments in response to selected questions about conversational topics, the importance of her husband's verbal and comprehension abilities at the present time, descriptions of communicative problems, and the impact of these problems on their relationship:

**Topics:** ...grandchildren, his mother, bridge, the news, well, not since he's been retired. But before that he had a very, very interesting job and he had a lot of conversation to talk about. Now that he's retired, he doesn't have as many outside interests to talk about.

**Importance of Verbal and Comprehension Abilities:** Oh, I think it's (verbal skills) very important, but not as important now as when he was working.

I think it's (comprehension abilities) very important, but not as important now that he is retired.

**Communication Problems and Their Impact:** I didn't see any problems up until a year and a half ago....I would have answered these questions a lot differently 2 years ago. Retirement has had a significant effect on my husband's talking.

Well, I don't think it's a problem for him. He enjoys this quiet part of his life. I find it a little lonely sometimes and less stimulating than it was before. I don't think others find him as interesting as he once was.

## Communication Changes First Observed for Individuals with DAT

All DAT family members were able to describe changes in communication they believed occurred near the onset of illness. Table 12.3 summarizes their observations.

All but one family member (14/15) first noticed communication problems within the semantic domain during the early course of the dementia. Whether they described word-finding difficulties in particular or used other terms to characterize disturbances in retrieval, recall, access, or organization of meaning relationship, family members were keenly aware of their relative's problems with semantic knowledge.

With regard to the two domains of discourse features and pragmatic functions, fewer family members (60 percent or 9/15) perceived disturbances associated with the estimated onset of DAT. This may not be surprising considering the subtle nature of contextually sensitive social interactive features. Family members were generally aware of interaction problems, although a few did not know why their relative had them or what the difficulties represented.

As has been previously documented, disturbances in syntax, morphology, and phonology normally are not early markers of communicative dysfunction in Alzheimer's disease.[1,2,3,14,21,22,28,33,34] Only one late-stage individual with DAT was reported to have exhibited word-order difficulties during onset.

Only one-half of the family members perceived early changes in auditory comprehension. Many commented that any declines in auditory function were subtle and gradual. General responses focused on the need for repetition, listening but tuning-out, and difficulty following simple directions.

In summary, family members' responses reveal that they are indeed able to perceive communication changes in relatives with DAT. Their comments demonstrate that they are sensitive to and able to describe in relative detail communicative changes that occurred presumably during the early phase of onset. Nearly all respondents observed disturbances in the semantic domain, and over half were acutely aware of subtle alterations in discourse features and pragmatic functions. Early changes in auditory comprehension were more difficult for family members to describe.

Family members' statements concerning the changes they first observed in their relative's verbal skills are best expressed by the following quotes from three different spouses of individuals with DAT.

**Early DAT:** He was starting to crawl into a shell kinda thing. I figured that he wasn't communicating with the people as much as he did before, and it really bothered me but I didn't know what it was.

**Early DAT:** He had trouble finishing sentences. He had trouble putting his thoughts into words. He just hesitated so much that you could be there and back before he got it all out.

**Early DAT:** ...wasn't initiating conversations. He wasn't talking that much around the house.

## Progressive Changes in Communication for Individuals with DAT

Responses describing progressive changes in verbal skills reflected increased involvement of the semantic domain, almost exclusively for word-finding problems (Table 12.4). Comments relating to discourse features and pragmatic functions included reduced participation in interactions, perseveration, use of stereotyped utterances, and disturbances in cohesion and coherence, i.e., problems with referencing and shared knowledge. A limit-

TABLE 12.3 **Family Members' Perceptions of Initial Changes in the Communicative Behavior of Relatives with DAT**

| | DAT (N=15) | | |
| --- | --- | --- | --- |
| | E (8)* | M (5) | L(2) |
| **INITIAL CHANGES IN VERBAL SKILLS**[†] | | | |
| **Semantics** | | | |
| Word-finding problems | 2 | 4 | 2 |
| Hesitations and pauses | 3 | 1 | 1 |
| Incomplete utterances | 1 | 2 | 1 |
| Circumlocutions | 0 | 1 | 1 |
| Decreased amount of utterances | 2 | 0 | 1 |
| **Pragmatics and Discourse** | | | |
| Critical comments, getting angry, and being argumentative | 1 | 1 | 1 |
| Fewer initiations of communication | 2 | 0 | 0 |
| Repeating topics and utterances | 1 | 0 | 1 |
| Speaking of past more often | 1 | 0 | 0 |
| Inappropriate utterances | 1 | 0 | 0 |
| Vagueness | 0 | 1 | 0 |
| Difficulty forming requests | 0 | 0 | 1 |
| **Syntax** | | | |
| Difficulty forming sentences | 0 | 0 | 1 |
| **General Comments** | | | |
| Cannot think of any changes | 1 | 0 | 0 |
| **INITIAL CHANGES IN COMPREHENSION ABILITIES**[†] | | | |
| Subtle and gradual changes | 3 | 3 | 1 |
| Could not follow simple directions | 1 | 2 | 0 |
| Needed utterances repeated | 2 | 0 | 1 |
| Listening but tuning out | 1 | 1 | 0 |
| Self-awareness of difficulties | 1 | 0 | 0 |
| Irrelevant responses | 1 | 0 | 0 |
| Work-related problems | 0 | 0 | 1 |

*Stage: E = early, M = middle, L = late
[†]Values represent multiple responses by family members

ed number of family members noted word-order problems and possible motor speech and verbal apraxia disturbances, especially for early-stage subjects. The motor speech and apraxic disturbances conflict with generally accepted knowledge that cortically demented individuals do not exhibit such problems until the advanced stages (see Chapter 5).

As was the case for recounting change during the onset of dementia, family members experienced difficulty describing specific progressive alterations in their relative's auditory comprehension abilities. Fully one-third did not notice any ongoing changes. Some respondents commented on their relatives' problems following conversations, instructions, and directions, while others noted that their relative actively covered up comprehension difficulties. A few made nonspecific statements indicating an insidious course of decline.

Outlined below are sage comments made by family members concerning perceived progressive changes in verbal skills.

Early DAT: Only this one where he starts to converse with people and it's more saying something by memory. It's stiff, as though he's searching for the right thing to say and is saying something that he has said so many times that he just says it, rather than... innovative isn't quite the word, creative isn't quite the word but saying something from his **memory rather than something from his heart.**

Middle DAT: He comes out with sentences but there's no connection between the thought and the words. Sometimes he doesn't really talk with any purpose.... I mean we were really connected. We should be and we always have been, but we've disconnected.

TABLE 12.4 **Family Members' Perceptions of Progressive Changes in the Communicative Behavior of Relatives with DAT**

| | DAT (N=15) | | |
|---|---|---|---|
| | E (8)* | M (5) | L (2) |
| **PROGRESSIVE CHANGES IN VERBAL SKILLS**[†] | | | |
| *Semantics* | | | |
| Increased word-finding difficulty | 6 | 2 | 1 |
| Hesitations and pauses | 2 | 1 | 0 |
| More incomplete and abandoned utterances | 1 | 1 | 0 |
| *Pragmatics and Discourse* | | | |
| Reduced participation | 2 | 1 | 2 |
| Use of stereotyped utterances | 1 | 1 | 2 |
| Coherence and cohesion disturbances | 1 | 2 | 0 |
| Increased output | 1 | 0 | 1 |
| Repetition of topics and utterances | 1 | 0 | 0 |
| *Motor Speech* | | | |
| Unintelligible utterances | 1 | 0 | 0 |
| Sound-sequencing difficulties | 1 | 0 | 0 |
| Stuttering (syllable repetition) | 0 | 1 | 0 |
| *Syntax* | | | |
| Word-order problems | 1 | 0 | 0 |
| *Nonverbal* | | | |
| Use of pantomime and gestures | 0 | 1 | 0 |
| **PROGRESSIVE CHANGES IN COMPREHENSION ABILITIES**[†] | | | |
| More difficulty following conversations and simple directions | 2 | 2 | 1 |
| General or gradual worsening | 1 | 2 | 1 |
| Simple directions required for comprehension | 1 | 0 | 0 |
| Actively covering up difficulty | 1 | 0 | 0 |
| More difficulty following complex directions | 1 | 0 | 0 |
| Reduced participation in conversations | 0 | 0 | 1 |
| No noticeable changes | 3 | 2 | 0 |

*Stage: E = early, M = middle, L = late
[†]Values represent multiple responses by family members

## Present Communication Abilities for Individuals with DAT

Family members perceived that relatives in the early stage exhibited a variety of verbal disturbances in the semantic domain. Continuing to show expressive problems with semantics, those in the middle and late stages had a limited array of semantic feature disorders (Table 12.5). Disruptions in pragmatic functions and discourse features were perceived by 80 percent (12/15) of family members across all stages, an increase of 20 percent from those who first noticed changes in these two domains. Comments describing present disturbances in pragmatic and discourse domains collapsed into a number of different clusters for all DAT individuals, regardless of stage, and suggest that family members are perceptive of impairments in subtle aspects of communication.

An overwhelming majority (14/15) of respondents stated that friends and family were now the primary communication partners for their relative with DAT, as a result of present communication problems. One-third (2/8 early and 3/5 middle stage) recounted that they and their relative suffered from a smaller social group and experienced fewer meaningful interactions. However, nearly all family members noted that their relative experienced no change in conversational topics (e.g., family activities, news and current affairs, sports, careers, personal accomplishments, television and music, hobbies, pets, and religion). These

TABLE 12.5 **Family Members' Perceptions of the Communicative Behavior of Relatives During the Present Stage of DAT**

|  | DAT (N=15) | | |
|---|---|---|---|
|  | E (8)* | M (5) | L (2) |
| **PRESENT VERBAL SKILLS**† | | | |
| **Semantics** | | | |
| Word-finding problems | 5 | 1 | 0 |
| Hesitations and pauses | 1 | 0 | 0 |
| Incomplete utterances | 1 | 0 | 0 |
| Decreased amount of utterances | 3 | 3 | 0 |
| Limited verbalizations | 0 | 1 | 2 |
| **Pragmatics and Discourse** | | | |
| Repetition of topics | 3 | 0 | 1 |
| Incoherent, nonsense | 2 | 2 | 1 |
| Communication attempted | 2 | 2 | 0 |
| Stereotype utterances | 1 | 0 | 1 |
| Limited initiation and impaired communicative intent | 1 | 1 | 2 |
| Inappropriate utterances | 1 | 0 | 1 |
| Selective topics only | 1 | 0 | 0 |
| **Nonverbal** | | | |
| Use of pantomime and gestures | 0 | 1 | 0 |
| **General Comments** | | | |
| Still good | 3 | 0 | 0 |
| Regression, poor talking skills | 1 | 1 | 1 |
| **PRESENT COMPREHENSION ABILITIES** | | | |
| Good listener, good comprehension | 1 | 2 | 0 |
| Good or average listener, misunderstands some things | 7 | 0 | 0 |
| Good listener, poor comprehension | 0 | 2 | 2 |
| Poor listener, poor comprehension | 0 | 1 | 0 |

*Stage: E = early, M = middle, L = late
†Values represent multiple responses by family members

topics do not differ substantially from those engaged in by the sample of older, normal adults in Shadden's study.[31]

Below is a collection of insightful comments made by family members describing their relative's present verbal skills. It is apparent from the respondents' remarks that their relatives' present expressive problems cause a great deal of suffering and lead to intense levels of frustration among family members.

**Early DAT:** I would say that it might be a little stiffer, stilted, saying the things that he thinks he's expected to say. His initial conversations with people, to me it sounds as though he is saying things by rote, "This is what I'm supposed to say, therefore I'm saying it."

**Early DAT:** He would make a statement out of the clear blue sky about something that we hadn't been talking about and I wouldn't be able to follow his train of thought and when I don't know what he's referring to he gets frustrated, which is understandable isn't it?

**Middle DAT:** Talks a lot but doesn't make much sense. Nothing hangs together. He just goes on and on and on and on. I can't communicate with him anymore and sit and tell him anything or discuss anything.

**Late DAT:** She doesn't talk at all. She doesn't start a conversation. She doesn't enter into one. Just sits. Everything [she says] is yes. It used to be 3 to 4 months ago you could get the "no" out of her, but it wouldn't be relative to what you were saying. It doesn't make any difference what you say to her it's "yes, yes." Everything I say to her is "yes, yes. . . ." Honestly it's quite frustrating at times.

Only 20 percent (1/8 early, 2/5 middle, and 0/2 late stage) of DAT individuals were described as currently having good listening and comprehension skills. Prior to the onset of dementia, 80 percent (7/8 early, 4/5 middle, 1/2 late stage) were described as good listeners with good comprehension. Although not all family members were able to explain in detail the nature of their relatives' present skills, some were able to describe aspects of length and utterance type best understood. Topics relating to the immediate family, personal and household activities (e.g., cleaning, cooking, eating, and washing), along with simple instructions were perceived as being the easiest to comprehend for over 85 percent of all subjects across all stages.

One-half of all DAT individuals (5/8 early and 2/5 middle stage) apparently exhibited frustration when they misunderstood what was said to them. Two of five middle- and all late-stage individuals did not exhibit frustration when they did not understand. For these individuals the dementia may have progressed to such a degree that it would preclude them from being cognitively aware of their comprehension deficits. Conversely, auditory comprehension skills may not be important to individuals in the advanced stages, especially as none of the family members for the middle- or late-stage subjects thought auditory comprehension was important for their relative then. As auditory skills become further compromised, individuals may rely more on visual input through written cues, pantomime, gestures, facial expressions, body postures, and exaggerations in paralinguistic features.

### Communication Problems Versus Other Selected Behaviors

Chenoweth and Spencer; Haley, Brown, and Levine; and Rabins et al described a number of behaviors that precipitated caregiving problems for family members.[4,11,25] Memory loss and disorientation caused 52 percent of the families in the Chenoweth and Spencer survey to seek out medical help. Haley et al determined that behaviors such as agitation, hallucinations, and dangerous or embarrassing actions were more of a concern for caregivers than were more common behaviors such as self-care deficits and disorientation. Physical violence, memory disturbance, incontinence, catastrophic reactions, hitting, and making accusations were cited by 50 percent or more of the families in the Rabins et al study as behaviors causing serious caregiving problems.

With these results in mind, family members were asked to rate their relatives' communication problems against 21 other troublesome behaviors often exhibited by individuals with DAT (e.g., outbursts of emotion, getting up at night, wandering, mismanaging money). This was undertaken to compare the relative contributions of communication disturbances and each selected behavior to overall problems in caregiving. In a paired comparison task, respondents identified the behavior that was more of a problem for them as caregivers.

Family members across all stages generated a broad range of responses. Each individual with DAT was perceived to exhibit a small cluster of troublesome behaviors. The most distinctive comparison was between memory disturbances and communication difficulties. Seven out of eight respondents for early-stage DAT individuals and both family members of the late-stage individuals rated memory difficulties as more of a caregiving problem than communication difficulties. Respondents for middle-stage DAT individuals were split in their ratings. Generally, comparisons among the other troublesome behaviors were evenly split, yielding few trends. Further detailed study is warranted to precisely establish the relative contribution of communicative disturbances on the impact of caregiving and to caregiving burden and strain.

### Psychosocial and Physical Environments Influencing Communication for Normal Elderly and Individuals with DAT

All family members were asked to describe the psychosocial and physical environments they perceived *interfered with* or *facilitated* communication for their relative. These conditions are outlined in Tables 12.6 and 12.7.

**Disruptive Conditions.** There were some differences between the responses of the DAT and control groups regarding conditions that contributed to communication difficulties. All DAT individuals were viewed as having difficulty talking and understanding in large groups, speaking or listening to strangers, and communicating when pressured to communicate. Background noise accentuated verbal and comprehension weaknesses. An overwhelming majority of the middle- and late-stage DAT individuals were perceived to have verbal and comprehension difficulties under most conditions.

For over 60 percent of the normal elderly, there were no conditions that appeared to contribute to communication difficulties. Those situations that did influence communication included large groups, strangers, noisy backgrounds, smoky places, discussion of unfamiliar topics, and small talk.

**Facilitating Conditions.** Table 12.7 summarizes responses describing conditions that facilitate communication for both subject groups. Again,

TABLE 12.6 **Psychosocial and Physical Environments That Contribute to Difficulties in Communication for Normal Elderly and Individuals with DAT**

| SITUATIONS AND PLACES | NORMAL CONTROLS (N=13) NC | DAT (N=15) E (8)* | M (5) | L (2) |
|---|---|---|---|---|
| **VERBAL SKILLS**† | | | | |
| *Psychosocial* | | | | |
| Large groups | 0 | 7 | 2 | 1 |
| Strangers | 3 | 1 | 1 | 0 |
| Some family members | 0 | 1 | 1 | 0 |
| Pressure to speak | 0 | 1 | 0 | 0 |
| No face-to-face contact | 0 | 0 | 0 | 1 |
| Unfamiliar topics | 2 | 0 | 0 | 0 |
| Small talk | 1 | 0 | 0 | 0 |
| *Physical Environment* | | | | |
| Noise | 0 | 4 | 0 | 0 |
| Smoky places | 1 | 0 | 0 | 0 |
| *Other* | | | | |
| All the time | 0 | 0 | 3 | 1 |
| No influence | 8 | 0 | 0 | 0 |
| **COMPREHENSION ABILITIES**† | | | | |
| *Psychosocial* | | | | |
| Large groups and strangers | 1 | 5 | 1 | 0 |
| Unfamiliar topics | 2 | 0 | 0 | 0 |
| Need to get attention | 1 | 0 | 0 | 0 |
| *Physical Environment* | | | | |
| Noise | 2 | 5 | 0 | 0 |
| Stores | 0 | 0 | 1 | 0 |
| *Other* | | | | |
| Most situations | 0 | 0 | 1 | 2 |
| No influence | 7 | 2 | 2 | 0 |

NC = Normal controls
*Stage: E = early, M = middle, L = late
†Values represent multiple responses by family members

there was a broad range of responses by all family members, regardless of subject classification.

The majority of DAT individuals were perceived to have minimal problems speaking or understanding when there were small groups of familiar, patient people, one-to-one contacts with conversational partners, interactions in familiar environments, and no pressure for them to contribute actively to conversations. These observations concur with comments made by health-care providers that dementia patients demonstrate better social functioning in environments where they are able to freely come and go and interact with small numbers of familiar people.[9,17,23] Reducing background noise, the number of people, and activities associated with confusion promoted comprehension regardless of stage.

Like the DAT individuals, the normal older controls were perceived to have minimal problems speaking and understanding when interacting with familiar people in small groups and discussing familiar topics under conditions of limited background noise. Slightly less than half (6/13) of the family members for the normals mentioned no specific environmental influences that facilitated communication.

TABLE 12.7 **Psychosocial and Physical Environments That Facilitate Communication for Normal Elderly and Individuals with DAT**

| SITUATIONS AND PLACES | NORMAL CONTROLS (N=13) NC | DAT (N=15) E (8)* | M (5) | L (2) |
|---|---|---|---|---|
| **VERBAL SKILLS**[†] | | | | |
| **Psychosocial** | | | | |
| Familiar people | 6 | 6 | 1 | 1 |
| Small groups | 1 | 4 | 2 | 1 |
| No pressure to speak, patient people | 0 | 4 | 3 | 0 |
| Children | 0 | 0 | 1 | 0 |
| Face-to-face contact | 0 | 0 | 0 | 1 |
| Large groups | 1 | 0 | 0 | 0 |
| Familiar topics | 1 | 0 | 0 | 0 |
| **Other** | | | | |
| No influence | 6 | 1 | 2 | 1 |
| **COMPREHENSION ABILITIES**[†] | | | | |
| **Psychosocial** | | | | |
| Small groups | 3 | 4 | 1 | 0 |
| Familiar people/places | 1 | 2 | 2 | 0 |
| One to one contact | 0 | 2 | 1 | 0 |
| Limited activity and confusion | 0 | 1 | 1 | 1 |
| **Paralinguistic** | | | | |
| Slow presentation of single utterances | 0 | 1 | 0 | 1 |
| **Physical Environment** | | | | |
| Limited noise | 2 | 5 | 1 | 0 |
| **Other** | | | | |
| Most situations | 0 | 1 | 0 | 0 |
| No influence | 8 | 1 | 2 | 1 |

NC = Normal controls
*Stage: E = early, M = middle, L = late
[†]Values represent multiple responses by family members

## Strategies That Minimize Communication Difficulties for Individuals with DAT

The majority of family members for the healthy elderly controls reported few communication problems in their relatives. Because of this, they were not questioned on the use of facilitative techniques.

**Verbal.** The commonly used and most effective strategies for the verbal difficulties of the DAT individuals were those where family members anticipated potential problems, made adjustments in their own utterances, and altered their style of interaction (Table 12.8). These included:

- Distracting the relative from his or her difficulties
- Using time-outs
- Ignoring verbal problems
- Supplying target words
- Controlling topics during conversations
- Remaining calm and not showing frustration
- Acting as translator and doing the talking for them

Only one family member, that of a middle-stage DAT individual, stated she routinely asks her husband to make adjustments in *his* mode and manner of expression, such as using pantomime and gestures, or writing out target words. Of added importance, none of the DAT family mem-

TABLE 12.8 **Family Members' Strategies for Verbal Difficulties of Relatives with DAT**

|  | DAT (N=15) | | |
|---|---|---|---|
|  | E (8)* | M (5) | L (2) |
| **Most Commonly Used Strategies**[†] | | | |
| Ignore or distract by engaging in other activities | 4 | 4 | 0 |
| Supply target word(s) during periods of difficulty | 3 | 1 | 0 |
| Anticipate difficulties and supply target word(s) | 1 | 1 | 0 |
| Ask questions or guess what was said | 3 | 1 | 1 |
| Act as translator, talk for subject | 1 | 1 | 1 |
| Wait until problem arises | 1 | 1 | 0 |
| Time-out or return to topic later | 0 | 1 | 0 |
| Have subject write target(s) | 0 | 1 | 0 |
| **Most Effective Strategies**[†] | | | |
| Ignore or distract by engaging in other activities | 5 | 2 | 0 |
| Supply target word(s) or guess | 3 | 3 | 0 |
| Remain calm, do not argue, use humor, give full attention | 2 | 2 | 0 |
| Initiate and control topics | 1 | 0 | 1 |
| Physical contact (hugging and kissing) | 1 | 0 | 0 |
| Have subject use pantomime/gestures | 0 | 1 | 0 |
| **Other** | | | |
| Nothing | 0 | 0 | 1 |
| Do not know | 1 | 0 | 0 |
| **Least Effective Strategies**[†] | | | |
| Show frustration, be impatient, hurry person | 7 | 4 | 0 |
| Point out errors or continually correct | 2 | 2 | 0 |
| Give or guess wrong word(s) | 2 | 0 | 0 |
| **Other** | | | |
| Do not know | 1 | 1 | 2 |

*Stage: E = early, M = middle, L = late
[†]Values represent multiple responses by family members

bers suggested reducing the number of participants in conversations or minimizing background noise, two strategies previously noted to positively influence the verbal output of individuals with DAT.

All family members of DAT individuals described adjustments they make in their verbal output and interactive styles to facilitate functional interaction. The strategies outlined in Table 12.8 may appear at first to be rather manipulative. However, on closer examination, responses demonstrate family member's sensitivity to their relatives' limited linguistic and communicative resources and illustrate the support they are willing to provide in order to maintain communication and interpersonal relations.

In terms of least effective strategies for verbal difficulties, caregiver respondents with early- and middle-stage DAT relatives were nearly unanimous in agreeing that: (1) showing frustration; (2) being impatient; (3) giving or guessing the wrong words; and (4) pointing out and continually correcting errors accentuated their relative's verbal weaknesses.

**Comprehension.** The most common and effective strategies for comprehension problems again illustrate DAT family members' insight and willingness to accommodate their relative's restricted competence (Table 12.9). Respondents described practical strategies addressing adjustments in content, manner, mode, and style of interaction. More specifically, these strategies include:

- Repetition, using same or different words
- Distracting the relative from their difficulties
- Using time-outs
- Ignoring problems
- Using nonverbal methods of communication
- Giving slow, detailed explanations
- Simplifying vocabulary and syntax
- Reducing the amount of information given at one time

TABLE 12.9 **Family Members' Strategies for Comprehension Difficulties of Relatives with DAT**

| | DAT (N=15) | | |
| --- | --- | --- | --- |
| | E (8)* | M (5) | L (2) |
| **Most Commonly Used Strategies**† | | | |
| Repetition with same or different word(s) | 5 | 2 | 1 |
| Ignore or distract by engaging in other activities | 3 | 4 | 1 |
| Use pantomime, gestures, writing, or physically assist | 0 | 3 | 1 |
| Time-outs and bring up later | 1 | 1 | 0 |
| Get eye contact | 1 | 0 | 1 |
| Use familiar style and vocabulary | 1 | 0 | 0 |
| Slow, detailed explanations | 1 | 0 | 0 |
| Short utterances, one-step directions | 1 | 0 | 0 |
| **Most Effective Strategies**† | | | |
| Repetition with same or different word(s) | 2 | 2 | 0 |
| Slow, detailed explanation | 2 | 0 | 0 |
| Ignore or distract by engaging in other activities, change topic | 1 | 1 | 1 |
| Pantomime, gestures or writing | 0 | 2 | 0 |
| Simplify vocabulary and syntax | 1 | 0 | 0 |
| Time-outs | 1 | 0 | 0 |
| Do not show frustration | 1 | 0 | 0 |
| Nothing works better | 0 | 0 | 1 |
| Do not know | 2 | 1 | 0 |
| **Least Effective Strategies**† | | | |
| Correcting or repeating too often, repeated attempts to make subject understand, pointing out errors | 4 | 1 | 0 |
| Show frustration and be impatient | 2 | 1 | 0 |
| Abandon attempts to improve comprehension | 1 | 1 | 0 |
| Too much information at once | 1 | 0 | 0 |
| Not face to face | 1 | 0 | 0 |
| Most everything | 0 | 0 | 1 |
| Nothing is ineffective | 3 | 2 | 1 |

*Stage: E = early, M = middle, L = late
†Values represent multiple responses by family members

- Remaining calm and not showing frustration

Albeit rather extensive, the list did not include comments such as reducing background noise or limiting the number of conversants, strategies that were previously cited as being particularly helpful. Response patterns show that relatively few family members across stages generated similar strategies. Almost all respondents however, were in agreement that showing frustration, being impatient, and repeatedly correcting and pointing out errors were the least effective measures for ensuring comprehension.

## Effects of Communication Problems on Relationship for Normal Elderly and Individuals with DAT

Each respondent was asked if his or her relative's verbal and comprehension difficulties affected their relationship in any way (see Table 12.10). Just over half of the DAT family members said there were no changes in their relationship. Those DAT family members noting changes in their relationship as a direct result of their partner communication problems described, in revealing detail, feeling the following:

- Frustration
- Loneliness
- Guilt
- Embarrassment
- Social isolation

One spouse of a middle-stage subject directly attributed the couple's lack of social life to her husband's communication difficulties. Both family members of the late-stage subjects reported assuming responsibility for and control of their relative's life. On a more positive level one DAT family member reported that her husband's communication problems brought them closer together.

Nearly 70 percent of respondents for the healthy elderly said there were no communication problems or no changes in their relationship. Those

TABLE 12.10 **Family Members' Descriptions of Changes in Relationship Because of Communication Difficulties for Normal Elderly and Relatives with DAT**

| IMPACT AND CHANGES | NORMAL CONTROLS (N=13) NC | DAT (N=15) E (8)* | M (5) | L (2) |
|---|---|---|---|---|
| **VERBAL DIFFICULTIES**† | | | | |
| **Negative Impact** | | | | |
| Isolated and lonely | 0 | 2 | 1 | 0 |
| Frustrated, short tempered, and impatient | 1 | 2 | 1 | 0 |
| Do not speak to one another because of frustration | 0 | 1 | 0 | 0 |
| Feel guilty about interacting with others | 0 | 0 | 1 | 0 |
| More embarrassed about going out because of spouse's poor skills | 0 | 0 | 1 | 0 |
| Get into more arguments | 1 | 0 | 0 | 0 |
| **Positive and Negative Impact** | | | | |
| Take control of spouse's life and make the decisions | 0 | 0 | 0 | 2 |
| Concern for relationship with others | 0 | 1 | 0 | 0 |
| Reduce outside activities to spend more time with spouse | 1 | 0 | 0 | 0 |
| Increase outside activities because of spouse's difficulties | 1 | 0 | 0 | 0 |
| **Positive Impact** | | | | |
| Makes them closer | 0 | 0 | 1 | 0 |
| **No Impact/No Changes** | | | | |
| No problems | 8 | 0 | 0 | 0 |
| No changes | 1 | 5 | 2 | 0 |
| **COMPREHENSION PROBLEMS**† | | | | |
| **Negative Impact** | | | | |
| Arguments and accusations (not listening or wanting to listen) | 2 | 0 | 0 | 0 |
| Isolated and lonely | 0 | 2 | 1 | 0 |
| Frustrated, short tempered, and impatient | 0 | 1 | 2 | 0 |
| Feels guilty about interacting with others | 0 | 0 | 1 | 0 |
| **Positive and Negative Impact** | | | | |
| Take control of spouse's life, make the decisions | 0 | 0 | 0 | 2 |
| Family member more of a helper now than in past | 0 | 1 | 0 | 0 |
| **No Impact/No Changes** | | | | |
| No problems | 8 | 0 | 0 | 0 |
| No changes | 3 | 4 | 2 | 0 |

NC = Normal controls
*Stage: E = early, M = middle, L = late
†Values represent multiple responses by family members

that did report changes acknowledged a downward shift in the number of contacts with family and friends. One family member noted increased outside activities because of the spouse's verbal difficulties. Another respondent reported being impatient and frustrated because of her relative's verbal problems.

DAT family members poignantly described changes in their relationships because of communication difficulties.

**Early stage:** Well naturally, it (verbal problem) has to have some impact. We have been not only husband and wife but the best of friends. I

**have always felt** that he was my best friend. I could tell him anything and work things out between us. But of course it's not the same and I do miss it.

**Early stage:** (Discussing comprehension problems) Well, not really our relationship. No it's just, I mourn the days when we could discuss anything and everything. That's the only thing.

**Early stage:** Well, yes, in that we don't have the good...rapport. I feel lonely sometimes because it's not the same. There is nothing coming back in the way of conversation...but it's the talking I miss. I miss the conversation. I miss discussing the why's and wherefore's and trying to figure out why those people did that or what's gonna happen down here. I miss that a whole lot.

**Middle stage:** I think it has maybe a bit, when you're in the house with a person and you can't talk to them, not that...it really doesn't bother me, I guess, but it's difficult when you haven't got somebody to talk to that understands what you're trying to say. We can go with the crowd (at church social functions) but the thing is, I find him sitting back in a corner not interacting. I feel rotten. I feel guilty. I think, now there he's sitting in the corner by himself, I should be sitting there too, but then, I mean I don't...

**Late stage:** Well it means I have to do everything. I have to think for her. She can't tell me when she has to go to the washroom so I have to think, When was the last time she went? so we won't have a problem. Because she doesn't talk to me I have to do everything. I have to think for her. Everything! She can't do anything by herself without being told or without being led or shown.

## Overview

The study of family members' perspectives of communication changes in normal, healthy relatives and relatives with DAT yielded a number of revealing facts. First, all family members were indeed able to describe in some detail the linguistic and communicative skills of their relative, when changes first occurred, what they were, and how their partner's abilities changed over time. Family members of DAT individuals first observed disruptions in the semantic domain and were sensitive to subtle shifts in pragmatic functions and discourse features during the estimated onset of DAT. Respondents perceived specific changes within each of these domains as the disease progressed. The potential for family members to act as sources of valuable and meaningful information about the communicative and linguistic performances in relatives with Alzheimer's disease has been demonstrated.

Second, respondents described psychosocial and physical conditions and specific communication strategies that supported and undermined their partner's communicative abilities. Family members of DAT individuals repeatedly stated how frustration and impatience shown by conversational partners interferes with their relatives' verbal and comprehension skills. They reported that their demented relatives communicated less effectively in environments with moderate amounts of noise and where there were large groups of unfamiliar people.

Finally, DAT family members eloquently described the impact their partner's communication problems had on their relationships. Recurring comments throughout the entire interview described how family members suffer frustration, loneliness, and both personal and social isolation as a result of their relative's communication disturbances. These emotions alone may have far-reaching implications for future studies examining outcome measures on caregiving burden and impact of care for family members.

## Clinical Implications of Communicative Changes

### NORMAL OLDER ADULTS

Communicative changes in healthy elders, as perceived by family members, have particular clinical importance to practitioners. Clinicians must be sensitive to family members' descriptions of deteriorations in auditory and visual performance. Concurrently, family members' observations of specific communicative changes may herald the presence of selective sensory deficits. Associations among family members' perceived changes in communication, sensory system acuity levels, normal aging processes, and pathologic conditions must be examined in detail by clinicians. Moreover, the impact of perceived and real changes in verbal and comprehension performance must be viewed from a broad perspective, especially as they may have consequences on interactions within the family structure.

Institutionalization of older adults has been shown to deleteriously affect qualitative and quantitative measures of communicative performance.[16] For the community-dwelling elderly, retirement appears to have a particularly negative impact on the range of conversational topics, number of communicative partners, and quality of interactions. Clinicians must be prepared to consider the influence of these factors on the perceptions of communicative competence and performance of older adults, especially when determining the need to establish intervention and support programs.

## INDIVIDUALS WITH DAT

Practitioners must consider family members' observations of early fluctuations in their relative's communicative performance, as these observations may augment and support interdisciplinary diagnostic information and may have certain relevance for management strategies. From a diagnostic point of view, it remains imperative that the knowledge base describing progressive changes in communicative problems and competencies within and across stages be expanded. Obler and Albert's and Bayles and Kaszniak's descriptions of linguistic and communicative features across stages of dementia form the foundation upon which many clinicians classify stages of performance.[3,22] Ongoing clinical programs that consider family members' perceptions of communicative change, in conjunction with standardized assessment measures and observations of interactions in natural contexts under spontaneous conditions, will extend that knowledge base.

Knowing the perceived declines in semantic, syntactic, discourse, and pragmatic domains, speech-language pathologists can compare and chart changes within each of these domains in relation to past performance levels on standardized instruments. With a clear understanding of perceived and measured changes, speech-language pathologists can provide appropriate strategies on how family members can most effectively respond to communicative distress during the progression of the syndrome. Clinicians have the responsibility to educate and counsel family members about the effects communicative and linguistic changes may have on their relationship with their demented relative. Family caregivers that are able to anticipate changes and employ productive management strategies may suffer reduced levels of caregiving burden and strain. This must be addressed empirically in future studies.

# Research Implications of Communicative Changes

## NORMAL OLDER ADULTS

To advance our understanding of the communicative and linguistic competence and performance of the healthy elderly, it is imperative that family members' perceptions of communicative change associated with normal aging be included in empirical investigations. Researchers must determine the correlations between perceived levels of performance and actual measures of achievement on standardized language and communication assessment instruments. Further, comprehensive research must consider the impact of cohort effects such as age, educational level, race, sex, socioeconomic status, health, and location of residence (e.g., in the community versus in an institution) on changes in linguistic and communicative performance. Such studies are best accomplished though longitudinal investigations. Finally, future research must be sensitive to the heterogeneity of communicative performance in the elderly and its influence on the dynamic interactions among older adults and family members. Family members' perceptions may have the greatest impact on how researchers view this heterogeneity.

## INDIVIDUALS WITH DAT

The research implications of family members' perceptions of communicative changes during the early onset of DAT are that investigators need to (1) differentiate perceived semantic knowledge disturbances related to normal aging processes from those perceived in pathologic conditions such as dementia; and (2) address discourse features and pragmatic aspects of functional communication, with weight given to interactions in natural contexts under spontaneous conditions. Ulatowska and Bond-Chapman (see Chapter 8) support contextually sensitive approaches to examine discourse features and pragmatic functions during the early course of dementia.

There is an urgent need to examine correlations among perceived changes and documented declines over time. That family members are sensitive to declines in communicative and linguistic abilities and are able to describe levels of function across all stages of DAT suggests that future research should include family members' observations. Knowing what family members observe during the progression of dementia may advance what is already known from the few scientific longitudinal studies that examined changes in linguistic and communicative performance. The ability of family members to provide reliable and valid data on early diagnostic changes and progressive deteriorations must be explored in greater depth, through future correlational studies employing objective measures of cognitive, linguistic, and communicative functions. Strong correlations may advance the development of more complete models describing the relationship among cognitive, linguistic, and communicative functions in dementia.

In future investigations, environmental and situational conditions that influence communication of older healthy adults and individuals with DAT must be empirically identified through rigorous, longitudinal clinical trials. The rising number of older adults in the United States and Canada, especially those with cognitive and communicative disorders, and the soaring costs of care compel researchers to identify these conditions. Until such time as they can be identified, clinicians cannot be absolutely certain which conditions facilitate or interfere with competent communication. Speech-language pathologists therefore must continue to rely on clinical experiences to guide their recommendations when advising contextually appropriate therapeutic intervention strategies.

In conclusion, future research on communicative behaviors of normal elders and individuals with dementia must not only continue to address performances in both experimental and natural social contexts but must include measures of the perceptions and influences of family caregivers. Serious consideration of these measures will undoubtedly advance the knowledge base describing theoretical constructs and clinical aspects of cognitive, linguistic, and communicative skills in older adults.

**References**

1. Bayles K. Language function in senile dementia. Brain Lang 1982; 16:265–280.
2. Bayles K. Communication in dementia. In: Ulatowska H, ed. The aging brain: Communication in the elderly. San Diego: College-Hill Press, 1985:157.
3. Bayles K, Kaszniak A. Communication and cognition in normal aging and dementia. San Diego: College-Hill Press, 1987.
4. Chenoweth B, Spencer B. Dementia: The experience of family caregivers. Gerontologist 1986; 26:267–272.
5. Deimling G, Bass D. Symptoms of mental impairment among elderly adults and their effects on family caregivers. J Gerontol 1986; 41:778–784.
6. Fischer L, Visintainer P, Schulz R. Reliable assessment of cognitive impairment in dementia patients by family caregivers. Gerontologist 1989; 29:333–335.
7. Fitting M, Rabins P, Lucas M, Eastham J. Caregivers for dementia patients: A comparison of husbands and wives. Gerontologist 1986; 26:248–252.
8. George L, Gwyther L. Caregiver well-being: A multidimensional examination of family caregivers of demented adults. Gerontologist 1986; 26:253–259.
9. Glickstein J. Therapeutic interventions in Alzheimer's disease: A program of functional communication skills for activities of daily living. Rockville, MD: Aspen Publishers, 1988.
10. Greene J, Smith R, Gardiner M, Timbury G. Measuring behavioral disturbance of elderly demented patients in the community and its effects on relatives: a factor analytic study. Age Ageing 1982; 11:121–126.
11. Haley W, Brown S, Levine E. Family caregiver appraisals of patient behavioral disturbance in senile dementia. Clin Gerontol 1987; 25:25–34.
12. Havelka J. Reflections and preoccupations. London, Ontario: Ergo Publications, 1980.
13. Helmick J, Watamori T, Palmer J. Spouses' understanding of the communication disabilities of aphasic patients. J Speech Hear Disord 1976; 41:238–243.
14. Kempler D, Curtiss S, Jackson D. Syntactic preservation in Alzheimer's disease. J Speech Hear Res 1987; 30:343–350.
15. Kinney J, Stephens MA. Caregiving hassles scale: Assessing the daily hassles of caring for a family member with dementia. Gerontologist 1989; 29:329–332.
16. Lubinski R, Morrison E, Rigrodsky S. Perception of spoken communication by elderly chronically ill patients in an institutional setting. J Speech Hear Disord 1981; 46:405–412.
17. Mace N, Rabbins P. The 36 hour day. Baltimore: Johns Hopkins Press, 1981.
18. Malone R. Expressed attitudes of families of aphasics. J Speech Hear Disord 1969; 34:146–150.
19. McKahnn G, Drachman D, Folstein M, et al. Clinical diagnosis of Alzheimer's disease: Report of the NINCDS-ADRDA work group under the auspices of the Department of Health and Human Services Task Force on Alzheimer's disease. Neurology 1984; 34:939–944.
20. Morycz R. Caregiving strain and the desire to institutionalize family members with Alzheimer's disease. Res Aging 1985; 7:329–361.
21. Obler L. Language and brain dysfunction in dementia. In: Segalowitz S, ed. Language functions and brain organization. New York: Academic Press, 1983:267.
22. Obler L, Albert M. Language in the elderly aphasic and in the dementing patient. In: Taylor Sarno M, ed. Acquired aphasia. New York: Academic Press, 1981:385.
23. Ostuni E, Santo Pietro MJ. Getting through: Communicating when someone you care for has Alzheimer's disease. Plainsboro: The Speech Bin, 1986.
24. Poulshock W, Deimling G. Families caring for elders in residence: Issues in the measurement of burden. J Gerontol 1984; 39:230–239.
25. Rabins P, Mace N, Lucas M. The impact of dementia on the family. JAMA 1982; 248:333–335.
26. Reisberg B, Ferris S, De Leon M, Crook T. The global deterioration scale for assessment of primary degenerative dementia. Am J Psychiatry 1983; 139:1136–1139.
27. Reveley J. One caregivers's view. In: Jarvik L, Hutner Winograd C, eds. Treatments for the Alzheimer patient: The long haul. New York: Springer Publishing, 1988:137–144.
28. Schwartz M, Marin O, Saffran E. Dissociations of language functions in dementia: A case study. Brain Lang 1979; 7:277–306.
29. Scott J, Roberto K, Hutton J. Families of Alzheimer's victims. J Am Geriatr Soc 1986; 34:348–354.
30. Shannas E. The family as a social support system in old age. Gerontologist 1979; 19:169–174.
31. Shadden B. Perceptions of daily communicative interactions with older persons. In: Shadden B, ed. Communicative behavior and aging. Baltimore: Williams & Wilkins, 1988:12.
32. Shewan C, Cameron H. Communication and related problems as perceived by aphasic individuals and their spouses. J Commun Disord 1984; 17:175–187.
33. Slauson T, Bayles K, Tomoeda C. Syntax production by Alzheimer's disease patients and the normal elderly. Paper presented at the Annual Convention of the American Speech-Language Hearing Association. Detroit, MI, 1986.
34. Ulatowska H, Allard L, Donnell A, et al. Discourse performance in Alzheimer subjects. Paper presented at the Annual Convention of the American Speech-Language Hearing Association. Detroit, MI, 1986.
35. Zarit S, Reever K, Bach-Peterson J. Relatives of the impaired elderly: Correlates of feelings of burden. Gerontologist 1980; 20:649–655.

# SECTION FOUR

*Dementia: Diagnostic and Rehabilitative Considerations*

# CHAPTER 13

# *Differential Diagnosis and Assessment*

DANIELLE N. RIPICH, Ph.D.

Despite our rapidly expanding knowledge of the dementias, the diagnosis and assessment of symptomatology in these syndromes remains a complex challenge. This complexity is reflected in the wide-ranging organization of topics in this chapter. First an overview of types of dementia and related disorders is presented to develop a frame of reference for diagnosis and assessment. Classification systems are included so that the differential diagnostic issues are made relevant. The premises for the diagnosis and assessment battery presented are discussed. Within this framework, a comprehensive diagnostic protocol and assessment plan with four major areas, as shown in Table 13.1, is constructed. Finally, future research in this emerging area of study is discussed.

Diagnosis and assessment of dementia have been complicated by a number of factors. Diagnosis is problematic in that presently a definitive diagnosis of dementia of the Alzheimer's type (DAT) can only be made based on histopathologic evidence of plaques and tangles found in the brain tissue after death.[74] Clinical intervention must precede from a presumptive or probable diagnosis based on a case history and clinical profile of medical and behavioral test results. The assessment of symptomatology of dementia is complicated by a number of factors, including the lack of well-developed instruments to study cognition in these syndromes, the overlap of common geriatric depression symptoms and dementia symptoms, and the paucity of clinical knowledge and criteria for description of certain symptoms with which dementia patients are likely to present.[91] Each of these complicating factors has been considered, and attempts have been made to minimize them in developing the approach to diagnosis and assessment presented in this chapter.

## Dementia Types and Related Disorders

Dementia is not a disease, it is a symptom complex caused by a disease. The term dementia will be used to refer to the impairment in short- and long-term memory associated with impairment in abstract thinking, impaired judgment, other disturbances of higher cortical function, or personality change. The disturbance is severe enough to interfere significantly with work or usual social activities or relationships with others.[37]

### REVERSIBLE AND IRREVERSIBLE DEMENTIAS

There are both reversible and irreversible dementias. All possible causes of reversible dementias must be ruled out in the diagnostic process before moving to an identification of irreversible dementia. Reversible or treatable dementias in-

---

TABLE 13.1 **Diagnosis and Assessment Model**

Case history interview
Neurologic and medical evaluation
Behavioral assessment
   Neuropsychological assessment
   Behavioral rating measures
Language and communication assessment
   Comprehensive language testing
   Pragmatics assessment
   Semantics assessment
   Syntax and phonology assessment
   Memory and language evaluation

---

This research was supported by the National Institute of Aging Grant #AG-0812-01 to the Alzheimer's Disease Research Center University Hospitals of Cleveland, Ohio.

clude dementias resulting from drug toxicity, metabolic imbalances, infections, tumors, normal measure hydrocephalus, alcohol abuse, neurosyphilis, and epilepsy. Geriatric depression (pseudodementia) is classified as a reversible dementia in some diagnostic models.[113] Irreversible dementias include DAT, multi-infarct dementia (MID), Pick's disease, and those associated with Parkinson's disease, Huntington's disease, Wilson's disease, supranuclear palsy, Creutzfeldt-Jakob disease, and Korsakoff's syndrome.

## CORTICAL AND SUBCORTICAL DEMENTIAS

One dichotomy used to distinguish dementia types is the cortical versus subcortical distinction. This classification system is controversial, and even its advocates acknowledge that the terms may be inappropriate and the concept of the dichotomy of functioning has yet to be documented.[122] The distinction made between cortical dementias (DAT and Pick's disease), the subcortical dementias (Huntington's disease, Parkinson's disease, Wilson's disease, and supranuclear palsy), and mixed or vascular dementias (MID, Creutzfeldt-Jakob disease, and Korsakoff's syndrome) emphasizes the separation of these anatomic regions but fails to account for neurochemical and neuropathologic relationships between areas.[122] Nevertheless, the cortical and subcortical distinction provides a neuroanatomic organization that is useful in sorting out the syndromes causing dementia. In the cortical dementias, the dementia is the primary dysfunction, whereas in the subcortical dementias the dementia occurs as a secondary feature of the symptom complex. Table 13.2 presents a chart outlining the characteristics of cortical, subcortical, and mixed dementias, as well as related disorders.

## CORTICAL DEMENTIAS

### Alzheimer's Disease

Of the irreversible dementias, Alzheimer's disease (DAT) is by far the most common, accounting for 65 percent of all dementias.[74] DAT refers to a classical clinical syndrome with a gradual and steady onset and course, accompanied by characteristic neuropathologic changes: helical neurofibrillary tangles, senile plaques, and grandulovascular degeneration.[123-125] Further, recent research has pointed to losses of neurons, neurotransmitters, and neuropeptides as significant indicators of DAT.[7,16,55,110]

In addition to the basic dementia criteria previously described, DAT or primary degenerative dementia, as labelled by the Diagnostic and Statistical Manual of Mental Disorders, third edition revised (DSM III), has two DSM III diagnostic criteria.[37] These are: (1) insidious onset with a generally progressive deteriorating course; and (2) exclusion of all other specific causes of dementia by history, physical examination, and laboratory studies.

It is estimated that 1 percent of the population over the age of 65 years and 2 percent of those over the age of 80 years has DAT.[50] This syndrome involves the loss of intellectual abilities such as memory, judgment, abstract thought, and other higher cortical functions and causes personality and behavioral changes. DAT may be accompanied by depression, delusions and/or, more rarely, delirium. First-degree biologic relatives of those with presenile DAT are more likely to develop the disease because it is believed to be inherited as an autosomal dominant trait.[53.] A confirmed diagnosis of DAT can presently only be made on autopsy. However, using the case history, medical, and behavioral tests discussed later in this chapter, a probable diagnosis can be concluded. For a discussion of language and discourse associated with changes in DAT, readers are referred to the descriptions in Chapters 7 and 8.

### Pick's Disease

This relatively rare progressive neurologic disease is characterized by marked frontotemporal-lobe atrophy as well as Pick bodies within the neurons and inflated and swollen neurons. The pattern of neuronal degeneration, i.e., primarily frontal-lobe atrophy, including the inferior motor area and anterior temporal lobes and sparing of the posterior cingulate gyrus and parietal lobes, differs from the diffuse pattern found in DAT. However, the amygdaloid nucleus and hippocampus are involved in both disorders.[21] Dementia of the frontal-lobe type (DFT) has been identified by Neary, Snoden, Northen, and Goulding as possibly representing a form of Pick's disease.[90] These authors contend that this form of dementia may be more common than presently recognized. Pick's disease occurs between 40 and 60 years of age, more often in women than men. As it proceeds, cognition, language, and memory decline, and patients become mute near the end of the disease course.[32]

## SUBCORTICAL DEMENTIAS

### Parkinson's Disease

The dementia syndrome occurs in approximately 40 percent of all Parkinson's disease patients; however, the mental status changes are ubiquitous, as in other subcortical dementias.[27] The changes include depression, bradyphrenia,

## TABLE 13.2 Dementia Types and Related Disorders

### CORTICAL DEMENTIAS

|  | **DAT** | **Pick's Disease** |
|---|---|---|
| Onset | Gradual | Gradual |
| Etiology | Diffuse damage:<br>    neurofibrillary tangles<br>    senile plaque<br>    granulovascular degeneration | Pick bodies<br>Inflated neurons<br>Atrophy of the anterior portions of the frontal and temporal lobes |
| Course | Progressive<br>Irreversible | Progressive<br>Irreversible |
| Language and speech | Semantics and pragmatics impaired early<br>Syntax and phonology impaired later<br>Speech impaired very late | Slow, deliberate speech<br>Anomia<br>Breakdowns in syntax<br>Defect in auditory comprehension |
| Memory | Impaired early<br>Worse for remote events | Impaired recent memory |
| Performance characteristics | Tries to perform<br>Alert<br>Consistent level of performance | Emotional lability and apathy<br>Loss of tact and judgement |
| Physical characteristics<br>Gait<br>Movement | Normal (some pacing) | Motor involvement in later stages |

### SUBCORTICAL DEMENTIAS

|  | **Parkinson's Disease** | **Huntington's Disease** |
|---|---|---|
| Onset | Sporadic | Insidious |
| Etiology | Autosomal dominant<br>Degenerative disease of the nervous system especially in the substantia nigra | Variety of causes:<br>    autosomal dominant trait<br>    idiopathic<br>    drug induced<br>    postencephalitic<br>    arteriosclerotic<br>    loss of Golgi cells in corpus striatum |
| Course | Progressive<br>Irreversible | Progressive<br>Irreversible |
| Language and speech | Language minimally impaired<br>Speech impaired<br>Weak, breathy voice<br>Abnormal pitch rate and loudness<br>Inappropriate silences | Dysarthria worsens<br>Language organization, sequencing, and naming abilities impaired as the disease progresses |
| Memory | Forgetful<br>Impaired recall<br>Slowed response | Impaired, especially for remote events early in the disease |
| Performance characteristics | Slowness of responses | Early stages:<br>    irritability<br>    apathy<br>    untidiness<br>    impulsiveness |

*Table continues on following page*

## TABLE 13.2 (continued)

### SUBCORTICAL DEMENTIAS

|  | Parkinson's Disease | Huntington's Disease |
|---|---|---|
| Physical characteristics | | |
| Gait | Abnormal | Abnormal |
| Movement | Slow | Shuffling gait |
|  | Tremor | Jerky gait |
|  | Rigidity | Festinating |
|  | Bradykinesia | Choreic |

### SUBCORTICAL DEMENTIAS

|  | Supranuclear Palsy | Wilson's Disease |
|---|---|---|
| Onset | Gradual | Gradual |
| Etiology | Related to changes in the reticular formation, thalamus, or hypothalamus | Inherited autosomal recessive trait<br>Basal ganglia<br>Excessive levels of copper in the brain and liver |
| Course | Progressive | Progressive<br>Rapid progression if untreated or undiagnosed |
| Language and speech | Dysarthria<br>Speech becomes inaudible and unintelligible with gurgling, harsh guttural sounds | Dysarthria<br>Irregular articulatory breakdown<br>Hypernasality<br>Inappropriate silences |
| Memory | Impaired | Impaired |
| Performance characteristics | | |
| Physical characteristics | Pseudobulbar palsy, dystonia, and severe rigidity of head/neck producing a backward retracted head position | Slowness<br>Tremors<br>Rigidity<br>Bradykinesia or involuntary movements<br>Later stages severe ataxia<br>Dysphagia<br>Mask-like face |

### MIXED DEMENTIAS

|  | Korsakoff's Disease | Creutzfeldt-Jakob Disease | MID |
|---|---|---|---|
| Onset | Gradual | Variable: gradual or sudden | Sudden |
| Etiology | Cortical atrophy resulting from chronic alcohol abuse | Infectious, transmissable, unconventional virus<br>Results in degenerative cortical tissue, i.e., spongiform encephalopathy and nonspecific atrophy | Multiple lesions<br>Softening of brain tissue<br>Alteration in cerebral blood vessels |
| Course | Stable or minimally progressive | Rapidly progressive | Stepwise<br>Irreversible |

*Table continues on following page*

## TABLE 13.2 (continued)

### MIXED DEMENTIAS

|  | Korsakoff's Disease | Creutzfeldt-Jakob Disease | MID |
|---|---|---|---|
| Language and speech |  | In stage 2: aphasia, apraxia, agnosia<br>In stage 3: mutism | Impaired pattern dependent on site of lesion |
| Memory | Decreased skills<br>Poor attention<br>Amnesia | Forgetfulness in initial phase | Impaired, depends on site of lesion |
| Performance characteristics | Affective lability | Apathetic | Variable performance based on focal lesions |
| Physical characteristics | May show disturbances | Sensory and visual impairments<br>Cranial nerve palsies, rigidity, myoclonus, tremor<br>Cerebellar disturbances | May be abnormal, dependent on site of lesion |

### RELATED DISORDERS

|  | Aphasia | Slowly Progressive Aphasia | Depression (Pseudodementia) |
|---|---|---|---|
| Onset | Sudden | Gradual | Can be dated with some precision |
| Etiology | CVA<br>Tumor<br>Trauma | Perisylvian region, left hemisphere degeneration | Unknown |
| Course | Reversible<br>Spontaneous recovery | Progressive<br>Irreversible | Rapid progression of symptoms<br>Reversible |
| Language and speech | Impaired across all levels of language<br>Speech not impaired | Anomia and pure word deafness<br>Speech not impaired | Word finding problems<br>Speech slowed<br>Reduced intonation contour and intensity |
| Memory | Not impaired | Not impaired | Impaired equally for remote and recent events |
| Performance characteristics | Poorer on language-based than nonlanguage tasks | Poorer on language than nonlanguage tasks | No effort to perform<br>Uneven performance<br>May do better on harder tasks |
| Physical characteristics<br>Gait<br>Movement | May show right hemiparesis<br>Hemiplegia | Not impaired | Gait slowed and shuffling<br>Movement slowed |

visuospatial disturbances, executive functioning deficits, and impaired recall (with other memory aspects relatively spared).[18,32,70,96] Results of a recent study by Cummings, Darkins, Mendez et al suggest that in Parkinson's disease the loss of speech and language abilities is a reflection of the overall cognitive loss.[31] In contrast, the loss of language in DAT correlates less strongly with severity of dementia and may result from pathologic changes specific to language areas of the cortex. Specifically, this study found four distinctions between speech and language in DAT and Parkinson's disease. First, DAT patients exhibit more language disturbances than equally demented Parkinson's disease dementia patients on the current assessment battery. Second, Parkinson's disease patients with and without overt dementia have more prominent speech and writing abnormalities than

DAT. Third, Parkinson's disease patients with overt dementia have more prominent abnormalities of the motor aspects of speech and writing, as well as select aspects of language function, than Parkinson's disease patients without dementia. Finally, Parkinson's disease patients with dementia may be distinguished from DAT on the basis of speech and language characteristics. These findings confirm earlier studies suggesting that language is relatively spared in this subcortical dementia.

### Huntington's Disease

Although choreic motor disturbances are the major characteristic of this autosomal-dominant progressive disease, cognitive and psychiatric disturbances are early manifestations.[69] Huntington's disease patients generally experience equally impaired recent and remote memory,[2] as well as problems in language organization and naming problems.[61] A case study by Moss, Mastri, and Schut of a patient with coexisting late-onset Huntington's disease and DAT, showed verbal skills relatively well preserved compared to other areas of cognitive functioning.[75]

### Supranuclear Palsy and Wilson's Disease

These rarely occurring dementias have symptoms common to the other subcortical dementias previously described.[29] These symptoms are attributable to dysfunction of the basal ganglia and frontal subcortical connections.[31]

## MIXED DEMENTIA

### Multi Infarct Dementia (MID)

The DSM III-Revised criteria for multi infact dementia (MID) include the basic dementia criteria with the addition of the following characteristics:[37]
1. Stepwise deteriorating course with "patchy" distribution of deficits (i.e., some functions affected but not others) early in the course
2. Focal neurologic signs and symptoms (e.g., exaggeration of deep tendon reflexes, extensor plantar response, pseudobulbar palsy, gait abnormalities, weakness of an extremity, etc.)
3. Evidence from history, physical examination, or laboratory tests of significant cerebrovascular disease that is judged to be etiologically related to the disturbance

MID is the second most common subtype of dementia but is much less frequently occurring than DAT. It accounts for approximately 20 percent of all dementia patients and occurs concurrently with DAT in another 15 percent.[112] This dementia, with its abrupt onset and stepwise course of "patchy" losses of function depending on the areas damaged by the infarcts, is presumed to result from vascular disease and is sometimes termed vascular dementia. MID results from multiple cerebral vascular accidents (CVA) occurring over time. The neurologic characteristics are multiple areas of softening of brain tissue and possibly also pathologic alterations in cerebral blood vessels.[112] In addition to the focal neurologic signs listed previously in item 2 of the listed criteria, cognitive functions such as memory, abstract thinking, judgment, impulse control, and personality are nearly always affected.[113] This disorder is more common in males and is without a documented familial pattern.[22] It appears to have arterial hypertension, extracranial vascular disease, and valvular disease of the heart as predisposing factors.[25]

Clinical evaluation may be the only means of distinguishing MID from DAT. There are no Weschler Adult Intelligence Scale-Revised data that serve to distinguish the two groups nor is there a standard battery of psychometric tests for differentiation.[117] Hachinski, Iliff, Zilhka et al developed ischemic scoring systems of 13 items (scored as 1 or 2 points each).[49] The system, shown in Table 13.3, is designed to create two distinct nonoverlapping groups. Patients scoring 7 or above are classified as MID and those scoring 4 or less as DAT. A study by Wagner, Oesterreich, and Hoyer evaluated the validity of the ischemic score as a differential diagnostic tool.[116] Results indicate that the ischemic score was of major importance in differentiating vascular type dementia (MID) from DAT and depression. Molsa, Paljarvi, Rinne, Rinne, and Sako also found good discrimination (70 percent

TABLE 13.3 **Ischemic Score**

| FEATURE | SCORE |
| --- | --- |
| Abrupt onset | 2 |
| Stepwise deterioration | 1 |
| Fluctuating course | 2 |
| Nocturnal confusion | 1 |
| Relative preservation of personality | 1 |
| Depression | 1 |
| Somatic complaints | 1 |
| Emotional incontinence | 1 |
| History of hypertension | 1 |
| History of strokes | 2 |
| Evidence of associated atherosclerosis | 1 |
| Focal neurologic symptoms | 2 |
| Focal neurologic signs | 2 |

From Hachinski VC, Iliff LD, Zilhka E, et al. Cerebral blood flow in dementia. Arch Neurol 1975; 32:632–637. Copyright 1975, American Medical Association.

accuracy) between DAT and MID patients, using the Hachinski scoring method.[73] Perhaps because of the heterogeneity of the language problems and the "patchy" nature of the loss of cognitive functioning in MID patients, there have been no large-scale studies of language loss in MID.[11] MID is a subtype of dementia that warrants additional research and documentation of patterns of loss as well as comparisons to other forms of dementia.

A recent comparison study of speech and language alterations between DAT and MID patients revealed that the verbal output of these two subject groups differed in several ways.[87] The MID patients demonstrated greater motor speech disruption, whereas the DAT patients showed more difficulty in language, i.e., empty speech and marked anomia. These results are noteworthy in that they revealed differences in these two syndromes despite the heterogeneity of the symptom complexes of DAT and especially MID.

## Creutzfeldt-Jakob Disease and Korsakoff's Syndrome

Dementia occurs in the syndromes of Creutzfeldt-Jakob disease, a rare viral degenerative disorder, and Korsakoff's syndrome, a disorder resulting from chronic alcohol abuse. Creutzfeldt-Jakob disease is fairly stereotypic and moves rapidly through three identifiable stages. First, for several weeks symptoms of neurologic decline emerge. Second, these diverse and widespread neurologic disturbances become evident, and aphasia, apraxia, and agnosia are present. Finally, the patient moves to a terminal vegetative state and is mute.[28] Korsakoff's syndrome is thought by some researchers to result in generalized dementia. However, this view is not universally held because of the stable or minimally progressive course of the symptoms.[113]

## RELATED DISORDERS

### Aphasia and Slowly Progressive Aphasia

The relation between aphasia and dementia has been debated in the literature. Cummings, Benson, Hill, and Read reported that all 30 DAT subjects they tested demonstrated aphasia and that aphasia should be included as a diagnostic criterion for DAT.[30] However, Bayles, Tomoeda, and Caffrey listed five criteria to differentiate aphasia and dementia.[13] First, the rate of onset is sudden in aphasia and slow in DAT. Second, decline is continuous in DAT but not in aphasia. Next, DAT results in diffuse brain atrophy, whereas aphasia results from focal lesions. Further, they contend that dementia affects a range of cognitive abilities and aphasia does not. Finally, aphasic patients' performance on verbal and nonverbal tasks is dissociated, but dementia patients show simultaneous decline in these performances. More recently Bayles and Kaszniak have acknowledged that it is difficult to develop strict criteria for this differentiation.[11] Au, Albert, and Obler hold that studying all language function impairments in ways that lead toward the development of a comprehensive model of brain-language relationships is more useful than using a differential approach.[6] These authors, in contrast to Bayles and Kaszniak,[11] Wertz,[121] Horner,[56] and others, propose that the language breakdown in dementia be viewed as a variation of the classical aphasia syndrome.[11,56,121] This view appears to come from the same broad theoretic basis as Whitehouse's argument against separating cortical and subcortical dementia.[122] In both cases the argument is that there is more to be gained from examining commonalities than from developing a differentiating perspective. Faber-Langendoen, Morris, Knesevich, et al studied aphasia in demented patients and concluded that aphasia is a common feature of DAT and identifies a subgroup with a more rapid progression of dementia.[39] Furthermore, they contend that aphasia represents a specific dysfunction beyond the global cognitive impairment of DAT. Both the differentiating and commonality perspectives are valid and depend on whether aphasia is defined as a result of "focal" brain damage or generalized brain damage. Shut reported cases in a which single vascular infarct, a homorganic stroke, produced part or all of the symptoms of the dementia complex.[102] The etiologic relationship between cerebrovascular disease and dementia warrants further study.

Bayles, Boone, Tomoeda et al reported on a group of neuropsychologic tests that differentiated DAT patients (early and middle stages) from fluent and nonfluent aphasics (classified on the basis of word-fluency measures).[10] Memory tasks such as delayed spatial recognition, delayed verbal recognition, and delayed story retelling showed significant differences between DAT patients and both groups of aphasics, with aphasics performing better. Mild DAT patients performed better than nonfluent aphasics on the word-fluency measure. Possibly the most difficult language differentiations among these language impairments are between early-stage DAT and the empty language of fluent and anomic aphasia.[82] Evaluation of memory performance can assist in this differentiation.

There was a group of six patients first identified by Mesulam as having slowly progressive aphasia (SPA) without generalized dementia.[72] This condition's initial presenting difficulties were anomia in five patients and pure word deafness in the sixth. These problems appeared similar to those of some early-DAT patients. However, results of neurodiagnostic tests suggest that in contrast to the diffuse damage in DAT, a relatively focal degeneration of the perisylvian region of the left hemisphere occurs in SPA. This language impairment is not well understood at present.

### Right-Hemisphere Damage

Right-hemisphere damage often results in a loss of orientation and thought disorders. These disturbances are evident in conversation tasks.[77] The communication impairments associated with right-hemisphere damage are described as disorders of "expression and reception of complex contextually based communicative events resulting from disturbance of the attentional and perceptual mechanisms underlying nonsymbolic, experiential processing."[77] These characteristics are found in DAT patients as well, and their presence can complicate a diagnosis of DAT. However, right-hemisphere-damaged patients do not exhibit the auditory comprehension problems found in dementia patients.[11]

TABLE 13.4 **Clinical Features Differentiating Pseudodementia from Dementia**

| PSEUDODEMENTIA | DEMENTIA |
|---|---|
| **Clinical Course and History** | |
| Family always aware of dysfunction and its severity | Family often unaware of dysfunction and its severity |
| Onset can be dated with some precision | Onset can be dated only within broad times |
| Symptoms of short duration before medical help is sought | Symptoms usually of long duration before medical help is sought |
| Rapid progression of symptoms after onset | Slow progression of symptoms throughout course |
| History of previous psychiatric dysfunction common | History of previous psychiatric dysfunction unusual |
| **Complaints and Clinical Behavior** | |
| Patients usually complain much of cognitive loss | Patients usually complain little of cognitive loss |
| Patient's complaint of cognitive dysfunction usually detailed | Patient's complaint of cognitive dysfunction usually vague |
| Patients emphasize disability | Patients conceal disability |
| Patients highlight failures | Patients delight in accomplishments, however trivial |
| Patients make little effort to perform even simple tasks | Patients struggle to perform tasks |
| Patients don't try to keep up | Patients rely on notes, calendars, etc. to keep up |
| Patients usually communicate strong sense of distress | Patients often appear unconcerned |
| Affective change often pervasive | Affect labile and shallow |
| Loss of social skills often early and prominent | Social skills often retained |
| Behavior often incongruent with severity of cognitive dysfunction | Behavior usually compatible with severity of cognitive dysfunction |
| Nocturnal accentuation of dysfunction uncommon | Nocturnal accentuation of dysfunction common |
| **Clinical Features Related to Memory, Cognitive, and Intellectual Dysfunctions** | |
| Attention and concentration often well preserved | Attention and concentration usually faulty |
| "Don't know" answers typical | "Near miss" answers frequent |
| On tests of orientation, patients often give "don't know" answers | On tests of orientation, patients often mistake unusual for usual |
| Memory loss for recent and remote events severe | Memory loss for recent events usually more severe than for remote events |
| Memory gaps for specific periods or events common | Memory gaps for specific periods unusual |
| Marked variability in performance on tasks of similar difficulty | Consistently poor performance on tasks of similar difficulty |

From Wells CE. The differential diagnosis of psychiatric disorders in the elderly. In: Cole J, Barrett J, eds. Psychopathology in the aged. New York: Raven Press, 1980:19.

## Dementia and Depression: Pseudodementia or Dementia Syndrome of Depression

Geriatric depression often co-occurs with dementia and is sometimes termed pseudodementia or dementia syndrome of depression because the symptoms exhibited are quite similar.[42,120] Differential diagnosis of these two disorders is sometimes difficult as a result of these similar symptoms. A comprehensive history, such as the one described later in this chapter, is useful in discriminating between these disorders. Based on a review of available literature, Wells developed a table (see Table 13.4) for comparing and contrasting dementia and pseudodementia based on the (1) history; (2) clinical behavior and complaints; and (3) memory and cognitive and intellectual performance.[119] Within the "Clinical Course and History" section of Table 13.4, the most discriminating factors are the *onset* (item 3) and the *progression of symptoms* (item 4). In pseudodementia there is a definitive onset with rapid occurrence of most symptoms. This is in contrast to true dementia with its gradual onset and slow progression of symptoms. In the "Complaints and Clinical Behavior" section, the easiest feature to note during assessment is the *patient's motivation* (item 5). Patients with pseudodementia make little effort to perform, whereas dementia patients in the early stages often make every effort to prove themselves adequate. In the final section, "Memory, Cognitive, and Intellectual Dysfunction," *performance variability* (item 6) reveals distinct differences in the two conditions. The pseudodementia patient's performance will be highly variable on tasks of similar difficulty. Dementia patients' poor performance is consistent across similar tasks.

## Summary

In summary, DAT is the most common type of dementia. It is classified as a cortical dementia, along with Pick's disease. Subcortical dementias (Parkinson's disease, Huntington's disease, Wilson's disease, and supranuclear palsy) occur as a part of a more extensive symptom complex. This cortical-subcortical distinction is not universally recognized but serves to organize the syndromes (see Chapter 2). Mixed or vascular dementia is a designation for multi infarct dementia. The relationship between aphasia and the communication features of dementia is an area of contention among researchers. The basis of disagreement appears to be whether aphasia is defined as resulting from focal brain damage or more broadly as resulting from any brain damage. Slowly progressive aphasia patients and patients with right-hemisphere damage have some language and spatial memory symptoms in common with dementia patients. It is important to note that these related disorders may co-occur with dementia. Careful comparisons across neuropsychologic and language measures are necessary for accurate diagnosis and assessment.

## Diagnosis and Assessment Premises

A correct diagnosis and comprehensive assessment of DAT and other forms of dementia are critical for prognosis, treatment, and case management. There are three premises that serve as the basis for the perspective taken in this chapter. First, the initial diagnostic work-up and assessment precedes intervention; however, assessment must be viewed as a dynamic and ongoing process.[105] Because the rate of change is variable and the symptom complex heterogeneous, systematic reassessment is required.

Second, because dementia is a symptom complex that includes physical, social, cognitive, and communication features, multiple perspectives are required for adequate diagnosis and assessment. These perspectives can only be provided by an interdisciplinary team of professionals from medicine, nursing, social work, psychology, speech-language pathology (SLP), and audiology. In addition, referral to a variety of other specialists may provide valuable information in a comprehensive evaluation. Referral should be made to those with geriatric expertise. Such professionals include but are not limited to: occupational therapists, physical therapists, ophthalmologists, optometrists, otologists, physiatrists, and nurses.

An overview of the appropriate case history, medical laboratory studies, and neuropsychological test and behavioral ratings as well as language and communication measures will be presented based on this collaborative perspective. As specialists in communication disorders, SLPs are often asked to provide consultation regarding communication competence of dementia patients. This consultation is generally sought by the primary-care physician, geriatrician, or neurologist who has made the diagnosis. Although the results of the communication assessment may be used for differential diagnosis, it is more likely that results will be used to evaluate the patient's progression in the course of the dementia. To this end, the communication assessment must be viewed in terms of other measures of psychological, cognitive, and medical status.

The third premise is that a communication assessment of dementia must be broadly based and move beyond traditional linguistic measures. There are several reasons that this premise is important. Communication is considered to be the most complex organizational and interactive behavior of human beings. Breakdowns in the ability to use language successfully and appropriately offer insight into the underlying cognitive decline of these persons.[95,114] Alzheimer's patients' communication abilities also may be closely tied to other abilities for functional living as well as to their rate of mortality.[60] Loss or disruption of abilities in communication frequently leads to institutionalization. For these reasons, understanding of communication abilities would better enable us to ascertain and predict the course of the patient care needs. A recommended battery for communication assessment that includes measures of language and functional communication abilities will be presented and its rationale discussed.

## Assessment and Initial Evaluation of Dementia

A complete evaluation for dementia should include (1) a careful and thorough case history; (2) neurologic and medical diagnostic studies and examination; (3) behavioral assessment; and (4) communication assessment. The selection of tests should be judiciously made by an interdisciplinary team based on the patient's cognitive skills and ability to participate and tolerate the testing situation. The following sections detail important considerations in each of these areas of assessment.

## CASE HISTORY INTERVIEW

The case history may be taken by the physician, nurse, social worker, neuropsychologist, SLP, audiologist, or other qualified health-care professional. If there is no case history or there is missing information at the time of the speech and language or audiologic evaluation, then a history should be completed by the SLP or audiologist. It is crucial that the history be fully developed because of the role the information plays in the diagnosis. Because no peripheral marker for DAT is presently known, diagnosis depends on a variety of different kinds of information that allows the exclusion of other possible causes for the presenting symptoms. Historical data are important to the SLP in the assessment process because they provide information describing the communication contexts and communicative demands encountered by the patient on a daily basis.

### Interviewing Considerations

History taking with demented patients is difficult because of the memory, attention, and language problems associated with this disorder. A family member, the caregiver, or close friend must serve as the informant or co-informant along with the patient. It may be helpful to have additional family members corroborate or expand on the essential information because of the various perspectives they may have on the patient's history and present problems.[1] Caregivers, family members, and friends should be interviewed separately from the patient. Otherwise, these persons may be reticent about revealing patient information important for diagnosis and assessment. Further, it is important to keep in mind that the interview may be a threatening experience for the patient, the family member, and the caregiver.[100] A friendly, accepting approach and a quiet, patient tone are essential. The basic considerations of the environment, e.g., low background noise levels, light on the face of the interviewer, comfortable seating, and privacy should be addressed. Readers are directed to Burnside for a full discussion of environmental factors to be considered in interviews with older adults.[23]

### Areas of Assessment

A complete history should include information in the areas of health, psychological, cognitive, social, and communication status, as well as any special problems that may be occurring. An *Alzheimer Dementia Risk Questionnaire* developed by Breitner and Folstein is a useful guide for conducting a full history of education, work, family, course of DAT, and present symptoms (see Appendix at the end of the chapter).[20]

**Health Status.** Health status information is generally available from medical reports; however, this is not always the case. The questions employed in this section of the interview are designed to clarify the patient's medical history and to provide a comprehensive picture of any present problems. Because older adults frequently have chronic health problems and often take medication to regulate these conditions, the health status questions must go beyond the presenting dementia symptoms and examine overall health.

**Cognitive-Psychological Status.** Obtaining a good cognitive history is difficult because although family and caregivers can provide general information, often they are not aware of small changes in cognitive abilities. In addition, they may not want to acknowledge or be aware of episodes such as forgetting which direction to hit the golf ball on the course as important case-history information. The loss of spatial awareness, for example, may not result directly from memory impairment and is an important indicator of cognitive status. A complete and thorough history of psychological and psychiatric problems is essential because symptoms of geriatric depression are similar to some observed in early-stage dementia. Feedback regarding onset and progression of symptoms helps assess what role, if any, depression may play in the patient's behavior. Wells' chart (see Table 13.4) for comparing and contrasting dementia and the dementia syndrome of depression, or pseudodementia as it is often termed, relies on information obtained from the case interview.[42,119,120]

**Social Status.** Three major areas need to be addressed in this section of the case interview: (1) daily living arrangements and interactions; (2) family attitudes toward and knowledge of the patient's situation; and (3) caregiver stress and burden resulting from and impacting on the patient.

A description of the patient's life-style, e.g., typical daily activities, living situation, and number of social contacts daily, provides a frame of reference for the social environment. The social status information regarding the patient's role in the family and the family's attitudes toward illness are particularly useful in that they can guide the interpretation of the rest of the case history report. By understanding the patient's family social culture we gain insight into the patient's communication context. For example, does the family deal with illness and problems through denial, blame, anger, or guilt? Some of the family's presenting attitudes may result from the role the patient previously played within the family unit. It is important to assess the caregivers' and family's level of knowledge of dementia. Their knowledge of the symptom complex of the dementia as well as its course may affect their interaction with and view of the patient. Haley, Brown, and Levine report that caregivers value knowledge regarding the symptom complex dementia.[51] They also value information regarding the coping skills that they as caregivers may need to deal with problems that arise from the dementia.

Assessing caregiver stress and burden can give insight into the impact of the patient's illness on the family.[126] Kinney and Stephens have developed a *Caregiving Hassles Scale*, a self-report rating questionnaire focused on the day-to-day experience of caregiving for demented patients.[64] Several of the items deal directly with communication (e.g., the care recipient asking repetitive questions or the care recipient talking about things that aren't real). This, or a similar rating scale, is a useful tool in the case interview, for it helps illuminate the social context in which the patient is living. Chapter 11 provides lists of other stress and burden measures and a detailed picture of the role of the caregiver with the demented patient.

**Communication Status.** The interview segment dealing with communication status involves questions regarding hearing, communication environment, speech and language abilities, and functional communication. The basic questions asked in speech and language adult case histories are appropriate for these patients.[24] Chapter 16 on environmental considerations provides additional questions to ask.

**Special Problems.** This section of the case interview provides an opportunity for patients and caregivers to raise questions that are of special concern for them, such as the patient getting up in the night or the patient pretending to take medication. Questioning during this phase of the interview should be open ended to allow for the richest responses. For example, "What concerns you most about the patient's behavior?," "What puzzles you most?"

## MEDICAL AND NEUROLOGIC EVALUATION

### Medical Evaluation

In combination with a careful history, a physical and neurologic examination should be completed by the patient's primary physician, geriatrician, or a neurologist. The examination should include a series of diagnostic laboratory studies with certain ancillary studies when appropriate.[78,79] These recommended studies are listed in Table 13.5. This list should serve as a guide to the SLP for the sorts of tests required initially to identify dementia and differentiate among the various disease bases for dementia. Interpretation of these test results can only lead to a presumptive clinical diagnosis.[71] However, these results serve to rule out a variety of systemic diseases and disorders, as well as cerebrovascular diseases and conditions that may produce symptoms similar to those associated with DAT.

A physical examination is important to establish the status of sensory abilities, i.e., vision and hearing, and to evaluate motor abilities. (See Chapters 4 and 14 for audiologic considerations.) Because subcortical dementia patients and some DAT patients demonstrate extrapyramidal problems, assessment of gait, posture, and movement is important in differentiating among DAT, Parkinson's disease, and other dementias.[14,74] Referral to a physiatrist, physical therapist, or occupational therapist for in-depth evaluation of motor abilities may be useful.

## TABLE 13.5 Medical and Neurologic Diagnostic Studies

**BLOOD STUDIES**

Complete blood cell count
Sedimentation rate
Glucose
Urea nitrogen
Electrolytes
Calcium and phosphorus
Bilirubin
Thyroid function
Vitamin $B_{12}$ and folate

**RADIOGRAPHIC STUDIES**

Chest x-ray
Computed tomography of the brain

**OTHER STUDIES**

Electrocardiogram (possibly Holter monitor)
Urinalysis
Tests for syphilis
Tests for AIDS
Electroencephalogram

**OPTIONAL STUDIES**

Magnetic resonance imaging
Regional cerebral blood flow-positron emission tomography
Lumbar puncture

Adapted from National Institute on Aging Task Force. Senility reconsidered: Treatment possibilities for mental impairment in the elderly. JAMA 1980; 244:259–263. Also adapted from the National Institutes of Health Consensus Conference. JAMA 1987; 258(23):3411–3416.

### Neurologic Evaluation

Test result information is valuable to SLPs and may guide their diagnostic assessment process. In return, language test results can prove valuable to neurologists and physicians in their diagnostic process. Recent research in neurologic aspects of DAT has indicated specific associations between loss of language abilities and neurologic alterations.[3,65,83,84] Kasznik et al indicated that poor expressive language scores may predict a poor prognosis for survival in DAT.[60] For some as yet unknown reason, early brain deterioration in the dominant hemisphere language areas appears to be a prognostically bleak sign. Improved specification of relationships between communication and neurologic changes may prove useful in the prediction of long-term care needs of DAT patients.

The neurologic examination can be valuable in differential diagnosis because neurologic tests explore the characteristics of cerebrovascular disease and can be crucial in differential diagnosis of MID and DAT. For example, the sudden onset and stepwise progression of MID can be contrasted with the insidiously slow and steady progression of DAT, so that the course indicates the type of dementia. Also, computed tomography (CT) studies of DAT reveal that enlargement of the ventricles is a reflection of the presence of DAT. In some cases, CT scans are useful to identify individuals with DAT.[5] In addition, relationships between CT scan patterns and neuropsychologic test and rating results are beginning to be identified.[74] The narrower the range of scoring choices on the measure (e.g., *Global Deterioration Scale* or *Mini Mental-State Examination*) the more difficult it is to produce robust correlations. The *Weschler Memory Scale* and other measures with a broader range of scores allow for better correlations between CT patterns and behavioral measures.[4] Regional cerebral blood flow (rCBF) and positron emission tomography (PET) studies have proved helpful in diagnosis of the different dementias. Advances in these techniques should allow for more precision in studying the biochemical markers of dementia.

### BEHAVIORAL ASSESSMENT

Behavioral assessment can best be completed using three approaches: (1) performance on neuropsychological tests; (2) observation of behavior in natural contexts; and (3) reports from family members, friends, and caregivers regarding the patient's behavior. These three approaches provide a multimodal perspective of behavior. They allow a comprehensive assessment as well as provide data for cross checking performance by looking for confirming evidence across multiple behavior assessment methods.

Behavior assessments conducted by neuropsychologists normally generate considerable direct information concerning memory, attention, orientation, etc. and more cursory information regarding communication, language, and speech. In contrast, SLPs comprehensively assess communication, language, and speech functions and more generally examine the domains of overall cognitive status. The overlap and separation of assessment domains should be acknowledged and discussed by the professionals and a working alliance developed to optimize patient care.[98]

Collaborative work among SLPs, medical, and social-work professionals is generally not problematic. Porch and Haaland, however, contend that neuropsychologists and SLPs are not well trained for interdisciplinary work, and the result is often duplication of efforts and a competitive

| TABLE 13.6 | Behavior Assessment Measures for Use with Dementia Patients |
|---|---|

### INTELLIGENCE
Weschler Adult Intelligence Scale-Revised[117]

### MEMORY
Weschler Memory Scale-Revised[97]
Fuld Object Memory Test[45]
California Verbal Learning Test[34]
Benton Visual Retention Test[15]

### ABSTRACTION
Picture Absurdities of Stanford-Binet[108]

### MENTAL STATUS
Blessed Orientation and Memory Examination[17]
Mini Mental-State Examination[41]
Mental Status Questionnaire[58]

### BEHAVIOR RATING SCALES
Brief Cognitive Rating Scale[89]
Mattis Dementia Rating Scale[68]
Global Deterioration Scale[92]
Functional Assessment Stages[90]
Clinical Dementia Rating[57]

---

rather than cooperative approach to working with adult brain-impaired patients.[86] In the disciplines of speech language pathology and neuropsychology, emphasis on the collaborative nature of diagnosis and assessment in dementia could prove beneficial both for the professionals and the patients involved.

It is important that SLPs and audiologists be knowledgeable about behavioral tests and ratings scales for three reasons. First, results from these evaluations can help predict the course of the dementia. Second, these measures describe the patient's full range of behavioral functioning to aid in communication assessment and intervention. Finally, these results can support and aid the interpretation of language, communication, speech, and/or hearing findings. Table 13.6 lists the behavioral assessment measures recommended for use with dementia patients.

## NEUROPSYCHOLOGICAL ASSESSMENT

Neuropsychological performance tests provide objective and precise measurement of cognitive function; however, a major problem with their use is that they do not relate directly to functioning in practical situations, i.e., they lack ecological validity. For this reason, behavioral rating scales that illustrate actual behavioral features are an important addition to the assessment protocol. A multimodal assessment provides various perspectives on the patient's behavioral abilities necessary for a comprehensive description of functional behavior.

Given the complex and diverse nature of cognitive disturbances in dementia, intelligence and memory should be assessed. At present there are no specific standardized comprehensive psychometric tests for dementia or DAT so that batteries of tests designed to assess cognitive functioning are most often used. Bayles and Kaszniak provide a comprehensive review of neuropsychologic tests.[11] A neuropsychological test battery should include assessments of all the domains of intelligence and memory functioning with additional assessments of abstraction abilities. The Wechsler Adult Intelligence Scale Revised (WAIS-R) is the most frequently used instrument for documenting intellectual functioning.[117] Breakdown between verbally based abilities (verbal scale) and visuospatial and visuomotor skills (performance scale) may reflect lateralized versus diffuse brain dysfunction.[105] Individual subtest scores may reveal discrete areas of impairment such as construction (WAIS block design subtest) or cognitive flexibility (WAIS similarities and comprehension subtests).[9]

Both the Wechsler Memory Scale (WMS)[118] and the Revised Wechsler Memory Scale[97] are used to assess memory functioning. The Revised WMS has been shown to differentiate normal and demented persons.[67] Haaland, Linn, Hunt, and Goodwin developed norms for ages 65 to 80 years for the Revised WMS.[48] Although there are certain limitations to the application of these norms in that the volunteer subjects were better educated than the general population, they provide much-needed, age-appropriate data for interpretation of memory performances.[11] Other commonly used memory assessments are shown in Table 13.6.

In addition to the assessment of intelligence and memory, a neuropsychological battery should include tests to examine skills of abstraction, e.g., comprehension of proverbs, picture absurdities, etc. Both DAT and Pick's disease demonstrate problems in this area of cognitive functioning early in their course.[74] A complete neuropsychological assessment will generally evaluate visual field acuity and perception, fine motor skills, hearing acuity and discrimination, and written and oral language skills. However, a comprehensive assessment of hearing and language requires the services of an audiologist and speech language pathologist.

## Rating Scales

Mental status assessment may be completed using the *Blessed Orientation and Memory Examination*,[17] or Fuld's modification of this examination,[44] the *Mini Mental-State Examination* *(MMS)*,[41] or the *Mental Status Questionnaire (MSQ)*.[46] In addition to mental status assessment, a series of cognitive functioning rating scales provide systematic guides for measuring loss and/or maintenance of abilities. Information from the Blessed Orientation and Memory Examination pro-

TABLE 13.7 **Brief Cognitive Rating Scale (BCRS)**

| AXIS | RATING | ITEM |
|---|---|---|
| I. Concentration and calculating ability | 1 | No objective or subjective evidence of deficit in concentration |
| | 2 | Subjective decrement on concentration ability |
| | 3 | Minor objective signs of poor concentration (e.g., on subtraction of serial 7s from 100) |
| | 4 | Definite concentration deficit for persons of their background (e.g., marked deficit on serial 7s, frequent deficit in subtraction of serial 4s from 40) |
| | 5 | Marked concentration deficit (e.g., giving months backwards or serial 2s from 20) |
| | 6 | Forgets the concentration task Frequently begins to count forward when asked to count backwards from 10 by 1s |
| | 7 | Marked difficulty counting forward to 10 by 1s |
| II. Recent memory | 1 | No objective or subjective evidence of deficit in recent memory |
| | 2 | Subjective impairment only (e.g., forgetting names more often than formerly) |
| | 3 | Deficit in recall of specific events evident upon detailed questioning. No deficit in the recall of major recent events |
| | 4 | Cannot recall major events of previous weekend or week. Scanty knowledge (not detailed) of things such as current events or favorite TV shows |
| | 5 | Unsure of weather; may not know current president or current address |
| | 6 | Occasional knowledge of some recent events. Little or no idea of current address or weather |
| | 7 | No knowledge of any recent events |
| III. Remote memory | 1 | No subjective or objective impairment in past memory |
| | 2 | Subjective impairment only. Can recall two or more primary school teachers |
| | 3 | Some gaps in past memory upon detailed questioning. Able to recall at least one childhood teacher and/or one childhood friend |
| | 4 | Clear-cut deficit. The spouse recalls more of patient's past than the patient. Cannot recall childhood friends and/or teachers but knows the names of most schools attended. Confuses chronology in reciting personal history |
| | 5 | Major past events sometimes not recalled (e.g., names of schools attended) |
| | 6 | Some residual memory of past (e.g., may recall country of birth or former occupation) |
| | 7 | No memory of past |
| IV. Orientation | 1 | No deficit in memory for time, place, identity of self or others |
| | 2 | Subjective impairment only. Knows time to nearest hour, location |
| | 3 | Any mistake in time: 2 hrs; day of week: 1 day; date: 3 days |
| | 4 | Mistakes in month: 10 days or year or month |
| | 5 | Unsure of month and/or year and/or season; unsure of locale |
| | 6 | No idea of date. Identifies spouse but may not recall name. Knows own name |
| | 7 | Cannot identify spouse. May be unsure of personal identity |

*Table continues on following page*

TABLE 13.7 (continued)

| AXIS | RATING | ITEM |
|---|---|---|
| V. Functioning and self-care | 1 | No difficulty, either subjectively or objctively |
| | 2 | Complains of forgetting location of objects. Subjective work difficulties |
| | 3 | Decreased job functioning evident to co-workers. Difficulty in traveling to new locations |
| | 4 | Decreased ability to perform complex tasks (e.g., planning dinner for guests, handling finances, marketing) |
| | 5 | Requires assistance in choosing proper clothing |
| | 6 | Requires assistance in feeding, toileting, bathing, or dressing |
| | 7 | Requires constant assistance in all activities of daily living |

From Reisberg B. Alzheimer's disease: The standard reference. New York: The Free Press, a division of Macmillan, Inc. 1983:178–179. Copyright 1983 by Barry Reisberg, M.D., with permission.

vides data regarding habits and everyday activities, sometimes termed activities of daily living.[17] The *Brief Cognitive Rating Scale (BCRS)*, shown in Table 13.7, is a rapid, structured instrument for assessing cognitive decline, regardless of etiology.[89] Items are organized into five categories or Axes: Axis I Concentration and Calculating Ability, Axis II Recent Memory, Axis III Remote Memory, Axis IV Orientation, and Axis V Functioning and Self Care. Within each axis behaviors are scored from one to seven, with one being the least impaired and seven being the most impaired. Each score is related to distinguishable levels of functioning within the category.

There are several observational rating scales designed specifically to evaluate the status of dementia patients. The *Mattis Dementia Rating Scale* is widely used.[68] Although it is not useful for differential diagnosis, it can be used through the late stages of the disease when patients often become untestable by other instruments.

The *Global Deterioration Scale (GDS) for Age Related Cognitive Decline and Alzheimer's Disease* shown in Table 13.8 is a scale of seven stages designed to parallel the seven levels within each of the five axis categories of the Brief Cognitive Rating Scale.[92] During Stage 1 there is no cognitive decline, and this rating should be supported by normal WAIS vocabulary and Mini Mental-State Exam scores. Stage 2, very mild cognitive decline and forgetfulness, should be supported by normal Mini Mental-State Exam, slightly depressed Wechsler Adult Intelligence Scale vocabulary scores, and, in the language area, the forgetting of names formerly well known. In Stage 3, the mild cognitive decline and early confusional phase, patients will still maintain at a borderline normal level on the Mini Mental-State Exam, but Wechsler Adult Intelligence Scale vocabulary scores are generally one standard deviation below normal. Word-finding and naming deficits are apparent to intimates, and memory for things read declines at this stage. Stage 4, the moderate cognitive decline and late confusional phase, is sometimes termed the "predementia" phase. Here the Mini Mental-State Exam will generally show a slightly depressed score (28 to 26). Stage 5 indicates moderately severe decline and early dementia. Almost all patients who reach this stage continue to decline. At Stage 6 patients show severe cognitive decline and middle dementia. In Stage 7, a very severe decline and late dementia generally correspond to the loss of all verbal abilities.

Although there is great variability in the presentation and progression of DAT, as well as difficulty differentiating the latter stages of symptoms, developing distinct stages of the illness has utility.[74] The Functional Assessment Stages (FAST) shown in Table 13.9 distinguish 15 distinct progressive characteristics of the disease.[90] These characteristics can be related to the seven stages within the Global Deterioration Scale and levels within Axis V, Functioning and Self Care, of the Brief Cognitive Rating Scale.

It is proposed that patients with uncomplicated DAT typically proceed on a linear course through the characteristics of decline. The authors contend that the linear progression of functional loss outlined in this scale can prove useful in the differential diagnosis process. For example, if patients show fecal incontinence (GDS Stage 6) but maintain the ability to plan marketing (GDS Stage 4), something other than DAT may be causing the incontinence. In contrast, a pattern of decline by stages outlined in the FAST suggests uncomplicated DAT. The recognition of these distinct stages of DAT is clearly an advance in enabling clinicians to identify the precise magnitude of the impair-

TABLE 13.8 **Global Deterioration Scale (GDS) for Age-Associated Cognitive Decline and Alzheimer's Disease**

| GDS STAGE | CLINICAL PHASE | CLINICAL CHARACTERISTICS |
|---|---|---|
| 1. No cognitive decline | Normal | No subjective complaints of memory deficit. No memory deficit evident on clinical interview |
| 2. Very mild cognitive decline | Forgetfulness | Subjective complaints of memory deficit, most frequently in following areas: (1) forgetting where one has placed familiar objects; and (2) forgetting names one formerly knew well. No objective evidence of memory deficit on clinical interview. No objective deficit in employment or social situations. Appropriate concern with respect to symptomatology. |
| 3. Mild cognitive decline | Early confusional | Earliest clear-cut deficits. Manifestations in more than one of the following areas: (1) patient may have gotten lost when traveling to an unfamiliar location; (2) co-workers become aware of patient's relatively poor performance; (3) word- and name-finding deficits become evident to intimates; (4) patient may read a passage or a book and retain relatively little material; (5) patient may demonstrate decreased facility in remembering names upon introduction to new people; (6) patient may have lost or misplaced an object of value; (7) concentration deficit may be evident in clinical testing |
| | | Objective evidence of memory deficit obtained only with an intensive interview conducted by a trained geriatric psychiatrist. Decreased performance in demanding employment and social settings. Denial begins to become manifest in patient. Mild to moderate anxiety accompanies symptoms |
| 4. Moderate cognitive decline | Late confusional | Clear-cut deficit on careful clinical interview. Deficit manifest in following areas: (1) decreased knowledge of current and recent events; (2) may exhibit some deficit in memory of one's personal history; (3) concentration deficit elicited on serial subtractions; (4) decreased ability to travel, handle finances, etc. |
| | | Frequently no deficit in following areas: (1) orientation to time and person; (2) recognition of familiar persons and faces; (3) ability to travel to familiar locations |
| | | Inability to perform complex tasks. Denial is dominant defense mechanism. Flattening of affect and withdrawal from challenging situations occur |
| 5. Moderately severe decline | Early dementia | Patient can no longer survive without some assistance. Patient is unable during interview to recall a major, relevant current aspect of their life, e.g., their address or telephone number of many years, the names of close members of their family (such as grandchildren), or the name of the high school or college from which they graduated |

*Table continues on following page*

| TABLE 13.8 (continued) | | |
|---|---|---|
| **GDS STAGE** | **CLINICAL PHASE** | **CLINICAL CHARACTERISTICS** |
| | | Frequently some disorientation to time (date, day of week, season) or to place. An educated person may have difficulty counting back from 40 by 4s or from 20 by 2s |
| | | Persons at this stage retain knowledge of many major facts regarding themselves and others. They invariably know their own names and generally know their spouses, and children's names. They require no assistance with toileting or eating, but may have some difficulty choosing the proper clothing to wear |
| 6. Severe cognitive decline | Middle dementia | May occasionally forget the name of the spouse upon whom they are entirely dependent for survival. Will be largely unaware of all recent events and experiences in their lives. Retain some knowledge of their past lives but this is very sketchy. Generally unaware of their surroundings, i.e., the year or the season. May have difficulty counting from 10, both backward and sometimes forward. Will require some assistance with activities of daily living, e.g., may become incontinent, will require travel assistance but occasionally will display ability to travel to familiar locations. Diurnal rhythm frequently disturbed. Almost always recall their own name. Frequently continue to be able to distinguish familiar from unfamiliar persons in their environment |
| | | Personality and emotional changes occur. These are quite variable and include: (1) delusional behavior, e.g., patients may accuse their spouse of being an impostor, may talk to imaginary figures in the environment or to their own reflection in the mirror; (2) obsessive symptoms, e.g., person may continually repeat simple cleaning activities; (3) anxiety symptoms, agitation and even previously nonexistent violent behavior may occur; (4) cognitive abulia, i.e., loss of willpower because an individual cannot carry a thought long enough to determine a purposeful course of action |
| 7. Very severe cognitive decline | Late dementia | All verbal abilities are lost. Frequently there is no speech at all—only grunting. Incontinence of urine, requires assistance toileting and feeding. Loses basic psychomotor skills, e.g., ability to walk. The brain no longer appears to be able to tell the body what to do |
| | | Generalized and cortical neurologic signs and symptoms |

From Reisberg B, Ferris SH, De Leon MJ, Crook T. The global deterioration scale for assessment of primary degenerative dementia. Am J Psychiatry 1982; 139:1136–1139.

ment as well as help in the differential diagnosis of DAT. FAST is particularly useful in the later stages of the disease when other measures may not carefully identify the magnitude of the breakdown.

The *Clinical Dementia Rating* (CDR) offers a rating from 0 (healthy), .5 (questionable), 1 (mild dementia), 2 (moderate dementia) to 3 (severe dementia) across six categories: Memory, Orientation, Judgment, Community Affairs, Home and Hobbies, and Personal Care.[57] This scale is frequently used to stage patients for subject groups in dementia research. However, it is

TABLE 13.9 **Functional Assessment Stages (FAST) in Normal Aging and Alzheimer's Disease**

| GLOBAL DETERIORATION SCALE | CLINICAL PHASE | FAST CHARACTERISTICS |
|---|---|---|
| No cognitive decline | Normal | No functional decrement either subjectively or objectively manifest |
| Very mild cognitive decline | Forgetfulness | Complains of forgetting locations of objects; subjective work difficulties |
| Mild cognitive decline | Early confusional | Decreased functioning in demanding employment settings evident to co-workers; difficulty in traveling to new locations |
| Moderate cognitive decline | Late confusional | Decreased ability to perform complex tasks such as planning dinner for guests, handling finances, and marketing |
| Moderately severe cognitive decline | Early dementia | Requires assistance in choosing proper clothing, may require coaxing to bathe properly |
| Severe cognitive decline* | Middle dementia | Difficulty putting on clothing properly; requires assistance bathing, may develop fear of bathing; inability to handle mechanics of toileting; urinary incontinence; fecal incontinence |
| Very severe cognitive decline* | Late dementia | Limited ability to speak; all intelligible vocabulary lost; all motoric abilities lost; stupor; comatose |

*Characteristics in Stages 6 and 7 correspond to Axis 5, functioning and self-care, in the Brief Cognitive Rating Scale. From Reisberg B, Ferris SH, Anand R, et al. Functional staging of dementia of the Alzheimer's type. Ann NY Acad Sci 1984; 435:481–486.

interesting to note that this scale does not include communication as a domain to be rated.

In summary, clinical assessment of behavior should include a comprehensive history and a series of recommended medical studies. In addition, neuropsychological instruments such as the Wechsler Adult Intelligence Scale-Revised, the Wechsler Memory Scale-Revised, as well as abstract thinking, visual, motor, and general hearing and language tests should be completed. Observational assessments of mental status are valuable. The Blessed Orientation and Memory Examination, the Mini Mental-State, Mental Status Questionnaire, and the Brief Cognitive Rating Scale all fulfill this requirement. Rating of stage of decline in dementia can be accomplished using the Mattis Dementia Scale, Global Deterioration Scale, Functional Assessment Stages, and Clinical Dementia Rating. These behavioral assessment tools provide information to complement the findings of the case histories and medical diagnostic studies.

## Language and Communication Assessment

Numerous investigations of aspects of language in dementia can be found in the literature. However, to date no comprehensive examinations of communication deficits or competence have been conducted.[11] Additionally, no normative data for evaluating the performance of individuals with dementia on functional communication tasks are available.[43,54] Although declines in phonology, syntax, and semantics have been well documented,[8,10,76,99] recent studies of communicative skills indicate that the degree of the decline in communication abilities seems to exceed the decline in specific language domains.[43,94,115] Therefore, a complete description of communication impairments in DAT would require a shift to a view of communicative competence encompassing more than simply linguistic competence. A comprehensive, valid, and reliable assessment of the breadth of communicative abilities should include evaluation of a range of pragmatic and discourse features (e.g., topic, repairs, cohesion and coherence, communicative acts, propositions, and organizational schemas) in addition to assessment of phonologic, syntactic, and semantic domains.[11]

## LANGUAGE AND COMMUNICATION MEASURES

### Conceptual Model and Rationale

The assessment battery presented here is designed to address the communication abilities of dementia patients based on conceptual models of language processing that includes "top down" (knowledge-driven) and "bottom up" (data-driven) organization.[33,66] These models are relevant to the study of dementia because they consider the language features more vulnerable to cognitive dissolution (i.e., knowledge-based pragmatics and semantics) as well as those that are better maintained (i.e., data-driven syntax and phonology).

The assessment battery presented in the following section is based on the principle that communication should be assessed across a variety of contexts or genres. In addition, it meets the present six principles for the composition of a test battery in dementia proposed by Bayles and Kaszniak: (1) measures should assess aspects of semantic memory (e.g., concepts, schemas, etc.); (2) the language tasks should include processing of inferences and generation of ideas; (3) the units of language analyzed should be longer than a sentence; (4) the assessment should include the study of discourse in an ecologically valid context such as conversation; (5) measures should test nonautomatic processes, such as pragmatics and semantics versus the more automatic processes of syntax and phonology; (6) the assessment should require active participation by the patient so that creative and generative communication occurs.[11] Using all of these principles as a guide, the following battery is recommended for assessing language and communication.

**Test Considerations**

A comprehensive evaluation of communication decline should include a standardized test of linguistic competence that assesses oral and written language production and comprehension, as well as additional tests for specific language problems in pragmatics, semantics, syntax and phonology, and finally a language memory task. Table 13.10 lists recommended assessment tools for measuring communication abilities.

The language and communication assessment battery described in this chapter is designed to be administered in approximately 2 hours. It may be completed across several sessions if necessary. The testing environment is critical to communication assessment. Consideration should be given to lighting, noise levels, temperature, and the comfort level of the seating arrangement. All of these fac-

TABLE 13.10 **Language and Communication Assessment Measures for Use with Dementia Patients**

| LEVEL | BEHAVIOR | MEASURE |
|---|---|---|
| I. Comprehensive | Receptive and expressive oral and written language | Arizona Battery for Communication Disorders of Dementia[11] Boston Diagnostic Aphasia Examination[47] Western Aphasia Battery[62] Porch Index of Communication Ability[85] |
| II. Pragmatics and discourse | Schemata Turn taking Topic management Conversational repair Speech act use Paralinguistic Nonlinguistic Cohesion and coherence | Discourse Abilities Profile[109] |
| III. Semantics | Lexical comprehension | Peabody Picture Vocabulary Test[38] |
| | Confrontation naming | Boston Naming Test[89] |
| | Word fluency | FAS Word Fluency Measure[19] |
| IV. Syntax | Sentence comprehension | Auditory Comprehension Test for Sentences[101] |
| | Sentence comprehension Sentence formulation | Token Test[35] Reporter's Test[36] |
| V. Phonology | Word production | Boston Diagnostic Aphasia Examination (Subtest III)[47] |
| VI. Memory and language | Delayed story retelling | Completeness of novel story retold after 1 hour |

tors can contribute to fatigue in the patient. It is also important that the patient is rested, nourished, and toileted so that internal distractions do not interfere with performance.

A critical consideration in testing older adults is their motivation to complete the test. DAT patients often require encouragement to respond. These patients, along with most normal elders, want to prove they can perform well but fear making errors. They may experience high test anxiety, particularly if they have insight into their own confusion and are unable to respond with confidence on many items. For these reasons, a supportive test atmosphere should be developed for dementia patients.

A hearing screening for pure tones and speech discrimination should be completed by the speech-language pathologist prior to any communication assessment. It is preferable to have hearing evaluated by an audiologist if possible. A vision screening may be completed by asking patients to recognize line drawings from practice items on the *Peabody Picture Vocabulary Test (PPVT)*.[38] Ideally, an ophthalmologist or optometrist specializing in testing demented patients should evaluate visual performance and identify the presence of visual problems such as cataracts, glaucoma, macular degeneration, and visual perception abnormalities.

## Comprehensive Language Tests

Although no standardized battery of measures of communication is presently available, the *Arizona Battery for Communication Disorders of Dementia (ABCD)* is in the process of being standardized.[11] This battery of linguistic and nonlinguistic based subtests examines communication problems in dementia and is outlined in Table 13.11. The *ABCD* expands the language measures of most standardized aphasia tests in that it evaluates memory, linguistic reasoning, and visuospatial abilities. The relationship of these tasks to those of primarily linguistic skills offers valuable information regarding language and cognitive status.

Standardized tests of aphasia (e.g., *Boston Diagnostic Aphasia Examination*,[47] *Western Aphasia Battery*,[62] and *Porch Index of Communicative Ability*[85]) provide an evaluation of breakdowns in linguistic functioning across domains in receptive and expressive contexts. A discussion of patterns of performance of DAT patients on these tests is found in Bayles and Kaszniak.[11] Aphasia tests are designed to assess the linguistic skills of individuals with focal brain damage and therefore may not address the more generalized cognitive deficits and disturbances in functioning of dementia patients. However, as pointed out in the discussion of the ABCD, measures of general linguistic abilities in dementia patients are useful when interpreted in light of other communication, neuropsychological, and behavioral performances.

## Pragmatics

A critical level of assessment is pragmatics, perhaps the most central and regulative portion of the language system.[88] This domain of communication is particularly relevant to the diagnosis and assessment of dementia in that a decline in pragmatics appears to affect functional communication. Assessment of pragmatics requires that SLPs incorporate into their protocols what is presently known about the requirements for successful discourse production.

The *Discourse Abilities Profile (DAP)* serves as a format for organizing and recording observa-

---

**TABLE 13.11 Arizona Battery for Communication Disorders (ABCD) of Dementia**

**SENSORY PERCEPTION**

Auditory Discrimination

**RECEPTIVE LANGUAGE**

Peabody Picture Vocabulary Test
Reading comprehension
   Words
   Sentences
   Paragraphs
Sentence disambiguation
   Nonoral

**EXPRESSIVE LANGUAGE**

Oral description of objects
Pantomime expression
Drawing
FAS verbal fluency
Sentence disambiguation
   Oral
Oral discourse
Written discourse

**RECEPTIVE AND EXPRESSIVE**

Repetition

**ORIENTATION AND MEMORY**

Mental Status Test (MST)
Story retelling
   Immediate
   Delayed
Recognition memory
   Spatial
   Verbal

Adapted from Bayles KA, Kaszniak AW. Communication and cognition in normal aging and dementia. Boston: College-Hill Press, 1987:185.

**TABLE 13.12 Discourse Abilities Profile**

Client _____ Date _____
Clinician _____
Co-participants* _____

**Introductory Interview***: "Tell me about (topic)." (Circle the topics introduced)
    Family        Health        Daily activities        Hobbies

**Narrative discourse**: "Tell me something interesting that happened to you when you were growing up."
Discourse Features

| | Present | Absent |
|---|---|---|
| Abstract | _____ | _____ |
| Setting | _____ | _____ |
| Episode | | |
|   Initiating Event | _____ | _____ |
|   Internal Response | _____ | _____ |
|   Plan | _____ | _____ |
|   Attempt | _____ | _____ |
|   Consequence | _____ | _____ |
|   Reaction | _____ | _____ |
| | # Features present | |

Overall rating of narrative ability (Circle one):
    Excellent        Good       Adequate       Fair       Poor

**Procedural discourse**: "Tell me how to make toast and jelly."
Discourse Features

| | Present | Absent |
|---|---|---|
| Essential Steps | | |
|   Get bread | _____ | _____ |
|   Get jelly | _____ | _____ |
|   Get toaster | _____ | _____ |
|   Toast bread | _____ | _____ |
| Target Step | | |
|   Put jelly on bread | _____ | _____ |
| Optional Steps | | |
| | # Features present | |

Overall rating of narrative ability (Circle one):
    Excellent        Good       Adequate       Fair       Poor

**Spontaneous conversation** (3 to 5 minutes): Initially, clinician should make statement (no direct yes/no questions) that introduces a common topic, e.g., weather, local sports. Clinician should also allow conversational space so the client has opportunity to introduce topics. Remember this is *interactive conversation*, not an interview
Discourse features

| | Present | Absent | No opportunity |
|---|---|---|---|
| Turn-taking skills | | | |
|   Takes turns | _____ | _____ | _____ |
|   Relinquishes turn | _____ | _____ | _____ |
|   Appropriate turn length | _____ | _____ | _____ |
| Topic skills | | | |
|   Initiation | _____ | _____ | _____ |
|   Maintenance | _____ | _____ | _____ |
|   Shift/Transitions | _____ | _____ | _____ |
| Conversational repair | | | |
|   Requests clarification | _____ | _____ | _____ |
|   Clarifies | _____ | _____ | _____ |
| Speech acts | | | |
|   Responses | _____ | _____ | _____ |
|   Requests | _____ | _____ | _____ |
|   Assertions | _____ | _____ | _____ |
| | # Features present | | |

Overall rating of narrative ability (Circle one):
    Excellent        Good       Adequate       Fair       Poor

*Table continues on following page*

## TABLE 13.12 (continued)

**General discourse rating:** Rate discourse abilities in each of the following areas based on performance in previous sections

Paralinguistic behavior, e.g., stress, intonation, and rate (Circle one):
    Excellent      Good      Adequate      Fair      Poor

Nonlinguistic behavior, e.g., eye contact and gestures (Circle one):
    Excellent      Good      Adequate      Fair      Poor

Coherence, e.g., appropriate use of pronouns, articles, or ellipsis (Circle one):
    Excellent      Good      Adequate      Fair      Poor

### Discourse Abilities Profile
### Scoring Summary

|  | # Features present | Overall rating | Quadrant |
|---|---|---|---|
| Narrative discourse | /8 | | |
| Procedural discourse | /5 | | |
| Spontaneous conversation | /11 | | |
| General discourse | | Rating | |
|   Paralinguistic | | | |
|   Nonlinguistic | | | |
|   Coherence | | | |

### Scoring Matrix

| 1 FEATURES<br>More than half present<br>RATING:<br>Adequate, good, excellent | 2 FEATURES<br>Half or less present<br>RATING:<br>Adequate, good, excellent |
|---|---|
| 3 FEATURES<br>More than half present<br>RATING:<br>Poor or fair | 4 FEATURES<br>Half or less present<br>RATING:<br>Poor or fair |

---

tions of patients during interactions.[109] The DAP form is shown in Table 13.12. The profile can serve as a quick way of structuring informal observations of naturally occurring interactions between patients and clinicians. In addition, the DAP can be used when observing interactions between the patient and his or her spouse, caregiver, or other persons. The DAP can be administered by SLPs or trained health professionals such as social workers, nurse clinicians, and psychologists. A comprehensive discussion of DAP can be found in Terrell and Ripich.[109]

**Organization.** The DAP is divided into four sections. Three of these sections correspond to three genres of discourse: narrative (Section I), procedures (Section II), and spontaneous conversation (Section III). In each of these sections specific discourse features of the genre are delineated. Space is provided on the profile form (Part A of each section) to indicate whether the discourse features were present or absent during the client's performance. In addition, the clinician may indicate his or her overall rating (Part B of each section) of the patient's performance for each genre (excellent, good, adequate, fair, poor).

Section IV of the DAP (general discourse rating) corresponds to those general discourse features (i.e., paralinguistic behavior, nonlinguistic behavior, and coherence) that are required for successful discourse regardless of genre. Performances within these domains are rated as excellent, good, adequate, fair, or poor. The rating of general discourse features is based on the clinician's judgment of adequacy across all three genres (narrative, procedures, and spontaneous conversation). A separate rating is given for each of the three dimensions.

**DAP Scores.** Results of a study comparing 12 normal elderly (NE) and 12 DAT (early and middle stage) patients on the DAP are shown in Table 13.13.[93] The DAT patients performed more poorly

TABLE 13.13 **Discourse Abilities Profile: Results Comparing Normal Elderly (NE) and Alzheimer's Disease (DAT) Subjects**

| Quadrant 1 | NE | DAT | Quadrant 2 | NE | DAT |
|---|---|---|---|---|---|
| Narrative | 8 | 4 | Narrative | 2 | 1 |
| Procedural | 12 | 5 | Procedural | 0 | 2 |
| Conversational | 12 | 9 | Conversational | 0 | 0 |
| Quadrant 3 | NE | DAT | Quadrant 4 | NE | DAT |
| Narrative | 0 | 0 | Narrative | (2)0 | (1)6 |
| Procedural | 0 | 0 | Procedural | 0 | (1)4 |
| Conversational | 0 | 3 | Conversational | 0 | 0 |

| General Discourse Ratings | | |
|---|---|---|
| | NE | AD |
| Excellent | 3 | 0 |
| Good | 9 | 3 |
| Adequate | 0 | 6 |
| Fair | 0 | 3 |
| Poor | 0 | 0 |

( ) Denotes number of clients who refused task

than the normals on all areas of assessment. Results show that performance of the NE subjects cluster in quadrant one (96 percent), and performance of DAT subjects is distributed across all four quadrants (quadrant 1: 52 percent, quadrant 2: 9 percent, quadrant 3: 9 percent, quadrant 4: 30 percent). (Note: Quadrant 1 represents the most competent performance and quadrant 4 indicates the least competent performance.) This pattern supports the view that DAT patients show a general decline in mental functions and a heterogeneity of performance.[52] Examination of specific tasks shows differing levels of performance across genres. Significant differences in performance by the two groups on the procedural instruction tasks were shown. The narratives showed a trend toward significant differences, and the conversation was the most similar. The conversation genre resulted in the best performances for both NE and DAT subjects.

Narrative tasks were the most difficult for both subject groups. The narrative was the only genre on which NE subjects showed less than adequate structure (i.e., half or fewer elements). The grammars and hierarchic structures of stories appear to be the most difficult genre for both subject groups to generate. More DAT subjects showed both incomplete structure and less than adequate ratings (i.e., quadrant 4) on the narrative task than on procedural or conversational tasks. In contrast to the narratives' hierarchical form, the organizing structure of procedures is linear; i.e., one act is sequentially tied to the next. Conversation requires a third interactive type of structure. The similarity of performance between groups on the conversation task may be a result of the dialogic structure of the interaction compared to the monologues used for narrative and procedures. In conversation, partners act jointly to generate and develop the exchange. One can speculate that DAT subjects may be able to follow the flow of ideas in dialogue but have difficulty generating features in a monologue (e.g., narratives and procedures). Several other distinctions between conversation and the other two genres are apparent. Conversational turns are normally brief, and, as such, attention and immediate and recent memories may be easier to maintain in this genre compared to the narrative and procedural genres. During conversations, DAT patients are not usually required to hold in mind a long set of instructions or a story plot. Instead they need to focus on the adjacent turns within the conversational topic immediately occurring. Related to this is the idea that conversations may be highly relevant and context specific for DAT patients. Conversations may be more engaging and provide more motivation for participation.[63] The conversational task, on which the two subject groups clearly did not differ, did not correlate with any of the standardized tests. Based on these distinctions and together with the narrative and procedural results, we can speculate that this conversation task may measure communication abilities different from those measured in either the narrative or procedural genres.

The general discourse ratings of paralinguistic, nonlinguistic, and coherence aspects showed all NE subjects to be good or excellent. Although no DAT subjects were judged excellent, none were judged poor. Fifty percent were judged as adequate, 25 percent good, and 25 percent fair. These subjective ratings appear to correspond with the discourse feature scores on the individual genres.

This study confirms the view that differing patterns of discourse features occur in NE and DAT speakers across genres. Further, these findings extend our knowledge of the patterns of disruption and maintenance of communicative functions in DAT patients. Not only are linguistic deficits present in the communication of DAT patients, but discourse deficits occur as well. Further systematic examination of patterns of language and discourse abilities may yield important information regarding the relative contributions of both linguistic and discourse impairments to the dissolution of functional communication in DAT.

The pattern shown by DAT patients on the DAP represents a communication performance and impairments profile. These data, together with information gained through assessment of other dimensions of language ability, can assist in planning intervention. Interventions can be implemented for the patient and their social-support systems (caregivers, family, and friends) so that the patient may live in environments that facilitate maximum communicative effectiveness.

### Semantics

Assessment of semantic abilities using the Peabody Picture Vocabulary Test (PPVT),[38] the Boston Naming Test (BNT),[59] and/or the FAS Word Fluency Measure[19] is recommended. The PPVT is a recognition task and is sensitive to the kinds of recognition difficulties DAT patients experience. Bayles and associates found the PPVT to be one of the most discriminating measures between normal and mild DAT patients.[10] Although this recognition task is less active than the word fluency and generative naming task found on the FAS Word Fluency Measure, it has value as a diagnostic and assessment tool.[9] The FAS Word Fluency Measure assesses generative naming of words beginning with the letters F, A, and S. Expressive naming difficulties are an early presenting and persistent problem in DAT.[11] However, the heterogeneity of DAT patients' performances suggests it is important to examine individual as well as group patterns of error types.[103,107] Confrontation naming as examined by the BNT necessitates the recognition of the stimulus, recall of its linguistic elements, and production of the target item. Research shows confrontation naming errors result from disruptions in the semantic network.[104] DAT patients demonstrate poor generative naming early in the course of their illness,[81] poorer than their confrontation naming ability.[12]

### Syntax and Phonology

Although syntax and phonology are relatively well preserved in the early stages of dementia, additional information regarding expression and comprehension performance on these levels may be useful for some patients.[26] DAT patients' comprehension at the syntactic level shows a greater deficit on the BDAE[47] subtests and the auditory comprehension test of sentences (ACTS),[101] both initially and over time, as compared to single word comprehension scores on the PPVT.[11] The ACTS systematically varies word frequency, sentence length, and syntactic complexity. The short version of the *Token Test*, also a measure of sentence comprehension, allows assessment of mild syntactic errors and can be administered quickly.[35,106] The Token Test is sensitive to the mild auditory comprehension problems demonstrated in early dementia. The *Reporters Test* (short version), an expressive language task, is a measure of language formulation abilities.[36] This test uses the test stimuli from the Token Test and can elicit mild syntactic errors. Phonology can be assessed in the context of the words and sentences from subtest III on the Boston Diagnostic Aphasia Examination.[47]

### Memory and Language

A delayed recall task is an excellent way to assess the extent to which memory problems are impinging on language functioning. Across a period of approximately 1 hour, patients may be asked to remember a list of ten common words or retell a 70- to 100-word story as a way of assessing functional memory. Bayles et al found that after a lapse of 1 hour, DAT subjects remembered only 2 percent of a novel story compared to 96 percent of story features recalled by normal elderly during a delayed story retelling task.[10] It is beyond the scope of this chapter to address the complex area of memory and language. However, Moss and Albert[74] and Bayles and Kaszniak[11] provide extensive discussions of this area. (See also Chapter 3 for discussion of memory.)

### Concluding Remarks

In summary, a comprehensive language and communication assessment should include a standardized comprehensive language test; additional tests of pragmatics, semantic, syntactic, and phonologic abilities; and as assessment of memory and language. Tapping all these levels of functioning provides an overview of communicative performance and of impairments in dementia patients.

The model of diagnosis and assessment presented has been based on three premises. Diagnosis and assessment of dementia are complex tasks. In progressive disorders such as dementia, assessments must be an ongoing, dynamic part of intervention and treatment. Further, diagnosis and assessment require a multiple-perspective approach that includes a careful case history, medical studies, neuropsychological tests, and behavior ratings, in addition to hearing, language, and communication measures. The language and communication assessment must be broadly based and move beyond traditional linguistic measures to encompass pragmatic aspects of discourse if it is to accurately reflect the competence and impairments of patients with dementia. The underlying cognitive decline in dementia makes this broad approach requisite for comprehensive assessment. If these three premises are used as a basis for approaching both diagnosis and assessment, a successful evaluation of the parameters of dementia and communication is within reach.

## Future Research

### MULTIDISCIPLINARY APPROACHES

The interdependence of language and other cognitive functions requires that the research into communication abilities and exploration of other related areas such as memory and attention go hand in hand.[52,83] A multidisciplinary approach can assist in the identification of subgroups within the DAT population, particularly based on pattern and progression of language and communication impairments. These subgroups may provide valuable insight into the underlying patterns of cognitive loss in the dementias.

### BASIC RESEARCH

As stressed throughout this chapter, careful attention must be paid to differential diagnosis and assessment of dementia when DAT is suspected. Much research is being done to isolate causal factors. Future research will undoubtedly focus on biologic markers and genetic determinants of DAT, and the ultimate advance will be prevention of dementing diseases.[111]

### LANGUAGE AND DEMENTIA

The literature on language assessment raises numerous questions. Can we develop a screening test that would be useful in early identification of dementia patients? Given the heterogeneity of language decline in these patients, this becomes a daunting task. Can current linguistically based aphasia tests be expanded or modified to assess language in dementia, or will new assessment tools such as the ABCD and DAP prove to be the most useful measures? Can we develop a reliable measure of pragmatic abilities in dementia patients? Can we resolve the questions surrounding "word store" disorganization versus retrieval at the semantic level? Will research show that the mild syntactic and phonologic errors in DAT patients support the view that these parts of language can be processed with little awareness or intent? Finally, can different forms of DAT be identified through differential patterns of language involvement? Answers to these questions would shed light on our knowledge of how language and communication abilities are organized and have implications for linguistic and cognitive theory.

### References

1. Albert MS. Assessment of cognitive dysfunction. In: Albert MS, Moss MB, ed. Geriatric neuropsychology. New York: Guilford Press, 1988:57.
2. Albert MS, Butters N, Brandt J. Patterns of remote memory in amnesic and demented patients. Arch Neurol 1981; 38:495–500.
3. Albert M, Naeser MA, Levine HL, Garvey AJ. CT density numbers in patients with senile dementia of the Alzheimer's type. Arch Neurol 1984; 41:1264–1269.
4. Albert MS, Stafford JL. CT scan and neuropsychological relationships in aging and dementia. In: Goldstein G, Tarter R, eds. Advances in clinical neuropsychology. vol. 3. New York: Plenum Publishing, 1986:31.
5. Albert MS, Stafford JL. Computed tomography studies. In: Albert MS, Moss MB, eds. Geriatric neuropsychology. New York: Guilford Press, 1988:211.
6. Au R, Albert ML, Obler LK. The relationship of aphasia to dementia. Aphasiology 1988; 2:161–173.
7. Bartus RT, Dean RL, Beer B, Lippa AS. The cholinergic hypothesis of geriatric memory dysfunction. Science 1983; 217:408–417.
8. Bayles KA. Language function in senile dementia. Brain Lang 1982; 16:265–280.
9. Bayles KA. Management of neurogenic communication disorders associated with dementia. In: Chapey R, ed. Language intervention strategies in adult aphasia. 2nd ed. Baltimore: Williams & Wilkins, 1986:462–473.
10. Bayles KA, Boone DR, Tomoeda CA, Slauson TJ, Kaszniak AW. Differentiating Alzheimer's patients from the normal elderly and stroke patients with aphasia. J Speech Hear Disord 1989; 54:74–87.
11. Bayles KA, Kaszniak AW. Communication and cognition in normal aging and dementia. Boston: College-Hill Press, 1987.
12. Bayles KA, Tomoeda CK. Confrontation and generative naming abilities of dementia patients. In: Brookshire RH, ed. Clinical aphasiology conference proceedings. Minneapolis: BRK Publishers, 1983:304.

13. Bayles KA, Tomoeda CK, Caffrey JT. Language in dementia producing diseases. Commun Disord 1983; 7:131-146.
14. Beck JC, Benson DF, Scheibel AB, Spar JE, Rubenstein LZ. UCLA Conference—Dementia in the elderly: The silent epidemic. Ann Intern Med 1982; 97:231-241.
15. Benton AL. Revised visual retention test: Clinical and experimental application. 4th ed. New York: The Psychological Corporation, 1974.
16. Bissette G, Reynold GP, Kilts CD, Widerlov E, Nemeroff CB. Corticotropin-releasing factor-like immunoreactivity in senile dementia of the Alzheimer's type: Reduced cortical and striatal concentrations. JAMA 1985; 254:3067-3069.
17. Blessed G, Tomlinson BE, Roth M. The association between quantitative measures of dementia and of senile changes in the cerebral grey matter of elderly subjects. J Psychiatry 1968; 114:797-811.
18. Boller F, Passafiume D, Keefe NC et al. Visuospatial impairment in Parkinson's disease: Role of perceptual and motor factors. Arch Neurol 1984; 41:485-490.
19. Borkowski JG, Benton AL, Spreen O. Word fluency and brain damage. Neuropsychologia 1967; 5:135-140.
20. Breitner JC, Folstein M. A prevalent disorder with specific clinical features. Psychol Med 1984; 14:63-80.
21. Brun A, Englude E. Regional pattern of degeneration in Alzheimer's disease: Neuronal loss and histopathological grading. Histopathology 1981; 5:549-564.
22. Butler RN, Lewis MI. Aging and Mental Health. New York: A Plume Book, 1983.
23. Burnside IM. Psychological nursing care of the aged. New York: McGraw-Hill, 1980.
24. Chapey R. The assessment of language disorders in adults. In: Chapey R, ed. Language intervention strategies in adult aphasia. 2nd ed. Baltimore: Williams & Wilkins, 1986:126.
25. Cohen D, Eisdorfer C. Risk factors in late life dementias. In: Wertheimer J, Marois M, eds. Senile dementia: Outlook for the future. New York: Alan R. Liss, 1984:221-237.
26. Constantinidis J. Is Alzheimer's disease a major form of senile dementia? Clinical, anatomical, and genetic data. In: Katzman R, Terry RD, Bick KL, ed. Alzheimer's disease: Senile dementia and related disorders. New York: Raven Press, 1978:15.
27. Cummings JL. The dementias of Parkinson's disease: Prevalence, characteristics, neurobiology, and comparison with dementia of the Alzheimer type. European Neurol 1988; 28:15-23.
28. Cummings JL, Benson DF. Dementia: A clinical approach. Boston: Butterworth, 1983.
29. Cummings JL, Benson DF. Subcortical dementia: Review of an emerging concept. Arch Neurol 1984; 41:874-879.
30. Cummings JL, Benson DF, Hill MA, Read S. Aphasia and dementia of the Alzheimer type. Neurology 1985; 35:394-397.
31. Cummings JL, Darkins A, Mendez M, et al. Alzheimer's disease and Parkinson's disease: Comparison of speech and language alterations. Neurology 1988; 38:680-684.
32. Cummings JL, Duchen L. Kliver-Bucy syndrome in Pick's disease: Clinical and pathologic correlations. Neurology 1981; 31:1415-1422.
33. Danks J, Glucksberg S. Experimental psycholinguistics. Ann Rev Psychol 1980; 31:391-417.
34. Delis DC, Kramer JH, Kaplan E. California verbal learning test. New York: The Psychological Corporation, 1987.
35. DeRenzi E, Faglioni P. Normative data and screening power of a shortened version of the token test. Cortex 1978; 14:41-49.
36. DeRenzi E, Ferrari C. The reporter's test: A sensitive test to detect expressive disturbances in aphasics. Cortex 1978; 14:279-293.
37. Diagnostic and statistical manual of mental disorders. 3rd ed. Revised. Washington, D.C.: The American Psychiatric Association, 1987.
38. Dunn LM, Dunn LM. Peabody picture vocabulary test-revised. Circle Pines, MN: American Guidance Service, 1981.
39. Faber-Langendoen K, Morris JC, Knesevich JW, et al. Aphasia in senile dementia of the Alzheimer type. Ann Neurol 1988; 23:365-370.
40. Flowers KA, Pearce I, Pearce JMS. Recognition memory in Parkinson's disease. J Neurol Neurosurg Psychiatry 1984; 47:1174-1181.
41. Folstein MF, Folstein SE, McHugh PR. Mini mental-state: A practical method for grading the cognitive state of patients for the clinician. J Psychiatr Res 1975; 12:189-198.
42. Folstein MF, McHugh PR. Dementia syndrome of depression. In: Katzman R, Terry RD, Bick K, eds. Alzheimer's disease: Senile dementia and related disorders. New York: Raven Press, 1978:87.
43. Fromm D, Holland A. Functional communication in Alzheimer's disease. Paper presented at the annual convention of the American Speech-Hearing-Language Association. New Orleans, November, 1987.
44. Fuld PA. Psychological testing in differential diagnosis of dementias. In: Katzman R, Terry RD, Bick KL, ed. Alzheimer's disease: Senile dementia and related disorders. New York: Raven Press, 1978:185.
45. Fuld PA. Guaranteed stimulus processing in the evaluation of memory and learning. Cortex 1980; 16:255-271.
46. Goldfarb AI. Memory and aging. In: Goldman R, Rockstein M, eds. The physiology and pathology of human aging. New York: Academic Press, 1975.
47. Goodglass H, Kaplan E. The assessment of aphasia and related disorders. 2nd ed. Philadelphia: Lea & Febiger, 1983.
48. Haaland KY, Linn RT, Hunt WC, Goodwin JS. A normative study of Russell's variant of the Wechsler Memory Scale in healthy elderly population. J Consult Clin Psychol 1983; 51:878-881.
49. Hachinski VC, Iliff LD, Zilhka E, et al. Cerebral blood flow in dementia. Arch Neurol 1975; 32:632-637.
50. Hagnell O, Lanke J, Rorsman B, et al. Current trends in the incidence of senile and multi-infarct dementia. A prospective study of a total population over 25 years: The Lundby study. Arch Psychiatrie Nervenkrankheiten 1983; 233:423-438.
51. Haley WE, Brown L, Levine EG. Experimental evaluation of the effectiveness of group intervention for dementia caregivers. Gerontologist 1987; 21:353-358.
52. Hart S. Language and dementia: A review. Psychol Med 1988; 18:99-112.
53. Heyman A, Wilkinson WE, Hurwitz BJ, et al. Alzheimer's disease: Genetic aspects and associated clinical disorders. Ann Neurol 1983; 14:507-515.
54. Holland A. Language disorders in adults. San Diego: College-Hill Press, 1984.
55. Hollander E, Mohs RC, Davis KL. Antemortem mark-

ers of Alzheimer's disease. Neurobiol Aging 1986; 7:367-387.
56. Horner J. Language disorder associated with Alzheimer's dementia, left hemisphere stroke, and progressive illness of uncertain etiology. In: Brookshire RH, ed. Proceedings of the clinical aphasiology conference. Minneapolis: BRK Publishers, 1985:149.
57. Hughes CP, Berg L, Danziger WL, Coben LA, Martin RL. A new clinical scale for staging of dementia. Br J Psychiatry 1982; 140:566-572.
58. Kahn R, Goldfarb A, Pollack M, Peck A. Brief objective measures for the determination of mental status in the aged. Am J Psychiatry 1960; 117:326-328.
59. Kaplan E, Goodglass H, Weintraub S. Boston Naming Test. Philadelphia: Lea & Febiger, 1983.
60. Kaszniak AW, Fox J, Gandell DL, et al. Predictors of mortality in presenile and senile dementia. Ann Neurol 1978; 3:246-252.
61. Kennedy J, Fisher J, Shoulson I, Caine E. Language impairment in Huntington's disease. Neurology 1981; 31:81-82.
62. Kertesz A. Western aphasia battery. New York: Grune & Stratton, 1982.
63. Kimbarow ML. The pragmatic paradox. Paper presented at the Clinical Aphasiology Conference, Incline Village, NV, June, 1989.
64. Kinney JM, Stephens MAP. Caregiving hassles scale: Assessing the daily hassles of caring for a family member with dementia. Gerontologist 1989; 29:328-332.
65. Kirshner HS, Webb WG, Kelly MP, Wells CE. Language disturbance: An initial symptom of cortical degenerations and dementia. Arch Neurol 1984; 41:491-496.
66. Lemme M, Danes N. Models of auditory linguistic processing. In: Lass N, McReynolds L, Northern J, Yoder D, eds. Speech, language and hearing, Vol. 1.: Normal Processes. Philadelphia: W.B. Saunders, 1982:348.
67. Logue P, Wyrick L. Initial validation of Russell's revised Weschler Memory Scale: A comparison of normal aging versus dementia. J Consult Clin Psychol 1979; 47:176-178.
68. Mattis S. Mental status examination for organic mental syndrome in the elderly patient. In: Bellack R, Karasu B, eds. Geriatric psychiatry. New York: Grune & Stratton, 1976:77.
69. Mayeux R. Behavioral manifestations of movement disorders: Parkinson's and Huntington's disease. Neurol Clin 1984; 2:527-540.
70. Mayeux R, Stern Y, Rosen J, Leventhal J. Depression, intellectual impairment, and Parkinson disease. Neurology 1981; 31:645-650.
71. McKhann G, Drachman D, Folstein M, et al. Clinical diagnosis of Alzheimer's disease: Report of the NINCDS-ADRDA Work Group under the auspices of Department of Health and Human Services Task Force on Alzheimer's Disease. Neurology 1984; 34:939-944.
72. Mesulam MM. Slowly progressive aphasia without generalized dementia. Ann Neurol 1982; 22:533-534.
73. Molsa PK, Paljarvi L, Rinne JO, Rinne UK, Sako E. Validity of clinical diagnosis in dementia: A prospective clinicopathological study. J Neurol Neurosurg Psychiatry 1985; 48:1085-1090.
74. Moss MB, Albert MS. Alzheimer's disease and other dementing disorders. In: Albert MS, Moss MB, eds. Geriatric neuropsychology. New York: Guilford Press, 1988:145.
75. Moss RJ, Mastri AR, Schut LJ. The coexistence and differentiation of late onset Huntington's disease and Alzheimer's disease. J Am Geriatr Soc 1988; 36:237-241.
76. Murdoch BE, Chenery HJ, Wilks V, Boyle RS. Language disorders in dementia of the Alzheimer's type. Brain Lang 1987; 31:122-137.
77. Myers PS. Right hemisphere communication impairment. In: Chapey R, ed. Language intervention strategies in adult aphasia. 2nd ed. Baltimore: Williams & Wilkins, 1986:444.
78. National Institute of Health Consensus Conference. JAMA 1987; 258:3411-3416.
79. National Institute on Aging Task Force. Senility reconsidered: Treatment possibilities for mental impairment in the elderly. JAMA 1980; 244:259-263.
80. Neary D, Snoden JS, Northen B, Goulding P. Dementia of frontal lobe type. J Neurol Neurosurg Psychiatry 1988; 51:353-361.
81. Nebes RD, Brady CB. Integrity of semantic fields in Alzheimer's disease. Cortex 1988; 24:291-299.
82. Nicholas M, Obler LK, Albert ML, Helm-Estabrooks N. Empty speech in Alzheimer's disease and fluent aphasia. J Speech Hear Res 1985; 28:405-410.
83. Obler LK. Language and brain dysfunction in dementia. In: Segalowitz S, ed. Language functions and brain organization. New York: Academic Press, 1983:267.
84. Obler LK, Albert ML. Language and aging: A neurobehavioral analysis: In: Beasley DS, Davis GA, eds. Aging: Communication processes and disorders. New York: Grune & Stratton, 1981:107-121.
85. Porch BE. Porch index of communicative abilities. Palo Alto, CA: Consulting Psychologists Press, 1967.
86. Porch BE, Haaland KY. Neuropsychology and speech pathology: An examination of professional relationships as they apply to aphasia. In: Logue PE, Schear JM, ed. Clinical neuropsychology: A multidisciplinary approach. Springfield, IL: Charles C Thomas, 1984:239.
87. Powell AL, Cummings JL, Hill MA, Benson DF. Speech and language alterations in multi infarct dementia. Neurology 1988; 38:717-719.
88. Prutting C, Kirchner D. Applied pragmatics. In: Gallagher T, Prutting C, ed. Pragmatic assessment and intervention issues in language. San Diego: College-Hill Press, 1983.
89. Reisberg B. Alzheimer's disease: The standard reference. New York: The Free Press, 1983:178-179.
90. Reisberg G, Ferris SH, Anand R, et al. Functional staging of dementia of the Alzheimer's type. Ann NY Acad Sci 1984; 435:481-486.
91. Reisberg B, Ferris SH, Borenstein J, et al. Assessment of presenting symptoms. In: Poon LW, ed. Handbook for clinical memory assessment of older adults. Washington, D.C.: American Psychological Association, 1986.
92. Reisberg B, Ferris SH, DeLeon MJ, Crook T. The global deterioration scale for assessment of primary degenerative dementia. Am J Psychiatry 1982; 139:1136-1139.
93. Ripich D. Differential diagnosis in the assessment of dementia. Short course presentation at New York Speech and Hearing Association. Buffalo, NY, 1988.
94. Ripich D, Terrell B. Patterns of discourse cohesion and coherence in Alzheimer's disease. J Speech Hear Disord 1988; 53:8-15.
95. Ripich D, Terrell B, Spinelli F. Discourse cohesion in senile dementia of the Alzheimer's type. In: Brookshire RH, ed. Proceedings of the clinical aphasiology conference. Minneapolis: BRK Publishers, 1983:316.
96. Rogers D. Bradyphrenia in Parkinsonian patients. Neurology 1986; 45:447-450.

97. Russell EW. A multiple scoring method for the assessment of complex memory functions. J Consult Clin Psychol 1975; 43:800–809.
98. Schear JM, Skenes LL. The interface between clinical neuropsychology and speech-language pathology in the assessment of the geriatric patient. In: Ripich D, ed. The handbook of geriatric communication disorders. Boston: College-Hill Press (In press).
99. Schwartz M, Marin O, Saffran E. Dissociations of language function in dementia: A case study. Brain Lang 1979; 7:277–306.
100. Shadden BB. Education, counseling and support for significant others. In: Shadden BB, ed. Communication behavior and aging: A sourcebook for clinicians. Baltimore: Williams & Wilkins, 1988:469.
101. Shewan CM. Auditory comprehension test for sentences. Chicago: Biolinguistics Clinical Institutes, 1979.
102. Shut LJ. Dementia following stroke. Clin Geriatr Med 1988; 4:767–784.
103. Shuttleworth EC, Huber SJ. The naming disorder of dementia of the Alzheimer type. Brain Lang 1988; 34:222–234.
104. Smith SR, Murdoch BE, Chenery HL. Semantic abilities in dementia of the Alzheimer type. Brain Lang 1989; 36:314–324.
105. Sohlberg MM, Mateer CA. Introduction to cognitive rehabilitation: Theory and practice. New York: Guilford Press, 1989.
106. Spellacy FJ, Spreen O. A short form of the token test. Cortex 1969; 5:390–397.
107. Stevens SJ. Differential naming difficulties in elderly dysphasic subjects with senile dementia of the Alzheimer type. Br J Disord Commun 1989; 24:77–92.
108. Terman LM, Merrill MA. Stanford-Binet intelligence scale. Manual for the third edition, form L-M. Boston: Houghton-Mifflin, 1973.
109. Terrell B, Ripich D. Discourse competence as a variable in intervention. Semin Speech Lang Disord 1989; 10:282–297.
110. Terry RD, Peck A, DeTeresa R, et al. Some morphometric aspects of the brain in senile dementia of the Alzheimer's type. Ann Neurol 1981; 10:184–192.
111. Thal LJ. Dementia update: Diagnosis and neuropsychiatric aspects. J Clin Psychiatry 1988; 49:5–7.
112. Tomlinson BE. The pathology of dementia. In: Wells CE, ed. Dementia. Philadelphia: F.A. Davis, 1977: 113.
113. Tonkovich JD. Communication disorders in the elderly. In: Shadden BB, ed. Communication behavior and aging: A sourcebook for clinicians. Baltimore: Williams & Wilkins, 1988:197.
114. Ulatowska HK, Cannito MP, Hyashi MM, Fleming SG. Language abilities in the elderly. In: Ulatowska HK, ed. The aging brain: Communication in the elderly. San Diego: College-Hill Press, 1985:125.
115. Ulatowska HK, Haynes SM, Donnell AJ, et al. Discourse abilities in dementia. Paper presented at the American Speech and Hearing Association Conference. Detroit, MI, November, 1986.
116. Wagner O, Oesterreich K, Hoyer S. Validity of the ischemic score in degenerative and vascular dementia and depression in old age. Arch Gerontol Geriatr 1985; 4:333–345.
117. Wechsler D. Wechsler Adult Intelligence Scale—Revised Manual. New York: The Psychological Corporation, 1981.
118. Wechsler D. A standardized memory scale for clinical use. J Psychol 1945; 19:87–95.
119. Wells CE. The differential diagnosis of psychiatric disorders in the elderly. In: Cole J, Barrett J, eds. Psychopathology in the aged. New York: Raven Press, 1980:19.
120. Wells CE. Pseudodementia. Am J Psychiatry 1979; 36:895–899.
121. Wertz RT. Neuropathologies of speech and language: An introduction to patient management. In: Johns DF, ed. Evaluation of appraisal techniques in speech and language pathology. Reading, MA: Addison-Wesley, 1978.
122. Whitehouse PJ. The concept of subcortical and cortical dementia: Another look. Ann Neurol 1986; 19:1–6.
123. Wisniewski HM, Merz GS. Neuropathology of the aging brain and dementia of the Alzheimer's type. In: Gaitz CM, Samorajski T, ed. Aging 2000: Our health care destiny: Vol. 1. Biomedical Issues. New York: Springer-Verlag, 1985:231.
124. Wisniewski HM, Narang HK, Terry RD. Neurofibrillary tangles of paired helical filaments. J Neurol Sci 1976; 17:173–181.
125. Woodward J. Clinico-pathological significance of granulovascular degeneration in Alzheimer's disease. J Neuropathol Exp Neurol 1962; 21:85–91.
126. Zarit SH, Reever KE, Bach-Peterson T. Relatives of the impaired elderly: Correlates of feelings of burden. Gerontologist 1980; 20:649–655.

# APPENDIX

## Alzheimer's Dementia and Risk to Family Member Questionnaire

Fact sheet
Subject: ..............................
Last known
address: ..............................
..............................
..............................
Informant: ..............................
Address: ..............................
..............................
Phone: ..............................
Additional
informant: ..............................
Address: ..............................
..............................
Phone: ..............................

Interviewer comments:
 1. Did the respondent seem to understand the questions?

 2. How confident are you about the accuracy of the respondent's answers?

 3. Any other comments?

Let me begin asking you a couple of questions about *subject*.
1. To the best of your knowledge, has *subject* ever had:

|  | Yes | No |
|---|---|---|
| a. High blood pressure? | 1 | 2 |
| b. A stroke? | 1 | 2 |
| c. Diabetes or "sugar"? | 1 | 2 |
| d. A drinking problem? | 1 | 2 |
| e. A head injury that resulted in loss of consciousness for more than a second or two? | 1 | 2 |
| f. A psychiatric illness that required hospitalization (other than the present problem)? | 1 | 2 |
| g. Any other neurological diseases or disorders of the brain such as a brain tumor, multiple sclerosis, or Parkinson's disease? | 1 | 2 |

IF YES TO ANY OF ABOVE, STOP INTERVIEW AT THIS POINT.

2. What was the last year of school that *subject* completed?
    1-12. Last grade completed
    14. Some college
    16. College graduate
    17. Graduate degree
3. Before he or she became ill, was *subject* able to read and write?  Yes  No
                                                                         1    2

IF NO, STOP INTERVIEW AT THIS POINT.

4. Could you tell me the last address where *subject* lived before he or she first entered a nursing home?

RECORD ON FACT SHEET.

5. What type of work did *subject* do before this illness began or before he or she retired? (IF MORE THAN ONE JOB, ASK FOR THE JOB SUBJECT HELD LONGEST)
    Homemaker
    Disabled
    Student
    Other

*Appendix continues on following page*

IF SUBJECT NEVER WORKED, ASK:                                              Yes   No

5a. Was *subject* ever married?                                             1    2

5b. IF YES: What type of work did *subject's* spouse do?
    (IF MORE THAN ONE JOB, ASK FOR THE JOB SPOUSE HELD
    LONGEST. IF MORE THAN ONE SPOUSE, CODE FOR SPOUSE
    WITH HIGHEST PRESTIGE JOB.)
    Homemaker
    Disabled
    Student
    Other

5c. IF NO: What type of work did *subject's* father do?
    (IF MORE THAN ONE JOB, ASK FOR JOB FATHER HELD
    LONGEST.)
    Disabled
    Other

6.  Now I'd like to ask you some questions about *subject's* recent illness
    and in particular about the time when you or your family first noticed
    some specific changes. Have you noticed:

|  |  | Yes | No | If yes mo/yr change began |
|---|---|---|---|---|
| a. | A change in *subject's* personality (e.g., a change in tidiness, restlessness, irritability, loss of concern for others)? | 1 | 2 | ___ / ___ |
| b. | Loss of memory? | 1 | 2 | ___ / ___ |
| c. | Difficulty in speech or finding words? | 1 | 2 | ___ / ___ |
| d. | Loss of ability to read (e.g., stopped reading books or newspapers)? | 1 | 2 | ___ / ___ |
| e. | Loss of ability to write (e.g., stopped writing notes or letters)? | 1 | 2 | ___ / ___ |
| f. | Loss of ability to cook or dress self? | 1 | 2 | ___ / ___ |
| g. | Loss of control of bladder or bowels? | 1 | 2 | ___ / ___ |

7.  To the best of your recollection, when was the last time *subject* was really well or his or her old self?                ___ / ___
                                                                         mo/yr

8.  When would you say you first noticed a change?                       ___ / ___
                                                                         mo/yr

9.  What was the first change (SYMPTOM) that you noticed?

Now I'd like to ask you a few questions about *subject's* children.

10a. How many children did *subject* have, including those who
     died in infancy or childhood, but not including stillbirths
     and abortions?

                                                                        _____
                                                                        no. children

IF NO CHILDREN, SKIP TO Q 11.

10b. Could you tell me the names of all these children, living or deceased, in order of their
     birth, starting with the oldest?

10c. What is the birthdate of *child*?

*Appendix continues on following page*

10d. What is the sex of *child*?

10e. Is *child* still alive?

10f. What is the current age of each child? (IF CHILD IS DECEASED, RECORD AGE AT DEATH.)

10g. IF DECEASED: What was the cause of *child's* death?

10h. Have any of these children suffered from any of the following?
1. Mental retardation (Down's syndrome, mongolism as a cause, if known)
2. Birth defects (e.g., congenital heart disease, spina bifida, etc.)
3. Malignancy of blood forming organs or lymphatics (e.g., leukemia or lymphoma, by type if possible, Hodgkin's disease, multiple myeloma, Waldenström's macroglobulinemia, etc.)
4. Central nervous system or brain disease (e.g., epilepsy, amyotrophic lateral sclerosis, Parkinson's disease, multiple sclerosis, etc. DO NOT INCLUDE "BAD NERVES," ETC.)
5. Symptoms of mental deterioration such as:
   a. Memory loss (ML)
   b. Loss of ability to read (RL) or write (WL)
   c. Difficulty finding words, speaking nonsense words, etc. (SL)
   d. Difficulty with cooking or dressing (due to apraxia) (CD)
   e. Loss of control of bowels or bladder (IN) (LIST ONLY IN PRESENCE OF OTHER ASSOCIATED SYMPTOMS OF DEMENTIA.)

IF NO SYMPTOMS OR CONDITIONS, SKIP TO Q 11.

| 10b<br>Name of child<br>(last name, first name;<br>if female, maiden name) | 10c<br>Birthdate<br>(mo/day/yr) | 10d<br>Sex<br>(M = 1;<br>F = 2) | 10e<br>Living?<br>(Yes = 1;<br>No = 2) | 10f<br>Age | 10g<br>Cause of<br>death |
|---|---|---|---|---|---|
| 1 | | | | | |
| 2 | | | | | |
| 3 | | | | | |
| 4 | | | | | |
| 5 | | | | | |
| 6 | | | | | |

10h
ALL APPLICABLE CONDITIONS OR SYMPTOMS WITH DATE OF ONSET (mo/yr). Be as specific as possible. (If positive response in 1-5, administer SUPPLEMENTAL FORM for relative with condition.)

1
2
3
4
5
6

Now I'd like to ask you the same questions about *subject's* brothers and sisters.

*Appendix continues on following page*

11a. How many brothers and sisters did *subject* have, including those who may have died at any time after birth? (DO NOT INCLUDE HALF-SIBLINGS OR STEP-SIBLINGS.)

_____ no. siblings

IF NO SIBLINGS, SKIP TO Q 12.

11b. Could you tell me the names of all brothers and sisters, living and deceased, from the oldest to the youngest? Please include subject but do not include any step-brothers or sisters or half-brothers or sisters.

11c. What is the birthdate of *sibling*?

11d. What is the sex of *sibling*?

11e. Is *sibling* still alive?

11f. What is the current age of each sibling? (IF SIBLING IS DECEASED, RECORD AGE AT DEATH.)

11g. IF DECEASED: What was the cause of *sibling's* death?

11h. Have any of these brothers or sisters suffered from any of the following?
   1. Mental retardation (Down's syndrome, mongolism as a cause, if known)
   2. Birth defects (e.g., congenital heart disease, spina bifida, etc.)
   3. Malignancy of blood forming organs or lymphatics (e.g., leukemia or lymphoma, by type if possible, Hodgkin's disease, multiple myeloma, Waldenström's macroglobulinemia, etc.)
   4. Central nervous system or brain disease (e.g., epilepsy, amyotrophic lateral sclerosis, Parkinson's disease, multiple sclerosis, etc. DO NOT INCLUDE "BAD NERVES," ETC.)
   5. Symptoms of mental deterioration such as:
      a. Memory loss (ML)
      b. Loss of ability to read (RL) or write (WL)
      c. Difficulty finding words, speaking nonsense words, etc. (SL)
      d. Difficulty with cooking or dressing (due to apraxia) (CD)
      e. Loss of control of bowels or bladder (IN) (LIST ONLY IN PRESENCE OF OTHER ASSOCIATED SYMPTOMS OF DEMENTIA.)

IF NO SYMPTOMS OR CONDITIONS, SKIP TO Q 12.

| 11b<br>Name of sibling<br>(last name, first name;<br>if female, maiden name) | 11c<br>Birthdate<br>(mo/day/yr) | 11d<br>Sex<br>(M = 1;<br>F = 2) | 11e<br>Living?<br>(Yes = 1;<br>No = 2) | 11f<br>Age | 11g<br>Cause of<br>death |
|---|---|---|---|---|---|
| 1 | | | | | |
| 2 | | | | | |
| 3 | | | | | |
| 4 | | | | | |
| 5 | | | | | |
| 6 | | | | | |

*Appendix continues on following page*

11h
ALL APPLICABLE CONDITIONS OR SYMPTOMS WITH DATE OF ONSET (mo/yr). Be as specific as possible. (If positive response in 1-5, administer SUPPLEMENTAL FORM for relative with condition.)

1
2
3
4
5
6

12a. What are the names of subject's biological parents, living or deceased?

12b. What was the birthdate of *parent*?

12c. FILL IN SEX.

12d. Is *parent* still alive?

12e. What is the current age of each parent? (IF DECEASED, RECORD AGE AT DEATH.)

12f. IF DECEASED: What was the cause of *parent's* death?

12g. Has either parent suffered from any of the following?
1. Mental retardation (Down's syndrome, mongolism as a cause, if known)
2. Birth defects (e.g., congenital heart disease, spina bifida, etc.)
3. Malignancy of blood forming organs or lymphatics (e.g., leukemia or lymphoma, by type if possible, Hodgkin's disease, multiple myeloma, Waldenström's macroglobulinemia, etc.)
4. Central nervous system or brain disease (e.g., epilepsy, amyotrophic lateral sclerosis, Parkinson's disease, multiple sclerosis, etc. DO NOT INCLUDE "BAD NERVES," ETC.)
5. Symptoms of mental deterioration such as:
   a. Memory loss (ML)
   b. Loss of ability to read (RL) or write (WL)
   c. Difficulty finding words, speaking nonsense words, etc. (SL)
   d. Difficulty with cooking or dressing (due to apraxia) (CD)
   e. Loss of control of bowels or bladder (IN) (LIST ONLY IN PRESENCE OF OTHER ASSOCIATED SYMPTOMS OF DEMENTIA.)

IF NO SYMPTOMS OR CONDITIONS, SKIP TO Q 13.

| 12b Name of parent (last name, first name; if female, maiden name) | 12c Birthdate (mo/day/yr) | 12d Sex (M = 1; F = 2) | 12e Living? (Yes = 1; No = 2) | 12f Age | 12g Cause of death |
|---|---|---|---|---|---|
| 1 | | | | | |
| 2 | | | | | |

*Appendix continues on following page*

12h
ALL APPLICABLE CONDITIONS OR SYMPTOMS WITH DATE OF ONSET (mo/yr). Be as specific as possible. (If positive response in 1-5, administer SUPPLEMENTAL FORM for relative with condition.)

1
2

---

13a. Was *subject* ever married? _____ (no. of times)

IF NO SKIP TO Q 14.

13b. What are the names of all of *subject's* marriage partners (INCLUDING COMMON LAW), whether living or deceased?

13c. What was the birthdate of *partner*?

13d. Is *partner* still living?

13e. What is the current age of each partner? (IF DECEASED, RECORD AGE AT DEATH.)

13f. When did this marriage (cohabitation) begin?

13g. IF APPLICABLE, When did *subject* separate from this partner? (Separation includes divorce, *de facto* or legal separation, death, institutional placement of partner or subject, etc.)

13h. IF DECEASED: What was the cause of *partner's* death?

13i. Have any of *subject's* partners suffered from the following?
   1. Mental retardation (Down's syndrome, mongolism)
   2. Birth defects (e.g., congenital heart disease, spina bifida, etc.)
   3. Malignancy of blood forming organs or lymphatics (e.g., leukemia or lymphoma, by type if possible, Hodgkin's disease, multiple myeloma, Waldenström's macroglobulinemia, etc.)
   4. Central nervous system or brain disease (e.g., epilepsy, amyotrophic lateral sclerosis, Parkinson's disease, multiple sclerosis, etc. DO NOT INCLUDE "BAD NERVES," ETC.)
   5. Symptoms of mental deterioration such as:
       a. Memory loss (ML)
       b. Loss of ability to read (RL) or write (WL)
       c. Difficulty finding words, speaking nonsense words, etc. (SL)
       d. Difficulty with cooking or dressing (due to apraxia) (CD)
       e. Loss of control of bowels or bladder (IN) (LIST ONLY IN PRESENCE OF OTHER ASSOCIATED SYMPTOMS OF DEMENTIA.)

| 13b<br>Name of partner<br>(last name, first name;<br>if female, maiden name) | 13c<br>Birthdate<br>(mo/day/yr) | 13d<br>Living?<br>(Yes = 1;<br>No = 2) | 13e<br>Age | 13f<br>Marriage<br>began? | 13g<br>Marriage<br>end? | 13h<br>Cause of<br>death |
|---|---|---|---|---|---|---|
| 1 | | | | | | |
| 2 | | | | | | |
| 3 | | | | | | |
| 4 | | | | | | |

*Appendix continues on following page*

13i
ALL APPLICABLE CONDITIONS OR SYMPTOMS WITH DATE OF ONSET (mo/yr). Be as specific as possible. (If positive response in 1-5, administer SUPPLEMENTAL FORM for relative with condition.)

1
2
3
4

14. Could you tell me the name of another family member who is knowledgeable about *subject's* family's medical history? (RECORD ON FACT SHEET.)

---

From Breitner JC, Folstein M. A prevalent disorder with specific clnical features. Psychol Med 1984; 14:63–80. Copyright 1984, Cambridge University Press. Reprinted with the permission of Cambridge University Press.

# CHAPTER 14

# *Auditory Testing and Rehabilitation of the Hearing Impaired*

BARBARA E. WEINSTEIN, Ph.D.

This chapter is divided into two sections. The goal of the first section is to establish a case for audiology in the physical diagnosis and management of individuals suspected of suffering from the symptom complex known as senile dementia. In short, the relevance of audiology to the diagnostic process grows out of the overlapping behavioral manifestations of hearing loss and senile dementia, the high prevalence and severity of hearing impairment in persons with dementia, and the impact of an unremediated hearing loss on performance on cognitive tasks. The second section will detail the testing techniques and rehabilitative technology used to uncover and remediate hearing loss in this population. The substance of the chapter is drawn from the research, albeit limited in this area.

## Behavioral Manifestations of Senile Dementia

Intellectual impairment sufficient to impair social or occupational function, disorientation, and confusion are hallmarks of senile dementia. Additional symptoms include social avoidance, fearfulness, irritability, agitation, failing attention, loss of sense of humor, increased speech irrelevance, and personality changes.[9] Older adults suffering from visual impairment and hearing loss exhibit similar symptoms. For example Luey, Belser, and Glaser reported that individuals with combined sensory deficits experience disorientation, difficulty coping with the environment, vulnerability, problems with communication, isolation, frustration, being misunderstood, helplessness, loss of ability to contribute, loss of dignity, and loss of competence and control.[8] The overlap in the behavioral manifestations of senile dementia and unidentified hearing loss has significant implications for correct diagnosis and management of persons with senile dementia.

## Hearing Loss in Senile Dementia

### PREVALENCE

A number of studies conducted in the United States and abroad have attempted to determine hearing status of older adults with a diagnosis of senile dementia. Uhlmann, Larson, Rees, et al conducted a case control study of 100 older adults with dementia and an age-, sex-, and education-matched group of nondemented individuals.[16] The clinical diagnosis of Alzheimer's disease was based on the criteria established by the National Institute of Neurologic and Communication Disorders and Stroke/Alzheimer's Disease and Related Disorders (NINCDS-ADRDA, see Chapter 1). In addition, control subjects had a score of more than 24 on the Mini-Mental State Examination (MMSE), while the cases with dementia had scores of 14 or greater. The prevalence of hearing impairment (weighted binaural average of thresholds at .5, 1, 2, and 3 kHz, $\geq 30$ dB) was 60 percent in the demented group and 40 percent in the nondemented group; with the differences statistically significant. Weinstein and Amsel reported the prevalence of hearing loss (PTA > 25 dBHL) to be 83 percent in a sample of institutionalized elderly individuals (N = 30) with an admitting diagnosis of senile dementia and 70 percent in an age-matched group of institutionalized older adults without a diagnosis of senile dementia.[19] Uhlmann, Rees, Psaty, and Duckert reported the prevalence of hearing loss based on the monaural average of thresholds at 500, 1000, 2000, and 3000 Hz to be significantly higher: 44 percent in their sample of older adults with mild to moderate dementia versus 26 percent in the nondemented control group.[17] Finally, Gilhome-Herbst and Humphrey reported that 79 percent of their sample of older adults with senile dementia also had a hearing loss, versus a prevalence of 60 percent in a sample of nondemented adults over 70 years of age.[2] The above research clearly indicates that hearing impairment is more prevalent in demented than in nondemented older adults living in the community and in institutions.

## SEVERITY

In addition to its high prevalence, the hearing loss characterizing persons with dementia tends to be more severe. Weinstein and Amsel found the severity of hearing loss to be greater in their subjects with a diagnosis of dementia than in an age-matched group of older adults free of cognitive impairments.[19] The majority of persons (55 percent) in the demented group had three frequency pure-tone averages in excess of 40 dBHL, while only 40 percent of those without dementia had pure-tone averages indicative of a moderate to profound hearing loss. Similarly, Uhlmann et al reported that the mean hearing level characterizing the individuals with a diagnosis of Alzheimer's disease was significantly greater than in the control group.[16] They also noted that the risk of dementia increased as a function of hearing loss. In short, there was a tendency for the risk of dementia to increase for mild and moderate hearing loss. The increased risk remained, after adjusting for such potentially confounding variables as depression, family history of dementia, and number of primary drug prescriptions. However, the increase in risk was statistically significant only for individuals with moderate/severe (>40 dB) hearing loss. Finally, Peters, Potter, and Scholer reported the mean hearing level (average of 1000 and 2000 Hz) of their elderly subjects with definite irreversible dementia to be 58 dBHL.[10]

In addition to the findings that hearing levels are more severe in demented than in nondemented older adults, evidence is beginning to mount that supports the hypothesis that hearing status bears a relationship to cognitive function/dysfunction as measured using tests of mental status. Uhlmann et al found that hearing loss was significantly correlated with the severity of cognitive dysfunction as measured using the Mini-Mental Status Examination (MMSE).[16] Although the correlation was weak (r=.26), it remained statistically significant when controlling for external variables including age, educational level, sex, medication use, and depression. Weinstein and Amsel reported a statistically significant, albeit weak (r=.34), relation between cognitive function and hearing level, according to scores on the Mental Status Questionnaire (MSQ).[19] A significant relation between the severity of dementia and severity of hearing loss also emerged in the study of Gilhome-Herbst and Humphrey.[2] However, in contrast to the findings of Uhlmann et al,[16] Gilhome-Herbst and Humphrey[2] found that once age was controlled for, the apparent relationship between hearing loss and dementia was lost. They concluded that hearing loss and dementia are merely contiguous medical conditions that occur as a function of age.

Peters et al followed 38 subjects longitudinally to determine if hearing impairment influences the change in cognition over time.[10] All subjects were diagnosed as presenting with definite irreversible dementia according to a complete battery of laboratory tests, physical examination, psychological tests, and neurologic examination. The Folstein Mini-Mental State Examination (MMSE) was administerd on two separate occasions over a 6-month to 16-month interval. Two trends emerged in the hearing-impaired subjects. First, decline in cognitive function at follow-up was greater in the hearing-impaired than in the unimpaired group. Second, the change in scores on the MMSE over time between the hearing-impaired and the unimpaired subjects was only significant for those individuals presenting with senile dementia of the Alzheimer's type. Peters et al concluded from that finding that there is a more rapid cognitive decline in the hearing impaired with SDAT, suggesting an interaction between hearing impairment and dementia.[10]

## DIAGNOSTIC SIGNIFICANCE

One possible implication of these findings is that an unrecognized hearing impairment may lower measured performance on verbally administered cognitive tests used to diagnose dementia, resulting in an underestimation of cognitive functioning. To test the hypothesis that hearing loss lowers measured cognitive performance, Weinstein and Amsel administered the MSQ under two conditions to a sample of 30 older adults with a diagnosis of senile dementia.[19] The MSQ was first administered face-to-face at the level of normal conversational speech (i.e., standard format) and then readministered face-to-face using an auditory trainer to amplify the signal. Interestingly, the statistically significant correlation (r=.34) that emerged under the standard administration was obliterated (r=.11) when an auditory trainer was used to amplify the questions. Similarly, amplification improved mental status test scores in approximately 30 percent of the subjects (predominantly those with moderately severe to severe hearing loss) in their sample. Weinstein and Amsel concluded that hearing status does in fact influence performance on orally administered cognitive tasks, especially in persons with moderate to moderately severe hearing loss.[19] As moderate to moderately severe hearing loss is not readily observable to the untrained eye, physicians administering mental status tests should be alerted to the risk and behavioral symptoms associated with hearing loss of this degree.

Uhlmann et al conducted a randomized trial comparing performance on written and standard versions of the MMSE to determine the impact of mild to moderate hearing loss on cognitive tests used in the diagnosis of dementia.[18] Two interesting trends emerged. The hearing-impaired subjects (mean hearing level = 34 dBHL based on sound field warble tone thresholds at .5, 1, 2, and 3 kHz) scored slightly more poorly on the MMSE (i.e., greater cognitive dysfunction) than the group without hearing impairment (mean hearing level = 18 dBHL). Further, performance on the written and verbally administered versions of the MMSE was similar for both groups of subjects with Alzheimer's type dementia. They therefore concluded that mild to moderate hearing impairment does not confound scores on verbally administered mental status tests.[18]

It is important to note that some of the hearing-impaired subjects wore their hearing aids when responding to the verbally administered MMSE, thereby enabling them to benefit from amplification. Further, in many cases, pure-tone thresholds were obtained using amplification; thus the thresholds do not reflect the true hearing loss. Finally, pure-tone thresholds were obtained in a sound field and therefore reflect the response of the better ear when a difference between ears exists. In light of these methodologic problems, the findings should be interpreted with some caution until, of course, the study is replicated. In light of the dearth of research on the interaction between hearing loss and performance on orally administered cognitive tasks, this area requires extensive investigation.

## Role of the Audiologist

Because the behavioral manifestations of hearing loss overlap with those of senile dementia, health-care professionals must be alert to the presence of hearing impairment in demented patients. Further, because hearing loss is prevalent in individuals with senile dementia, is a treatable cause of dementia, contributes to cognitive dysfunction in older adults, and may confound performance on verbally administered cognitive tests, the audiologist must be integrally involved in all aspects of interdisciplinary assessment and management. Specifically, audiologists play an important role in identifying persons with hearing impairment, evaluating hearing status, and designing treatment regimens that minimize the impact of hearing loss on an individual's daily function.

The audiologist can administer a formal hearing screening at the time of the initial patient and family interview, can train the professional administering the initial interview to recognize hearing impairments in persons suspected of presenting with senile dementia, and can offer suggestions for minimizing the confounding effect of an unremediated hearing loss on the geropsychological assessment. The dementia work-up includes an extensive battery of laboratory and radiologic tests that are designed to rule out any medical illness that may precipitate a cognitive loss. As sensory deprivation has been identified as a potential treatable cause of dementia, a complete audiologic evaluation conducted by an audiologist should be included among the battery of diagnostic tests administered to diagnose senile dementia. Maintenance of orientation and social interaction are primary management goals, and provision of a hearing aid and/or assistive listening device to the hearing impaired with senile dementia is an important part of their rehabilitation program. The audiologist is uniquely trained to provide each of the above services, and, thus, he or she must be aggressive in convincing medical personnel of the integral role played by audiology.

## SCREENING FOR HEARING LOSS

The high prevalence and severity of hearing loss among individuals with Alzheimer's disease, the correlation between hearing loss and cognitive dysfunction, the similarity in the behavioral manifestations of the two conditions, coupled with the fact that technology is available to facilitate communication in the hearing impaired suffering from senile dementia, would suggest that hearing impairment should be uncovered early in the differential diagnostic process.[15] A first step in identifying individuals with undetected hearing loss is the application of sensitive and specific screening tests. Researchers have been reluctant to evaluate the validity of hearing screening tests in demented individuals because of the time necessary to condition and screen these individuals and because of the questionable reliability and validity of responses of individuals with senile dementia. Thus, data from which to develop a screening protocol are limited.

Uhlmann et al evaluated the performance of four hearing screening tests on a sample of 34 individuals with mild to moderate dementia and an age-matched group of 31 nondemented individuals.[17] They assessed the reliability, sensitivity, and specificity of a tuning-fork test, a pure-tone screening test, the finger rub, and whispered voice tests utilizing pure-tone audiometry as the "gold standard." Specifically, they evaluated the ability of each screening test to detect an average hearing loss at 500, 1000, 2000, and 3000 Hz in excess of 40 dBHL. Their findings were as follows:

1. Inability to hear any 2 or more of 4 of the above frequencies at 40 dBHL is highly sensitive (.97) and moderately specific (.72)
2. The tuning fork test was highly specific (.82 to .95) and sensitive (.80) in the demented subjects.
3. The finger rub and whispered voice test were sensitive (.80) and specific (.89 to .95) in the demented subjects.

The authors concluded that although the pure-tone screen was a valid technique in this population, the technologically less sophisticated physical examination tests (e.g., finger rub) are comparably accurate and less expensive and thus should be pursued in this population. They did, however, caution that the tests were performed by different examiners, perhaps rendering comparisons premature. An additional limitation of the study was that the standard against which Uhlmann et al judged the validity of the screening procedures was a monaural, four-frequency, pure-tone average (500, 1000, 2000, and 3000 Hz) of 40 dBHL.[17] The adequacy of this operational definition of hearing loss for individuals with senile dementia has not been subjected to rigorous analysis. Finally, interobserver reliability of the physical examination tests used for screening (i.e., tuning fork, finger rub, and whispered voice) and the correlations with pure-tone thresholds at selected frequencies were low, jeopardizing the validity of these procedures. Given the aforementioned procedural limitations, the data of Uhlmann et al should be interpreted with some caution.[17]

Irrespective of the validity of their sensitivity and specificity values, an important conclusion reached by Uhlmann et al is that individuals with mild to moderate dementia can perform a pure-tone screening test.[17] Although their data lend support to the feasibility of screening persons with mild to moderate senile dementia, some caveats are in order, as are some recommendations for organizing a screening program. The major considerations in designing an identification program include: (1) time necessary for the screening; (2) examiner; (3) setting; (4) scheduling; (5) procedure and availability of a mechanism for follow-up; and (6) referral sources to ensure follow through on the screener's recommendations.

**Procedures**

It is of utmost importance that the procedure be quick and easy to administer and, of course, valid. The technique chosen to screen this population for hearing impairment should require no more than 10 minutes to administer. Accordingly, time constraints may preclude the screening of those with moderate to severe dementia, especially persons wherein a concentration deficit may be evident or in persons unable to perform complex tasks. Clinical judgment and experience rather than the patient's medical chart may be the only vehicle available to assist in the decision regarding eligibility for screening. For example, individuals who cannot be conditioned and screened within the allotted time period should be referred for a complete audiologic evaluation. Often, utilizing a number of trial periods, an experienced audiologist can condition individuals with moderate cognitive decline to respond to the audiometric tasks required of them. To reiterate, it is incumbent on the professional performing the screening test to adopt as a referral criterion all persons who, because of physical or cognitive factors, are unable to perform the screening test.

A major issue involved in screening persons with dementia is the credentials of the professional charged with the task. Ideally, clinicians experienced in working with persons with senile dementia and persons with hearing impairment are the most appropriate professionals to perform hearing screenings. Unfortunately, few professionals have a background in these areas because of the constraints imposed by professional education and practice. Accordingly, the type of facility in which the screening takes place and the professionals involved in the multidisciplinary assessment will dictate the clinician who will perform the screen, as well as the feasibility of conducting a hearing screen on patients suspected of suffering from dementia. For example, the majority of nursing homes do not routinely employ audiologists, hence speech-language pathologists often find themselves in the position of screening for hearing impairment and subsequent referral to an audiologist. Further, formal hearing screening is not routine in the majority of nursing homes. Thus, physicians or nurses who represent the primary referral source to audiology may choose to administer screenings. If the latter is the case, the audiologist should educate these professionals regarding techniques and procedures for conducting a valid screening. In an acute-care setting, the audiologist should be part of the team conducting the multidisciplinary assessment of persons with possible senile dementia and is the professional of choice to administer the screening. Irrespective of the professional conducting the screening, an audiologist should be consulted initially to select the protocol and to train individuals in the art of screening difficult-to-test patients.

The screening should be conducted on the patient's floor or in a context familiar to the patient, whenever possible. A new setting, an unfamiliar examiner, and unfamiliar procedures can further disorient persons suffering from dementia. Similarly, transporting the patient a long distance is fatiguing and can confound the validity of the screening. Screening tests should be conducted in the morning, as patients are most alert and least fatigued at this time.

With regard to the screening protocol, two major issues that remain unresolved are the procedures and instrumentation to be used. Most would agree that pure-tone testing rather than a self-report of hearing problems is the technique of choice with this population. However, the instrumentation (e.g., portable audiometer versus hand-held audioscope) that delivers the most valid outcome in the shortest period of time and with the least discomfort to the patient has not been determined. Similarly, the pure-tone criteria, including the frequencies, appropriate hearing levels, and pass/fail criteria, have not been delineated. When selecting hearing levels, frequencies, and pass-fail criteria, one must remember that the goal of screening is to identify those individuals whose hearing impairment is significant and those individuals who will be amenable and responsive to audiologic intervention. Further, overreferrals to audiology must be avoided because of the physical, cognitive, and economic constraints of persons with senile dementia and the limited availability of audiologists in settings where many persons with dementia reside (e.g., nursing homes).

As regards the latter, given the dearth of audiologists in nursing homes, screening failures are often referred to an outside clinic or hospital for a complete audiologic evaluation and possible hearing-aid fitting.[7] Often several visits to the audiologist are required to obtain valid results. As the travel time and repeated testing place a physical burden on the demented individual, efforts should be made to conduct on-site testing. Despite the fact that most nursing homes do not maintain a sound-treated booth, valid thresholds that reflect the patient's functional communication abilities can be obtained by the audiologist.

## THE AUDIOLOGIC EVALUATION

According to Uhlmann et al, hearing impairment may reduce input from the environment, thereby decreasing one's level of orientation.[16] Further, hearing status affects responsiveness and memory storage. Mental acuity depends in part on the accessibility of audiovisual stimuli and social interaction. Accordingly, the audiologist should be available to offer techniques that will minimize the confounding effects of an unremediated hearing loss on cognitive task performance. For example, the use of an inexpensive hardwire assistive listening device that will enable amplification of the items comprising the mental status test is a simple yet effective way of ensuring that hearing loss will not lower performance on verbally administered cognitive tests.

Given the aforementioned implications of unremediated hearing loss in persons at risk for senile dementia, the audiologic evaluation should be integral to the differential diagnosis of senile dementia. The test battery should include, at the very least: a case-history, a hearing handicap assessment, air and bone conduction testing, speech audiometry, and immittance testing. Although it is preferable for most of the testing to be conducted in a sound-treated room, clinical experience suggests that the data obtained in a quiet room provide ample information on which to base most diagnostic and management decisions.

The purpose of the case history is to elicit information about the patient's hearing status, communicative difficulties, and hearing-aid history. Further, pertinent nonaudiometric factors that may influence management decisions should be obtained. For example, information on such variables as the patient's cognitive status, living arrangements, level of dependence, and visual status should be explored. As the majority of patients will be unable to provide a valid history, a primary and familiar caregiver should be available to answer pertinent questions.

The goal of the hearing handicap assessment is to determine the perceived emotional and social effects of the hearing loss on patient function. Often, the patient will not offer valid responses to the questions. In the latter case, the caregiver's impressions of the handicap experienced by the demented individual can be of considerable import in determining treatment options. Pure-tone air and bone conduction testing should be attempted to determine: (1) the patient's hearing sensitivity, (2) the nature and type of hearing loss if one exists; and (3) the configuration of the hearing loss. Although data are not available regarding the reliability/validity of test results obtained from persons with senile dementia, clinical experience suggests that the vast majority can be conditioned over several sessions and ultimately offer reliable pure-tone thresholds. Despite time constraints, it is imperative that the intratest and intertest reliability of results be assessed as a check on the accuracy of results. If it initially appears fruitless to obtain pure-tone data, brief sessions wherein the patient is acquainted with auditory input may facilitate testing. Following these sessions, a final attempt should be made to obtain threshold data.

Speech testing, depending on the individual's cognitive status, may include a speech awareness threshold and word recognition threshold. In addition, speech recognition ability should be attempted to obtain an objective assessment of the patient's communicative abilities. The assessment of communicative ability should be functional, reflecting the environment in which the patient resides. Immittance testing is administered primarily to determine the status of the middle ear because the audiologist frequently will be unable to mask the nontest ear to determine valid bone conduction thresholds. Tympanometry and acoustic stapedial reflex testing should be attempted when valid pure-tone thresholds cannot be obtained and when there is a history of middle ear involvement.

### Procedural Modifications for Pure-Tone and Speech Testing

Clinical experience suggests that the majority of patients with mild to moderate dementia can be tested reliably. However, as the severity of the cognitive impairment increases, the probability of obtaining reliable and valid test results decreases. It is imperative that the clinician routinely check the reliability of thresholds obtained using test retest data at 1000 Hz and pure-tone/word recognition threshold data. Keep in mind that the validity of thresholds may be jeopardized by severity of dementia. For example, although persons undergoing threshold testing are instructed to respond to the softest sound they hear, persons with dementia may not comprehend this concept and may reliably respond to sounds that are most comfortable to them. The same trend may be apparent for speech testing as well.

Persons with severe dementia who may be noncommunicative because of the dementing process and/or a hearing loss may require several trial periods before obtaining reliable responses to pure-tone stimuli. Occasionally, brief hearing-awareness sessions, wherein the patient is gradually reintroduced to auditory stimuli via an auditory trainer or the speech audiometer, are necessary as part of the conditioning process. When reliable threshold data cannot be obtained, informal rehabilitation sessions using low levels of amplification delivered via an auditory trainer should be instituted to provide exposure to the external environment and ultimately to determine responsiveness to auditory input.

It is important to note that, in light of the behavioral manifestations and cognitive correlates of dementia, certain modifications in the routine test battery are often indicated. For example, it may be necessary to begin the test session by obtaining speech information, as speech is a more realistic and more natural message than pure tones. A speech awareness threshold can usually be elicited using the patient's name as the stimulus. The speech and language problems that often accompany dementia may preclude obtaining a speech reception threshold or word recognition scores in general or using routine stimuli such as spondee or monosyllabic words, in particular. The client's chart should be reviewed to reveal patient history that can be used as stimuli for speech testing. For example, simple questions that tap remote memory (which tends to be preserved to a greater degree than recent memory) may be useful as material for speech testing. Asking the patient to repeat a short series of words or numbers when varying the decibel level of the audiometer may also prove efficacious. A simple picture-pointing task or object identification may also be used successfully to elicit information about functional communication. When picture-pointing or object identification tasks are employed, the client's visual status must be considered.

Further, objective tests such as tympanometry and acoustic stapedial reflex testing may be invaluable when valid air and bone conduction thresholds cannot be obtained. The validity of brainstem auditory evoked response testing with this population has been discussed in Chapter 4. When evaluating patients with dementia, an important point to remember is that repeated trials are often necessary before obtaining a complete picture of the individual's hearing status. Further, inflexibility and strict adherence to traditional procedures will most likely hinder efforts at defining the individual's auditory sensitivity.

Additional modifications in the instructions, response criteria, and the test technique are listed in Table 14.1. Table 14.1 lists the behaviors characteristic of individuals with dementia and suggested modifications.

The information gleaned from the audiometric evaluation coupled with input from the caregiver will be used to make some management decisions including necessity for an ENT examination, candidacy for a hearing aid and/or assistive listening device, and appropriateness of motivational, informational, and family counseling.

TABLE 14.1 **Modifications in the Standard Test Battery**

| BEHAVIOR | TEST MODIFICATION |
|---|---|
| Poor memory | Repetition and simplification of test instructions |
| | Use of gestures to facilitate understanding of instructions |
| | Extended opportunity for practice |
| | Frequent conditioning/reconditioning trials |
| | Verbal reinforcement and verbal reassurances |
| Movement deficits | Evaluate different strategies before initiating testing and select response that requires the least effort and is the most natural. Try to select responses from the patient's behavioral repertoire (e.g., hand raising, waving tissue, knocking cane on floor in response to tonal presentation) |
| | Be consistent in choice of response behavior to avoid confusion and frustration |
| Disorientation | Allow patient the opportunity to listen to the spoken voice before initiating testing, because persons with severe dementia and/or moderately severe to profound losses have often been denied sensory input for extended periods of time. A simple procedure is to adjust the hearing level dial of the audiometer to 65–70 dBHL and speak to the patient through the speech audiometer. |
| | Alternatively, an auditory trainer can be adjusted to the patient's most comfortable listening level |
| Failing attention, distractable | Reduce length of test session keeping it to a maximum of 20 to 30 minutes. Oftentimes, two to three sessions are required to successfully complete the test battery |
| Slower response time | Slow down rate of tonal presentation, allowing the patient's behavior to dictate the pace of the examination |
| Speech and language | Evaluate speech reception and word recognition abilities, using relevant materials such as asking the patient to follow simple commands and asking questions about daily life. As verbal repetition skills remain intact in less severe cases, the Central Institutes for the Deaf everyday sentences may be useful in selected cases. In light of word-finding difficulties, failing memory for recent events, and reduced vocabulary, speech tests requiring verbal responses may be inappropriate in more advanced stages of dementia |

## Management of Individuals with Senile Dementia

According to Katzman, the major goals of care for individuals with dementia include maintenance of socialization and provision of support for the family.[3] Similarly, Wondolowski and Chartock contend that the intervention efforts should be designed to maximize the patient's residual assets/strengths and to relieve the emotional distress associated with cognitive decline.[21] Rehabilitation efforts should be client-centered and instituted early to prevent secondary disabilities related to the hearing loss.[6] In order to help the patient realize his or her maximum communicative potential, the audiologist must earn the confidence and trust of the patient and caregiver and strive to preserve the dignity of the disabled individual.[6]

Audiologists have at their disposal tools that can help professionals realize the previous management goals. The intervention strategies include (1) provision of a personal hearing aid and/or assistive listening device (ALD); (2) training in the use of amplification; (3) counseling of the hearing impaired and significant others; (4) environmental manipulation; and (5) in-service training. Some or all of these rehabilitative procedures must be implemented simultaneously to ensure that the clinician maximizes the individual's communication

## Sound Enhancement Technology

### PERSONAL HEARING AIDS

Myths abound regarding the efficacy of amplification with the hearing impaired with senile dementia. Although empirical data are not available, clinical experience suggests that candidacy and success are contingent on a number of factors that are both extrinsic and intrinsic to the individual. The sociologic, physical, psychological, and cognitive variables that must be factored into the decision to fit a hearing aid are listed in Table 14.2. The most influential of the sociologic considerations is level of independence and availability of a significant other. Individuals with senile dementia are limited to a certain extent in performance of activities of daily living (ADLs) and instrumental activities of daily living (IADLs). Further, they have difficulty remembering recent events, frequently misplace objects, and may have difficulty forming new memories.[12] Persons in the more advanced stages tend to be oblivious to the environment.[12] Accordingly, they may have difficulty: (1) locating their hearing aid to position it in their ear; (2) maintaining the hearing aid; (3) regularly positioning and repositioning the hearing aid in the ear; and (4) adjusting the unit to a comfortable level. Further, the memory deficit, that is, the tendency to forget where objects have been placed, increases the likelihood that the hearing aid will be lost. Informal and formal caregivers must assume responsibility for these tasks if a hearing aid is to be used successfully. Further, the caregiver must modify his or her communicative style and adapt the environment to facilitate adjustment to the hearing aid and to enhance speech understanding.

The psychological factors include motivational level and perception and acceptance of the hearing loss. The severity of the senile dementia will determine the extent to which these variables can be assessed directly from the patient or indirectly from a caregiver. Similarly, knowledge of the client's hearing-aid history may help uncover his or her attitude toward hearing-aid use. Central auditory processing abilities, manual dexterity, and visual status are the primary considerations influencing hearing-aid candidacy. With regard to central auditory processing ability, evidence is beginning to mount that enhanced signal-to-noise ratio, such as that provided by an FM auditory trainer, is preferable to a hearing aid. The latter devices are most helpful in the presence of competing noise, in reverberant rooms, and in large listening areas. Manual dexterity is an important consideration not only influencing the level of independent use of the unit, but dictating the style of the unit to recommend. Finally, when the visual system is compromised by disease or the aging process, the individual is deprived of other important sensory input. This deprivation has been associated with disorientation and confusion. Accordingly, the auditory input provided by a hearing aid can be invaluable in compensating for the loss of sensory stimulation resulting from visual problems.

Each of the cognitive factors listed in Table 14.2 plays an integral role in hearing-aid satisfaction and hence influences hearing-aid candidacy. The more severe the dementing illness, the great-

TABLE 14.2 **Variables Affecting Hearing-Aid Candidacy in Individuals Suffering from Senile Dementia**

| SOCIOLOGIC | PSYCHOLOGICAL | COGNITIVE | PHYSIOLOGIC |
| --- | --- | --- | --- |
| Economics | Motivational level | Mental status | Age |
| Lifestyle | Perception and acceptance of the hearing loss | Memory capacity | Hearing status |
| Level of independence/ dependence | | Ability to learn new tasks | Manual dexterity |
| Availability of a caregiver | | Ability to perform complex tasks | Visual status |
| | | Ability to concentrate | Central auditory processing abilities |
| | | | Hearing aid history |

er the cognitive decline and the less likely the individual is to use the hearing aid successfully. In the presence of significant cognitive decline, however, the individual's hearing-aid history may be a factor in the decision to proceed with a hearing aid. For example, if a resident of a nursing home with moderate dementia has been using the same hearing aid on a regular basis for several years (e.g., 5 to 8 years) and the audiologist notes that it is malfunctioning, the unit should most likely be replaced. The new unit should be identical in terms of the style and controls to the old unit so that minimal adaptation is necessary. Further, the person should continue to wear a hearing aid until the replacement aid is dispensed to ensure immediate carryover. A loaner hearing aid with similar specifications and controls would be preferable; however, if one is not available, the old unit should be used until a replacement arrives. In the latter case, a personal amplifier or auditory trainer should be used simultaneously as a means of delivering an amplified signal.

Conversely, if a resident of a nursing home presents with a moderately severe hearing loss and moderate dementia, a brief treatment trial with the recommended hearing aid would facilitate a decision regarding prognosis for an effective response to a hearing aid. The speech-language pathologist or audiologist should work with the resident and a nursing assistant for a period of 3 to 4 weeks to determine the use patterns, the stimulability of the patient, the responsiveness of the individual to the new unit, and the capabilities of the caregiver. After the brief trial period, a decision should be made about dispensing the hearing aid or considering an alternate form of amplification. It is important to note that as mental status fluctuates in many persons with senile dementia and is integrally related to acceptance or rejection of a hearing aid, it is imperative that the audiologist administer a simple mental status test to assist in a decision regarding amplification. Further, the client's mental status should be monitored for the duration of hearing-aid use, because of its tendency to fluctuate. Finally, memory also tends to fluctuate so that it is imperative that instructions be reiterated during each rehabilitative session and during ongoing use.

If a hearing aid is recommended, a number of adaptations should be made by the audiologist to maximize acceptance and to minimize the probability of loss of the unit. With regard to style, the audiologist should avoid fitting canal units because of their small size and the size of their batteries. Body aids are advantageous because of the ease of manipulation of the controls, although they are typically cosmetically unappealing. In-the-ear or behind-the-ear aids are equally appropriate for this population. The major disadvantage of an in-the ear unit, however, is their tendency to malfunction and the corresponding need for frequent repairs, leaving the patient without an aid for extended periods of time. Typically, if a behind-the-ear unit malfunctions, a loaner aid can be used in the interim, allowing for continued auditory stimulation that is so critical to persons with senile dementia. Irrespective of the style unit, controls should be preset and kept to a minimum. For example, an on-off switch is unnecessary, the client-operated tone control should be eliminated, and the volume control preset. In light of the tendency for hearing aids to be misplaced, the client's name should be engraved on the hearing aid and the serial number recorded in the client's chart for those in institutions.[20] Similarly, as hearing aids frequently are found in clothing, all pockets should be checked prior to cleaning all garments. An extended warranty that covers loss and damage should be recommended for all new hearing-aid users.[20] Most manufacturers make 2- or 3-year warranties available to the consumer through the hearing-aid dispenser. To minimize the expense associated with repeated loss of hearing aids, the use of calibrated loaner hearing aids should be considered, or use of a hearing aid under the supervision of a family member or caregiver should be encouraged.

**Hearing Aid Orientation**

To maximize rehabilitation efforts, the audiologist should incorporate the following intervention strategies. Instructions should be simple, repetitive, and to the point. The individual's habits and routines should be maintained. Every effort to promote a sense of competence despite the presence of impairments should be made. One should be wary of signs of frustration or agitation. Finally, each accomplishment should be reinforced, pictorial or written memory aids should be adopted, and family members should be integral to the sessions.[21]

A number of essential points should be covered with the caregiver and new hearing-aid user at the time of dispensing and during the hearing-aid orientation sessions. As stated in an earlier section, it is imperative that hearing-aid placement become a part of the routine of the individual's daily life. The unit should therefore be inserted at the same time daily (e.g., in the morning when dispensing medication, when dressing, etc.). The steps to be reviewed for hearing aid insertion include the following:

1. The earmold or hearing aid should be checked daily for wax build-up, prior to inserting the unit in the client's ear. The caregiver or client should be given a wax loop to remove excess wax from the mold

or hearing aid and the client's ear should be checked for impacted cerumen.

2. Battery insertion should be explained and demonstrated at each hearing-aid orientation session. Weekly battery changes are essential to ensure that the hearing aid is operating to its potential. Signs of a weak battery (e.g., no feedback when turning volume control up before placing in ear or insufficient loudness at routine volume control setting) should be discussed, and the use of a battery tester should be encouraged. The battery type and number should be written into the instructional brochure that accompanies the hearing aid, along with sources for obtaining the appropriate battery. The date of battery change should be noted on a person's calendar and/or in the individual's medical chart.

3. Proper insertion of the hearing aid must be reviewed repeatedly. The client or caregiver should demonstrate proper hearing-aid insertion at each orientation session. It is best if the volume control is set prior to placement in the client's ear. If the volume control is not preset, the client should be introduced to increasing amounts of amplification gradually, to allow for adaptation to the unit. The clinician should keep in mind that some dementia patients are unaccustomed to auditory input because of long-term deprivation, and therefore may not accept a unit that provides too much amplification. Accordingly, gain and output controls should also be adjusted incrementally to facilitate adjustment to the sensory stimulation provided by the hearing aid.

4. A schedule for inserting the hearing aid and battery should be established and adhered to so as to establish a routine for the patient. For example, each morning when medications are dispensed, the hearing aid should be inserted, and the unit should ideally be removed prior to going to sleep. When shorter use periods are desired, the schedule should be monitored accordingly. For persons in nursing homes or homebound persons relying on home-health aides, a schedule is imperative if hearing-aid use is to become a reality.

5. Proper care and maintenance of the unit must be explained in detail orally and in writing to the caregiver and, when appropriate, to the client. For example, the unit should be handled gently (never thrown on the floor), should not be exposed to excessive heat or moisture, and should be removed prior to sleep.

6. The new hearing-aid user should be monitored for signs of rejection of the hearing aid during the orientation session. For example, the patient should wear the unit for increasing periods of time both during the orientation and during the day. If the client is unwilling or unable to gradually become acclimated, then the clinician should consider an alternative unit or an assistive listening device.

## ASSISTIVE LISTENING DEVICES

The term assistive listening devices (ALDs) refers to groups of products that are specially designed to enhance the signal-to-noise ratio for the hearing-impaired listener and to decrease the deterioration in the clarity of the speech message attributable to distance.[1,11] ALDs are able to perform this function by picking up the signal from as close as possible to the sound source and transmitting it directly to the ear of the listener. During the transmission process, the integrity of the signal, regardless of distance or the presence of noise in the environment, is maintained.[1] ALDs can be used alone or in conjunction with personal hearing aids. They are helpful in a variety of situations, including listening to the television or radio, communicating on a one-to-one basis with another person, in small group situations such as during occupational, recreational, or physical therapy sessions, and in large group situations such as when attending religious services.

Functionally, the four main categories of ALDs include: (1) sound enhancement technology that can be used to facilitate one-to-one and large group communication; (2) television enhancement technology that interfaces with the television to promote understanding; (3) signal alerting technology that alerts the hearing impaired to the presence of environmental signals; and (4) telephone enhancement technology that enables telephone communication.[5] Each of these technologies enhances the signal-to-noise ratio by way of hardwired or wireless transmission of the auditory signal. Wireless technologies make use of radio frequencies (frequency modulated signals), infrared light, and magnetic induction, while hardwired technology uses direct electrical connection to transmit the electrical signal.[1] Each technology has specific features, advantages, and disadvantages when considering the applicability to the hearing-impaired individual presenting with senile dementia.

The sound enhancement technology most applicable to the demented population includes the hardwired amplification systems that carry the auditory signal from the sound source via a wire connection to the hearing-impaired listener. As the electrical hardwire connection limits mobility, hardwired systems are preferable for one-to-one communication (e.g., television viewing or interpersonal interactions with family or health-care workers). Hardwire systems that resemble a portable radio are comprised of a microphone, amplifier, receiver, and controls that are easy to operate.[1] These battery-operated devices are inexpensive, easy to manipulate, and commercially available at prices ranging from $40 to $100. Hardwired systems are ideal as an alternative to a personal hearing aid or can be used to provide temporary amplification when a hearing aid is malfunctioning. When used as a personal amplifier, the speaker talks directly into the microphone, and the message is delivered to the listener through a set of headphones. A particularly appealing feature is the fact that they can be coupled directly and easily to the television for viewing, or to a radio or stereo system for listening. When coupling a hardwired system to the television, the device is plugged into the earphone jack of the television, or the microphone is positioned near the loudspeaker of the television. The signal from the television is then delivered to the listener through personal headphones. In light of the accessibility of the controls, hardwired systems provide persons with "the benefits of amplification without having to depend on others to assist with their hearing needs."[1] Another hidden advantage of a hardwired system is that it alerts others to the fact that the user has a hearing impairment necessitating the speaker to make special efforts or modifications to enhance communication.

Wireless systems, including infrared systems that use infrared light or FM systems that use frequency modulated (FM) broadcast technology, provide excellent fidelity and are among the most versatile for transmitting an auditory signal. However, the cost of these devices is substantially higher than the hardwired systems. Similarly, these systems are more sophisticated than the hardwired devices and accordingly may be threatening and difficult to operate. Despite these disadvantages, the infrared system, which transmits the auditory signal to the listener by way of modulated infrared light, conveys a high-quality signal from the television or stereo. The infrared user is equipped with a receiver that is individually tuned to enable listening at a most comfortable listening level. The FM system that conveys the audio signal via radio waves is ideal for interpersonal communication in a noisy environment. It can be used to supplement the performance of a hearing aid or to assist persons who cannot benefit from hearing aids due to auditory processing problems.[1]

### Signal Alerting Technology

Signal alerting devices are used to notify the hearing-impaired individual of the presence of environmental signals such as telephone ring, doorbell ring, smoke alarm, baby cry, and wake-up alarm.[4] Given their physical and cognitive limitations, persons with senile dementia should be most concerned about their ability to hear those environmental stimuli. Because personal safety is an overriding concern of the interdisciplinary team working with persons suffering from senile dementia, audiologists should play a role in analyzing the environment and making the following recommendations as they relate to alerting devices.[4]

1. The number and type of sounds to be monitored
2. The way in which the sound should be monitored and transmitted
3. The alerting mode to be employed

Table 14.3 lists the variables to be considered in selecting alerting devices designed to meet the specific needs of the hearing impaired with senile dementia. The choice of location for monitoring the signal will, of course, depend on the individual's living arrangements (i.e., in own home, child's home, or nursing home). Along with a decision regarding the location of the sound source, the audiologist must consider the optimal method for detecting the presence of the sound and transmitting it to the hearing-impaired person.[4] The three options include a sound-activated pick-up, a direct connect sound pick-up, and an induction sound pick-up.[4] The sound activated pick-up that is portable detects the presence of the sound via a microphone that is connected to an electronic switching mechanism.[4] Once the switching mechanism is activated, the hearing-impaired person is alerted to the presence of the sound. The direct connect sound pick-up devices are directly connected to the signal source, thereby limiting the portability of the system.[4] Finally, an induction sound pick-up uses electromagnetic energy as the mechanism for activating the system. Although this mode of activation is portable, it is limited to use with the telephone and doorbell.[4] The audiologist will be able to arrive at a decision regarding the best system after consulting with the parties of interest and after surveying the location of the monitored sound.

Finally, the alerting mode to be used to signify the presence of sound can be visual (e.g., flashing light), auditory (e.g., telephone ringers),

TABLE 14.3 **Variables to Consider in Selecting Alerting Devices**

| SIGNAL | SOURCE LOCATION | PICK-UP MODE | ALERTING MODE |
| --- | --- | --- | --- |
| Telephone | Residence | Sound activated | Visual |
| Doorbell | Nursing home | Direct connection | Auditory |
| Smoke alarm | | Induction | Vibrotactile |
| Alarm clock | | | |

Modified from Larose G, Evans M, Larose R. Alerting devices: Available options. In: Compton C, ed. Seminars in hearing. New York: Thieme Medical Publishers, 1988:66.

vibrotactile (e.g., vibrating indicators), or any combination of the above.[4] For persons with senile dementia, a system that combines an auditory and visual mode should be employed in the person's residence although a visual mode may be more appropriate in a nursing home to prevent annoyance to other residents and staff. It is important to note that persons with mild to moderate dementia will require considerable conditioning to utilize alerting devices. In light of their confused state, only the most important sounds that will ensure the individual's safety should be monitored. For a person who resides in a nursing home and cannot be conditioned, a system should be adopted by the staff to ensure that the hearing impaired with dementia are alerted to an emergency when one arises (e.g., a red circle on top of the door should inform the nurse that the patient is hearing impaired and is unable to hear an alarm). To determine the signaling equipment that best meets the needs of the individual, a number of resource centers can be consulted (see Appendix at the end of this chapter).

## Telephone Enhancement Technology

The most popular and efficient form of telephone enhancement technology includes amplified replacement handsets that essentially add amplification to the telephone.[14] For the most part, the handsets are compatible with modular, carbon, bell-ring telephones with detachable receivers, as these systems have enough power to drive the amplifier of the handset.[14] Handsets are available in a variety of styles and colors. Some of the handsets have a rotary volume-control wheel that maintains a set loudness until the volume control is adjusted; other handsets automatically return to the normal volume level when one hangs up the telephone.[14] Given cognitive and physical considerations, the former mechanism is preferable for those with senile dementia. As receiver mouthpieces on most telephones are sensitive to extraneous noise, a noise-canceling mouthpiece is an option to consider to promote understanding in a noisy environment such as a nursing home.[14] Other options for amplifying telephone conversations are available such as portable audio amplifiers or telephones with built-in amplifiers. The portable amplifier that straps onto most telephones generates an adequate message; however, it would be difficult for the individual with senile dementia to position and manipulate. The AT&T National Special Needs Center in Parsippany, NJ provides information about telephone technology.

## CONCLUSIONS REGARDING ASSISTIVE LISTENING DEVICES

ALDs are important therapeutic tools for the hearing impaired with senile dementia. The sound-enhancement technology provides coupling to the environment, thus facilitating orientation and promoting awareness of individuals and events surrounding them. Television-enhancement technology is an effective solution for persons with difficulty hearing and understanding television. Available devices, including the hardwired devices that provide a direct connection between the user and the television, and wireless devices such as the infrared system deliver a clear, undistorted message, enabling the hearing impaired to enjoy this important leisure activity. Alerting devices and telephone-enhancement technology enable audiologists to make an invaluable contribution to the safety and well-being of persons with senile dementia. Some of the devices, such as the telephone ring, the smoke alarm, and replacement telephone handsets, can contribute to making the home environment safe and comfortable, thereby helping to promote the possibility that the individual can remain at home for as long as it is physically and psychosocially possible. Since some audiologists may not be familiar with available technology, professionals should explore these options before making a decision regarding the technology most suitable to the needs of persons with senile dementia.

## Educating the Caregiver

For a person with dementia, the caregiver assumes a number of important roles as they relate to the rehabilitation process. These include:
1. Providing information to the audiologist or speech-language pathologist regarding communication difficulties and demands
2. Facilitating carryover of goals and activities to the home environment or within the nursing home
3. Assisting in the operation and manipulation of hearing aids and assistive listening devices
4. Providing information about the physical environment with regard to safety, acoustics, and lighting
5. Serving as a primary communication partner[13]

Given the aforementioned responsibilities of the caregiver, he or she requires information regarding the nature of hearing loss, the symptoms of hearing impairment, the difficulties experienced by the hearing impaired, and the interaction between the symptoms of hearing impairment and the behavioral manifestations of senile dementia. The caregiver must understand the situations that will be most problematic for the hearing impaired as well as emotional reactions to some of their difficulties.[11] Specific strategies for communicating with the hearing impaired with senile dementia should be reviewed, as well as the resources and technology available for promoting communication.[13] Increased awareness of resources will enable the caregiver to become an advocate for the demented individual. Caregivers must have access to technology that facilitates communication and promotes the safety of the individual. Similarly, environmental modifications necessary for communication (e.g., adequate lighting and acoustics) and the role of nonauditory as well as tactile cues in communication must be emphasized. (See Chapter 16 about environmental manipulations.) Specialized training in the operation, manipulation, and maintenance of amplification devices is critical. Further, the caregiver's expectations regarding the benefits of amplification must be realistic if the individual with dementia is to become a successful hearing-aid user.

The format of educational sessions with caregivers should be flexible, with each session being modified to best meet the needs of those persons in attendance. Further, opportunities for hands-on experiences with available devices are critical for carryover into the daily lives of the hearing impaired with dementia. Whenever possible, the hearing-impaired individual should be present during the educational sessions to ensure that the caregiver is effective in carrying out his or her roles. Caring for an individual with senile dementia is extremely stressful; therefore all instructions and counseling tips should be written down, and sessions should be repetitive, with ample opportunity for practice. The number of sessions should be kept to a minimum as the demands on the caregiver are great and hearing loss is only one of many conditions afflicting the person with dementia. Finally, it is important to remember that caregivers play a decisive role in the rehabilitation process, and thus every effort should be made to design educational sessions that will maximize the learning experience.[13]

## Implications for Future Research

The dearth of research on the evaluation and management of the hearing impaired with senile dementia and the impact of hearing loss on diagnosis renders this area an exciting and fruitful one to explore. With regard to the latter, a large-scale multidisciplinary study of the extent to which unidentified or unremediated hearing loss confounds mental status testing and the ultimate diagnosis of dementia is essential. A study of this nature should explore the impact of all levels of hearing loss and all levels of dementia on diagnosis. The severity of hearing loss sufficient to confound mental status testing should be delineated.[16] If a large proportion of individuals are falsely diagnosed, reliable and valid methods for overcoming auditory mental status artifact should be investigated.

The extent of the relationship between cognitive status, as measured using a variety of mental status tests, and hearing loss severity (i.e., ranging from normal hearing to profound) remains somewhat controversial because of methodologic problems of earlier studies. A related question that requires an answer is whether there is a causal link between hearing loss and dementia or the extent to which hearing loss exacerbates dementia. If a definite relationship is noted, this finding would have profound implications for the role of the audiologist in the multidisciplinary assessment. Additionally, if a relationship emerges, the importance of auditory interventions would be underscored.

The effect of short-term or long-term amplification use on performance on selected cognitive tasks and on patient function should be explored to determine the efficacy of this treatment approach. For example, what are the effects of consistent use of amplification on level of orientation, memory, communicative function, and performance of activities of daily living?

As mental status tends to fluctuate, the reliability of pure-tone and speech tests over time should be explored. Further, the influence of severity of dementia on the reliability and validity of pure-tone and speech tests requires investigation. The severity and prevalence of hearing loss in a large sample of individuals should be determined and compared to that of a nondemented population. Depending on the outcome, the findings may assist in underlining the importance of the audiologist in the assessment of persons with dementia. Answers to some or all of the above questions will help define a more extensive research agenda for the future.

## Concluding Remarks

Persons with senile dementia suffer from a unique set of cognitive, physical, and psychosocial problems that are often compounded by an unidentified hearing loss. The goal of this chapter was to provide convincing evidence for the importance of uncovering hearing loss in persons with senile dementia and to offer techniques for identifying and reliably testing the hearing of persons with dementia. The interventions available for managing the hearing impaired, including hearing aids and assistive listening devices, were discussed, with special emphasis placed on the technology most appropriate for persons with dementia. The critical role of the caregiver in helping to overcome the difficulties created by hearing loss were acknowledged and strategies for promoting adjustment to new technologies outlined. Finally, it should be reiterated that management of persons with senile dementia is typically interdisciplinary. The audiologist or speech-language pathologist must therefore be diligent in attempting to become part of the team that assesses and ultimately decides on the management of persons with dementia. Once communication disorders specialists gain recognition as part of the team, it will become apparent that the ability to communicate is integral to the well-being of persons with dementia and to their families.

## References

1. Beaulac M, Pehringer J, Shough L. Assistive listening devices: Available options. In: Compton C, ed. Seminars in hearing. New York: Thieme Medical Publishers, 1988:1.
2. Gilhome-Herbst KG, Humphrey C. Hearing impairment and mental state in the elderly living at home. Br Med J 1980; 281:903–905.
3. Katzman R. Medical progress. N Engl J Med 1986; 314:964–973.
4. Larose G, Evans M, Larose R. Alerting devices: Available options. In: Compton C, ed. Seminars in hearing. New York: Thieme Medical Publishers, 1988:66.
5. Leavitt R. Considerations for use of rehabilitation technology by the hearing impaired person. In: Compton C, ed. Seminars in hearing. New York: Thieme Medical Publishers, 1988:1.
6. Locke S. Neurological disorders of the elderly. In: Reichel W, ed. Clinical aspects of aging. 2nd ed. Baltimore: Williams & Wilkins, 1983:151–166.
7. Lubinski R, Weinstein B. Status of communication services in nursing homes in New York State. ASHA 1988; 30:69–72.
8. Luey H, Belser D, Glass L. Beyond refuge: Coping with losses of vision and hearing in late life. San Francisco: University of California, 1989.
9. National Institute on Aging. Senility reconsidered. JAMA 1980; 244:259–263.
10. Peters CA, Potter JF, Scholer SG. Hearing impairment as a predictor of cognitive decline in dementia. J Am Geriatr Soc 1988; 36:981–986.
11. Raiford C. Treatment of the hearing impaired older individual: A gerontological perspective. In: Shadden G, ed. Communication behavior and aging. Baltimore: Williams & Wilkins, 1988:237.
12. Reichel W. The evaluation and management of the confused, disoriented, or demented elderly patient. In: Reichel W, ed. Clinical aspects of aging. 2nd ed. Baltimore: Williams & Wilkins, 1983:151.
13. Shadden B. Education, counseling, and support for significant others. In: Shadden B, ed. Communication behavior and aging. Baltimore: Williams & Wilkins, 1988:309.
14. Slager R. Romancing the phone: The adventure continues. In: Compton C, ed. Seminars in hearing. New York: Thieme Medical Publishers, 1988:66.
15. Uhlmann R, Larson B, Koepsell T. Hearing impairment and cognitive decline in senile dementia of the Alzheimer's type. J Am Geriatr Soc 1986; 32:207–210.
16. Uhlmann R, Larson E, Rees T, et al. Relationship of hearing impairment to dementia and cognitive dysfunction in older adults. JAMA 1989; 261:1961–1969.
17. Uhlmann R, Rees T, Psaty B, Duckert L. Validity and reliability of auditory screening tests in demented and non-demented older adults. J Gen Intern Med 1989; 4:90–96.
18. Uhlmann R, Teri L, Rees T, et al. Impact of mild to moderate hearing loss on mental status testing: comparability of standard and written Mini-Mental State Examinations. J Am Geriatr Soc 1989; 37:223–228.
19. Weinstein B, Amsel L. Hearing loss and senile dementia in the institutionalized elderly. Clin Gerontol 1986; 4:3–15.
20. Witte K. Hearing impairment and cognitive decline among aging nursing home patients. Hear J 1989; 42:17–20.
21. Wondolowski C, Chartock P. Guidelines for nursing management in Alzheimer's care. J Adv Surg Nurs 1989; 1:76–87.

# APPENDIX

*Resource Centers for Information on Alerting Devices**

Sound Resources Inc.
201 E. Ogden Ave. #126
Hinsdale, IL 60521
(312) 325-6133

National Information
Center on Deafness
Gallaudet University
800 Florida Ave NE
Washington, DC 20002
1-800-672-6720 (ext. 5051)

HARC Mercantile, Ltd.
Div. HAC of America, Inc.
3130 Portage Road
P.O. Box 3055
Kalamazoo, MI 49003-3055
1-800-962-6634

---

*From Larose G, Evans M, Larose R. Alerting devices: Available options. In: Compton C, ed. Seminars in hearing. New York: Thieme Medical Publishers, 1988:66–78.

# CHAPTER 15

# Nature and Efficacy of Communication Management in Alzheimer's Disease

LYNNE W. CLARK, Ph.D.
KASSIE WITTE, M.S.

Alzheimer's disease is one of the most serious health care concerns associated with the growing elderly population and is the major form of the irreversible and progressive forms of dementia.[8,32] Presently, 1.5 to 2 million Americans suffer from this devastating disease, which erodes personality and cognition and communicative and daily functioning.[49,71]

With our current professional knowledge of Alzheimer's disease, there is no definitive medical treatment that can reverse or arrest the course of the disease. Consequently, once an accurate clinical diagnosis is reached, health-care professionals are charged with the responsibility of planning management approaches directed toward providing a safe, structured, supportive, consistent, and predictable environment for symptomatic relief of the physical and psychosocial discomforts associated with the advancing illness. Most speech-language pathologists would agree that they have an important professional role in the diagnosis of the communication impairments associated with Alzheimer's disease. However, professional disagreement exists as to what the role of the speech-language pathologist should be in the management of a person with Alzheimer's disease and that person's caregivers.

For professionals in speech-language pathology, there exists a paucity of empirically derived communication management approaches for Alzheimer's disease. The lack of communication management approaches for Alzheimer's disease may arise for several reasons. The speech-language pathologist may adopt an adverse view of Alzheimer's disease patient care management because of the progressive nature of the disease. The absence of communication management programs may derive from the lack of adequate academic and clinical preparation concerning the aging in general and, more specifically, those with Alzheimer's disease. At present, only a handful of graduate programs across the United States provide academic and clinical training in aging.[65,77] Speech-language pathologists may be less inclined to participate as professionals in continuing-education programs offered in aging and dementia because more traditional academic and clinical preparation views treatment as an option for those who will likely be able to improve and stabilize their communication functions. Speech-language pathologists may avoid management of this population because some private insurance companies refuse reimbursement for communication services.

The American Speech-Language-Hearing Association's position statement on the roles of speech-language pathologists and audiologists who work with older persons details the need for:

*Increasing involvement in the evaluation and management of the patient with Alzheimer's disease and related disorders through such assessment of level of communication skills, control of the potential confounding effects of unrecognized communication disorders on the diagnosis of dementia, interdisciplinary participation in program development, provision of specific treatment programs designed to facilitate and maintain functional commu-*

TABLE 15.1 Direct Nonmedical Management Approaches and Benefits

| | ENVIRONMENTAL AWARENESS | EMOTIONAL SECURITY | COGNITIVE FUNCTIONING (MEMORY) | COMMUNICATION SKILLS | APPROPRIATE BEHAVIOR | PHYSICAL FUNCTIONING | SOCIAL SKILLS | CLINICAL STAGE |
|---|---|---|---|---|---|---|---|---|
| Reality orientation*[33] | X | | X | X | | | X | Early |
| Psychotherapy[27] | | X | | X | | | | Early |
| Resocialization[10] | X | | X | X | | | X | All |
| Remotivation[22] | X | X | X | X | X | X | X | Early and middle |
| Pet program[9] | X | X | | | | | X | Middle |
| Reminiscence[19] | | X | X | X | | | X | Middle |
| Validation therapy[30] | X | X | | X | X | | X | Advanced |
| Operant conditioning[45] | X | | | X | X | | | Advanced |
| Behavioral contingency therapy[27] | X | | X | X | | | | Middle and advanced |
| Memory retraining[53,102] | | | X | X | | | | Early |
| External memory aids[38] | | | X | | | | | Early and middle |
| Direct cognitive stimulation[70] | | | X | X | | | | Early and middle |
| Sensory training[81] | X | | | X | | | X | Middle and advanced |
| Music therapy[74] | X | X | | X | | | | All |
| Art therapy[91] | | X | X | X | | | | All |
| Dance movement therapy[17] | X | X | | X | | X | X | All |

*Superscript numbers indicate reference for these approaches

nication for as long as possible, and assistance to families in understanding communication breakdown, specific deficits, and needs.[18]

This chapter begins with an historical review of the nonmedical management approaches directed toward maintaining or enhancing daily functioning in persons with Alzheimer's disease. Within this historical review, direct management approaches for communication disturbances associated with Alzheimer's disease are highlighted. The chapter also provides suggestions for direct, patient-oriented communication management. Finally, efficacy issues and methodologic considerations for future communication management studies are discussed.

## Direct Management Approaches of Various Health-Care Disciplines

A variety of management approaches have been developed by professionals in the disciplines of social work, nursing, occupational therapy, movement and dance, art and music therapies, psychology, and psychiatry for directly managing persons with Alzheimer's disease.[47] Table 15.1 outlines the major direct patient management approaches. As listed in Table 15.1, the therapeutic benefits for each approach include the primary benefits initially intended by an investigator, as well as unintended additional benefits. What follows is a brief description of these major approaches.

Reality orientation (RO) is a relearning process that involves reorienting individuals to the physical environment, time, persons, and past events through environmental and interpersonal cues. This process informs persons about significant factors in their environment.[2,24,33,37,44] Psychotherapy attempts to establish a "therapeutic communication" milieu for reducing the stress and feelings of helplessness that Alzheimer's patients experience when they first learn of the diagnosis of their condition.[27,89] Psychotherapy also attempts to prevent additional maladaptive defenses from occurring that exacerbate the degree of patients' clinical impairments.[54,57]

During resocialization, patients experience a secure, personal, and supportive atmosphere for maintaining self-esteem and social interaction skills.[10,62,95] Remotivation therapy provides a structured discussion-group format for stimulating and revitalizing persons' interest and involvement with the immediate environment.[7,22] Similar to the intended benefits of remotivation therapy, pet therapy has been used to combat social withdrawal and loneliness.[9] Reminiscence groups provide members with an opportunity to socialize and communicate where members are allowed to recall and share their memories without being labeled as "living in the past."[19,26,60] Validation therapy is designed to assist the moderately to severely disoriented demented elderly in learning that they can replace their confused thinking with cogent emotional memories.[28-30] In this way, patients regain self-worth, reduce emotional stress, feel satisfied with their lives, and help resolve unfinished conflicts with the past. Operant conditioning techniques are used to decrease withdrawn, nonverbal, and regressive behavior in Alzheimer's disease patients.[45,75,85]

A variety of approaches has been developed to improve the memory abilities of Alzheimer's disease patients in the early stages of the disease. However, the reported results of many of these approaches have been less beneficial than those reported for aforementioned approaches that are designed to create a healthier living environment for the person with Alzheimer's disease. Behavioral contingency therapy in the form of tokens earned with a reward has been employed to increase patients' attention to the environment and memory for daily activities (e.g., when to take medications, recalling nursing-home activities, and when visitors are expected).[27,40] Visual imagery techniques, alphabetical cueing, and first letter mnemonics have been used to stimulate the memory abilities of patients in the early stages of Alzheimer's disease.[53,61,63,97,102] Pictures of concrete objects, daily symbols (e.g., toilet for bathroom), and other external memory devices have been used to aid memory.[38,98] For example, Kurlycheck used a digital alarm watch to remind patients of their daily programs.[52] In addition, word games and Piagetian cognitive tasks have been used to stimulate general cognitive functioning in Alzheimer's patients.[70] Sensory training is designed to stimulate cognitive functioning and to increase the person's ability to interact with the environment through the five senses (i.e., tactile, kinesthetic, proprioceptive, olfactory, auditory, and visual).[23,81,92]

Nonverbal management approaches for persons with Alzheimer's disease include music, art, and dance therapies. Music therapy is designed to maintain remaining nonverbal communication abilities and responsiveness to the environment, to experience emotions, and to enhance relaxation.[74] Dance and movement therapies are intended to stimulate nonverbal communication and social awareness in Alzheimer's patients while decreasing the physical and emotional stress that often takes the form of agitation and restlessness.[17,96] In addition, these therapies are aimed at increasing overall physical and cardiovascular functioning and regulating normal appetite and digestion.[86] Similarly, art therapy provides a nonverbal means for emotional expression and thought.[91]

As highlighted in Table 15.1, a majority of the direct patient management approaches provide temporary therapeutic benefits. In the early stages of the disease, patients' social skills are enhanced and environmental awareness is enhanced through reality orientation, psychotherapy, resocialization, remotivation, and reminiscence therapies. Patients' remaining cognitive abilities are stimulated through memory and sensory training, direct cognitive stimulation activities, and use of external memory aids. Patients in later stages receive benefits that include the maintenance of socially appropriate behavior and emotional security through validation therapy, operant conditioning, behavioral contingency, and art and music therapies. Physical functioning is enhanced through dance and movement therapies.

Communication, whether nonverbal or verbal, is an unstated theme in many, if not all, of these direct patient management approaches. In these approaches, communication serves as an important vehicle for expressing emotion, sharing memories, interacting socially, developing a supportive emotional atmosphere, stimulating awareness and responsiveness to the physical and human environment, and maintaining body awareness for activities of daily living. Further, as reported anecdotally by various investigators, communication abilities of persons with Alzheimer's disease are enhanced by these approaches. Nonverbal, withdrawn persons begin verbalizing or begin using gestures with persons in their environment and become responsive to spoken information.[28] Communicatively impaired persons increase the amount of their verbal output and use more socially appropriate verbal expressions with familiar persons in their environment.[10] Thus, the speech-language pathologist must have a clear understanding of these approaches so that he or she can work more effectively with other members of a health-care team (e.g., occupational and recreational therapists) and help establish therapeutically valid and reliable methods for direct patient care management practiced by the other care professions.[21]

## Studies on Communication Management

In the speech-language pathology literature there have been few direct patient care communication management studies reported. Many of the communication approaches used with Alzheimer's patients are adaptations of approaches used with classical aphasic patients and the normal elderly.[31]

Ratusnik, Lascoe, Herbon, and Wolfe used group sessions to attempt to improve demented patients' awareness of themselves and others, their social behavior, and their orientation to time and place.[78] This approach was also intended to decrease patients' word-finding difficulties while increasing their appropriate verbal responses and gestural communication abilities. The program included traditional stimulus-response activities and group discussion. Groups included persons with varying types of dementia and at varying stages of the dementing process. Following approximately 2 months (four 40-minute sessions weekly) of treatment, Ratusnik et al reported that over half of the 16 patients, and more specifically those with senile dementia, had improved receptive and expressive language abilities and were better oriented to time and place. The degree of patients' improvement was based on the combined subjective clinical observations of a nurse and two speech-language pathologists.

Schwartz, Marin, and Saffran were unsuccessful in their attempts to teach a moderately impaired Alzheimer's patient to use her unimpaired syntactical abilities to aid her lexical semantic deficits.[87] By combining written with auditory information for 13 comprehension subtests of the Boston Diagnostic Aphasia Examination, Obler, Oberman, Samuel, and Albert showed that eight of their nine mild to moderate Alzheimer's disease patients' comprehension abilities could be enhanced.[36,69] As Obler and her colleagues point out, patients' comprehension abilities were most enhanced by this approach for more lengthy and more syntactically complex material. Harris and Ivory used reality orientation activities over a 5-month treatment period.[39] They noted that the verbal behaviors of treated demented patients (e.g., spontaneous verbal interactions, correctly using their own and the other patients' names, and following simple verbal requests) were significantly better than the verbal behaviors of nontreated patients. Witte reported maintaining the level of conversational pragmatic and discourse abilities for over 1 year in a group of eight institutionalized patients in the more advanced stages of Alzheimer's disease.[99] Her approach utilized communication facilitation programs previously employed with normal institutionalized adults, reality orientation procedures, aphasia stimulation therapy techniques, and group dynamic skills. Patients maintained the ability to self-initiate conversational turns and to embellish topics by providing new and related ideas to the conversation during group sessions. There was, however, no apparent carryover of these conversational skills to the patients' own daily situations.

In Clark's study, eight mild- to moderate-stage, community-dwelling Alzheimer's patients practiced adaptive coping communication strategies (i.e., patient-generated phrases to externally manipulate the communication environment, such as asking the speaker to repeat the message to aid comprehension) and facilitatory communication strategies (i.e., conscious use of remaining communication strengths such as circumlocution when word-finding difficulties occur) during group sessions over a 6-month period.[15] Results of her study showed that both patients and caregivers reported that patients had maintained or, in some instances, even improved the adequacy of their daily functional communication. Although their actual linguistic skills (i.e., naming, discourse, and auditory comprehension) as measured by formal aphasic test batteries (i.e., Boston Diagnostic Aphasia Exam and Boston Naming Test) did not improve, the treated patients actually maintained their naming and auditory comprehension skills for longer periods than did the nontreated demented patients.

Glickstein designed a communication treatment approach for individual patients in the mild and moderate stages of Alzheimer's disease.[34] Although no actual treatment data are available, her approach focuses on enhancing the patient's interpersonal communication skills in daily situations. Her approach utilizes multimodality sensory stimulation and cueing techniques. Both the patient and caregiver are provided with communication-oriented activities of daily living. For example, during the activity of unpacking groceries in the kitchen, the patient must read the shopping list and identify for the caregiver whether all items on the list were purchased.

These communication management studies need to be empirically validated. Among the methodologic flaws in most of these studies are the lack of adequate control groups, the use of inappropriate or inadequate measures, and poor sampling procedures. Thus, the results cannot be generalized. Further, management approaches that purport to require learning of new behaviors or to stimulate previously learned communicative abilities may be undermined by disturbances in memory, attention, and learning. These and other methodologic considerations will be addressed in more detail in a later section of this chapter.

## Communication Management Principles: State of the Art

Although many of the communication management principles apply throughout the disease process, the specific therapeutic approaches will vary according to the severity of the presenting clinical communication symptoms. As a general management principle, health-care professionals must recognize and accept the fact that all demented patients have the right to maintain optimal use of their functional residual communication abilities. For Alzheimer's patients, this principle will enhance their quality of life at all stages and will also reduce the communication stress and burden imposed on their caregivers. Emphasizing the use of remaining communicative functions, regardless of how primitive and regressive they may be, demonstrates respect for personhood and the notion of adding quality and not just years to life. This is an ethical and obligatory consideration for all health-care providers. The authors, as do all speech-language pathologists, accept that communication is the essence of human socialization. Therefore, by managing the functional communication abilities of Alzheimer's patients, we have complied with the two prerequisites for the quality of life—having a purpose for living and deriving pleasure from life through social interaction.

The following points outline more specific communication principles. These principles should guide the communication disorders specialists' direct and indirect communication management of individuals with dementia.

### Promotion of Communication Competency

Patients in all but the final stages of the disease must experience continued social communication adequacy within the constraints of the communication impairments that are directly related to the disease. In this way, premature and excessive functional communication disability may be prevented.

Functional communication disability is beyond what is a direct consequence of the disease itself.[100] For example, a patient often withdraws from communication interactions when he or she is experiencing feelings of inadequacy as a successful communicator (see Chapter 10 on helplessness). Further, patients in the early stages may use inappropriate verbal cover-up strategies that interfere with the natural flow of conversation such as stating: "I know all that, I just don't want to talk about it now." By maintaining existing use of functional and residual linguistic abilities for as long as possible, patients may reduce the risk of premature loss of such capabilities.

### Promotion of Normal Adaptive and Facilitative Communication Behaviors

Patients in the early stages of Alzheimer's disease must be encouraged to use normal adaptive and facilitative communication strategies to prevent their existing communication impairments from interfering with competent interpersonal communication.

### Promotion of Communication Opportunities

Patients at all stages of the disease must be provided with a variety of communication opportunities in their own daily environments. Opportunities for communication during activities of daily living, leisure, recreation, and social pursuits may encourage Alzheimer's patients to achieve their maximum levels of communication. In the institutional setting, communication interaction groups may be the primary situation where patients have the opportunity to communicate. Moreover, such groups provide the necessary communicative and linguistic structure for patients to communicate at their maximum level. (See Chapter 16 on the environment for more details on communication opportunities.)

### Control Over Communication Interactions

During the early stages of Alzheimer's disease when patients first experience a general loss of control of their own lives, they must have opportunities to demonstrate self-directedness over their own social communicative interactions.

### Enhancement of Communication Interactions Between Patient and Caregiver

Patients at all stages of the disease experience communication deficits (see Chapters 7 and 8). These irreversible changes become more disabling over time. Yet, without professional guidance, their communication partners rarely modify the lexical, syntactic, and pragmatic components of verbal exchange to help patients compensate for their ensuing deficits. Consequently, programs designed to enhance the communication skills of caregivers with Alzheimer's patients are warranted.

### Maintenance of Self-Esteem and Dignity Through Promotion of Communication Exchange

Patients at all stages of the disease experience a multiplicity of losses, not the least of which is the ability to share thoughts, feelings, and ideas with others. Patients' self-esteem and dignity are promoted by creating a communication environment that fosters adult-to-adult exchange at the patients' functional level.

### Reduction of Emotional Communicative Stress

Patients in the early stages of the disease often deny the communication changes associated with the disease. In an effort to try to hide these changes, patients experience anxiety and stress. Patients must share their anxiety about these changes with others and at the same time experience communication success.

### Maintenance of Emotional Security

Alzheimer's patients in the middle and late stages of the disease may have the need to belong and to feel comforted and emotionally secure.[83] These very basic needs continue long after the patient can express them. Effective verbal and nonverbal communication strategies convey feelings of continued caring, love, and respect for patients at the latter end of the disease continuum.

## Communication Management Approaches

Two major approaches to communication management of Alzheimer's patients are direct and indirect patient care. In the first, the speech-language pathologist works directly with the patient to maintain as many communication strengths as possible. In the second, the speech-language pathologist works with caregivers to develop strategies for better interpersonal communication between the patient and caregivers. This latter approach includes communication techniques that are designed to benefit both the patient and caregivers. The specific techniques within these broad approaches vary depending on the severity of the patient's clinical communication symptoms and the caregivers' ability to adapt strategies that are appropriate along the disease continuum. Further, these approaches are not mutually exclusive but, in fact, complement each other throughout the stages of Alzheimer's disease. Thus, it is imperative that the speech-language pathologist know the communication changes associated with each specific clinical stage and appreciate all the other clinical symptoms associated with the disease.

### DIRECT PATIENT CARE APPROACHES FOR THE EARLY STAGES

Direct communication approaches during the early stage of Alzheimer's disease are based on the clinically diagnosed communication and cognitive strengths and weaknesses of the patient, assessment of the emotional impact these changes have on the patient and caregiver, and a general knowledge of stress management techniques.[101]

In accordance with Reisberg's Global Deterioration Scale, patients in the clinical stages 2 and 3 and those beginning stage 4 demonstrate mild to bordering moderate cognitive impairments.[79] Patients exhibit some abstract and problem-solving capabilities, are fairly well oriented to person and place, and retain some ability to manipulate concrete information. Communicatively, patients at the early stage still understand the meaning of most lexical items and possess good expressive syntactic and phonologic skills.[67] Pragmatic abilities of these patients are still fairly well intact, although they may experience some difficulty with self-initiated as opposed to responsive speech acts.[16] Conversationally, they can still maintain turn taking and self-revisions.[82]

Despite these communication strengths, patients display communication weaknesses that may require direct patient management. Patients display expressive difficulty in finding correct words and receptive difficulty in fully comprehending lengthy and syntactically complex auditory material.[73] Patients may provide pronouns without referents and focus on the secondary rather than primary details of the conversational topic so that topic maintenance and cohesion are mildly disrupted.[68] Patients at these earlier stages express concern over the communication changes they are experiencing in social situations.

With knowledge of the cognitive and communicative changes associated with the early stage of Alzheimer's disease, the following direct patient management strategies are proposed to assist in managing patients' communicative competency, naming, comprehension, and conversational skills. Although these strategies are based on present knowledge of the cognitive and linguistic processes and may prove helpful, they need to be empirically tested for validity and reliability.

Communication *adaptive strategies* are patient-generated strategies that are to be used consistently by the patient to manipulate the communicative environment externally so as to gain control as a communicator. Use of such strategies is intended to prevent the patient's *communication weaknesses* (i.e., naming, comprehension, and conversational topic-maintenance difficulties) from interfering with the person's ability to be a competent communicator. In addition, the use of such strategies alerts the other communicators in the speaking situation to the immediate nature of the person's communication difficulties.

The following examples illustrate the use of such strategies. The patient who has difficulty comprehending the speaker might say "Please repeat exactly what you just said" or "Say what you said more slowly." When the patient has difficulty finding the correct words and does not want assistance or interruption from the listener, the patient might state, "Give me a little time, I'm having trouble finding the exact words to describe what I want to tell you." For conversational topic maintenance and cohesion, the patient might inform the listener by stating "I forgot what we were discussing."

With communication *facilitation strategies*, patients consciously use their remaining avenues of *communication strengths* to assist in enhancing their expressive abilities as a communicator. As outlined below, different strategies are used to assist patients in finding target words, in maintaining cohesiveness of conversation topics, and in relating the idea of an abstract message to the listener.

1. Circumlocutions and semantically related word strategies. During the early stages of the disease, Alzheimer's patients still benefit from lexical semantic (and phonemic) cueing to elicit the name of an object or its action.[67] Therefore, patients are encouraged to use circumlocution or a semantically related word for the intended word as strategies to facilitate the eventual retrieval of the correct word. For example, Mary had difficulty saying "movies" in response to Joe's question, "What did you do last night?" Mary then stated, "I saw a story, an adventure story. It was on a large screen. There were lots of people sitting. Oh you know, I went to the *movies*."

2. Phonemically related word strategies. Often, Alzheimer's patients experience the "tip of the tongue" phenomenon. Phonemic cueing strategies such as saying a word that rhymes with the intended word, saying the first sound of the intended word, or silently spelling the word may facilitate the patient's production of the word. For example, Jim could not say the word "tea" in response to Betsy's question, "What do you want to drink with your dinner?" Jim then responded, "I want the thing that starts with the letter [t] and rhymes with 'flea' and 'pea.' Oh, I want *tea*."

3. Script strategy. For topic maintenance and cohesion during conversation, patients are instructed to design a script strategy prior to sharing their story. This requires that the patient state the conversational theme, setting, main characters, events, actions, consequences, or outcomes. For example, in discussing a recent vacation, Sue said, "I went on a *vacation* (theme). My

husband, *Joe*, went with *me* (characters). We flew to *Hawaii* (setting). In Hawaii, we went *swimming* and *sight-seeing* (events). Although it was a delightful vacation, it *cost a lot of money* (consequence)!"

4. Life experience strategy. When patients experience difficulty expressing an abstract idea, they are encouraged to use their life experiences to explain the idea. In this way, patients are able to convey the intent of their abstract message to the listener. For example, Mr. Smith's grandson asked him what the word democracy meant when doing his social studies assignment for school. Mr. Smith explained, "It's like when I decided to go alone to Alaska last year to see your Uncle Jim. Your grandmother argued with me and said I couldn't go alone. Don't you remember that in the end, I did fly there on my own and had a great trip."

### Group Therapy for Early Stages

For persons in the early stages of the disease, a group setting is an ideal design for patients to practice their communication *adaptive and facilitative strategies*. Group activities should be designed to stimulate patients' active use of these strategies. For example, an object-barrier task can be used to facilitate patients' active *use of circumlocution* and semantically related words. To *maintain topic coherence*, patients can be asked to create a story from a Norman Rockwell picture using the script structure outlined above. To *express the intent of an abstract idea*, a task using idioms can be utilized. Patients who keep a notebook that lists the adaptive and facilitative strategies are able to review the strategies for use in their own environment and to report to the other patients in the group which strategies are the most beneficial.

The group setting provides a context for demonstrating social communicative confidence. Discussion of patients' communication difficulties associated with the disease is one of the major focuses of the group. In the group, patients can share their feelings regarding their communication difficulties and come to realize that their problems are not unique. By no longer denying their communication impairments, patients' communicative stresses and anxieties may be reduced. By achieving functional communication successes in the nonthreatening atmosphere of the group, patients come to accept that although the communication changes associated with the disease are occurring, they still can be vital and successful communicators. In doing so, patients build self-esteem by developing a sense of being helped as well as helping others.

The speech-language pathologist must act as the group's facilitator. The facilitator must have skills in manipulating turn taking, sustaining the group's interest, knowing when to offer cognitive challenge for eliciting group participation, and maintaining attention in a nonthreatening and nonjudgmental emotional climate. Such an atmosphere fosters positive reinforcement of patients' participation and establishes an optimal number of communication successes.

Group programs for patients in the early stages of Alzheimer's disease are likely to be found in outpatient speech-language and hearing centers and adult day-care settings. Eight to 10 patients with Alzheimer's disease who display similar levels of cognitive and communicative functions make an ideal grouping. Two 45 to 60 minute group sessions should be scheduled weekly. Group programs for patients in the early stages have a limited duration of 3 to 6 months. By this time, group members will have had sufficient time and opportunity to learn and practice the communication strategies so as to use them successfully in their environment to regain a measure of self-esteem as a communicator and to better cope emotionally with their communication changes.

The physical setting of the group program is important. A private area with good lighting, devoid of acoustic interference and visual distractions, and with temperature control is ideal. Semicircular seating for the group is recommended. The facilitator then can move within the enclosed space to encourage attention and interaction. The group also provides an ideal setting for professional caregivers and family to observe various facilitating communication techniques used by the group's leader. Although most caregivers will better understand these techniques after description, explanation of the rationale, observation, and practice, the astute caregiver will be able to learn to use these techniques through observation alone.

## APPROACHES FOR THE ADVANCED STAGES

During more advanced stages of dementia (GDS stages 6 and 7), the earlier communicative problems are further compounded by comprehension, lexical, syntactic, and pragmatic deficits. Patients in this phase of the disease process demonstrate difficulty following one-step verbal requests, have difficulty understanding simple conversations, and cannot maintain topical cohesion. Increased anomia, disorganized and incomplete syntactical constructions, and lack of communication initiative become characteristic of patients' communication attempts. These patient's demonstrate extremely poor topical cohesion, which results in an overabundance of inappropriate responses.[66] As the disease progresses, comprehension may be limited to intermittent recognition of simple, familiar phrases. Severe anomia contributes to vacuous speech. Utterances are perseverative and for the most part egocentric. Output may be severely limited, or characterized by paraphasias (i.e., substitution of a semantically or phonemically related word for the intended word) and speech dysfluencies, confounding the analysis of syntax and phonology.[68] For the most part, the pragmatics of adult discourse are no longer functional.[46] There may be no evidence of discourse tracking except for very rudimentary social greetings. By the end of stage 7, the patient may either be mute, vocalize only in response to pain, or engage in self-stimulation phonatory behavior.[80]

In light of the functional limitations of patients at the more advanced stages of the disease, a direct patient-care management approach for the preservation of communication function is not designed to promote new learning or relearning. Rather, the intent of any direct patient care management program during the advanced stages is to provide a structured format that supplies the linguistic constructs, vocabulary options, and social opportunities for self-expression similar to the daily adult-to-adult conversations that persons experienced during their lives. Because these patients lack utterance initiative and the ability to sustain conversation, they require a structured format provided by a facilitator in order to converse and use their remaining communication skills to their maximal ability.

## Group Therapy for Advanced Stages

Group programs for persons in more advanced stages of the disease depend on the group facilitator's ability to encourage the use of patients' residual communication strengths. The facilitator focuses on communication as a task-oriented activity. Treatment principles applicable to group communication management can be extrapolated from Schuell's stimulation therapy[25] and Chapey's divergent semantic intervention therapy.[12] Group communication management principles for the advanced stages of Alzheimer's disease are summarized in Table 15.2.

It is a challenge to the group facilitator when working with a group of advanced-stage Alzheimer's patients to maintain topical cohesion and ensuing discourse. By actually manipulating the conversational turn taking and by refocusing the topic when topic maintenance is disrupted, the facilitator is able to sustain dialogue and enable the patients to exercise their communication strengths. One very important consideration is the level of abstraction and conceptualization required for auditory comprehension. Topics must be presented at the appropriate conceptual level to maintain attention, interest, and to ensure maxi-

TABLE 15.2 **Group Communication Management Principles for the Advanced Stages of Alzheimer's Disease**

Use intensive auditory stimulation

Stimuli must be tangible, adequate, and of genuine interest to the group. Each stimulus should elicit a response

The facilitator provides reinforcement and positive feedback. No responses are forced or corrected

The group progresses from less to more challenging, from simple to more complex, from real to possible responses

Facilitator elicits the maximum number of participant responses in a systematic fashion

New information should be extensions of the familiar

Work systematically and intensively

Develop a theme

Allow the patients' responses to dictate the thematic flow

Summarize and restate points under discussion to ensure a unified and coordinated discussion

Present participation opportunities to each member of the group at their own level of communicative ability

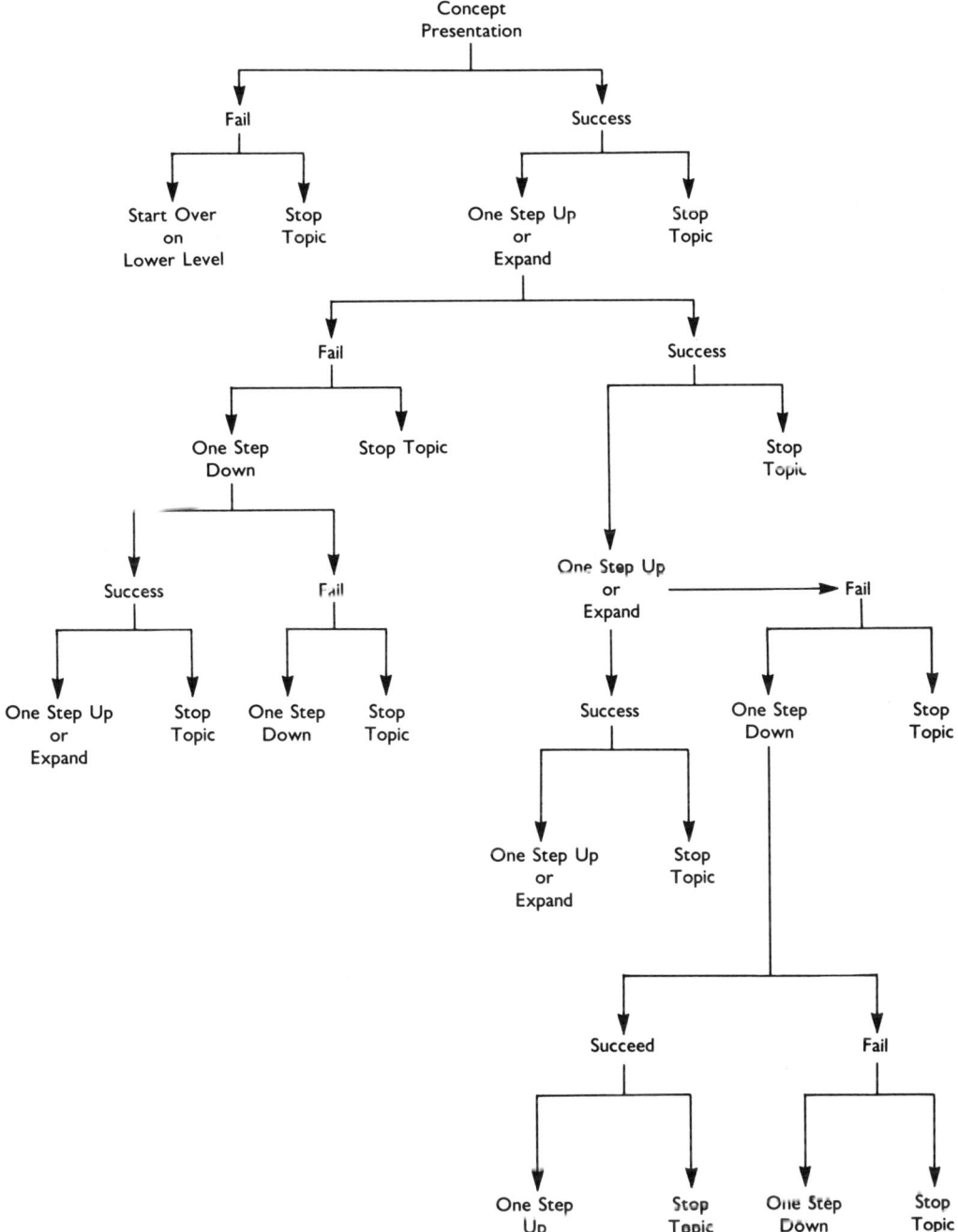

Figure 15.1 Probe technique. From Witte K. Discourse and dialogue. Am J Alzheimer's Care Res 1987; 2:30–39.

mum verbal participation. Without dynamic maintenance of the level of conceptualization, there is little opportunity for group cohesion or topic maintenance.

The facilitator depends on the group members' responses to maintain an appropriate and stimulating level of conceptual difficulty. The probe technique, illustrated in Figure 15.1, is a technique designed to identify and maintain the appropriate level of conceptual difficulty throughout the group session. As each new topic is introduced, the facilitator uses the probing technique to determine if the group members can respond to what is being said. If they cannot, then the facilitator retrenches and presents the same idea more simply. If unsuccessful, the facilitator simplifies the concept still further or abandons it. Similarly, the facilitator uses the probe technique to successfully expand topics in order to maintain attention and interest and to provide opportunities for self-expression. The probe technique allows the facilitator to monitor subtle gradations of increasing or decreasing levels of cognitive complexity so that the verbal challenges can be presented and swiftly simplified if they are beyond the ability of the group members.

For example, the group facilitator might choose to encourage group discussion on the topic of Thanksgiving meal preparation. In doing so, an initial probe might be "Does anyone know which holiday is coming up?" If there is no response, a lower level probe is introduced such as "Thanksgiving is next week. What do you do to celebrate?" If there is still no response, the facilitator would lower the conceptual level of the probe and state "Thanksgiving is next week. What do we eat on this holiday?"

Group programs for patients in the advanced stages of Alzheimer's disease are likely to be found in institutional settings or adult day-care programs. Recognizing that these settings have intrinsic limitations to creating and coordinating the "ideal" group therapy experience, the following suggestions are offered. Manage the group membership so that during each group session no more than eight participants are present. Select the group members with care. The greater the degree of common life experiences, personal life-styles and interests, and common heritage among the group members, the easier it is for the facilitator to maintain group cohesion. Select group members within a narrow range of communication disability. The group can tolerate two or three lower functioning members, but more than that will contribute to the disintegration of group cohesion. When these variables are considered, group sessions can continue for approximately 30 to 45 minutes. Conditions of the physical setting are similar to those outlined for earlier stage Alzheimer's group programs. Group sessions provide excellent opportunities to illustrate facilitating communication techniques to caregivers.

## INDIRECT PATIENT CARE APPROACHES

Indirect patient care management strategies attempt to modify the patient's "communication environment" in order to promote the person's maximal level of communication function. Indirect strategies include such interventions as communication skills training, supportive counseling, and a referral source for caregivers, in-service training for health-care professionals, and management of the physical, psychosocial environment.[76,90]

Most indirect patient-care management strategies focus on the caregiver, who may be a family member, volunteer, or paid professional.[88] It is important for the speech-language pathologist to be knowledgeable and sensitive to the impact that the person's deteriorating communication ability has on the caregiver. Family caregivers find their relative's communication deficits to be devastating (see Chapter 12). The disease insidiously deteriorates the person's lifelong communication patterns because of irreversible changes in cognitive and linguistic functions. The person's ability to compensate for these losses decreases in efficiency and effectiveness, rendering the person a handicapped and frustrated communicator. Further, these communication and cognitive changes generate feelings of frustration, agitation, stress, and despair in the caregiver.[101] Often caregivers unknowingly exacerbate the situation by continuing to use the same communication tactics that were appropriate before the onset of the disease. Modifications of lifelong patterns of verbal interactions are difficult to effect without emotional support and practical skill-development training.

Communication skill training for the family caregivers is one way to meet this need. Training focuses on educating caregivers regarding the communication changes associated with the progression of Alzheimer's disease. It also stresses implementation of appropriate caregiver communication strategies. (See Chapter 11 for further suggestions.)

The specific communication strategies taught to caregivers are linked to the implicit and explicit needs of the patient: the basic biological needs, the need for security, the need to belong, and the need for self-esteem. Caregivers require training and practice to better integrate the situational, contextual, lexical, and suprasegmental components of the message. If these elements are in any way discordant for Alzheimer's disease patients, they may become confused and thus more likely to create a behavioral disturbance (i.e., wandering, shouting, and other mood changes).

At the very least, caregivers require training to integrate the basic guidelines given in Table 15.3. For further suggestions to maximize effective communication by the caregiver at each of the various stages of the disease, refer to Beame;[5] Bollinger, Waugh, and Zatz;[6] Carroll;[11] Clark;[13] Golper and Rau;[35] and Ostuni and Santo Pietro.[72]

In-service training for staff incorporates many of the same objectives as communication skills training for home caregivers. Staff need education-

**TABLE 15.3 Guidelines to Maximize Caregiver Communication Effectiveness**

Use calm and inviting facial expressions

Assume calm and non-threatening body postures

Approach the patient within his or her visual field

Use touch to reassure

Listen for the patient's perspective and the feelings being expressed

Facilitate with nondirective comments
Use: "Let's do this together."
   "May I work with you on this one?"
   "Would you give me a hand and help?"

Use praise and compliments that are fitting for an adult

Share information one point at a time. Wait for evidence of comprehension before continuing

Use the same spoken phrases to signal routine daily activities
Use: "Your food is ready."
   When it is time to eat

   "Let's go to bed."
   When it is time to retire

   "Put your coat on."
   When it is time to go outside

Make sure the situational, contextual, and verbal cues are harmonious so they contribute to the redundancy of information within the situation

Speak slowly

---

al opportunities to understand the cognitive, behavioral, and linguistic changes observed in the Alzheimer's patient. Practical skill-development training, often in the form of an in-depth workshop series, is appropriate. Program emphasis should include how the various appropriate communication approaches commonly used with the dementia patient can facilitate patient care management during all activities of daily living, as well as how specific communication techniques can reduce the intensity or frequency of behavioral problems associated with the disease. In addition, staff need to form a support group to help them cope with the ongoing stress and frustrations of caring for Alzheimer's patients. It is recommended that a social worker be involved in this latter type of intervention. (See Chapter 17 for more details on in-service training.)

Counseling and referral to other resources are other indirect approaches that the speech-language pathologist should include in the armamentarium of services to benefit the person with Alzheimer's disease and their caregivers. Although the speech-language pathologist is not expected to provide the counseling services offered by psychologists and social workers, there is a need to be open and sensitive to the holistic concerns of the Alzheimer's family. The speech-language pathologist should be familiar with: (1) resources such as the regional chapter of the Alzheimer's Disease and Related Disorders Association; (2) the time and place of family support groups in the community; (3) resources for respite care; and (4) sources for home-health services.

In Chapter 16 Lubinski discusses the role of the speech-language pathologist in environmental intervention. This is yet another indirect-patient management approach. She suggests maintaining a positive communicative atmosphere through intensive staff training, family-caregiver counseling, and management of the physical and psychosocial environment.[55,56,84]

## Efficacy Issues

### DEFINING EFFECTIVENESS

The results of previous studies on management of communication disturbance in dementia raise compelling issues regarding how we define effectiveness and what factors should be considered when designing future investigations. Despite the obvious clinical need for both direct and indirect patient management programs, few studies document the efficacy of these approaches. If speech-language pathologists are to have a viable role with dementia patients and their families, research efforts and funding must be directed toward well-designed clinical studies.

How speech-language pathologists delineate their roles in the communication management of persons with Alzheimer's disease will depend on how they define effectiveness. Effectiveness can be defined in three ways. The most traditional method of defining improvement is to document steady increase in communication skill(s) over time. It is unrealistic, however, to expect improvement when persons with Alzheimer's disease experience difficulty learning new information or even relearning old information. The speech-language pathologist must go beyond the traditional rehabilitative paradigm and pose the effectiveness question again to professionally define what is meant by "effective."

A second option when defining effectiveness is to describe it as the maintenance of existing communication skill(s) without expectation of improvement. This may be possible in some communication areas of Alzheimer's disease, particularly during the early and middle stages.

A third option is to define effectiveness in terms of how well caregivers are able to maintain conversational adequacy with Alzheimer's patients. Effectiveness might be documented by the quality and quantity of the strategies used to facilitate meaningful exchange of information. Further, effectiveness might be measured in the level of frustration caregivers experience in communicating with the demented patient and the change in caregiver burden and stress that is experienced. This may apply to Alzheimer's patients at all stages of the disease, particularly if communication management includes caregiver communication strategies. Clinicians and researchers will find effectiveness possible if management contributes to a consistent, supportive, predictable, and structured environment that meets the patient's physiologic and psychosocial needs and those of the caregiver throughout the disease.

## METHODOLOGIC CONSIDERATIONS

Studies of direct and indirect communication management programs are complex in design and implementation. Such studies should answer the questions: (1) Is communication management effective? (2) For whom is it effective? (3) When is it effective? and (4) What techniques and strategies are effective?

In order to conduct management studies, fundamental patient selection criteria and other methodologic considerations must be taken into account. Failure to consider these factors will lead to results that are ambiguous and lack generalization.

1. The *presence and type of dementia* must be documented and well controlled. Numerous studies have used inadequate diagnostic criteria to establish the presence and type of dementia. Studies have demonstrated that communication changes differ in nature according to type and stage of dementia.[4,43]
2. Subjects should be grouped according to *similar levels of cognitive functioning*. Several studies have demonstrated that the cognitive level and not the duration of the disease correlates better with the communication changes associated with Alzheimer's disease.[1,20,64] Thus, the study should include a homogeneous group of subjects based on cognitive level.
3. An equal representation of patients at various age levels is required to *minimize cohort effect*. The literature shows that even some normal elderly adults, particularly those age 80 years and above, demonstrate communication changes, e.g., naming and discourse.[4,58,68] It is beneficial to cluster age groups such as 60 to 65 years, 66 to 70 years, 71 to 74 years, etc.
4. Psychotropic *drugs* are often used with dementia patients to decrease depression and hyperactive behavior. Although it is known that one of the negative side effects of certain psychotropic drugs is tardive dyskinesia, it is possible that these and other drugs used by the elderly may affect other communication functions.[14] It is advisable that patients be as drug-free as possible.
5. The researcher runs the risk of having the *institutional setting* act as an independent confounding factor if both noninstitutionalized and institutionalized subjects are grouped together in the study.
6. The *targets* or *goals* of the communication therapy must be *operationally defined*. Clear identification of target communication behavior(s) leads to well-chosen measuring tools. For example, if the goal is to maintain existing residual linguistic strengths such as naming, formal aphasia tests might be chosen.[36,48,50] The development of the Bayles Arizona Battery for Communication in Dementia will prove a powerful tool for this goal.[3] Should functional communication be the goal, the Scale of Communication Adequacy in

Daily Situations (CADS) might be useful (see Appendix at the end of this chapter). Finally, if the goal is adequate exchange of information between dementia patient and caregiver, observation and detailed video analysis of effective versus ineffective strategies should be used.

7. Management *procedures and rationale must be detailed* for analysis and replication purposes. Materials used in management must be relevant to patient's needs, interests, and communication level and be presented in a systematic manner. The intensity and duration of management must be examined, as that which is appropriate at one stage may not be at another stage.
8. The researcher faces an ethical dilemma when matched *control subjects* not receiving therapy are used because these subjects might also benefit from a management program. Consider using subjects who choose not to have treatment or who are unable to participate in therapy for a number of reasons (e.g., physically too remote to travel to the clinic or having insufficient income to pay for treatment). In addition, when normal or other neurologically impaired groups are used, subjects should be carefully screened and matched.
9. Other factors that must be controlled because they may affect subjects' quantitative performance include *handedness, socioeconomic level, education and occupational levels, visual and auditory acuity, primary spoken language and bilingualism, and general physical status*.[93,94] Each of these factors should be controlled, and when measuring sensory functioning, vision and hearing screenings should be performed on all subjects.
10. When considering whether the study should use a *group or single-subject design*, the researcher must remember that the results of studies using a single-subject design only show whether management is effective for one specific person. Results cannot be generalized to the population at large as they can be with a group-design study. Single-subject studies help to refine methodology and explore new and complex approaches to direct or indirect communication management. See Hartman and Hall, Kirk, Hersen and Barlow, and McReynolds and Kearns for further information on design and methodology.[41,42,51,59]

# Need For Future Clinical Research

This chapter reviewed some of the current research findings about communication management in Alzheimer's disease and the efficacy of management in general. As demonstrated, there are more questions than there are answers. The professional role of the speech-language pathologist with Alzheimer's patients will continue to be undefined until we can answer questions relating to the efficacy of communication management. Future communication management studies need to focus on several issues. First, researchers must define effectiveness. Second, studies must explore for whom management is effective and at what stages. It may well turn out that direct patient care management is not effective for patients at all stages of Alzheimer's disease. Rather, indirect patient management may be more effective at certain stages of the disease. Third, studies need to determine what specific communication behaviors are best suited for management and at what stages. Fourth, studies must determine what, when, and for whom direct and indirect approaches are appropriate. Fifth, longitudinal studies of management are needed to determine whether long-term intervention proves beneficial to patients and caregivers. Sixth, studies should explore whether the newer experimental treatment drugs for Alzheimer's disease, such as THA, oxiracetam, and piracetam have therapeutic benefits on patients' communication skills. Finally, studies need to assess whether the systematic inclusion of communication management principles and strategies into the other health-management approaches can enhance the therapeutic benefits of these approaches.

Obviously, it will be difficult to design adequate studies that examine the effectiveness of communication management in Alzheimer's disease. It is hoped that the methodologic considerations and management suggestions outlined in this chapter will assist future researchers by helping speech-language pathologists to define their role more clearly with respect to the communication management of patients with Alzheimer's disease.

### References

1. Appell J, Kertesz A, Fisman M. A study of language functioning in Alzheimer patients. Brain Lang 1982; 17:73–91.
2. Barnes J. Effect of reality orientation classroom on memory loss, confusions, and disorientation in geriatric patients. Gerontologist 1974; 14:138–142.
3. Bayles K, Boone D, Tomoeda C, et al. Differentiating Alzheimer's patients from the normal elderly and

stroke patients with aphasia. J Speech Hear Disord 1989; 54:74–87.
4. Bayles K, Kaszniak A. Communication and cognition in normal aging and dementia. Boston: College-Hill Press, 1987:35.
5. Beam J. Helping families survive. Am J Nurs 1984; 84:229–232.
6. Bollinger R, Waugh P, Zatz A. Communication management of the geriatric patient. Danville, IL: Interstate Printers & Publishers, 1977.
7. Bowers M, Anderson G, Blomeier E, Pelz K. Brain syndrome and behavior in geriatric remotivation groups. J Gerontol 1967; 22:348–352.
8. Brody J. An epidemiologist's view of the senile dementias: Pieces of the puzzle. In: Wertheimer J, Marois M. eds. Senile dementia: Outlook for the future. New York: Alan R. Liss, 1984:383.
9. Burton B. To care while waiting for cure. People, animals and environment 1989; Winter:26–31.
10. Carey B, Hansen S. Social support groups with institutionalized Alzheimer's disease victims. J Gerontol Soc Work 1985/86; 9:15–26.
11. Carroll D. When your loved one has Alzheimer's disease. New York: Harper and Row, 1989.
12. Chapey R. Cognitive intervention: Stimulation of cognition, memory, convergent thinking, divergent thinking and evaluative thinking. In: Chapey R, ed. Language intervention strategies in adult aphasia. Baltimore: Williams & Wilkins, 1981:215.
13. Clark L. Enhancing communication. In: Tanner F, Shaw S, eds. Caring: A family guide to managing the Alzheimer's patient at home. New York: New York City Alzheimer's Resource Center, 1985:20.
14. Clark L. Positive effects of physostigmine on the language deficits associated with Alzheimer's disease. Research paper presented at Albert Einstein College of Medicine. Bronx, New York, 1982.
15. Clark L. Enhancement of communication adequacy in early stage Alzheimer's disease patients. Unpublished research paper, Hunter College of CUNY. New York, 1988.
16. Clark L, Witte K, Macchia C. Pragmatic abilities in Alzheimer's disease: A pilot study. Unpublished research paper, Hunter College of CUNY. New York, 1989.
17. Cohen I, Segall J. Using dance therapy in the extended care facility. Nurs Homes 1974; 23:28–30.
18. Committee on Communication Problems of the Aging. The roles of speech-language pathologists and audiologists in working with older persons. ASHA 1988; 30:80–84.
19. Cook JB. Reminiscing: How it can help confused nursing home residents. J Contemp Soc Work 1984; 2:90–93.
20. Cummings J, Benson DF, Hill M, Read S. Aphasia in dementia of Alzheimer's type. Neurology 1985; 35:394–397.
21. Davis C. The role of the physical and occupational therapists in caring for victims of Alzheimer's disease. In: Taira E, ed. Therapeutic interventions for the person with dementia. New York: The Haworth Press, 1986:15.
22. Dennis H. Remotivation therapy. J Gerontol Nurs 1976; 2:28–30.
23. Downey J. Sensory training reawakens patients to life. Modern Nursing Home 1971; 24:62.
24. Drummond L, Kirchhoff L, Scarbrough D. A practical guide to reality orientations: A treatment approach for confusion and disorientation. Gerontologist 1978; 18:568–573.
25. Duffy J. Schuell's stimulation approach to rehabilitation. In: Chapey R, ed. Language intervention strategies in adult aphasia. Baltimore: Williams & Wilkins, 1981:105.
26. Ebersole P. Problems of group reminiscing with institutionalized aged. J Gerontol Nurs 1976; 2:23–27.
27. Eisdorfer C, Cohen D, Preston C. Behavioral and psychological therapies for the older patient with cognitive impairment. In: Miller N, Cohen G, eds. Clinical aspects of Alzheimer's disease and senile dementia. New York: Raven Press, 1981:209.
28. Feil N. Group therapy in a home for the aged. Gerontologist 1967; 7:192–195.
29. Feil N. A new approach to group therapy, research findings. Unpublished paper presented at the 25th Annual Meeting of the Gerontological Society. San Juan, Puerto Rico, December 1972.
30. Feil N. V/F validation: The Feil method. Cleveland, Ohio. Edward Feil Productions, 1982.
31. Feier C, Leight G. A communication-cognition program for elderly nursing home residents. Gerontologist 1981; 21:408–415.
32. Finch C. Alzheimer's disease: A biologist's perspective. Science 1985; 230:1109.
33. Folsom J. Reality orientation for the elderly mental patient. J Geriatr Psychiatry 1968; 1:291–307.
34. Glickstein J. Therapeutic interventions in Alzheimer's disease: A program of functional communication skills for activities of daily living. Rockville, MD: Aspen, 1988.
35. Golper L, Rau M. Treatment of communication disorders associated with generalized intellectual deficits in adults. In: Perkins W, eds. Language handicaps in adults. New York: Thieme-Stratton, 1983:119.
36. Goodglass H, Kaplan G. Examination of aphasia and related disorders. Philadelphia: Lea & Febiger, 1983.
37. Greene JC, Timbury GC, Smith R, Gardiner M. Reality orientation with elderly patients in the community: An empirical evaluation. Age Aging 1983; 12:38–43.
38. Hanley J. The use of sign posts and active training to modify ward disorientation in elderly patients. J Behav Ther Exp Psychiatry 1981; 12:241–247.
39. Harris C, Ivory P. An outcome evaluation of reality orientation therapy with geriatric patients in a state mental hospital. Gerontologist 1976; 16:496–503.
40. Harris S, Snyder B, Snyder R, Magraw B. Behavior modification therapy with elderly demented patients: Implementation and ethical considerations. J Chronic Dis 1977; 30:129–134.
41. Hartman D, Hall R. The changing criterion design. J Appl Behav Anal 1976; 9:527–532.
42. Hersen H, Barlow D. Single case experimental designs. New York: Pergamon Press, 1976.
43. Hier D, Hagenlocker K, Shindler A. Language disintegration in dementia: Effects of etiology and severity. Brain Lang 1985; 25:117–133.
44. Holden U, Sinebruchow A. Reality orientation therapy: A study investigating the value of this therapy in the rehabilitation of elderly people. Age Aging 1978; 7:83–90.
45. Hoyer W. Application of operant techniques to the modification of elderly behavior. Gerontologist 1974; 13:18–22.
46. Hutchinson J, Jensen M. A pragmatic evaluation of

discoure communication in normal and senile elderly in a nursing home. In: Obler L. and Albert M, eds. Language and communication in the elderly. Lexington, MA: Lexington Books, 1980:34.
47. Kahn RL, Zaring SH. Evaluation of mental health programs for the aged. In: Davidson PO, Clark FW, Hamerlynck LA, eds. Evaluation of behavioral programs in community, residential and school settings. Champaign, IL: Research Press, 1974:51.
48. Kaplan E, Goodglass H, Weintraub S. Boston Naming Test. Philadelphia: Lea & Febiger, 1983.
49. Katzman R. The prevalence and malignancy of Alzheimer's disease. Arch Neurol 1976; 33:217–218.
50. Kertesz A. Western Aphasia Battery. New York: Grune & Stratton, 1982.
51. Kirk R. Experimental design. Monterey, CA: Brooks/Cole, 1982.
52. Kurlycheck R. Use of a digital alarm chronograph as a memory aid in early dementia. Clin Gerontol 1983; 1:93–94.
53. Lewinsohn P, Danaher B, Kikel S. Visual imagery as a mnemonic aid for brain-injured persons. J Consult Clin Psychol 1977; 45:717–723.
54. Linden ME. Group psychotherapy with institutionalized senile women: Study in gerontologic human relations. Int J Group Psychother 1953; 3:150–170.
55. Lubinski R. Geriatric communication in institutional settings: Communicative disorders. Audio J Continuing Education, Vol. 3, 1978.
56. Lubinski R. Speech, language, and audiology programs in home health care agencies nd nursing homes. In: Beasley D, Davis G, eds. Aging communication processes and disorders. New York: Grune & Stratton, 1981:339.
57. Manaster A. Therapy with the senile geriatric patient. Int J Group Psychother 1972; 22:250–257.
58. Martin A, Fedio P. Word production and comprehension in Alzheimer's disease: The breakdown of semantic knowledge. Brain Lang 1983; 19:124–141.
59. McReynolds L, Kearns K. Single-subject designs in communicative disorders. Baltimore: University Park Press, 1983.
60. Merriam S. The concept and function of reminiscences: A review of the research. Gerontologist 1980; 20:604–609.
61. Miller E. Impaired recall and the memory disturbance in presenile dementia. Br J Soc Clin Psychol 1975; 14:73–79.
62. Mueller DJ, Atlas L. Resocialization of regressed elderly residents: A behavioral management approach. J Gerontol 1972; 27:390–392.
63. Morris R, Wheatley T, Britton P. Retrieval from long-term memory in senile dementia: Cued recall revisited. Br J Clin Psychol 1983; 22:141–142.
64. Murdoch B, Chenery H, Wills V, Boyle R. Language disorders in dementia of the Alzheimer type. Brain Lang 1987; 31:122–137.
65. Nerbonne M, Show R, Hutchinson T. Gerontologic training in communication disorders. ASHA 1980; 22:404–408.
66. Nicholas M, Obler L, Albert M, Helm-Estabrooks N. Empty speech in Alzheimer's disease and fluent aphasia. J Speech Hear Res 1985; 28:405–410.
67. Obler L, Albert M. Language in elderly aphasic and in the dementing patient. In: Sarno MT, ed. Acquired aphasia. New York: Academic Press, 1981:385.
68. Obler L, Albert M. Language and aging: A neurobehavioral analysis. In: Aging communication processes and disorders. New York: Grune & Stratton, 1981:394.
69. Obler L, Obermann L, Samuel I, Albert M. Written input to enhance comprehension in dementia of the Alzheimer's type. Paper presented at the Annual Convention of the American Speech-Language-Hearing Association. Washington, DC, 1985.
70. Old S. The effectiveness of stimulation on therapy for the cognitively impaired institutionalized elderly. Paper presented at Annual Meeting of American Psychology Association. Washington, DC, 1986.
71. Oriol W. Getting the story on aging: A sourcebook in gerontology for journalists. New York: Brookdale Institute on Aging and Human Development, 1984.
72. Ostuni E, Santo Pietro M. Getting through: Communicating when someone you care for has Alzheimer's disease. Plainsboro, NJ: The Speech Bin, 1986.
73. Overman C, Geoffrey V. Alzheimer's disease and other dementias. In: Mueller H, Geoffrey V, eds. Communication disorders in aging: Assessment and management. Washington, DC: Gallaudet University Press, 1987:271.
74. Panella T Jr, McDowell F. Day care for dementia: A manual of instruction for developing a program. White Plains, NY: The Burke Rehabilitation Center, Dementia Research Service, 1983:25.
75. Perez FI. Behavior studies of dementia: Methods of investigation and analysis. In: Cole JO, Barrett JE, eds. Psychopathology in the aged. New York: Raven Press, 1980:81.
76. Quayhagen M, Quayhagen M. Alzheimer's stress: Coping with the caregiving role. Gerontologist 1988; 28:396–401.
77. Raiford C, Shadden B. Graduate education in gerontology. ASHA 1985; 27:37–41.
78. Ratusnik D, Lascoe D, Herbon M, Wolfe V. Group language stimulation for patients with senile dementia. Aphasia, Apraxia and Agnosia 1979; 1:14–29.
79. Reisberg B, Ferris S, DeLeon MJ, Crook T. The Global Deterioration Scale (GDS): An instrument for the assessment of primary degenerative dementia. Am J Psychiatry 1982; 139:1136–1138.
80. Reisberg B. Clinical presentation, diagnosis and symptomatology of age-associated cognitive decline and Alzheimer's disease. In: Reisberg B, ed. Alzheimer's disease: The standard reference. New York: The Free Press, 1983:93.
81. Richman L. Sensory training for geriatric patients. Am J Occupational Therapy 1969; 23:254–257.
82. Ripich DN, Terrell BY. Patterns of discourse cohension and coherence in Alzheimer's disease. J Speech Hear Disord 1988; 53:8–15.
83. Ronch J. Practical guide for those who help others. New York: Crossroads, 1989.
84. Rosin A, Abramowitz L, Diamond L, Tesselson P. Environmental management of senile dementia. Soc Work Health Care 1985; 11:33–43.
85. Sachs D. Behavioral techniques in a residential nursing home facility. Behav Modif 1981; 5:417–427.
86. Sandel S. Movement therapy with geriatric patients in a convalescent hospital. Hosp Community Psychiatry 1978; 19:738–741.
87. Schwartz M, Marin O, Saffran E. Dissociation of language function in dementia: A case study. Brain Lang 1979; 7:277–306.
88. Shadden B. Education, counseling and support for sig-

nificant others. In: Shadden B, ed. Communication behavior and aging: A sourcebook for clinicians. Baltimore: Williams & Wilkins, 1988:309.
89. Verwoerdt A. Individual psychotherapy in senile dementia. In: Miller N, Cohen G, eds. Clinical aspects of Alzheimer's disease and senile dementia. New York: Raven Press, 1981:187.
90. Volicer L, Fabiszeski K, Rehaume Y, Lasch K, eds. Clinical management of Alzheimer's disease. Rockville, MD: Aspen, 1988.
91. Wald T. Alzheimer's disease and the role of art therapy in its treatment. Am J Art Ther 1983; 22:2–5.
92. Weiner M, Brok A, Snadowsky A. Working with the aged. Englewood Cliffs, NJ: Prentice-Hall, 1978:34.
93. Weinstein B, Amsel L. Hearing loss and senile dementia. Clin Gerontol 1986; 4:3–15.
94. Weinstein B, Amsel L. Hearing impairment and cognitive function in Alzheimer's disease. J Am Geriatr Soc 1979; 35:274–275.
95. Weisberg R. Raiding the self-esteem of mentally impaired nursing home residents. Soc Work 1983; 28:163–164.
96. Welden S, Yesavage J. Behavioral improvement with relaxation on training in senile dementia. Clin Gerontol 1982; 1:45–59.
97. Weston J. Effects of training on severe memory loss. Paper presentation at 33rd Annual Scientific Meeting of the Gerontology Society. San Diego, CA, 1980.
98. Wilson B, Moffat N. Clinical management of memory problems. Rockville, MD: Aspen, 1984:35.
99. Witte K. Discourse and dialogue: Prolonging adult conversation in the Alzheimer's patient. Am J Alzheimer's Care Res 1987; 2:30–39.
100. Zarit S, Anthony Z. Interventions with dementia patients and their families. In: Gilhooly N, Zarit S, Birren J, eds. The dementias: Policy and management. Englewood Cliffs, NJ: Prentice-Hall, 1986, 66.
101. Zarit SH, Orr NK, Zarit JM. The hidden victims of Alzheimer's disease: Families under stress. New York: New York University Press, 1985.
102. Zarit SH, Zarit MJ, Reever KE. Memory training for severe memory loss: Effects on senile dementia patients and their families. Gerontologist 1982; 22:373–377.

# APPENDIX

## Communication Adequacy in Daily Situations (CADS)

### Individual's Perspective

Answer these questions according to the following ratings:

        5 – Almost always        2 – Rarely
        4 – Usually               1 – Almost never
        3 – Sometimes

1. During conversations, does your family member appear to lose patience with you? _____
2. Do you lack enjoyment in talking to friends and family members? _____
3. Do you withdraw from speaking in familiar situations? _____
4. Do you feel upset when you fail to understand what has been said? _____
5. During conversation, do you experience difficulty getting your message across to the listener? _____
6. When you do not understand what the speaker has said, do you fail to let the speaker know or fail to ask them to repeat? _____
7. Do you refrain from speaking on the phone? _____
8. During conversation, does your family member have difficulty understanding when you change the topic of conversation? _____
9. When you cannot find the exact word(s), do you fail to find another way to get your idea across? _____
10. Do you experience difficulty following your family member's conversation? _____
11. During conversation, do you give up speaking when you cannot find the exact word(s) to express what you want to say? _____
12. Do you become annoyed if you lose your train of thought while speaking? _____
13. In general, how often do you think you experience communication difficulties? _____

### Caregiver's Perspective

Answer these questions according to the following ratings:

        5 – Almost always        3 – Sometimes
        4 – Usually               2 – Rarely
                                           1 – Almost never

1. During conversation, do you become impatient with your family member? _____
2. Does your family member now appear to lack enjoyment in talking to friends and family members? _____
3. Does your family member now appear to withdraw from speaking in unfamiliar situations? _____
4. Does your family member appear upset when you fail to understand what they have said? _____
5. During conversations, do you misunderstand what your family member is saying? _____

6. Does your family member fail to ask you to repeat what you have said or fail to tell you that they did not understand? _____
7. Does your family member now refrain from speaking on the phone? _____
8. During conversations, do you become annoyed when your family member abruptly changes the topic? _____
9. Does your family member appear upset when they cannot find the exact word(s) to express their thoughts? _____
10. Does your family member appear to experience difficulty following what is being said? _____
11. During conversation, does your family member give up speaking when they cannot find the exact words they want to express their thoughts? _____
12. Does your family member show annoyance when they lose their train of thought while speaking? _____
13. In general, how often do you think your family member experiences communication difficulties? _____

# CHAPTER 16

# *Environmental Considerations for Elderly Patients*

ROSEMARY LUBINSKI, Ed.D.

This chapter emanates from three premises: (1) the ability to communicate is the single most important skill for the elderly to maintain, if not improve, to a functional level; (2) the physical and social environment where communication occurs influences the availability of partners, topics, and activities that generate conversations; and (3) the environment of those with dementia is a crucial determinant of their well-being. Indeed, this chapter stems from Lawton's hypothesis that "The less competent the individual, the greater the impact of environmental factors on that individual."[47] These three concepts form the core philosophy of working with older demented persons, particularly those in institutional settings, in order to improve their communication lives. The first part of the chapter discusses the value of communication to all elderly individuals and underscores its critical importance to those with dementia, their family, or caregivers. The second part of the chapter provides a theoretic basis for understanding the environment and how it affects communication. The final part of the chapter provides clinical and research implications.

## Value of Communication

Communication is a basic ingredient in successful living across the life span. At a time of life that may be influenced by negative stereotyping and filled with unparalleled changes, including those involved with health, mental, and social status, communication assumes a prominent role in the well-being of all older persons. Being able to communicate effectively is important in maintaining independence, forestalling further deterioration, and preventing isolation and withdrawal. Communication is important for the elderly with dementia for at least eight reasons.

Communication helps everyone develop and maintain a sense of identity. Throughout the life span each of us assumes a variety of roles from childhood through old age. Our roles are established and demonstrated through our interactions with others in the family and wider social environments. Unfortunately, aging frequently means change, if not a reduction, in roles available for the elderly. These changes may be overt such as retirement, widowhood, and institutionalization. Rosow states that with the exception of widowhood, the rites of passage to old age are not publicly observed by the rest of society.[68] Gradual, subtle loss of roles also arises from societal misconceptions about older persons. Society may generalize that the elderly are physically infirm, mentally incompetent, sexually inactive, isolated, useless, and unhappy.[6] This societal misconception results in reduction of expectations for participation and performance by the elderly in a variety of familial, work, social, and leisure roles. Considering the fact that daily activities and roles help lay a foundation for communication topics and partners, lack of such opportunities for role actualization has a negative effect on communication.

Communication also helps the elderly transmit and receive information that will keep them active participants in their own care. Elderly individuals who can tell physicians or other care providers about their health or physical needs undoubtedly will receive more accurate diagnosis of their problems. Communication plays an important role in elderly persons describing symptoms and in providing feedback about the effects of medications, therapy, and other procedures prescribed for them. Gray suggests that health-care professionals may be "hostile" toward the elderly because of their higher prevalence of visual, speech, and hearing impairments.[24] She states: "The frustration which may result may lead to a loss of interest in the person's problems or even angry dismissal of the old person as being 'too knocked off' or 'impossible to talk to.' " Thus, when older persons communicate effectively, good care is enhanced.

Communication also has a therapeutic role for the elderly. Through both verbal and nonverbal communication older persons can vent anxieties, relieve loneliness, and diminish depression. Communication has a cathartic effect in that by discussing a real or perceived problem, feelings are released, and solutions may be explored and found. In some cases, discussion of problems even without solution will be helpful in restoring the older person to a more healthy state.

There is yet another therapeutic role in communication for the elderly. They may not only relieve their own distress through communication but also help others through listening, reflecting feelings, and offering alternatives and solutions. Older persons bring a special perspective to the helping situation: They can often sort through problems in ways younger individuals cannot. Many younger persons refrain from discussing their own problems for fear of burdening the elderly. In fact, many elderly, through their own experiences and values, are uniquely capable of being sensitive communication partners. The "helper" role may be a critically important one for the elderly.

Through communication, older persons also express one of the most basic human needs: to exert influence or power. Part of the maturing process during infancy and childhood is learning how to influence those around us. This role is also vital for the elderly, particularly at a time characterized by changes in social roles within the family and community.

Communication plays another life-span role by allowing the elderly to reflect on the continuity of their past, present, and future. Reminiscence or "life review" helps to cope with the future by reviewing the past. This can aid in the natural process of aging while building self-esteem and stimulating thinking. Life review can generate both positive and negative memories and feelings and therefore must be facilitated through careful communication.

Inherent in the communication process is the cognitive stimulation of such interaction. Cognitive stimulation means the availability of and interaction with sensory and interpersonal stimuli. Each verbal and nonverbal interaction becomes a source of information about the physical and social environment. For those elderly individuals with visual and/or auditory losses, communication input, and hence cognitive stimulation, becomes more difficult. For those with dementia, the availability of cognitive stimulation through sensory avenues and communicative interaction is essential.

Finally, communication has aesthetic and entertainment roles for elderly demented persons. Music, dance, theatre, and other forms of art can be important sources of communication for the elderly. In addition, humor may play a powerful role in the everyday lives, the healing process, and the rehabilitation of older adults.

## Definition of the Environment

It has become well recognized in the past 20 years that elderly individuals and their environments are dynamic interdependent variables: The environment affects individuals, and individuals affect their surroundings.[48,61,63] The environment is not simply a passive backdrop in which older people live, but an active contributor to what older persons will do and how well they will function. Ittelson describes the environment as an "open system which is seen as a total, active, continuous process involving the participation of all aspects."[33] Thus, the "total environment" is comprised of the physical background, the individual, and the relationship of the individual to others. It should be noted that each of these components changes over time and as a consequence of its relationship with other components.[52]

### PHYSICAL ENVIRONMENT

It is easier, but by no means simple, to define the physical setting of the environment. The physical setting is composed of the objective physical surroundings including natural phenomena, manmade objects, space utilization, and sensory characteristics such as visual, auditory, olfactory, and tactile information. Moos states that the physical environment surrounds behavior,[61] while Barker calls it the "circumjacent milieu."[4] Two of the primary functions of the physical environment are to provide the physical setting for our daily functions and interactions and to stimulate our thinking processes. The physical environment defines the space that individuals and groups will use. Pfeiffer postulates that communication is the key to "regulating interaction with others with whom we share space."[65]

The physical environment helps to build the "raw material of reality."[34] Wohlwill states that the physical environment stimulates individuals through its intensity, novelty, complexity, temporal variation, and surprisingness and incongruity.[80]

Ideally, the environment will provide just the right amount of stimulation because both sensory deprivation and sensory overload have been found to have serious psychological effects.[34]

## THE INDIVIDUAL

The environment also comprises the individual and all of his or her personal lifelong characteristics and resources, as well as present needs, desires, and perceptions. Thus, older persons bring a history of personal characteristics such as physical attributes and abilities, family roles, education, occupation, social, political, and religious beliefs, and leisure preferences. Perhaps more important, older persons contribute their problem-solving abilities acquired over a lifetime of positive and negative experiences. In addition, older individuals bring their current needs to any environment, including those related to age changes and physical and psychological disabilities. Finally, each time older persons enter an environment they add their own perception of the situation.

Itteleson, Proshansky, Rivlin, and Winkel believe that perception is the crucial element in person and environment interchange.[34] Perception is determined by the person's sensory, cognitive, and emotional abilities, personal history, experiences, and information received from others in the environment. Reduced vision or hearing will limit or distort information input for perception. Emotional problems such as depression and cognitive changes in dementia including memory difficulties will similarly provide insufficient or distorted raw data for perception building and verification. Input from others in the environment is also likely to affect perception. Input may affect how the physical environment can be used, expected role performance, rules about interaction, and positive and negative performance feedback. Koffka posits that a person's perception of the environment may bear little resemblance to the objective surroundings.[44]

## TOPOGRAPHIC ISSUES

**Space.** The living and working space of demented individuals is likely to decrease dramatically as the disorder progresses. Working space is eliminated when the individual no longer enters the work force. Thus, even when the individual remains in the community, space becomes increasingly curtailed, usually by family members who distrust the demented individual's ability to function independently in unlimited and unsupervised space. Institutionalization diminishes space even more to the point where the individual has access only to public areas within the setting that can be monitored by staff. Some individuals become nonambulatory or are restrained from independently ambulating and thus have even less personal choice in the space they are to occupy and use. Finally, interpersonal space may become more limited simply by the nature of the stigmatizing label given to demented individuals.[15,43]

The issue of space with regard to social interaction is yet more complicated. Jones found that close physical proximity does not ensure that positive interaction will occur among nursing-home patients.[36] Thus, a delicate balance between respecting the individual's spatial needs and providing physical opportunities is necessary in order for social interaction to occur.

**Privacy.** The two concepts of privacy and territoriality repeatedly emerge in the environment literature that describes how individuals relate to their physical environment. Calkins defines privacy as "the degree to which the environment inhibits or facilitates opportunities for a person to control amounts of privacy between people."[11] This definition reflects Altman's theoretic orientation that privacy functions to control social interactions and hence communication.[2]

Westin and Pastalan describes four states of privacy and their functions.[64,77] Solitude is that situation where there is deliberate physical separation from visual observation that provides a person with opportunity for reflection and personal functions. Intimacy provides opportunity for a close relationship with others, again free of observation. Anonymity is achieved when individuals can participate in public activities without attention being called to themselves. Finally, reserve is the internal need to limit disclosures about oneself.

Although these may be well-established, lifelong needs, they appear to be concepts that may be violated for those with dementia. Family and institutional caregivers may design environments that promote continued visual and auditory monitoring and deprive the individual of any opportunity for solitude or intimacy. Anonymity may also be discouraged because active participation in activities is considered a sign of adaptation and integration in family life or long-term care facilities. Reserve may also be difficult to achieve because of cognitive and communicative difficulties. For example, when caregivers answer for demented patients in interviews or complete biographical forms for outside agencies, the natural lifelong reserve of the individual may be violated. The response by the demented patient to these violations of privacy may range from social withdrawal to extreme socially unacceptable behavior. Both reactions result in fewer opportunities to exhibit intact appropriate skills.

**Territoriality.** The second concept of territoriality has been well developed in both the animal and human literature. Altman defines territorial behavior as a "self/other boundary-regulation mechanism that involves personalization of, or marking of, a place or object, and communication that it is 'owned' by a person or group."[2] Individuals want to have space they call their own and will demarcate it with physical signs and possessions or verbally defend it. It becomes more difficult for those with dementia to determine their own territory. Personal space steadily decreases and the ability to demarcate space may also decline as a result of cognitive, communicative, and physical problems. Caregivers need to be aware of the lifelong internal need for personal space. Although there is no research documenting how the demented react to unwarranted use of their possessions or blatant intrusion into their personal areas, it can be assumed that their privacy and territorial needs are the same, if not greater, as other individuals. For a detailed description of the concepts of privacy and territoriality see references by Altman,[2] Heinstra and McFarling,[29] Engebretson,[20] and Roberts.[66]

**Physical Activity.** Recent research indicates that increasing the physical activity of elderly individuals has positive benefits including increasing sociability and improving some aspects of cognitive performance.[60] Thus, when elderly demented individuals have opportunities for physical movement in their environment, there may be residual benefits in the realms of cognition and communication.

## SOCIAL ENVIRONMENT

The individual interacting with other individuals in the physical environment creates the social environment. The social environment is defined by Insel and Moos as "people and their interactions with each other."[32] Through verbal and nonverbal communication, individuals learn the attitudes and expectations of the groups to which they belong and gradually establish roles for themselves and for each other.[7] Individuals with their inherent characteristics become stimuli for each other.[71]

Social environments can be characterized in a variety of ways and on a number of dimensions. Kirtz and Moos state that although environments are unique, they can be characterized according to how individuals help and support each other (relationship dimension), how well an individual achieves autonomy and independence (personal dimension), and a dimension called system maintenance and system change.[42]

All individuals need psychological support from their social environment. Elderly persons undergoing dramatic changes in their social environment through the loss of spouse or relocation may be particularly vulnerable in their need for psychological support from family and caregivers. Similarly, they may benefit from living in an environment where individuals feel close to each other, what Kirtz and Moos call cohesion, affiliation, and involvement.[42] They state that a supportive environment may counteract numerous problems. Numerous authors postulate that older persons also benefit from a social environment where they can maximize their independence and achieve some sense of personal autonomy over their physical environment.[11,14,17,18,31,35,46–50,72–75]

## ENVIRONMENTAL FIT

When environmental characteristics and expectations and the individual's characteristics and perceptions do not fit, there will be a loss of environmental congruence or fit.[40,46] Deutschman calls this a loss of environmental competence.[18] Elderly individuals, particularly those with dementia, come to their environment with a wide range of special characteristics and needs. First, they come as elderly individuals with all that that might entail. Ittelson et al state that "environmental failure is often common for the elderly."[34] Lawton suggests that the environment for the elderly needs to accommodate life-maintenance needs, perceptual changes, cognitive changes, self-maintenance skills, and effectual behavior.[50]

Second, the demented bring their special cognitive changes above and beyond those of aging itself. Calkins states that the environment of those with dementia should be designed with respect to their memory difficulties, orientation problems, loss of ability to do complex tasks, increased activity levels, and agitation.[11] Thus, the environment in which the elderly demented person lives must take many factors into consideration if there is to be "person-environment" fit. Further, considering the progressive deterioration of the problem, evaluation of the environment needs to be continuing. An environment that is supportive, competence enhancing, independence nurturing, and cognitively stimulating at one point of the disorder may not be so at other stages. The physical and psychosocial variables must be reassessed along with the individual's needs and perceptions. Deutschman states that the physical environment must be "continually changed if it is to remain effective and therapeutic ... or [it will] result in ineffective communication and unnecessary stress."[17] An excellent source on environmental competence during old age is the reference by Windley and Scheidt.[79]

## CAREGIVER NEEDS AND ATTITUDES

In this model of environmental fit, not only must the characteristics, needs, and perceptions of the elderly demented person be considered but also those of their caregivers. Most, if not all, elderly demented will live with at least one family caregiver or in a long-term care setting cared for by staff outside the family. The environment must also meet the caregivers' characteristics and needs both in its physical design and psychosocial structure. Caregivers must understand how the physical and social environment creates opportunities and barriers for communication. In addition, they must realize how their own awareness of environmental factors and willingness to modify the environment may be crucial in maximizing communication skills and opportunities of the demented patient. Further, caregivers' own needs must be considered and met when possible. Caregivers who are under unrelenting stress from "36-hour days"[55] may need continuing counseling and education as well as respite. Caregivers who understand the nature of the problems of the demented individual and who realize that their own needs must be met simultaneously will undoubtedly create a more positive communicative environment. This will result in more willingness to experiment with environmental modification and to create communication opportunities. (See Chapters 11, 12, and 17 for further discussion of in-service education and family burden.)

## Communication-Impaired Environment

Lubinski, in a variety of publications on the elderly and those with aphasia, introduced the concept of a communication-impaired environment.[52,53] A communication-impaired environment is one where there are few opportunities for successful, meaningful communication. Although this concept has been applied primarily to institutional settings, it has relevance for other settings. Both home and institutional settings may be communicatively impoverished and thus limit opportunities for demonstrating intact communication skills. Both qualify as communication-impaired environments. Further, any setting that is overtly or covertly insensitive to the communications needs, styles, and desires of its participants can represent a communication impoverished environment. Ten points characterize such a setting:

1. *Lack of sensitivity* exists to the value of interpersonal communication as the cornerstone of effective functioning and self-realization. This insensitivity may be demonstrated by communication partners who speak for the demented individual, restrict social activities where communication might occur, and dismiss communication difficulties as unimportant or insurmountable. It is also demonstrated by caregivers and professionals who knowingly limit communication opportunities during their daily interaction. Patients and staff both agree that staff have little time for communication.[53] Lack of sensitivity is inherent in the modicum of referrals by staff for hearing evaluations in long-term care settings, despite the high prevalence of hearing loss among the institutionalized demented elderly.[54] Similarly, communication disorders professionals who refuse to test or readily dismiss the demented as too difficult to assess also show a lack of sensitivity to the importance of communication. Professionals and family who adopt such an attitude believe that communication is a byproduct of care rather than a primary dimension of quality care and quality of life.

2. *Restrictive rules* inhibit communication. Lubinski et al, in a study of communication on a long-term care setting, found that patients were able to identify features of the physical and psychosocial milieu that they perceived as restricting their communication.[53] Although these "rules" were not stated or officially endorsed by the staff, patients perceived that they should not complain, that they were expected to exchange pleasantries with others and not talk with those with severe communication problems. In addition, they stated that any statements they made in public places were likely to be grist for gossip. Thus, they should limit what they should talk about, where, and with whom.

3. *Few or no partners of choice are present.* The presence of others in the environment does not ensure that they are willing or qualified communication partners. The issue is one of perceived characteristics of partners. Although individuals with dementia eventually have severe problems in remembering names, they may respond to the nonverbal characteristics of those around them. For example, they may respond positively to those who take the time to interact, those who soothingly touch them, and those whose voice and body language convey warmth and acceptance.[45]

4. *Few reasons to talk* emanate from internal needs or activities of choice. Coupled with the changing cognitive skills is an environment that becomes more restrictive. Thus, there is less opportunity for a variety of social encounters that reflect lifelong interests and friends. Eventually there is little to talk about. Although demented individuals do become more dependent on having communication partners who are willing to assume topic direction, it cannot be assumed that the demented do not have topics about which they want to talk.
5. *Individuals perceive themselves as having little meaningful contribution* to their environment through their communication. Because it is frequently difficult to follow the content flow of the conversations of demented individuals, a natural reaction is to promptly dismiss their comments. Further, those in the environment do not expect the demented individual to make a contribution through their social role or their communication. Chapter 16 on helplessness discusses how this vicious spiral may lead to imposed learned helplessness of the demented individual.
6. *A lack of private places inhibits conversation.* This characteristic is derived from the concepts of privacy and territoriality along with patient perceptions that private conversations are difficult to consummate. Although it is most evident in institutional settings where privacy is at a premium, it can also occur in home settings where the demented individual is constantly monitored.
7. *Accessibility is limited* to activities and communication partners of choice. Individuals with dementia may depend on personal assistance in getting to places where activities occur and where others congregate. For those who are ambulatory, the environment must meet their wayfinding difficulties.
8. *The environment is sensory-confusing and depriving.* Although anyone can be confused in an unfamiliar and complex environment such as an institutional setting, those with cognitive and/or perceptual disorders are likely to find them particularly disconcerting.[38] If the environment's sensory dimensions of light, sound, and tactile and kinesthetic information are insufficient or bombarding, confusion is likely to result. The environment needs to meet the demented individual's sensory needs related to aging and cognitive impairment. Further, an environment that is confusing to the senses is likely to aggravate these needs. For example, an individual who is agitated, has memory problems, and visual perceptual difficulties may be more confused when navigating within an environment that has not accommodated to these needs. Calkins states that wayfinding in one's environment is linked to "feelings of autonomy, independence, and self-sufficiency."[11] Thus, a sensory-confusing environment will contribute to a decrease in the demented individual's ability to access chosen communication partners and activities.
9. *The communication-impaired environment is socially stagnant.* Individuals are not only stimulated by the physical aspects of their environment but also through the interpersonal exchange among participants in the environment. The family caregiver who is enmeshed in providing total care and monitoring, in addition to other home and family duties, may not consider interpersonal communication a priority. The same is true for professional caregivers. It takes skill, time, and deliberate effort to communicate with demented individuals. Staff who are busy, unskilled in communication techniques, and unaware of the importance of communication, may not make the effort to stimulate the patient through communication.
10. *The environment does not support the particular needs of the caregivers.* Family and professional caregivers often face unrelenting hours of mental and physical exertion in caring for the demented individual. Elderly spouses bound to the home may carry an especially heavy burden that reflects itself in communication. What does a wife talk about with a husband who does not recognize her or whose comments are disjointed and inappropriate? Adult children caught between the demands of their own families and careers and the needs of their elderly demented parent may have little time and place little priority on "just talking" with their parent. Similarly, staff who are underpaid, overworked, and often uneducated as to the nature of dementia are unlikely to expend much effort in communication.

## Identification Strategies

Assessment of the environment in which demented individuals live should be an interdisciplinary activity. Professionals trained in architecture, human engineering, and environmental psychology have a strong theoretic basis for understanding the nature of environments and their impact on individuals. Health-care providers including nurses, physicians, and social workers have practical knowledge based on their everyday experiences with demented individuals. Speech-language pathologists and audiologists bring a special realization of the relationship of the environment and communication skills and opportunities. Indeed, in many settings lacking access to environmental psychologists, it may be the communication disorders specialist who plays a leading role in sensitizing others to the powerful effects of the environment on quality of life and quality of care. Further, the communication disorders specialist may be instrumental in helping families understand how their home and the social interaction in that setting influence the communication behavior of the demented individual. The bottom line remains, however, that someone must assume responsibility for assessing the physical and psychosocial dimensions of the environment in which demented individuals live.

## IDENTIFICATION TOOLS

Environmental checklists and audits are available for evaluating a variety of dimensions of the environment. The Ebenezer Center for Aging in Minneapolis, MN publishes specific environmental checklists for vision, hearing, memory and orientation, and accessibility and safety.[13] These lists delineate particular characteristics of the environment that can be identified on a yes-no basis. For example, in the Hearing Environmental Checklist, there are questions such as "Has there been an effort to limit background noise in the area where the residents spend much of their time?" The National Council on Aging publishes the *Sixth Sense* that also includes checklists to evaluate lighting, colors, lettering, hearing, communication, touch, and dangerous areas.[62] Other excellent sources on identification of environmental factors include articles and books by Calkins,[11] Deutschman,[17,18] and Snyder.[72-75] Lubinski, in a chapter on environmental considerations in aphasia, also presents an environmental assessment tool.[52]

These environmental assessment tools, and the one presented in the Appendix at the end of this chapter, can be used for several purposes. First, they can be used to directly identify physical and psychosocial aspects of a setting that promote or minimize communication skills and opportunities. Second, they can be used more indirectly through in-service training and counseling as a means of sensitizing caregivers to the influence of the environment. Third, they can be used as research tools to identify the impact of environmental programming on the improvement of communication skills and opportunities.

### Communication Environment Checklist

The Communication Environmental Assessment and Planning Guide (CEAP) presented in this chapter (see this chapter's Appendix) incorporates many items included in other environmental checklists. This tool is different, however, in that the focus is on the impact of the environment on communication opportunities and on the needs of each individual. General checklists such as those mentioned above provide a global picture of the environment but do not focus on individual needs. A second difference in the instrument is the inclusion of a planning section where remedial steps can be outlined.

The CEAP is divided into two main sections. Part I focuses on the physical environment, with sections devoted to the visual, auditory, tactile and olfactory environment, and the physical setting. Part II is directed toward the psychosocial environment. In both sections, there is opportunity to evaluate both the general environment and the individual's needs. For any items marked "No," the assessor should specify what actions might be taken to remediate the problem.

It should be remembered that even one negative item may have a great effect on any one demented individual, considering his or her characteristics and needs. Thus, although an increasing number of "No's" may clearly demarcate a severely communication-impaired setting, specific item analysis is crucial to meet the needs of any individual. Finally, the CEAP should be used as a monitoring tool over time. The progressive nature of dementia and the changing aspects of home and institutional environments necessitate repeated observation and modification of the environment.

### Enhancing the Environment

The suggestions proposed in this chapter to enhance the communicative environment have been gleaned from observation and numerous research studies. There are two types of suggestions given: (1) those that focus on passive environmental enrichment; and (2) those that require active interaction between the dementia patients and their physical and social surroundings.[60] In the first case, the environment is deliberately manipulated by caregivers with the hope that these changes translate to better quality of life for the dementia patient. In the second, the dementia patient becomes more active in the selection and manipulation of environmental factors. A selective combination of both types of suggestions will undoubtedly enhance the communication opportunities of the elderly dementia patient.

## CAREGIVER COOPERATION

Once the environment is evaluated, the questions then focus on what changes are realistic and how these changes can be accomplished. The first and most crucial step in making any changes in an institutional or home environment is to ensure that those in decision-making positions within that setting understand the nature and importance of communication and its relationship to the physical and psychosocial environment. Although there is a growing awareness on the part of federal and state funding agencies regarding "quality of life issues," their priorities still primarily focus on traditional health, physical care, and housekeeping features. Bowker states that the sicker an individual is, the more his medical needs dominate institutional life.[8] Thus, long-term care settings for the demented elderly are likely to be governed by a medical model that will subordinate social needs of patients in order to meet medical goals.

Similarly, family caregivers may not understand the relationship of communication, functional behavior, and the environment. Thus, before any changes are attempted, the decision makers must be thoroughly grounded in the concept of a communication-impaired environment and its relationship to effective overall functioning of the demented person. To impose changes without the concurrence of the decision makers and caregivers will have less than optimum results.

Discussion with decision makers should focus on answering the following questions regarding the proposed environmental changes:
1. What specifically needs to be done?
2. What expected and measurable effect(s) will changes have on the demented individual or others in the environment?
3. How many individuals might benefit from these changes?
4. What are the financial costs in materials and personnel time?
5. What can be modified in the present setting to accommodate the identified needs?
6. Who will be responsible for the changes and who will monitor them in the future?

Decision makers, be they nursing-home administrators, medical, nursing, rehabilitation staff, or family caregivers will benefit from continuing-education programs and counseling aimed at the themes of the value of communication for demented individuals, characteristics of a communication-impaired environment, the relationship of dementia and communication, and strategies for enhancing communication through conversational and environmental manipulation. Communication disorders specialists and others interested in environmental psychology should not assume that caregivers naturally understand these concepts and incorporate them in their daily interactions with demented persons. The general thesis of these discussions should be the need to balance meeting the medical and custodial needs of the demented individuals with their human, social, and communicative needs. This philosophy is in keeping with Bowker's suggestion that institutional services need to be reconceptualized through maximizing patient freedom of choice, humanizing the institutional environment for patients and staff, and maximizing institutional permeability.[8] See Chapter 17 for suggestions on in-service training.

## PRIORITIZING GOALS

The second step in improving the communication environment is to prioritize the features of the general physical and social environment and the individual's communication environment. It is unrealistic to enter a nursing home or an individual's community residence and totally redesign the setting to meet all the physical, sensory, and social needs of everyone residing there. Although there are unique opportunities for environmental consultants in the design of new facilities or the remodeling of existing ones, it is more likely that changes will need to be made within existing structures. Changes that are easily incorporated in the existing structure may be less threatening to caregivers and more easily assimilated by the demented individual.

Similarly, it is unrealistic to expect that all caregivers within a setting will simultaneously and completely change their approach to communicating with demented individuals. In fact, the physical environment may actually be easier to modify than the deeply rooted attitudes and behavior patterns of professional and family caregivers.

## GENERAL PHYSICAL ENVIRONMENT

The physical environment should be designed to maximize the individual's current abilities while accommodating the progressive nature of the disorder. Whenever possible, the environment should provide opportunities for individual control, personalization, choice, and interpersonal communication.[28] The general environment needs to balance the amount of support it offers with the individual's need for self-management and self-direction.

### Topographic Issues

Perhaps what becomes most important in spatial considerations for the demented individual is not how much space is available but how much choice the individual has in using and maneuvering in that space. Deutschman hypothesizes that it is one's personal choices in the use of space that are critical.[17] Calkins similarly states that the individual needs to "feel in control" and this can usually be done through personalization of the environment.[11] Further, institutional caregivers should be aware of the differences regarding interpersonal use of space for various cultural and ethnic groups.[5] Thus, caregivers should allow demented individuals to have personal choice in their space and how it is designed and utilized.

Personalization of the environment will have several benefits for the demented individual, including enhancing personal choice, increasing personal responsibility, reflecting a home-like atmosphere, and increasing familiarity with the environment.[17,18] Personalization also visually reminds caregivers that the resident is more than an anonymous patient. Caregivers may be less likely to encroach on a personalized environment than on one that is institutionally neutral. Further, Millard and Smith found that when elderly persons are surrounded by personal items, they are perceived in a more positive way.[59]

Personalization can be achieved through:
1. Increasing the caregivers' understanding that personalization is important through in-service training and counseling.
2. Encouraging the demented individual to make choices in room design, color, furniture, and decorative elements.
3. Encouraging the individual to be responsible for as long as possible for some physical maintenance of the environment.

**Privacy.** An additional benefit of personalization of the environment is that privacy is likely to be enhanced. All humans crave some degree of privacy throughout the day (see earlier discussion of types of privacy). Although caregivers may be hesitant to allow privacy, there may be ways of balancing the need for safety and privacy. Several researchers have found that increased opportunities for privacy yield more social interaction.[11,51,64] Some suggestions for increasing privacy include:
1. Increasing caregivers' understanding that privacy is important through counseling and in-service training
2. Allowing and encouraging patients to use some areas that are not constantly visually and auditorially monitored, such as quiet rooms and chapels[11]
3. Encouraging patients to observe activities without having to participate[11]
4. Decreasing staff or family members' unwarranted and intrusive invasion and use of the demented individual's room, space, or possessions

**Accessibility.** If communicative interaction is to occur, people need to have reliable and frequent access to partners and activities of their choice. Accessibility can be enhanced through:
1. Increasing caregivers' understanding that the demented individual may need assistance in getting to communication partners and activities and that the physical environment must meet their cognitive and physical abilities to traverse their physical surroundings.
2. The environment must be perceived as accessible by the demented individual. Long corridors with shiny floors may appear threatening and impassable.[11,17,18]
3. The environment must be visually coded to enhance way-finding. For example, Calkins states that way-finding is helped through multi-cueing of visual, auditory, tactile, and olfactory sensory information.[11]
4. Caregivers must be mindful that patients in wheelchairs may not be able to move their chairs independently and may require assistance to get to activities and partners.
5. Areas must be wheelchair accessible. Furniture in public places should be moveable so that wheelchairs can be easily moved in and out. Public places in institutional settings include corridors, nurses' station, day rooms, dining areas, and activities centers. Major public areas in home settings include living and dining areas.

**Design Considerations.** Calkins suggests that environments for the demented be as homelike as possible with the addition of physical and social prosthetic supports that allow the demented individual to function as independently as possible for as long as possible.[11] Whatever environment the demented individual resides in, it should reflect personal taste and lifelong furniture and possessions. Physical prosthetic supports include those items added to the environment to help the individual "compensate for limited physical or other capabilities." These can be incorporated in the actual physical design of the environment or can be additions or modifications of existing ones. Undoubtedly more considerations concerning communication skills and opportunities can be incorporated into newly designed facilities if management design planners and architects regard them as important.

Social supports stem from the understanding and attitude of the caregivers that independent functioning should be encouraged. Social supports are given basically through the communication of the caregivers. These include verbal reminders and directions, redirection of conversation topics, and encouragements to verbally or nonverbally interact with those around them. The area of social supports will be discussed in greater detail later in the chapter.

**Physical Props.** Physical props can be easily incorporated into existing living areas and should be considered as priorities for new facilities. The following list includes basic considerations for the use of such props.

1. Encourage caregivers to use the physical environment as a dynamic tool in caring for the demented.[26] Physical props can enhance the existing abilities of the demented individual while helping to compensate for diminishing skills.
2. Develop or encourage the use of areas of focal interest where activities occur and individuals naturally congregate. In a home setting these include increasing the demented individual's access to the kitchen and living room and family room areas where families naturally join together for meal preparation, eating, and other social activities. In a nursing home, the major areas where patients tend to congregate are entrances and nurses' stations. Congregation in these areas should be considered normal and should be capitalized upon. Similarly, dayrooms would be better utilized if they incorporated several small activity centers for games, activities, visiting, arts and crafts, etc. Simply putting a television and chairs around the periphery of the room will not maximize cognitive abilities or encourage conversations. Acoustically treated moveable room dividers can help section large multi-purpose rooms into more homelike, manageable areas. Brent suggests that fireplaces, plants, murals, fountains, and art work can all be used as focal points within nursing home settings.[9]
3. Encourage the use of sociopetal seating arrangements during meal times and activities. The use of round tables that are high enough for a wheel chair to slide under or angled seating facilitates face-to-face communication.[9,17,18] Generally, seating arrangements that place pairs of individuals at 90-degree angles encourage interaction, while side-by-side seating discourages it.[57]
4. Comfortable and accessible seating will encourage patients to sit near each other. Patients slumped down and tied in wheel chairs are unable to see adequately what is going on or with whom they are communicating.[9]
5. Visual access to activities occurring outside the setting.[11] These activities can be sources of cognitive stimulation and conversational topics. Visual access to changing seasons and activities of daily living helps strengthen temporal, spatial, and person orientation.
6. Access to a bathroom or call system.[73] Demented and elderly persons may have frequent need to go to the bathroom and may refrain from going to activities because of this. Clearly marked facilities near major activity centers may encourage patients to attend. For those individuals with way-finding problems, clearly marked call systems or visual access to someone who can help them may also encourage participation in activities.
7. Access to rest areas on the way to activities. Ambulatory demented individuals may not be able to traverse long corridors without rests. Again, clearly available rest stops may encourage activity participation.

## SENSORY ENVIRONMENT

Elderly demented individuals are likely to incur some degree of change in their sensory abilities associated with aging itself. The ability to see and hear one's communication partners is vital in effective communication. Other sensory avenues of touch, taste, and smell also become information sources for communicative interaction and "making sense" from the physical, perceptual, and psychosocial environment.[58] Thus, improving the sensory environment becomes crucial when encouraging communicative success for demented individuals.

## Visual Environment

Elderly demented individuals are likely to evidence such visual difficulties as glaucoma, cataracts, retinitis pigmentosa, macular degeneration, diabetic retinopathy, homonymous hemianopsia, and retinal detachment.[13] These disorders can result in blurred vision, decreasing peripheral or central vision, and blindness. In addition, older individuals will generally require two to three times more light, will tend to move toward light, will have visual foreground and background discrimination difficulties, and difficulties distinguishing among pastel colors and among dark colors.[11,15,17,18,72,73] Visually impaired individuals may range from those with relatively good functional vision to those who are completely blind. Carroll provides an excellent discussion of the characteristics and needs of each of these groups.[13] Suggestions for improving the visual environment of the demented include:

1. Referral for complete optometric and ophthalmologic evaluations. Caregivers should seek guidance from local medical societies and dementia family groups for referrals to physicians who specialize in the evaluation of those with dementia.
2. Ensuring that glasses and visual assistive devices are readily accessible to demented individuals. These may include reading aids such magnifying glasses and magnifying sheets. Large-print newspapers, books, and magazines as well as talking books may stimulate cognitive skills and serve as a source of conversational topics.
3. Improving visual contrasts within the environment.[11] Examples of visual contrasts include dark printing against light backgrounds, white dishes placed against darker tablecloths, and furniture and walls of opposite contrasts. An environment of color oppositions rather than color coordinates may be more effective for elderly demented persons with visual problems and orientation difficulties.
4. Using color to enhance orientation. Brent suggests that warm, medium-intensity, contrasting colors facilitate orientation.[9] She also suggests that color coding be used for handrails, hallways, and information boards. Other color factors to consider include the amount and nature of light available, the juxtaposition of colors, and the quantity of surfaces covered. For a detailed discussion of color in nursing-home settings, see the reference by Brent.[9]
5. Eliminating shiny, slick surfaces that reflect glare to the demented person's visual field. Matte surfaces on furniture and walls, indirect fluorescent lighting, and controllable, filtering window treatments all help to reduce glare.[11] Glare can also be reduced through the use of shades and nonreflective tiles and floor coverings.[30,73] Brent also suggests that window treatments should be changed periodically to provide seasonal information.
6. Having communication partners come face to-face with the demented person when communicating. This allows the demented individual to see the partner clearly, take advantage of natural lip-reading cues and expression of body-language cues, and provide feedback to the partner. For the individual in a wheelchair, this may entail the partner stooping down, in effect sending a clear and positive message to the demented individual that their participation in communication is wanted. Generally, this simple act also encourages the caregiver to speak slower, more carefully, and to monitor communicative meaningfulness. Face-to-face communication has the added benefit of reducing the authority role differences between careprovider and patient. Encouraging family or staff caregivers to come clearly into the visual field of the dementia patient is one of the simplest techniques to facilitate communication.
7. Placement of important visual information and decorative items at eye level. Items such as bulletin boards, photographs, calendars, clocks, announcements, and any other items of possible interest to the demented individual should be placed at the eye level of someone sitting in a wheelchair. What may be appropriate visual height for caregivers will be too high and consequently meaningless to those who spend much time in a wheelchair or other seating arrangement. Lawton suggests that orientation is enhanced when there is "environmental legibility."[48,49] Windley and Scheidt define this concept as "the extent to which a setting is perceptually understandable and facilitates orientation, predictability, and direction finding."[79]

8. Making the environment as visually interesting as possible without provoking sensory overload. Items that are visually interesting include abstract and realistic art work, arts and crafts projects of varying colors and textures, family photographs, photographs depicting an earlier period such as the Depression or World War II, famous people, mobiles, sculptures, holiday or religious decorations, and personal mementos. Snyder suggests using hallways as art galleries that can serve as topics for conversation.[73]
9. Providing opportunity for lumination control of the visual environment. Hayward suggests that both demented individuals and their caregivers should have the ability to control the lumination within their environment to meet their own visual needs, activities, and preferences.[28] Effective control of overhead and window illumination is especially important.

## Auditory Environment

With aging there are likely to be some changes in both the ability to receive sounds (peripheral hearing) and the ability to interpret sound (central hearing). For instance, elderly individuals may have specific difficulty understanding in a background of noise and distinguishing high-frequency sounds such as [s] and [z] and may respond slowly to auditory information. For the individual with dementia, these difficulties exacerbate existing and progressive cognitive and orientation difficulties. In addition, fatigue, stress, and pressure to communicate quickly and accurately further reduce opportunities for communicative effectiveness.

Maurer states that unfortunately most nursing-home settings were not designed with these factors in mind.[56] He maintains that some institutions "constitute the ultimate for poor speech comprehension with linoleum floors, walls that are hard and flat, and poor insulation from outside noise." In fact, a person's own home filled with furniture, carpeting, and memorabilia may actually be more auditorially conducive. For more complete discussion of hearing characteristics of aging and dementia, see Chapters 4 and 14.

Consider the following to help improve the auditory environment:

1. Provide a complete otologic and audiologic evaluation by a professional specializing in evaluation of those with dementia.
2. Encourage patients to use hearing aids if prescribed. Dementia patients are likely to need daily assistance in inserting and removing the aid and adjusting controls. Further, caregivers should assume the responsibility of battery changes and general maintenance of the aid. When not being worn, hearing aids should be kept in a constant and safe place to avoid misplacement by the dementia patient.
3. Encourage the use of assistive hearing devices when possible. Portable assistive listening devices may be especially useful for those patients who cannot be fitted with an aid or who refuse to wear one. The use of hearing aids and assistive devices is discussed in more detail in Chapter 14.
4. Reduce interior noise sources by placing noisy areas such as elevators, heating and cooling units, food preparation, and ice machines away from areas where communication is likely to occur.
5. Reduce interior noise through carpeting, matte surfaces on walls and floors, and sound-absorbent ceilings. In fact, sound-absorbent materials should be used on the walls of areas where communication occurs frequently, including near the nurses' station, day rooms, dining rooms, and activity centers. Again, portable screens constructed of sound-absorbent materials provide increased flexibility and are cost effective because they can be moved to areas where communication occurs. In hospital-like settings, corridors are the noisiest places.[69] Thus, these areas should receive special attention in interior noise control.
6. Use sound-absorbent materials in patients' rooms. This allows patients to use radios, televisions, stereos, and tape recorders more freely. In some cases, patients should be provided with individual earphones.
7. Reduce extraneous sounds such as unattended radios and television and uncontrolled and continuous loudspeaker music.
8. Encourage caregivers to monitor background noises when communicating with the demented individual. This may be done by turning down the volume of television, radio, or stereo, closing the door during conversations to eliminate corridor or other noise, monitoring the noise level of air conditioners, fans, and heaters during conversations. Caregivers will find that communication will be more effective if extraneous noise is monitored, reduced, or eliminated. This aids in au-

ditory comprehension, attention, and orientation.

9. Speak within handshake distance of the patient, slightly loudly, and articulate clearly while facing the patient.[73] Again, face-to-face positioning facilitates hearing and promotes carefully modulated articulation and volume. Shouting generally results in frustration for both parties.
10. Avoid creating anechoic rooms that are maximally sound proofed. Rooms that are "sound dead" may also create confusion.
11. Avoid using public-address systems for transmitting crucial information. Demented individuals may not attend carefully to this media, may have a hearing loss that distorts reception, and may need a face-to-face communication partner to monitor communication effectiveness. Snyder states that ideal public-address systems should have control of bass tones that facilitates hearing among the elderly.[72-74]

### Tactile/Kinesthetic and Olfactory Environment

In addition to the visual and auditory environment, other sensory avenues such as touch provide concrete information. Langland and Panicucci found that elderly confused women improved their attention when nurses provided touch along with verbal requests.[45] Lawton cautions, however, that touch is a complicated social issue between staff and patients.[48,49] Caregivers should monitor cues given by the patient as requesting or refusing touch overtures.

Further, textures and smells may generate topics for conversations. For example, the pungent aroma of ethnic foods, the scent of growing flowers, and the fibrous texture of garden loam may all stimulate thinking and conversations. A sensory-stimulating environment is rich in its textures and smells. The growing emphasis on multisensory cues in environmental engineering for the demented requires that the environment stimulate all senses. In fact, for those demented individuals with visual and/or hearing problems, other sensory avenues may become increasingly important in receiving information from the environment.

## COGNITIVE ENVIRONMENT

It is artificial to separate out the cognitive environment from either the sensory or the social environment because both provide information for the individual's cognitive abilities. For the purposes of this chapter, the cognitive environment includes the sensory and social environment, but, in particular, the objective of environmental designers and caregivers is to stimulate the thinking abilities of the demented individuals and meet their difficulties in time, place, and person orientation. A stimulating cognitive environment considers the person's past history, interests, and abilities while matching current and changing abilities to allow for maximum competence. Hiatt states that the environment must deal creatively with paradoxes such as: "the need for stimulation versus the problem of overstimulation, the need for predictability versus the value of prompting curious inquiry through change, the need for social interaction versus the importance of time out or one-li-ness."[30] Feier and Leight remind us that "all stimulation occurs in a meaningful context."[22] Thus, a cognitively stimulating environment should encompass the following:

1. Reflect the demented person's history, interests, and abilities. This can be done through incorporating the individual's suggestions and personalizing the environment.
2. Provide the individual with maximum multisensory cueing regarding time and place. This might be done by placing large, easily perceived clocks and calendars at eye level, periodically changing physical props such as pictures and posters to reflect seasonal and holiday changes, and bringing time and place into discussion during the course of natural interaction.
3. Balance the need for a consistent cognitive environment without creating a static, dull one. This can be done by introducing changes in the physical environment slowly, orienting the demented individual to those changes, and monitoring ability to cope successfully with them. Hiatt and Feier and Leight also suggest that continuity be achieved through the use of themes throughout the environment.[22,30] For example, they suggest that a clergyman's visit can be followed through with visual slides of religious sites, activities related to the Mediterranean, etc.
4. Adapt to the demented individual's time and pace. Cognitively impaired individuals are likely to take longer to do simple, lifelong activities of daily living, yet are also likely to react impulsively when concentration is needed. This is particularly true in conversations that may require that communication partners provide ample time for exchange.
5. Provide a menu of activities that reflects

the demented individual's interests rather than that of the caregivers. Activities need to be cognitively stimulating, matched to the patient's abilities, and conducive to communicative interaction. What the demented individual does all day can provide topics for communication with caregivers and possibly other patients.
6. Provide opportunities for the demented individual to contribute to the functioning of the environment. For example, activities can be adapted that allow the individual to help care for him- or herself, to assist with food preparation and clean up, and to participate in other chores. These activities should foster the use of existing problem solving and other cognitive skills and a sense of contribution to the environment.

## SOCIAL ENVIRONMENT

As dementia progresses, it is axiomatic that the social life of the patient decreases. The social identity of the individual becomes increasingly and singularly that of a demented patient. Chapter 10 on learned helplessness details this phenomenon. Although it is unrealistic to assume that lifelong social roles can be completely retained, it is possible to cultivate a social environment that encourages self-sufficiency, independence, contribution, and self-expression to the degree possible for the individual. Coons, in her discussion of milieu therapy, states that "a humanistic, affirmative posture is essential to therapeutic treatment and to wholesome environments in general."[16] This is first and foremost accomplished through working with the significant caregivers in the environment because they will comprise the major social and communication partners of those with dementia. Excellent references concerning the establishment of a therapeutic milieu have been provided.[1,3,10,12,16,23,37,67,76] The following are suggestions for improving the social environment.

1. Increase caregivers' understanding that they are crucial in creating a positive social and communicative environment. Family caregivers carry an oppressive burden of being the constant primary social partner for the demented person. Institutional caregivers weighted with the ceaseless job of caring for several demented patients are not likely to consider communication an important part of their work. Understanding and strategies for improving the social environment can be achieved through long-term counseling and support for families through peer-support groups such as the Alzheimer's Disease and Related Disorders Association, community-agency counseling programs, and specialized counseling with professionals including social workers, nurses, and communication disorders specialists. Staff will benefit from in-service programs geared toward understanding the nature of dementia, its impact on the individual and family, and the relationship of dementia and institutionalization. See Chapters 11 and 12 on families and Chapter 17 on in-service training.
2. Provide appropriate reading materials to families and institutional caregivers on the nature of dementia and institutionalization to possibly augment in-service training and counseling. Two suggested readings include *The Thirty-Six Hour Day*[55] and *Alzheimer's: A Caregiver's Guide and Sourcebook*.[25]
3. Provide every opportunity for the dignity of the individual to be preserved. Communication partners may assume that the demented individual does not comprehend. Communication thoughtfulness and discretion should always be a priority.
4. Encourage individuals other than the primary caregivers to play an active role in communicating with the demented individual. Family and professional caregivers cannot provide constant socialization opportunities. Others should be enlisted in these activities including former friends, other family members, children, volunteers, and other patients when possible. These individuals should also be given informal training in how to communicate with the demented individual and should be positively reinforced for their efforts. Eichler et al observed dramatic success in the use of well-trained volunteer counselors as relationship therapists for institutionalized geriatric patients.[19]
5. Create opportunities for demented individuals to interact frequently with those in their environment. Snyder suggests that conversations may not be the focus of organized activities such as reality orientation and crafts, while less formal

ones including puzzles and reading may serve as conversational props.[72,73] Although dementia patients will have difficulty remembering names, activities adapted to their abilities and based on mutual interest may increase the process and value of acquaintanceship.

6. Encourage dementia patients to observe activities even if they are reluctant to participate. Sideline observation can be a productive social role for some individuals, mimicking that of fans at sporting or entertainment events.
7. Encourage dementia patients to help others in some way. Some dementia patients, particularly in the early and mid stages, can be given the responsibility of talking to a new patient, assisting in an activity, or helping with activities of daily living.
8. Provide ample social events that have as their primary goal communicative interchange. These include social hours, coffee hours, cocktail parties, welcoming parties, discussion groups, and special theme meals.[41]
9. Develop cross-generational access between children and dementia patients.[70,78] Foster grandparent programs, on-site staff day care and nursery programs, and family programs and visits are three examples of linking generations, particularly for the institutionalized dementia patient.
10. Encourage communication partners to appreciate the cultural and historic background of the demented individual.[21] Include topics related to the individual's personal history to possibly facilitate orientation and communication. Individuals who speak English as a second language should have opportunities to converse in their primary language. The opportunity to communicate in one's native language is culturally sensitive and stimulating for the demented individual.
11. Promote participation in activities outside the home and institutional setting. Broadening the scope of the demented individual's environment is likely to kindle some interaction and stimulate topics for conversation.
12. Encourage family members of institutionalized dementia patients to visit and participate in activities whenever possible. Families, however, need help and reinforcement in planning and implementing visits so that they are profitable for both parties.[27,39,81]

## Research Needs

Considerable research needs to be done to determine what aspects of the environment will facilitate the best communication opportunities for those with dementia. For example, four primary questions that need to be asked include:

1. What stages of dementia appear to respond best to an enhanced physical environment versus a social environment?
2. How can we best measure the positive effects of an enhanced communicative environment? Should this be in terms of improvement or maintenance of skills or slowing of the progression of the deterioration?
3. What is the effect of an improved communicative environment on the caregivers?
4. How does an improved communicative environment translate to cost effectiveness of service delivery to demented patients?

These are difficult questions to answer considering the complicated, multi-faceted, and dynamic nature of the environment and the progressive nature of dementia. The environment, in contrast to laboratory conditions, is not controllable.

## Concluding Remarks

This chapter explored the theoretic framework of the physical and psychosocial environment as it pertains to those individuals with dementia. Identification strategies as well as intervention suggestions were provided. The discussion of this chapter, combined with suggestions provided in the other chapters, provides a holistic approach to dementia and communication. Dementia, the environment, and communication considered individually or in combination are very complex. Improving the communicative environment of demented persons requires that we challenge ourselves to original and productive thinking.

## References

1. Abrams GM. Defining milieu therapy. Arch Gen Psychiatry 1969; 21:553–560.
2. Altman I. The environment and social behavior. Monterey, CA: Brooks/Cole, 1975.
3. Arnetz B, Theorell T. Psychological, sociological and health behavior: Aspects of a long term activation

programme for institutionalized elderly people. Soc Sci Med 1983; 17:449–456.
4. Barker RG. Ecological psychology: Concepts and methods for studying the environment of human behavior. Stanford, CA: Stanford University Press, 1968.
5. Baxter JC. Interpersonal spacing in natural settings. Sociometry 1970; 33:444–456.
6. Benedict R, Ganikos M. Coming to terms with ageism in rehabilitation. J Rehabil 1981; 47:10–18.
7. Bernard J, Thompson L. Sociology: Nurses and their patients in a modern society. 8th ed. St. Louis: C.V. Mosby, 1970:246.
8. Bowker LH. The humanization of geriatric facilities. Int J Rehabil Res 1981; 4:553–554.
9. Brent R. Advocacy design in the nursing home: Cultivating public and private spaces for the newly admitted resident. In: Spicker S, Ingman S, eds. Vitalizing long-term care. New York: Springer Publishing, 1984:159.
10. Brodsky C, Platt R. The rehabilitation environment. Lexington, MA: D.C. Heath and Company, 1978:1.
11. Calkins MP. Design for dementia: Planning environments for the elderly and confused. Owings Mills, MD: National Health Publishing, 1988.
12. Canter D, Canter S. Designing for therapeutic environments. New York: John Wiley and Sons, 1979.
13. Carroll K. Human development in aging: Compensating for sensory loss. Minneapolis: Ebenezer Center for Aging and Human Development, 1978.
14. Carroll K. Human development in aging: The nursing home environment. Minneapolis: Ebenezer Center for Aging and Human Development, 1978.
15. Comer R, Piliavin J. The effects of physical deviance upon face-to-face interaction: The other side. J Pers Soc Psychol 1975; 23:33–39.
16. Coons DH. Milieu therapy. In: Reichel W, ed. Topics in aging and long-term care. Baltimore: Williams & Wilkins, 1981:53.
17. Deutschman M. Environmental competence and environmental management. J Long-Term Care Admin 1985; 13:78–84.
18. Deutschman M. Environmental settings and environmental competence. Gerontol Geriatr Education 1981; 2:237–242.
19. Eichler M, McCuan L, Berdit L. Volunteers as relationship therapists for institutionalized geriatric patients. Mental Health Soc 1976; 3:212–222.
20. Engebretson DE. Human territorial behavior: The role of intervention distance in therapeutic interventions. Am J Orthopsychiatry 1973; 43:108–116.
21. Engram BE. Communication skills training for rehabilitation counselors working with older persons. J Rehabil 1981; 47:51–56.
22. Feier CD, Leight G. A communication-cognition program for elderly nursing home residents. Gerontologist 1981; 21:408–416.
23. Gottesman LE. Milieu treatment of the aged in institutions. Gerontologist 1973; 13:23–26.
24. Gray M. Communicating with elderly people. In: Pendleton D, Hasler J, eds. Doctor-patient communication. London, New York: Academic Press, 1983:193.
25. Gruetzner H. Alzheimer's: A caregiver's guide and sourcebook. New York: John Wiley and Sons, 1988.
26. Gunzberg H, Gunzberg A, eds. Mental handicap and the physical environment. London: Baillière Tindall, 1973.
27. Haley W. A family-behavioral approach to the treatment of the cognitively impaired elderly. Gerontologist 1983; 23:18–20.
28. Hayward DG. Psychological factors in the use of light and lighting in buildings. In: Lang J, Burnette C, Moleski W, Vachon D, eds. Designing for human behavior. Stroudsburg, PA: Dowden, Hutchinson and Ross, 1974:120.
29. Heinstra NW, McFarling LH. Environmental psychology. 2nd ed. Belmont, CA.: Wadsworth Publishing, 1978.
30. Hiatt LG. Architecture for the aged: Design for living. Inland Architect 1978; 22:6–18.
31. Hiatt LG. Designing for mentally impaired persons: Integrating knowledge of people with programs, architecture and interior design. Paper presented at the American Association of Homes for the Aging annual meeting. Los Angeles, CA, November, 1985.
32. Insel PM, Moos RH. The social environment. In: Insel PM, Moos RH, eds. Health and the social environment. Lexington, MA: Lexington Books, 1974:3.
33. Ittelson W. Environmental perception and contemporary perceptual theory. In: Ittelson W, ed. Environment and cognition. New York: Seminar Press, 1973:1.
34. Ittelson WH, Proshansky M, Rivlin L, Winkel G, eds. An introduction to environmental psychology. New York: Holt, Rinehart and Winston, 1974.
35. Jones DC. Social isolation, intervention and conflict in two nursing homes. Gerontologist 1972; 12:230–234.
36. Jones DC. Spatial proximity, interpersonal conflict, and friendship formation in the intermediate-care facility. Gerontologist 1975; 15:150–154.
37. Jones M. The therapeutic community. New York: Basic Books, 1953.
38. Jones MA, Catlin JH. Design for access. In: Spiegel A, Simon P, Fiorito E, eds. Rehabilitating people with disabilities into the mainstream of society. Park Ridge: Noyes Medical Publications, 1981:175.
39. Kahana E. The humane treatment of old people in institutions. Gerontologist 1973; 13:282–289.
40. Kahana E. A congruence model of person-environment interaction. In: Windley P, Buerts T, Ernst F, eds. Theory development in environment and aging. Washington, DC.: Gerontological Society, 1975.
41. King AP. Cocktail hour in a nursing home. Nurs Care 1977; 10:26.
42. Kirtz S, Moos RH. Physiological effects of the social environment. In: Insel PM, Moos RH, eds. Health and the social environment. Lexington, MA: Lexington Books, 1974:13.
43. Kleck R, Buck P, Goller W, et al. Effect of stigmatizing conditions on the use of personal space. Psychol Rep 1968; 23:111–118.
44. Koffka K. Principles of gestalt psychology. New York: Harcourt Brace, 1935, cited in Chenin I. The environment as a determinant of behavior. J Soc Psychol 1954; 39:115–127.
45. Langland R, Panicucci C. Effects of touch on communication with elderly confused clients. J Gerontol Nurs 1982; 8:152–155.
46. Lawton MP. Assessment, integration and environments for older people. Gerontologist 1970; 10:38–46.
47. Lawton MP. Environment and aging. Monterey, CA: Brooks/Cole Publishing, 1980.
48. Lawton MP. Environment as a communication mode. Bull Audiophonol 1983; 8:17–31.
49. Lawton MP. Environmental and other determinants of well-being in older people. Gerontologist 1983; 23:349–357.
50. Lawton MP. Social rehabilitation of the aged. J Am Geriatr Soc 1968; 16:1346–1363.
51. Lawton MP, Badar J. Wish for privacy by young and old. J Gerontol 1970; 25:48–54.
52. Lubinski R. Environmental language intervention. In:

Chapey R. Language intervention for adult aphasia. Baltimore: Williams & Wilkins, 1981.
53. Lubinski R, Morrison EB, Rigrodsky S. Perception of spoken communication by elderly chronically ill patients in an institutional setting. J Speech Hear Dis 1981; 46:405–412.
54. Lubinski R, Weinstein B. States of communication services in nursing homes in New York State. ASHA 1988; 30:69–72.
55. Mace N, Robins P. The thirty-six hour day. Baltimore: Johns Hopkins University Press, 1981.
56. Maurer JF. Auditory impairment and aging. In: Jacobs B, ed. Working with the impaired elderly. Washington, DC: The National Council on the Aging, Inc., 1976.
57. Mehrabian A, Diamond S. Effects of furniture arrangement, props and personality on social interaction. J Pers Soc Psychol 1971; 20:18–30.
58. Michigan State Housing Development Authority. Housing for the elderly development process. Lansing, MI: 1974:46–49.
59. Millard P, Smith C. Personal belongings—A positive effect? Gerontologist 1981; 21:85–90.
60. Mirmiran M, Van Gool W, Van Haaren F, Polak CE. Environmental influences on brain and behavior in aging and Alzheimer's disease. In: Swaab DF, Fliers E, Mirmiran M, et al, eds. Progress in brain research. New York: Elsevier Science Publishers, 1986:443.
61. Moos RH. The human context. New York: John Wiley and Sons, 1976.
62. National Council on the Aging. The sixth sense: Understanding sensory changes and aging. Washington, DC, 1985:4–9.
63. Parr J. The interaction of persons and living environments. In: Poon LW, ed. Aging in the 1980s: Psychological issues. Washington, DC: American Psychological Association, 1980:393.
64. Pastalan LA. Privacy as an expression of human territoriality. In: Pastalon LA, Carson DH, eds. Spatial behaviors of older people. Ann Arbor, MI: University of Michigan Press, 1970:88.
65. Pfeiffer TS. Behavior and interaction in built space. Built Environment 1980; 6:35–50.
66. Roberts S. Territoriality: Space and the aged patient in the critical care unit. In: Burnside I, ed. Psychological nursing care of the aged. New York: McGraw-Hill, 1980:195.
67. Rosenstock F, Goldman M, Rothenberg R. Rehabilitation of the long-term patient: An action research program in milieu therapy. J Chronic Dis 1969; 22:493–503.
68. Rosow I. The social context of the aging self. Gerontologist 1973; 13:82–87.
69. Sabine H. Less noise better hearing. Chicago: Celatex Co., 1950:64.
70. Sherman SR, Newman ES. Foster-family care for the elderly in New York State. Gerontologist 1977; 17:513–522.
71. Skinner BF. Science and human behavior. New York: Macmillan, 1953:299.
72. Snyder LH. An exploratory study of patterns of social interaction, organization, and facility design in three nursing homes. Int J Aging Human Dev 1973; 4:319–333.
73. Snyder LH. Design promotes self-reliance. H.U.D. Challenge 1973; 4:10–12.
74. Snyder LH. Environmental changes for socialization. J Nurs Adm 1978; 1:44–30.
75. Snyder LH, Pyrek J, Smith KC. Vision and mental function in older residents of health facilities. Unpublished research report. Minneapolis: Ebenezer Center for Aging and Human Development, January 1976.
76. Stubblebine JM. The therapeutic community—A further formulation. In: Rossi J, Filstead W, eds. The therapeutic community. New York: Behavioral Publications, 1973:47.
77. Westin A. Privacy and freedom. New York: Atheneum Publishers, 1970.
78. Wilson L, Titus ME. Communication across four generations. Reading Horizons 1978; 19:82–84.
79. Windley P, Scheidt R. Person-environment dialects: Implications for competent functioning in old age. In: Poon LW, ed. Aging in the 1980s: Psychological issues. Washington, DC: American Psychological Association, 1980:407.
80. Wohlwill JF. The physical environment: A problem for a psychology of stimulation. J Soc Issues 1966; 22:29–38.
81. York J, Calsyn R. Family involvement in nursing homes. Gerontologist 1977; 17:500–505.

# APPENDIX

## Communication/Environment Assessment and Planning Guide

### Physical Environment

**GENERAL VISUAL ENVIRONMENT**

| | Yes | No | Action plan |
|---|---|---|---|
| 1. Is there sufficient, diffuse lighting to clearly see communication partners? | | | |
| 2. Can lighting from windows and lamps be easily controlled? | | | |
| 3. Is indirect lighting available? | | | |
| 4. Does area contain glare-resistant furniture, floors, and surfaces? | | | |
| 5. Is printed information presented clearly on contrasting background? | | | |
| 6. Are areas color or pattern coded by function (e.g., bedroom, toilet)? | | | |
| 7. Is the setting visually interesting in color, design, and topic? | | | |
| 8. Is visually stimulating material placed at eye level for most patients? | | | |

**PERSONAL VISUAL ENVIRONMENT NEEDS**

| | Yes | No | Action plan |
|---|---|---|---|
| 1. Has the person's vision been tested within the past 2 years? | | | |
| 2. Does the person wear corrective lenses or use an assistive vision device? | | | |
| 3. Is the person given daily assistance and encouragement to use glasses or visual assistive devices? | | | |
| 4. Do caregivers communicate at eye level with the individual? | | | |
| 5. Does the person have access to large-print reading material or talking books? | | | |

*Appendix continues on following page*

## GENERAL AUDITORY ENVIRONMENT

|   | Yes | No | Action plan |
|---|---|---|---|
| 1. Does area contain sound-absorbent materials? | | | |
| 2. Can background noise be controlled during conversations? | | | |
| 3. Do caregivers control background noise during conversations and care? | | | |
| 4. Is information presented via intercoms or loudspeakers intelligible to patients? | | | |
| 5. Are there noise-reduced areas available for conversations with caregivers, friends? | | | |
| 6. Do caregivers come close enough to patients to facilitate hearing and visual cues? | | | |

## PERSONAL AUDITORY ENVIRONMENT NEEDS

|   | Yes | No | Action plan |
|---|---|---|---|
| 1. Has the person's hearing been tested within the past 2 years? | | | |
| 2. Does person have a hearing aid for one or both ears? An assistive listening device? | | | |
| 3. Does person wear hearing aid or assistive listening device during conversations and activities? | | | |
| 4. Do caregivers know how to insert, control, and maintain hearing aid or assistive listening device? | | | |
| 5. Are assistive listening devices easily available for use with caregivers? | | | |
| 6. Have caregivers been instructed in techniques for facilitating auditory reception/comprehension? | | | |
| 7. Do caregivers speak clearly and with moderate volume while facing the individual? | | | |

## GENERAL TACTILE AND OLFACTORY ENVIRONMENT

|   | Yes | No | Action plan |
|---|---|---|---|
| 1. Does the setting contain a variety of textures? | | | |
| 2. Does the setting contain a variety of appropriate odors? | | | |
| 3. Does the setting appear to maximize multisensory cueing to facilitate orientation and thinking? | | | |

*Appendix continues on following page*

## PERSONAL TACTILE/ OLFACTORY NEEDS

|  | Yes | No | Action plan |
|---|---|---|---|
| 1. Do caregivers frequently and appropriately touch person during conversations and care? | | | |
| 2. Does the individual appear to benefit from touching people and objects? | | | |

## GENERAL SPATIAL ENVIRONMENT

|  | Yes | No | Action plan |
|---|---|---|---|
| 1. Do patients have access to a variety of sites to pursue activities and conversations? | | | |
| 2. Is physical accessibility to activities easily available to all patients? | | | |
| 3. Are a majority of activities held on the patient's own floor? | | | |
| 4. Is there a bathroom easily accessible at activity sites? | | | |
| 5. Can furniture be grouped to facilitate communication? | | | |
| 6. Are there private places available for conversations? | | | |
| 7. Are patients' territorial needs respected by caregivers? | | | |
| 8. Do caregivers respect patients' private possessions? | | | |

## PERSONAL SPATIAL ENVIRONMENT

|  | Yes | No | Action plan |
|---|---|---|---|
| 1. Does the individual have clearly identified personal space? | | | |
| 2. Does the individual personalize his or her personal space? | | | |
| 3. Does the individual's room reflect a personal identity? | | | |
| 4. Is there ample seating available for individual's visitors? | | | |
| 5. Is the individual's room conducive to privacy? | | | |

*Appendix continues on following page*

## Psychosocial Environment

### GENERAL PSYCHOSOCIAL ENVIRONMENT

|  | Yes | No | Action plan |
|---|---|---|---|

1. Do caregivers respect the dignity of the individual in care and conversations?
2. Are patients encouraged to be decision makers in their activities of daily living?
3. Are all forms of communication including complaining responded to appropriately?
4. Is communication an integral part of all interactions and activities?
5. Do caregivers monitor nonverbal cues they send during care and conversations?
6. Does the setting reflect season changes, holidays, special events?
7. Are staff made aware of patients' former interests, vocations, lifestyle?
8. Are patients given responsibilities that reflect a contribution to their environment?
9. Are patients encouraged to be both participant and observer of activities?
10. Are families encouraged to include patients in outside social activities?
11. Do caregivers have opportunities to discuss their perceptions, frustrations, and strategies for communication?

### PERSONAL PSYCHOSOCIAL ENVIRONMENT NEEDS

|  | Yes | No | Action plan |
|---|---|---|---|

1. Do activities meet the individual's present and changing cognitive abilities?
2. Are daily activities reflective of patient's personal interests and abilities?
3. Do caregivers inform and individually invite person to activities?
4. Does individual have access to activities outside the home or institution?
5. Does the individual have at least one person of choice who is a primary communication partner?

*Appendix continues on following page*

|  | Yes | No | Action plan |
|---|---|---|---|
| 6. Do caregivers use special techniques to facilitate comprehension and expression? | | | |
| 7. Do caregivers take special time to converse with the individual on a daily basis? | | | |
| 8. Do caregivers understand the nature of the patient's communication abilities and disabilities? | | | |

# CHAPTER 17

# *Effective In-Service Training for Staff Working with Communication-Impaired Patients*

LAURIE NASH KOURY, M.A.
ROSEMARY LUBINSKI, Ed.D.

In the next 30 years there is expected to be a dramatic increase in the number of elderly. The number of elderly individuals 65 years of age and older has risen from 3 million in 1900 to 27 million (11.3 percent of the population) in 1982.[32] Current figures indicate that approximately 2.2 million of the elderly are over age 85, and the U.S. Bureau of the Census predicts that this number is likely to rise to 15 million people by the year 2030.[32] Although the majority of the elderly reside in the community, Hickey states that at least 10 percent of them will spend some time in an institution during the course of a year.[17] For the age group over 85 years, this percentage will triple.[17] In order to meet these institutional needs, the number of nursing-home beds is increasing and will continue to increase for some time.[4,22] In 1976 there were 23,000 nursing homes in the United States, providing about 1,235,404 beds.[33]

Surveys have indicated that from 60 to 92.5 percent of nursing home residents have communication impairments requiring speech and hearing services.[4,26] Mueller and Peters indicate that approximately 11 percent of residents are diagnosed with aphasia, 19 percent with dysarthria, and 21 percent with voice problems.[26] The prevalence of hearing disorders among residents was determined to range up to 90 percent of the population.[4] A survey of the prevalence of senile dementia indicated an occurrence of 50 to 63 percent of the resident population.[34] These numbers indicate that the potential need for rehabilitation services for communication impairments is remarkable given the growth projection of the elderly population. Between the years 1980 and 2050, the number of persons with communication disorders will increase faster than the total U.S. population, as a direct result of the aging of the population.[11]

Treatment of communication disorders associated with dementia has traditionally been neglected. In the past, the attitudes held by physicians and other health-care professionals have been "Why try to teach people who are incapable of learning?" and "These people are only going to get worse." Current data suggest, however, that demented patients can and do retain selected items of knowledge.[6,8,25] The demented patient is often able to learn communication behaviors that improve function and activities of daily living (ADLs) and hence improve the quality of life for the patient and the family.[14]

As speech-language pathologists provide a service to demented patients where none existed before, an opportunity will be created to develop an interdisciplinary team that will make quality care a reality. The speech-language pathologist may identify communication deficits and retained abilities of the demented patient that can be stabilized and managed. Progress depends, however, on the understanding and commitment on the part of the patients' communication partners. This is especially true in nursing-home settings where patients may have limited opportunity to communicate frequently with supportive family and friends.[23]

Nursing staff, particularly nurses' aides or nursing assistants, are presented with the greatest number of opportunities to communicate with the demented patients during their everyday interactions. Nursing assistants have the opportunity to reinforce functional communication skills. In addition, nursing assistants have an important role in setting a positive communication atmosphere for all patients, not only those with dementia.[23] Thus, the goals of effective carryover of functional communication skills and the improvement of the communication environment in this setting may be enhanced by providing nursing assistants with selective and focused continuing educational opportunities.

Many authors have pointed to a need for providing education and guidance to nursing home staff working with communication-impaired patients.[19] There is, however, little specific information on how patient goals derived by the speech-language pathologist should be translated effectively to staff other than through summary reports, progress notes, and in-service training. Current literature provides us with limited information on (1) what nursing assistants know about communication problems associated with dementia; (2) effective approaches to providing in-service; or (3) studies of in-service effectiveness. Therefore, the purposes of this chapter are the following:

1. Describe traditional approaches to in-service
2. Discuss goals of in-service in long-term care settings
3. Discuss results of a study comparing three approaches to in-service training in a nursing home setting
4. Provide clinical examples for improved in-service training with nursing assistants

## In-Service Training

In-service training in nursing homes is a systematic and continuing process of providing job-related learning experiences for all personnel responsible for direct and indirect care and services to resident patients.[31] In the nursing home, the ultimate goal of in-service training is to improve the quality of life for the residents; therefore, in-service training should focus on increasing the technical proficiency and communication skills of the nursing-home staff, as well as keeping the staff up-to-date on new techniques, equipment, and concepts of care.[10] In-service training should also focus on increasing the sensitivity of the staff to the residents' frustration and feelings of isolation associated with their decreased communication skills. Although in-service training is generally thought of as being directed toward the nursing staff, there are actually four beneficiaries: the nursing staff, the patients, the nursing-home administration, and the speech-language pathologist.

In-service training benefits the nursing assistant in that it improves problem-solving skills concerning communicating with the demented patient. In-service training provides the nursing assistant with the skills to spontaneously and independently manage communication breakdowns commonly encountered with demented patients. As communication breakdowns are avoided or swiftly repaired, nursing assistants' attitudes toward patients change, and hence, personal growth and improved job satisfaction are positive outcomes.

The benefits to the patients with dementia include an increased number of willing communication partners and an availability of communication partners who have skills to facilitate communication or repair communication breakdowns. Thus, the quality of patient life will most likely be improved. As indicated by Lubinski, communication for the patient becomes the "crucial difference between isolation and social connectedness, between dependence and independence, and between withdrawal and fulfillment."[23]

Nursing-home administrators benefit from in-service training through improved employee performance and job satisfaction. In-service training helps create a setting that provides an environment for better patient care. This results in better operating efficiency of the nursing home. Reduced staff turnover rates for nursing assistants and patients who are more receptive to care may lower costs of service delivery.

Lastly, in-service training benefits the speech-language pathologist and the profession, in general. Conducting in-service training increases visibility and may result in more referrals. In addition, the opportunity to train other health-care professionals on the interdisciplinary team approach may ultimately improve job satisfaction and enhance professional self-esteem. More important, by helping to create more positive communication environments, all patients may have a greater number of opportunities to experience quality communication. An enhanced communication environment facilitates carryover of skills developed in therapy.

Although there exists a great deal of literature on in-service training, the majority focuses on the development of in-service programs by nurses. Lutenegger states that the basic elements of the development of in-service programs are ostensibly the same regardless of the groups involved; therefore, the considerations would apply to the development of in-service programs by speech-language pathologists or other health-care providers.[24]

Researchers and educators have generally identified three elements necessary for the development of a successful in-service program:[10]

1. Identification of the learning needs and objectives of the individuals to be trained
2. Selection and implementation of an appropriate learning experience
3. Follow-up to evaluate whether or not desired outcomes are achieved

## IDENTIFICATION OF LEARNING NEEDS

The term "learning need" is used in the job context as meaning a lack of knowledge, skill, or attitude that prevents the nursing assistant from giving a satisfactory job performance.[18] There are many ways to recognize learning needs and many places to look for evidence of them.[15,18]

1. *Observation.* A great deal of employee knowledge can be gained by walking through the various areas of the nursing home and observing staff and residents carrying out their daily activities. For example, observe staff and patient interaction in the day room, the hall around the nursing station, or the dining room.
2. *Interview.* This is an effective way to assess the learning needs of nursing assistants by interviewing the supervisor, either formally or informally. Ask the supervisor, "Who are your best employees? What do these employees do specifically that makes them effective with demented patients? Could these traits be taught to other employees? and How could this teaching best be done?"
3. *Survey/skills inventory.* This approach presents the nursing assistants with a listing of learning needs. The assistants are instructed to circle "Yes" or "No" to items such as "I would like to learn how to help my demented patients understand what it is that I want them to do without provoking a fight." There should be space on the survey for the nursing assistant to write additional items of interest that have not been included.
4. *Group consensus/committee.* This is another way to amplify enthusiasm for the whole personnel development process through sharing program suggestions and educational experiences. Create a committee of nursing assistants and have them assign a chairperson. The committee should develop a plan to gather learning-needs information. Once in-service training has been implemented by the speech-language pathologist and the committee is in working order, the committee can work with the speech-language pathologist to develop orientation plans for new employees. They can assign experienced "coaches" to instruct new employees and to develop plans for maintaining employees' skills and knowledge.

It should be noted that none of these approaches should be viewed as complete enough to use alone. A combination of approaches provides crosschecks on the information collected by each means.[18]

## IDENTIFICATION OF LEARNING OBJECTIVES

Once learning needs have been established, it follows that objectives to remedy learning deficiencies should be developed. A learning objective is a statement of what the nursing assistant should know as a result of the learning experience.[18] Because learning is demonstrated by some degree of behavioral change at the end of the learning experience, it is important that objectives be stated in performance terms that can be quantified ("will be able to"; "will know"). The outcomes reveal whether learning has resulted in improving specific aspects of the nursing assistant's performance.

An objective criterion or set of criteria must be established by which performance will be evaluated. Deciding on criteria should be an integral part of the planning process for any learning experience. The following is an example of a learning objective developed by a speech-language pathologist for training nursing assistants:

> The nursing assistant will use gesture to facilitate a demented patient's ability to follow single-stage motor commands. Improvement will be measured by: (1) observation of gesture 100 percent of the time when appropriate in role-playing scenarios, and (2) follow-up interview with supervisors. Supervisors will be instructed to observe assistants on the job and to document percentage of gesture used in appropriate interactions.

## SELECTION OF LEARNING EXPERIENCES

Selection of an appropriate instructional methodology or in-service strategy is the step that naturally follows the determination of learning needs and learning objectives. As a result of educational research, there is a growing awareness that no one in-service strategy succeeds in all situations or with all types of staff. In general, the speech-language pathologist should consider: (1) the background knowledge and experiences of the nursing assistants; (2) previous in-service training given by the speech-language pathologist; (3) what the assistants want to know; and (4) what is reasonable for the assistant to know and do given the work environment of a specific nursing home.

Three broad categories of instructional methodology to consider are: (1) telling methods; (2) showing methods; and (3) doing methods. In general, the selection of the learning experience should be related to the type of established learning objectives. The Hospital Continuing Education Project of the Hospital Research and Educational Trust correlated the following generalized objectives with a variety of telling, showing, and doing methods:[18]

1. If the principal intent of in-service training is to increase knowledge, then assigned readings, lectures, discussions, field trips, and written tests are appropriate.
2. If the principal intent of in-service training is to improve skills, then demonstrations, case study discussions, problem-solving groups and role plays are appropriate.
3. If the principal intent of in-service training is to change attitudes, then relatively intense use of action methods (role plays and forceful motion pictures combined with discussion) is appropriate.

### Lecture

The lecture is the widely accepted approach in telling learning situations. In this method the speaker presents a series of related ideas and facts. The speaker is active while the listeners are passive, being expected to listen and to perhaps take notes.

The lecture has been utilized extensively as an instructional method because it has the advantages of being efficient, economical, and versatile.[18] The lecture is efficient because the speaker can cover a specified quantity of material in a short period of time and a great number of people can be reached at one time. It is economical because it generally requires less preparation time than other approaches and bypasses time-consuming discussions. The lecture is versatile because other instructional methods may be incorporated into it. Discussions, demonstrations, and role plays are often introduced by brief lectures to provide needed terminology or instructions.

The Hospital Continuing Education Project of the Hospital Research and Educational Trust developed the following suggestions for improving the content and presentation of lectures:[18]

1. Choose the extent and complexity of the material to be presented based on the education and experience of the intended audience. Deliver the information, then summarize what was presented.
2. Practice the presentation in front of a qualified observer or record the presentation to assess the organization of the talk, the speaking rate and voice quality, the nature of any speaking mannerisms or gestures, and the length of time taken.
3. Use notes, but try not to read a lecture in full. Reading for more than a few minutes may result in loss of listener attention. If large amounts of material must be read, the listeners should be provided with copies to read themselves.
4. Establish and maintain eye contact with members of the group. Making visual contact with various listeners will provide some information as to how well the materials are being received.
5. Vary the pace of the presentation. Concentrated listening for 30 minutes is hard work. The speaker should consider incorporating a variety of audiovisual aids such as slides, movies, overheads, or models to provide variety and to achieve an impact greater than could be achieved by voice alone.

### Role Playing

The Ohio Department of Education identified that the most common methodologies of instruction, lecture, and demonstration were rated low in effecting changes in staff behaviors, whereas role playing was rated high in both behavior and attitude change.[27] The role-play technique is a widely accepted approach in showing and doing learning situations.[7] Shadden, Raiford, and Shadden state that in-service role playing probably has a greater and longer lasting impact on the participants than a full hour of lecture.[29]

Role playing provides an action-oriented technique for group instruction. Nursing assistants, who generally have limited knowledge of speech-language and hearing facts, and who have limited knowledge of the complex and dynamic nature of the interaction between cognition and language deficits of dementia patients, would greatly benefit from the visualization and active participation of in-service role playing. The objective is to develop more effective on-the-job behavior. The nursing assistant's creativity and problem-solving skills are maximized as the participants are left on their own to cope with a situation as it is described to them.

The role play encourages the participants to "think on their feet," and involves observers in the interactions that could not be achieved through lectures, discussions, or hand-outs. Mistakes have no lasting penalties; they occur in an informal, protected environment and serve to reinforce appropriate behavior.

## IMPLEMENTATION OF LEARNING EXPERIENCES

Once the learning experience is selected to meet the learning objective, the in-service environment must be carefully selected. Selecting an appropriate time, a suitable room, hand-outs, and preparing a clear, unambiguous announcement for in-service presentations are not trivial considerations. A mid-afternoon in-service period (1:30 to 2:30 PM) is usually appropriate as it crosses the day and evening shifts, occurs after the busy periods of morning ADLs and lunch, and still allows time for regular conferencing and staffing of patients between the staff of the day and evening shifts. It has been shown that room arrangements can promote or handicap the learning process.[15,18] The quality of the setting reflects the importance of the topic and the speaker to the listeners. The in-service room should be quiet, well lighted, and adequately ventilated. In addition, semicircular or open-ended rectangular seating arrangements make it easy for each participant to see and hear the other members of the group. Hand-outs should be used only if deemed absolutely necessary. When constructing a hand-out the following should be considered:
1. Use only one page per hand-out
2. Use colored paper if possible to attract attention
3. Use simple, easy-to-understand language
4. Avoid jargon and too much information
5. List practical suggestions
6. Include your name, department name, telephone number, office number, and date of presentation
7. Include an invitation with material presented in the hand-out or in-service training for the participants to discuss any patients or problems

Every effort should be made to announce in-service programs about 1 week in advance, with interesting posters placed strategically on each nursing unit, in the staff work room, in the staff locker room, and in the staff dining room. A note to the nursing supervisor to remind staff and public address announcements the day of the in-service program will also improve attendance. If attendance is poor for in-service programs at a given nursing home, those who attend can be asked to sign an attendance sheet.[5] With administrative support, attendance at in-service programs might become part of the nursing-service file and be considered at a nursing assistant's evaluation time. This may be negotiable with the assistant's supervisor.

In addition, the communication-disorders specialist should provide the administrator with a summary of the in-service program when it is completed. Include the in-service title, learning objectives, number of attendees, comments, and a listing of future in-service program dates and topics. This informs the administration of the importance of communication to dementia patients, increases visibility for the speech-language pathologist, and possibly increases staff numbers and dollars spent on patient care.

## FOLLOW-UP EVALUATION

The in-service program has been conducted. Was it successful? Within an in-service frame of reference, the term "evaluation" means the determination of the value of a training or educational activity, as seen and as measured by the program participants, the instructor, supervisors, or by a combination of these groups.[18] Follow-up evaluations are important because they provide visibility and accountability to administration; they provide documentation of what has been done and for whom; and they promote the field of communication disorders within the nursing home setting. Speech-language pathologists will likely place emphasis on program evaluations from the nursing assistants immediately following the in-service program. In most instances, the evaluation needs to be completed quickly; hence, checklists, rating scales, and quizzes are appropriate evaluation tools. The rating scale that forces a choice is useful because it provides the speech-language pathologist systematic coverage of topic comprehension and ease of tabulation. Loss of individualized expression may be a disadvantage of forced choices, but this negative feature may be compensated for by providing a space at the bottom of the evaluation form for comments. Evaluations should be brief, no longer than one page. The following are two examples of forced-choice rating scales.

### Sample 1

Which of the following statements describes this in-service program? Check all that apply.

_____ It provided a welcome change from the everyday job.

_____ The material covered will have a high degree of value to me on the job.

_____ It was attended by people with practical experience who could learn from each other.

_____ It was held in pleasant surroundings.

Sample 2

Rate each of the following on a scale of 1 to 5.
1. Enthusiasm and clarity of speaker
   | 1 | 2 | 3 | 4 | 5 |
   |---|---|---|---|---|
   | poor | fair | average | good | excellent |
2. Practicality of examples given
   | 1 | 2 | 3 | 4 | 5 |
   |---|---|---|---|---|
   | poor | fair | average | good | excellent |
3. Effectiveness of group discussion
   | 1 | 2 | 3 | 4 | 5 |
   |---|---|---|---|---|
   | poor | fair | average | good | excellent |

Suggestions and comments:

Post–in-service evaluation should be an ongoing activity. It should not end with the written evaluation. The participants should be encouraged to consider the speech-language pathologist as a readily available resource concerning their patients' communication characteristics and needs. Giving positive feedback to nursing staff working with demented patients will reinforce behavioral changes, enhance job satisfaction, and ultimately improve the quality of patient care.

## AVAILABLE IN-SERVICE PROGRAMS

To date, no in-service programs have been empirically derived, tested, and published that specifically relate to the communicative disorders of patients with dementia. An increasing number of commercially available texts have been recently published related to communicative disorders of the elderly in general. The American Speech-Language-Hearing Association (ASHA) published an in-service training module, *Breaking the Silence Barrier: An Inservice Program for Nursing Home Staff Working with Communicatively Handicapped Geriatric Patients*.[2] The manual includes suggested visual aids and helpful suggestions for in-service activities. ASHA also published a program entitled *Communication Disorders and Aging*, which was designed for speech-language pathologists to use in an in-service workshop for staff or those working with geriatric patients.[3] The program provides booklets containing definitions of common communicative disorders of the elderly and color slides with audiotapes of speech-language pathologists and audiologists appropriately interacting with elderly patients. Shadden, Raiford, and Shadden published an in-service manual, *Coping with Communication Disorders in Aging*, that integrates training material with training experience.[29] The programs tend to be didactic in nature, focusing on the nature of communication disorders, the role of the speech-language pathologist, and lists of techniques for improved communicative interaction.

## Effective In-Service Training for Staff Working with Demented Patients

Generally speaking, if speech-language pathologists have conducted in-service training for nursing home staff, they have traditionally lectured on common speech, language, and hearing disorders associated with dementia. This was probably due to the fact that speech-language pathologists receive extensive theoretic background about the nature of communication disorders. The communication disorders literature, however, has failed to provide a rationale and/or evidence to suggest what type and how much knowledge is necessary for health-care staff to acquire in order to effectively provide optimal care for the communication-impaired, demented patient. In developing a successful in-service program, the previously cited literature advocates the first step of identifying and assessing the needs of the nursing-home staff. A question that needs to be addressed is whether knowledge of communication disorders of the demented patient is in fact a learning need of nursing assistants; and if so, is it sufficient to improve the quality of care of the demented patient. Ideally, the speech-language pathologist could accomplish this task by developing a tool to make direct behavioral observations. Research to date has had difficulty translating observations into behavioral rating scores. Hatton found support for the assumption that a nurse with a favorable disposition toward patients exhibits a high percentage of positive interactions.[16] Her study was limited by a small sample size and difficulties in collecting and categorizing the data. Adelson et al developed the Interaction Behavior Rating Code to quantify interpersonal behaviors of doctors and nurses with bedridden geriatric patients.[1] Assuming a valid and reliable tool could be developed in a similar fashion to identify specific overt behaviors contributing to the development of a communication-impaired environment, its use for in-service development would be impractical. In lieu of the numbers of speech-language pathologists who are employed part time or as consultants, it would be time and cost inefficient to administer such a scale in context with each staff member.

A paper-and-pencil tool that could be administered to a large number of staff members at one time and that could effectively predict overt behaviors would be ideal for the development of communication in-service training for nursing assistants. Such a tool could assess if knowledge of communication disorders of the demented is an appropriate learning need for nursing assistants. In addition, such a tool that could effectively predict behaviors might be used to measure differences between various in-service methodologies in effecting positive changes in nursing assistants' interactions with their demented patients.

The idea that in-service education can positively influence negative attitudes implies that a person's behavior might be predicted from his attitudes. The concept of "attitude" denotes the degree of positive or negative effect associated with some psychological object.[30] Based on this assumption, a speech-language pathologist might develop an attitude scale toward the communication-impaired elderly, administer it to determine the needs of staff for in-service training, and determine in-service effectiveness by administering the scale after in-service training. The psychological literature, however, after more than 75 years of attitude research, has found little consistent evidence supporting the hypothesis that knowledge of an individual's attitude toward some object will allow one to predict the way he will behave with respect to the object.[12,13]

Within this same psychological literature on attitude research, the concept of "behavioral intent" was hypothesized to be a predictor of overt behavior. A behavioral intent is defined as an individual's intention to perform a given action in a particular situation.[12] Dulany developed the Theory of Propositional Control that evolved from psychological studies of verbal conditioning and is concerned with predicting the probability with which an individual will make a particular verbal response.[9] According to Dulany's theory, a behavioral intent is the antecedent of overt behavior. Whereas the attitude measurement literature dealt with a subject's intention to engage in an action "in general," Dulany's theory is concerned with a more precise and specific type of behavioral intention—namely, an individual's intention to perform a given action in a particular situation. Statistical analysis reveals the correlation between the measure of behavioral intent toward a particular context and the actual overt behavior to be near perfect—about .95.

The material presented in this chapter thus far set the groundwork for two companion studies conducted by Koury and Koury and Lubinski, in which a paper-and-pencil measuring tool was developed to: (1) aid the speech-language pathologist to identify and assess the learning needs of nursing-home staff working with the communicatively impaired elderly; and (2) measure the effectiveness of three types of in-service learning experiences of nursing assistants.[20,21]

## STUDY I

For the first study a two-part instrument, entitled "Protocol for Assessing Nursing Aides' Knowledge and Behavioral Intents Toward the Communication-Impaired Elderly," was developed. It was designed to (1) utilize the concept of "behavioral intent" to assess strategies that nursing assistants use when communicating with elderly patients in a long-term care facility, and (2) assess nursing assistants' general knowledge of geriatric communication disorders.

The behavioral intent portion of the measuring tool was designed as 14 written scenarios depicting probable nursing assistant and patient communication interactions. These scenarios described eight types of communication problems including communication impairment associated with dementia.

*Example:* When you ask Mrs. Caldwell, an 80-year-old patient, what happened to her dentures she says, "Teeth, teeth, teeth...oh, if only my hair were combed, combed....Brush my hair, now!" What would you do?

The second part of the measuring tool consisted of 20 multiple-choice items evaluating knowledge of geriatric communication disorders. These questions focused on specific knowledge related to the eight communication areas depicted in the behavioral intents portion of the instrument including communication impairment associated with dementia.

*Example:* A patient with early stages of Alzheimer's disease:

1. Has trouble remembering what you said to him 5 minutes ago
2. Has slurred, unclear speech
3. Has trouble forming sentences
4. Uses nonsense or jibberish
5. Shows no interest in communicating

The measuring tool of Study I was administered to a group of experienced, ASHA-certified speech-language pathologists working in long-term care facilities and a group of nursing assistants in their place of employment. The responses of the speech-language pathologists to the behavioral intents portion of the measuring tool were used as a scale for evaluating the fluency and quality of responses generated by nursing assistants. Fluency was defined as the number of behavioral intents generated by a subject. Quality was defined as the response rank of how well nursing assistants' responses matched the most commonly given responses of speech-language pathologists. For each question on the knowledge portion of the measuring tool, there was one correct response that was generated from the communication disorders literature. The knowledge measure was scored on a percentage correct basis. A comparison of results between the two groups revealed the following major findings:

1. Speech-language pathologists generated a significantly greater number and higher quality of behavioral intents concerning the communication-impaired demented patient than did nursing assistants.
2. Nursing assistants had little knowledge of the nature of communication disorders associated with dementia.
3. As the number of responses given by a nursing assistant increased, the quality of responses increased as well.
4. There appeared to be no relationship or predictive nature between what a nursing assistant knows about communication disorders and the quality of behavioral intents generated in scenarios dealing with demented patients.

The findings of the first study lent strong support to the nursing and education literature that suggests that solely presenting knowledge about a topic is an ineffectual method for changing staff behaviors. It seemed apparent that in-service role playing might be an alternative training method to improve nursing assistant interactions with patients and to increase problem-solving techniques. With this in mind, a second study was conducted to compare the effectiveness of three in-service learning strategies for nursing assistants working with the communication-impaired elderly.

## STUDY II

Students from nursing assistant training programs were utilized for the second study to prevent job experience and/or previous in-service programs focusing on communication problems of the elderly from biasing the results. The nursing assistant students were divided into three groups: Group 1 received traditional in-service training, Group 2 received in-service role-playing, and Group 3 received no in-service training. The traditional in-service program was a 1-hour-lecture format. It focused on (1) the role of the speech-language pathologist with elderly and demented patients; (2) the importance of communication to the elderly; (3) a description of communication problems among the elderly, including communication disorders associated with dementia; and (4) a list of common do's and don'ts in communicating with individuals who have these types of communication problems.

The in-service role playing was given to Group 2. This was also 1 hour in length, with the content focusing briefly on the same topics given in the traditional in-service program with the exclusion of what assistants should do in communicating. The instructor and volunteer students then engaged in five role-playing situations that were similar but not identical to those in the measuring tool. The students were given specific tasks to complete while the instructor portrayed communicatively disordered patients. Students were encouraged to "think on their feet" and try different techniques that they thought would facilitate communication. Students remaining in the audience were encouraged to critique the interaction and offer suggestions for improved communication during and after the interaction. All students were verbally reinforced for active participation in the role-playing scenarios and the critique (see this chapter's Appendix).

All three groups completed the measuring tool at the beginning of a 12-week training program. The traditional and role-playing groups received an in-service program during the middle of their training program. All three groups completed the measuring tool at the conclusion of their nursing assistant training program.

A comparison of results between groups revealed the following major findings:

1. The number and quality of strategies generated by nursing assistants increased for both traditional in-service and role-playing in-service groups; however, the increase in quality was significant only for the role-playing group.
2. There was no significant difference in the amount of knowledge gained on the nature of communication disorders associated with dementia between the traditional in-service and role-playing in-service.
3. The role-playing group consistently outperformed the other two research groups in number of responses generated, quality of responses, and knowledge subtest.

In summary, the results of the second study support the literature that states that in-service training, in general, is necessary to elicit change in employee behavior. The study clearly demonstrated that role playing was the most effective in-service strategy and should be employed more often by speech-language pathologists. Role playing encourages nursing assistants to spontaneously and independently manage the communication problems they face in interacting with demented patients.

## Clinical Content for Improved In-Service Training with Nursing Assistants

This chapter has attempted to build a case for role playing as the most effective in-service learning experience for nursing assistants working with patients with communication disorders associated with dementia. Koury and Lubinski, in their study discussed above, designed the in-service role-playing to include a brief, 5-minute lecture.[21] The emphasis of the lecture was not to provide volumes of facts on dementia or give lists of "Do's and Don'ts." The lecture was designed to set the stage and provide a reference for behavioral characteristics of patients with dementia that the role-playing participants and observers would see in the actual role-play experiences to follow

The following is a sample outline for the lecture portion of a role-play learning experience:

I. Introduce yourself. Give your name, position, and roles in the nursing home. It is important to print your name and title on a board so that the nursing assistants can identify you.

II. Talk about the importance of communication to the elderly. Encourage the nursing assistants to offer the following values of communication: self-expression, stimulation of thinking skills, socialization, emotional expression, expression of needs, humor, and reducing feelings of isolation and frustration.

III. Talk about what nursing assistants need to know about dementia. The instructor should realize that many nursing assistants will not know the term "dementia." A brief description of the following dementia characteristics may be useful:

  A. "Brain disorder" that progressively gets worse, not better; it has been found that patients can learn or have skills maintained and that ADLs can be managed more efficiently.

  B. Impairment of recent, short-term memory, and remote, long-term memory. Give nursing assistants examples of each in mild and severe cases such as, "You go into Mr. Jones' room after he has finished eating. He demands that you bring him his lunch and wants to know why it hasn't arrived yet."

  C. Impairment of understanding (comprehension). Give nursing assistants examples in mild and severe cases such as, "You ask Mrs. Smith to stand up and you find yourself repeating this command 2 to 3 times before she does it."

  D. Impairment of expression (linguistic and pragmatic skills). Give nursing assistants examples in mild and severe cases such as, "Mr. Roberts wants something out of his reach on the shelf. He keeps repeating the word 'sugar' while he is pointing, but there is no sugar to be found. He nods his head 'yes' and becomes angry with you."

The role-play technique that was used in the Koury and Lubinski study was open-ended.[21] That is, the participants (speech-language pathologist and the volunteer nursing assistants) had maximum freedom for creativity. The nursing assistant played himself or herself and was given a specific duty to do with the patient (played by the speech-language pathologist). Whom to call on as volunteers, and how long to let the role playing go on are left to the judgment of the speech-language pathologist. Generally, the following guidelines were found to be helpful:

1. Stop the action if the player is too anxious or runs out of ideas.
2. Ask the audience to make suggestions to help the player.
3. Give the player and the audience hints if they are having trouble coming up with appropriate ideas.
4. Restart the role play to give the player a second chance to provide him or her with a positive experience. If video recording equipment is available, use it to give the volunteer visual feedback.
5. Emphasize actions and attitudes by requiring the player to cope with emotionally charged statements. For example, "You're frustrated, even angry by now. She hit you."
6. Summarize communication-repair strategies frequently for the group each time the action stops.
7. At the end of the in-service program, have the audience help you to derive a list of common strategies useful in the role plays that fostered successful communication, such as:[28]
   - Orient patient to upcoming situations
   - Keep patient on subject by asking relevant questions
   - Remind patient what he was talking about
   - Repeat message frequently
   - Use short sentences (noun-verb-object)
   - Avoid competing messages (t.v., radio, etc.)
   - Enhance your message with pictures, objects, gestures, body language, or manual guidance
   - Encourage communication through any means
   - Don't stop talking to the patient

## Research Implications

The literature presented indicates that in-service training does improve nursing assistants' behavioral intents toward communicating with elderly patients, thus underscoring the value of in-service programs for this group of staff members. This finding, however, is based on the psychology literature that states behavioral intents are highly correlated with or are the antecedents of overt behavior. Although these results may be "apparent," direct behavioral evidence is also needed for administrators and nursing supervisors as a rationale for speech-language pathologists to conduct communication in-service programs with nursing assistants. The fundamental objective of all in-service training for nursing assistants is to change employee behavior in some desired direction. Finding out whether change took place, and if so, whether it was desirable, is difficult. Research to date has been limited because of the difficulty translating direct observations into behavioral rating tools.[1,16] If the profession of speech-language pathology is committed to the delivery of quality care, then there is a need for research to develop a direct method for evaluating the impact of in-service training on nursing assistants or on the patients themselves. This might be done through video/audio tape analysis of nursing assistants' actual communication exchanges during activities of daily living, through structured observations, or in naturalistic contexts. The focus of this chapter has been on changing the behaviors of nursing assistants, because this group has the most contact on a day-to-day basis with patients. There are, however, several other groups in the nursing-home setting where communication skills are crucial for delivery of care. These include physicians, nurses, and physical and occupational therapists. Thus, future areas to be investigated include: (1) the development of standardized measures to be correlated with observed behaviors in the nursing home; (2) comparisons after in-service programs of subsequent observed behaviors with dementia patients and with patients exhibiting other types of communication disorders; and (3) types of staff where in-service training is most effective (physicians, R.N.s, nursing assistants, physical therapists, or occupational therapists).

# References

1. Adelson R, Nasti B, Sprafkin J, et al. Behavioral ratings of health professionals' interactions with the geriatric patient. Gerontologist 1982; 22:277–281.
2. American Speech-Language-Hearing Association. Breaking the silence barrier: An inservice program for nursing home staff working with communicatively handicapped geriatric patients. ASHA, 1977.
3. American Speech-Language-Hearing Association. Communication disorders and aging. ASHA, 1985.
4. Chafee CE. Rehabilitation needs of nursing home patients: A report of a survey. Rehabil Literature 1967; 28:377.
5. Convenuto S. Giving zest to inservice. Am J Nurs 1974; 74(10):1835.
6. Corkin S, Growdon JH, Sullivan EV, Shedlack K. Lecithin and cognitive function in aging and dementia. In: Kidman AD, Tomkins JK, Westerman RA, eds. Proceedings of the second symposium of the foundation for life sciences. Sydney: Excerpta Medica, 1981:229.
7. Corsini RJ. The role-playing technique in business and industry. Chicago: University of Chicago, Industrial Relations Center, 1957.
8. Davis CM. The role of the physical and occupational therapist in caring for the victim of Alzheimer's disease. In: Taira ED, ed. Therapeutic interventions for the person with dementia. New York: Haworth Press, 1986:15–28.
9. Dulany DE. Hypothesis and habits in verbal operant conditioning. J Abnormal Soc Psychol 1961; 63:251–263.
10. Ernst NS, West HL. Nursing home staff development: A guide for inservice programs. New York: Springer Publishing, 1983.
11. Fein DJ. Projections of health care spending to 1990. Health Care Financing Rev 1986; Spring, 20.
12. Fishbein M. Attitude and the prediction of behavior. In: Fishbein M, ed. Readings in attitude theory and measurement. New York: John Wiley and Sons, 1967.
13. Fishbein M. A consideration of beliefs and their role in attitude measurement. In: Fishbein M, ed. Readings in attitude theory and measurement. New York: John Wiley and Sons, 1967:493.
14. Glickstein JK. Therapeutic intervention in Alzheimer's disease: A program of functional communication skills for activities of daily living. Rockville, MD: Aspen, 1988.
15. Grubb R, Mueller C. Designing hospital training programs. Springfield, IL: Charles C Thomas, 1975.
16. Hatton J. Nurses' attitudes toward the aged relationship to nursing care. J Gerontol Nurs 1977; 3:21–26.
17. Hickey T. Health and aging. Monterey, CA: Brooks/Cole, 1980.
18. Hospital Continuing Education Project of the Hospital Research and Educational Trust. Training and continuing education: A handbook for health care institutions. Chicago: Hospital Research and Educational Trust, 1970.
19. Jacobs-Condit L, ed. Gerontology and communication disorders. Rockville, MD: ASHA, 1985.
20. Koury LN. Assessing nursing home aides' knowledge and behavioral intents toward the communication impaired elderly. Unpublished masters thesis, State University of New York at Buffalo, 1987.
21. Koury LN, Lubinski R. Effective inservice for staff working with communication-impaired patients. (In preparation).
22. Lohmann R, Lohmann W. Medicare, Medicaid—Geriatric residential environments. Minneapolis: Institute for Interdisciplinary Studies American Rehabilitation Foundation, 1971:23–32.
23. Lubinski R. Speech, language and audiology programs in home health care agencies and nursing homes. In: Beasley D, Davis G, eds. Aging: Communication processes and disorders. New York: Grune & Stratton, 1981:339.
24. Lutenegger RR. Patient care and rehabilitation of communicative-impaired adults. Chicago: Charles C Thomas, 1975.
25. McEvoy C, Patterson R. Behavioral treatment of deficit skills in dementia patients. Gerontologist 1986; 26:475–478.

26. Meuller PB, Peters TJ. Needs and services in geriatric speech-language pathology and audiology. ASHA 1981; 23:627.
27. Ohio State Department of Education. Focus on inservice education. Columbus, OH, 1978.
28. Ostuni E, Santo Pietro M. Getting through: Communicating when someone you care for has Alzheimer's disease. Plainsboro, NJ: Speech Bin, 1986.
29. Shadden BB, Raiford CA, Shadden HS. Coping with communication disorders in aging. Tigaard, OR: C.C. Publications, 1983.
30. Thurstone LL. Theory of attitude measurement. Psychol Rev 1929; 36:222–241.
31. United Hospital Fund of New York. A concept in inservice education in nursing homes. New York: Nursing Home Trainer Program NYM/RMP Project #2061-70A, 1972.
32. United States Bureau of the Census. America in transition: An aging society. Current population reports. Series p-23, No. 128. Washington, DC.: U.S. Government Printing Office, 1983.
33. United States Department of Health, Education, and Welfare. Health resources statistics. Rockville, MD: Health Resources Administration, 1976.
34. Wang MS, Busse EW. Dementia in old age. In: Wells CE, ed. Dementia. Philadelphia: F.A. Davis, 1971:151.

# APPENDIX

## Example of Role-Play Procedure

1. Prepare five different cards with an example of a likely nursing assistant and patient interaction printed on each card. Provide appropriate props necessary for each role play (e.g., washcloth, toothbrush, comb, plate, spoon, cup, etc.). ADL activities are good to use. Example of instructions on card: "The patient's name is Mrs. Cooper. She needs to brush her teeth, then wash her face."
2. For each role play, choose several common behaviors characteristic of dementia for the patient that you are playing. Plan ahead of time how you will act out the part of each patient. Make sure that you cover the major cognitive, linguistic, and pragmatic deficits to ensure a comprehensive summary of "communication tips" for the nursing assistants to utilize with their real patients. Some behavioral characteristics might include: (1) being hostile at times; (2) exhibiting word-finding deficits; (3) exhibiting perseveration; (4) exhibiting comprehension deficits; and (5) exhibiting memory deficits.
3. Enlist a volunteer for the role play. Say, "I'd like you to read out loud to the group the following description of a patient you are likely to encounter in a nursing home. I will act like that patient and you are to carry out the assignment given on the card."
4. *Role play.* The ADL activity will be for the nursing assistant to have the "patient" brush her teeth and wash her face.
   *Props.* Chair and table, toothbrush, toothpaste, washcloth, and wash basin are placed in front of the "patient" on a table. Radio playing music.
   *Scene.* Following is an example of how a typical role play might develop.

| | |
|---|---|
| Nursing assistant (Bob): | "Brush your teeth, honey." |
| Patient (speech path): | "Brush, brush, brush..." (patient's voice trails off and patient is looking off in another direction). "This is *not* the hairdresser" (becomes mildly agitated). |
| Assistant: | "Brush your teeth, Mrs. Cooper." |
| Patient: | Scans table. Slowly picks up wash cloth and puts it in mouth. |
| Assistant: | Pulls wash cloth from patient's mouth, hands toothbrush and toothpaste to patient, "Brush your teeth. Put on some toothpaste." |
| Patient: | Mumbles, "teeth, teeth..." |
| Assistant: | Takes brush from patient, puts on toothpaste and attempts to brush patient's teeth for her. |
| Patient: | Becomes hostile. Screams! |
| Assistant: | Attempts to soothe patient, no luck. Turns to audience for help. |
| Speech path: | "Was this a good interaction? Let's look at the kind of troubles Bob was having. Who has a suggestion for him? Let's try this again." |
| Participant one: | "He never got your attention." |
| Speech path: | "That's right. You need to get your patient so that she can see you if possible. Get in front of her—even better, stoop down to her sitting level. What about distractions?" |
| Participant two: | "The radio might be a problem?" |

| | |
|---|---|
| Speech path: | "Yes, turn it off. You don't want to have your message to the patient competing with the newscaster! What else? (Silence.) The patient got the idea that Bob wanted her to do something, but she put the wash cloth in her mouth instead of the toothbrush. What could he have done to possibly prevent this?" |
| Participant three: | "Show her what to do?" |
| Speech path: | "Sure. He could gesture or pantomime 'brushing teeth,' he could have used the actual item to demonstrate, he could have pointed to the items. O.K., let's go back and try this again, Bob. Try these new hints and let's see what else might happen." |

Repeat the role play until the communication interaction is successful. If you play a patient who is unmanageable this would be the time to talk about the role of the head nurse, speech pathologist, or audiologist in helping the nursing assistant.

| | |
|---|---|
| Speech path: | "O.K. You all did a great job. Let's summarize the techniques you used to communicate effectively with these patients." |

# *Index*

**A**

Abstract thinking, 38
Accessibility, 265
Acoustic reflex, 53
Acoustic stapedial reflex testing, 228
Acquired dysfluency, 72–73
Acquired knowledge manipulation, 28
Adaptive strategies, 244
Adult children as caregivers, 2
Adult day-care programs, 13–14
Advocacy groups, 17
Age bias, 148
Aging. *See also* Elderly persons
   academic training in, 238
   language in normal, 84–85. *See also* Language changes in normal aging
   rights of passage, 257
Agnosia, 28
Agrammatism, 100
AIDS (acquired immunodeficiency syndrome)
   CANS impairment in, 65
   cause of dementia, as, 3
AIDS dementia complex, 6
Alphabetic cueing, 240
Alzheimer's Association, 152
Alzheimer's Dementia and Risk to Family Member Questionnaire, 197, 216–222
Alzheimer's disease. *See* Dementia of Alzheimer's type (DAT)
Alzheimer's Disease and Related Disorders Association (ADRDA), 17. *See also* Alzheimer's Association
   support group, 13
   Work Group, 3, 4, 22
American Speech-Language-Hearing Association, 238, 240
Amplification, 229
Amyotrophic lateral sclerosis (ALS), 77
Anatomy of dementia
   approaches to study of, 23, 24
   comparative neuropsychology and, 32–33
   neuroanatomic approach to, 23, 31–32
   neurobehavioral approach to, 23–29
   neurochemical approach to, 23, 29–31
Angular gyrus syndrome (AGS), 109 Anomia, 98, 99, 101–102, 104–106
Anonymity, 259
Anterograde memory, 24, 39
Aphasia
   DAT, in, 101
   differential diagnosis, 192, 194–195
   relationship between dementia and, 194–195
   test batteries, 107, 207
Aphasics, bilingual, 133
Aphonia, 70
Apraxia, 27–28, 70
Arizona Battery for Communication Disorders of Dementia, 10, 107, 207

Art therapy, 241
Assertiveness training, 94
Assessment. *See* Dementia assessment
Assistive listening devices (ALD), 229, 232–235. *See also* Auditory impairment management
Audiologist, 225
Auditory brainstem response (ABR), 52–54
Auditory Comprehension Test for Sentences (ACTS), 211
Auditory environment, 268–269
Auditory impairment
   behavioral manifestation of, 223
   central auditory function in elderly and demented, 58–65
   central auditory function in non Alzheimer dementias, 65–67
   dementia, in, 47–49
   evaluation of, 11, 47, 48, 65–66, 227–229
   neural, 53–54
   prevalence of, 90, 223–224
   rehabilitative implications of, 66
   research needs of, 66–67, 235–236
   screening techniques for, 225–227
   severity of, 224
   temporal lobe and, 54–58
Auditory impairment management
   assistive listening devices, 232–235
   explanation of, 229–230, 234
   hearing aids, 230–232. *See also* Hearing-aid use
Auditory processing, 48
Auditory system
   conductive mechanism, 49
   effects of aging on, 67
   neural mechanism, 52–54
   sensory mechanism, 49–52
   temporal lobe, 54–58

**B**

Behavior
   assessment of, 199–200
   manifestations of, 223
Behavior and Mood Disturbance Scale, 157
Behavioral contingency theory, 240
Bilingual dementia
   clinical and research implications, 138
   discussion of, 137–138
   future research, 139
   methodology, 134–135
   results, 135–137
   review of literature, 133–134
Bilingualism, 133
Binswanger's encephalopathy, 75
Blessed Orientation and Memory Examination, 201–202
Boston Diagnostic Aphasia Examination (BDAE), 10, 93, 99, 119, 211
Boston Naming Test (BNT), 38, 211
Brain-behavior relationships, 105–106

Brainstem auditory nuclei, 52
Brief Cognitive Rating Scale (BCRS), 201–202

## C

Caregiver burden
  concept of, 159–160
  correlates of perceived, 161–162
Caregivers
  assessing stress of, 198
  communication-impaired environment, in, 262
  environmental needs of, 261
  family. See Family caregivers
  formal versus informal, 153–154
  in-service education of, 111, 148–149, 235, 248–249. See also In-service training
  management strategies for, 248
  role in environmental enhancement, 264
  spouse, 158
Caregiving Hassles Scale, 198
Case history interview, 197–198
Category fluency, 38
Central auditory function
  assessment of, 54–58
  elderly and demented, in, 47, 58–65
  non-Alzheimer's dementias, in, 65
Central auditory nervous system (CANS)
  age-related changes in, 54
  function of, 47–48
Central auditory-processing disorder, 48
Cerebellar dysfunction, 73
Cerebellar lesions, 73
Cerebral cortex, 26
Cerebral hemisphere, 23, 24
Cerebrum, 29
Cerumen accumulation, 49
Cholinergic systems, 29–31
Chomsky Test of Syntax, 103
Circumlocutions, 244, 245
Clinical Dementia Rating (CDR), 11, 204–205
Cochlea, 49–53
Cochlear conductive presbycusis, 50, 51
Cochlear lesions, 52, 53
Code-switching
  between familiar and relative stranger, 138
  breakdown in, 133. See also Bilingual dementia
  linguistic appropriateness of, 134, 137–138
  types of errors in, 134–137
Cognitive environment, 269–270
Cognitive impairment. See also Abstract thinking; Language impairment; Memory impairment; Visuospatial functions
  Alzheimer's disease, in, See Dementia of Alzheimer type (DAT)
  role of cholinergic system in, 30–31
  role of dopamine loss in, 31
Coherence impairment, 116–117, 125
Cohesion impairment, 116–117
Cohort effect, 250
Committee on Hearing, Bioacoustics, and Biomechanics (CHABA), 48, 58
Communication. See also Discourse; Discourse studies in Alzheimer's patients
  assessment, 93, 205–211. See also Language and communication assessment
  environment and, 91–92
  gestural, 110
  individual differences and, 90–91

  methods to improve, 147. See also Communication management in DAT
  patient-aide, 146
  social-cognitive model of, 89–90
  value of, 257–258
  with elderly, 84–85, 93. See also Language changes in normal aging
Communication Adequacy in Daily Situations (CADS), 255–256
Communication disorders specialist, 263
Communication/Environment Assessment and Planning Guide, 263, 274–278
Communication management in DAT
  approaches, 243–250
  direct, 239–241
  methodologic considerations, 250–251
  need for future clinical research in, 251
  overview of, 238, 240
  principles of, 242–243
  studies on, 241–242
Communication skill training, 248. See also Family caregivers
Communication-impaired environment, 261–262
Communicative Abilities in Daily Living (CADL), 10, 107
Communicative changes
  DAT, in, 185
  normal elderly adults, in, 184–185
  perceptions of family caregivers regarding DAT relatives, 170–184
  research implications of, 185–186
Comparative neuropsychology, 32–33
Computerized tomography, 11
Confrontation naming, 38
Content analysis, 124
Control, 148
Conversation skills, 87–88
Cortical dementia, 22–23, 33. See also Dementia of Alzheimer type (DAT); Pick's disease
  amyotrophic, 76
  differential diagnosis, 108, 189, 190
  dysarthrias in, 71
  language impairment, 25, 27
  memory loss in, 24–25. See also Memory; Memory impairment
Cortical stuttering, 76
Corticodentatonigral degeneration, 76
Counseling, 163, 248, 249
Cranial nerve
  eighth, 52–54
  nuclei and, 73
Creutzfeldt-Jakob disease, 65, 76
  differential diagnosis, 191–193
  language impairment in, 108
Cues
  alphabetic, 240
  lexical semantic, 244
  outcome, 144
  phonemic, 244
  situational, 144

## D

Dance and movement therapies, 240–241
DAT. See Dementia of Alzheimer's type (DAT)
Delayed recall task, 211
Dementia
  anatomy of. See Anatomy of dementia

Dementia (*Continued*)
  aphasia and relationship to, 194–195
  assessment. *See* Dementia assessment
  behavioral manifestations of, 223
  cortical. *See* Cortical dementia
  dangers in labeling, 144
  definition of, 3, 22
  diagnosis problems of, 70–71, 143–144, 196–197
  differential diagnosis of, 107–109. *See also* Differential diagnosis
  education and advocacy issues regarding, 16–17
  etiology and risk factors, 8
  evaluation of, 10–11
  financial concerns, 15–16
  impact of, 2
  incidence of, 6–7
  institutionalization for, 14–15. *See also* institutionalization
  irreversible, 188–189
  management of, 11, 12
  mixed. *See* Creutzfeldt-Jakob disease; Multi-infarct dementia
  mortality, 7–8
  motor system and, 71–72
  neuropsychological evaluation, 10
  pharmacotherapy for, 12, 13. *See also* Medication
  policy issues of, 15
  prevalence of, 6–7
  research needs, 17
  reversible. *See* Reversible dementia
  scope of evaluation of, 10
  service delivery of, 16
  staging, 11
  subcortical. *See* Subcortical dementia
  types of, 3, 4, 190–192. *See also individual types*
Dementia of Alzheimer's type (DAT)
  Abstract and problem-solving processes in, 38
  agnosia in, 28
  apraxia in, 27–28, 70
  auditory brainstem response in, 54, 55
  brain imaging to diagnose, 11
  central auditory function in, 58–65
  cholinergic system and, 30, 31
  clinical and research implications for, 44
  communication management in. *See* Communication management in Alzheimer's disease
  comparative neuropsychology and, 32–33
  criteria for diagnosis of, 4, 5
  differential diagnosis, 108, 188–190. *See also* Differential diagnosis
  discourse studies in. *See* Discourse studies in Alzheimer patients
  familial, 109
  language impairment, 25, 27, 37–38. *See also* Language changes in dementia of Alzheimer type
  memory in, 24, 25, 37, 39. *See also* Memory; Memory impairment
    explicit, 39–42
    implicit, 42–43
  neuroanatomic changes in, 31, 32
  pathophysiology of, 8–9
  prevalence of, 2–4, 189
  risk factors of, 8, 9
  study of family caregiver's perceptions of relatives with, 170–184
  symptomatology of, 4–5
  temporal lobe impairment and, 58–62
  treatment implications, 109–111

visuospatial function in, 28, 38–39
Dementia assessment
  behavioral, 199–200
  case history interview, 197–198
  language and communication, 93, 205–211
  medical and neurologic evaluation, 198–199
  neurophysical, 200–205
  premises, 196–197
Dementia patients
  nursing homes, in, 14. *See also* Institutionalization; Nursing homes
  receiving informal care, 154
  stresses of caring for, 155–157
Dependency development, 144–146
Depression
  caregivers, in, 158–159
  communicative performance and, 90
  dementia syndrome accompanying. *See* Pseudodementia
  geriatric, 189
  Parkinson's disease, in, 73
Descriptive discourse, 124–125
Design, environmental, 265–266. *See also* Environment
Diagnosis
  differential. *See* Differential diagnosis
  problems in, 70–71, 143–144, 147, 196–197
Diagnostic imaging, 11
Dichotic assessment, 56, 58–63
Dichotic listening, 56, 57
Dichotic sentence task, 58
Differential diagnosis
  aphasia, 192, 194–195
  cortical dementias, 108, 189, 190
  explanation of, 107, 188
  irreversible, 188–189
  mixed dementias, 109, 191–194, 199
  pseudodementias, 107–108, 188–189
  right hemisphere damage, 195
  subcortical dementias, 108, 189–193
  tables, 190–192
  treatment and, 117–118
Digressions, 117
Discourse
  analysis of, 124–127
  assessment of, 207–211
  changes in normal aging, 87–88
  deficits in, 115–117
  descriptive, 124–125
  explanation of, 115
  genre types, 124–125
  narrative, 88, 120, 124–125
Discourse Abilities Profile (DAP), 207–211
Discourse studies in Alzheimer patients
  clinical and research implications, 128–129
  explanation of findings in, 117–119
  methodology, 119–123
  overview of, 115
  results and discussion, 123–127
  sample of subjects' language, 131–132
Dissociations, 118
Divergent semantic intervention therapy, 246
Dopaminergic system, 31
Dorsolateral frontal system, 32
Down's syndrome, 9
Drug therapy. *See* Medication
Dysarthrias, 25
  early in dementia, 72
  explanation of, 70, 79

Dysarthrias (*Continued*)
  focal lesions, in, 74–75
  identifying types of, 71, 72
  loci of lesions in dementing, 73–74
  types of dementia causing, 72
Dysphasia, 70, 79
Dysprosodias, 74
Dysprosody, 74

# E

Ebenezer Center for Aging, 263
Echolalia, 100
Education
  family members, of, 149
  in-service. *See* In-service training
  public, of, 16–17
Effectiveness, 249–250
Eighth cranial nerve, 52–54
Elderly persons. *See also* Aging
  conversation skills of, 87–88
  family perceptions of communicative changes in normal, 184–185
  language in normal, 84–85. *See also* Language
    changes in normal aging statistics, 2, 22, 279
  syntax changes in, 86–87
  value of communication to, 257–258
Electrophysiologic testing, 53
English-language proficiency, 143
Environment
  caregiver needs and attitudes regarding, 261
  caregiver's role in enhancement of, 264
  cognitive, 269–270
  communication-impaired, 261–262
  identification strategies, 263
  immediate, 92
  individual, and the, 259
  language and, 89
  living arrangements and activities, 92
  physical, 258–259, 265–266
  research needs regarding, 271
  sensory, 267–269
  social, 260–271
  social expectations, and, 91–92
  topographic issues and, 259–260
Environmental fit, 260
Episodic memory, 39
Eustachian tube, 49
Explicit memory, 39–42
Extrapyramidal lesions, 73–74

# F

Facilitation strategies, 244
False starts, 127
Familial myoclonic dementia, 77
Familial non-Alzheimer's dementia, 78
Familial olivopontocerebellar degeneration, 77
Familial spino-cerebellar degeneration and dementia, 30, 31
Family caregivers. *See also* Caregivers
  adult children as, 2
  assessment of, 164
  burden of, 159–162
  communication skill training for, 248
  impact of dementia on, 152–153
  interventions, 162–164
  perceptions of caregiving role by, 162
  spouse as, 158
  statistics regarding, 153–154
  study of perceptions of communication changes in relatives with DAT, 170–184
Family caregiving, 12–14. *See also* Caregivers
  clinical implications of, 164
  dimensions of, 154–155
  impact of, 157–159
  research issues and questions regarding, 164–165
  stresses of, 155–157
Family counseling, 163
Family history, 9
Family members
  caregivers, as, 12–14
  perceptions on communication changes in dementia, 146, 169–170
  perspectives of, 168–169
Family support groups, 13, 163
FAS Word Fluency Measure, 211
Financial concerns, 2, 15–16
First letter mnemonics, 240
Focal lesions, 74–75
Formal caregivers, 153
Frontal-lobe, 28
  dysfunction, 75
  syndrome, 25
  type of dementia, 189
Functional Assessment Stages (FAST) in Normal Aging and Alzheimer's Diseases, 202, 205

# G

Geriatric depression, 189
Gerstmann-Sträussler dementia (familial spino-cerebellar degeneration and dementia), 30, 31
Gerstmann-Sträussler-Scheinckler disease, 76
Gestural communication, 110
Grammatic ability, 103
Grief process, 164
Group therapy
  advanced stage, 246–248
  early stage, 245

# H

Hachinski scale, 11
Head trauma, 9
Health care costs, 2, 15–16
Hearing loss. *See* Auditory impairment
Hearing-aid use, 229. *See also* Auditory impairment
  management
  explanation of, 230–231
  orientation of, 231–232
  prior to becoming demented, 65–66
  with peripheral hearing loss, 66
Hedges, 127
Helplessness
  innate, 145
  labeling problems and, 143–144
  learned, 144–146
  methods to minimize, 147–149
  research needs and, 149
Hesitations, 127
Hippocampus, 31
Home care, 13. *See also* Family caregivers; Family caregiving
Huntington's disease, 22
  differential diagnosis, 190–191, 193
  language deficits in, 108
  memory in, 25
Hydrocephalic dementia, 107

## I

Ideational apraxia, 27-28
Ideomotor apraxia, 27
Implicit memory, 42-43
Incompetence cycle, 144-146
Indirect patient care strategies, 248-249
Individual life history, 89, 90
Informal caregivers, 153-154
Information, 116, 126-127
Information processing
  hesitation phenomena in, 127
  normal aging, in, 90-91
Innate helplessness, 145
In-service training, 111, 148-149, 235
  effective, 284-285
  evaluation of, 283-284
  identifying learning needs for, 281
  identifying learning objectives for, 281
  learning experiences, implications for, 283
  manuals for, 284
  nursing assistants, for, 280, 282, 286-287
  objectives for, 248-249
  overview of, 280-281
  research implications, 287-288
  strategy selection for, 281-283
  studies, 285-286
Institutionalization. *See also* Long-term care; Nursing homes
  decision-making process for, 14-15
  effects of, 142, 184-185
Intellectual competence assessment, 144
Intimacy, 259
Ipsilateral noise, 57-58
IQ assessment, 59-61
Irreversible dementias, 188-189

## K

Korsakoff's syndrome, 30, 31
  differential diagnosis, 191-193

## L

Language, 10-11
Language changes in dementia of Alzheimer type
  clinical issues, 106-109
  future research needs, 111
  research on, 101-106
  stages of, 98-101
  treatment implications, 109-111
Language changes in normal aging
  age-associated differences, 85-89
  clinical implications, 93-94
  health-promotion interventions, 94
  overview of, 84-85
  performance in specific situations, 92-93
  variability in aged communication, 89-93
Language and communication assessment, 93
  conceptual model and rationale, 205-206
  language tests, 207
  memory and language, 211
  overview of, 205, 211-212
  pragmatics, 207-211
  semantics, 211
  test considerations, 206-207
Language history inventory, 138
Language impairment
  Alzheimer's disease, in, 37-38
  differentiating cortical from subcortical dementia, in, 25, 27
Language therapy, 109. *See also* Communication management in DAT
Learned helplessness, 144-146. *See also* Helplessness
Lecture, 282
Lesions, 73-75
Life experience strategy, 245
Life history, individual, 89, 90
Limbic system lesions, 73
Long-term care, 16. *See also* Institutionalizations; Nursing homes

## M

Magnetic resonance imaging (MRI), 11
Masking level difference, 53
Mattis Dementia Rating Scale, 202
Mechanical conductive presbycusis, 50, 51
Medicaid, 15
Medical evaluation, 198-199
Medicare, 15
Medication
  effects on motor speech, 74
  experimental, 251
  psychotropic, 250
  treating Alzheimer's disease with, 13
Memory
  anterograde, 24, 39
  discourse study, in, 125
  episodic, 107
  explicit, 39-42
  implicit, 42-43
Memory impairment
  Alzheimer's disease, in, 24, 25, 37, 39-43
  assessment of, 211
  differentiating cortical from subcortical dementias, in, 24-26
  effect on communication, 90-91
Metabolic presbycusis, 50, 51
Mental health, 158, 159
Mental processing, 90-91
Mental Status Questionnaire (MSQ), 143, 201, 224-225
Metaphoric titles, 126
Micrographia, 27
MID. *See* Multi-infarct dementia
Middle ear, 49
Middle-latency responses, 64
Milieu therapy, 270
Mini-Mental Status examination (MMSE), 119, 199, 201, 202, 223-225
Mixed dementias, 109, 191-194, 199. *See also* Creutzfeldt-Jakob disease; Multi-infarct dementia
Mortality, 7-8
Motor speech
  changes in, 70, 75
  effects of medications on, 74
  features of, 72
Motor speech dysfunction
  case presentations, 78
  causes of, 72-73
  therapeutic intervention, 78-79
Motor system, 71-72
Multidisciplinary approaches, 212
Multi-infarct dementia (MID)
  differential diagnosis, 109, 191-194, 199
  dysarthria and, 74
  etiology of, 9
  impaired CANS performance in, 65

Multi-infarct dementia (MID) *(Continued)*
   mortality rate of, 8
   overview of, 6
   prevalence of, 3
   staging of, 11
Multiple sclerosis (MS), 53
Music therapy, 240
Mutism, 70

## N

Narrative discourse
   descriptive versus, 124–125
   explanation of, 120
   production of, 88
National Council on Aging, 263
National Institute of Neurological and Communicative Disorders and Stroke (NINCDS) Work Groups, 3, 4, 22
Neocortical system lesions, 73
Neural presbycusis, 50, 53
Neuroanatomical perspective, 23, 31–32
Neurobehavioral perspective, 23
   gnosia, 28
   language impairment, 25, 27
   manipulation of acquired knowledge, 29
   memory, 24–26
   praxis, 27–28
   visuospatial functions, 29, 30
Neurochemistry
   cholinergic system, 29–31
   dopaminergic system, 31
Neurologic evaluation, 198–199
Neuropsychological assessment, 10, 200–205
Neurotransmitters, 73, 75
NINCDS-ADRDA Work Group, 3, 4, 22
Non-Alzheimer amyloid plaques, 77
Nonverbal communication
   changes in normal aging, 88
   music therapy to maintain, 240
Normalization needs, 147–148
Nosoacusis, 51
Nucleus basalis of Meynert, 29–31, 37
Nursing assistant in-service training, 280, 282, 286–287
Nursing homes. *See also* Institutionalization
   characteristics of patients in, 14, 154
   effects of, 142
   factors in choice of, 14–15
   in-service training in, 280–281
   legislation, 16
   overcare in, 144–145
Nursing-home administrators, 280

## O

Olfactory environment, 269
Olivopontocerebellar degeneration, 77
Omnibus Budget Reconciliation Act of 1987, 16
Operant conditioning, 240, 241
Orbitofrontal system, 32
Ossicular chain, 49
Otitis media, 49
Otosclerosis, 49
Outcome cues, 144
Outer ear, 49

## P

Palilalia, 100
Parkinson's disease, 22
   amyotrophic lateral sclerosis with, 77
   cholinergic system and, 30
   co-existence of DAT and, 70–71
   depression in, 73
   differential diagnosis, 189–193
   dopamine reduction in, 31
   dysarthria in, 72–74
   language impairment in, 25, 27
   memory in, 24, 25
   visuospatial impairment in, 28
   with non-Alzheimer's amyloid plaques, 77
Pathophysiology of Alzheimer's disease, 8–9
Peabody Picture Vocabulary Test (PPVT), 207, 211
Perception, environment and, 259
Performance-intensity function, 52, 53
Peripheral hearing loss, 47, 48, 58, 66–67
Perseverations, 117
Personal communication devices, 66
Personalization, 265
Pet therapy, 240
Phonemic cueing, 244
Phonology
   assessment, 211
   studies, 117
Physical activity, 260
Physical environment, 258–259, 265–266
Physical health, effects of caregiving on, 157–158
Physical props, 266
Pick's disease, 31, 65
   differential diagnosis, 108, 189, 190
   motor system and, 71, 72, 75
Positron emission tomography (PET)
   assessment of auditory function and, 61
   diagnosis of dementia and, 11
Pragmatic deficits
   assessment of, 207–211
   in DAT, 104–105
Presbycusis, 50–53, 143
Prevalence, 6–7
Privacy, 259, 265
Probe technique, 247–248
Problem-solving impairment, 38
Procedural memory, 25
Progressive supranuclear palsy (PSP), 75–76, 79, 108. *See also* Supranuclear palsy
Prose comprehension and recall, 87
Pseudodementia, 108, 143. *See also* Depression
   description of, 189
   differential diagnosis, 195, 196
Psychotherapy, 240, 241
Psychotropic medications, 250
Public policy issues, 15, 16
Pure-tone testing, 227, 228

## R

Reading comprehension, 27
Reality orientation therapy, 110, 240, 241
Reminiscence therapy, 240, 241, 258
Remotivation therapy, 240, 241
Reporters Test, 211
Reserve, 259
Resocialization, 240, 241
Reticular system lesions, 73
Retrograde memory, 24, 39
Reversible dementias
   differential diagnosis, 107–108, 188–189
   incidence of, 3
Revised Weschler Memory Scale, 200

Right-hemisphere damage, 194
Role playing
　example of, 290–291
　explanation of, 282–283
　used for in-service training of nursing assistants, 286–287

## S

Scopolamine, 58
Script strategy, 244–245
Second-language functioning, 90
Self-esteem, 243
Semantic impairment
　assessment of, 211
　in DAT, 101–102
Semantic language systems, 118
Semantic memory, 25, 38, 39
Semantic priming, 102
Sensory environment, 267–269
Sensory presbycusis, 50
Sensory training, 240
Sentence processing, 86–87
Sentential analysis, 122–124
Service delivery, 16
Shewan Spontaneous Language Analysis System, 93
Signal alerting technology, 233–234, 237
Single photon scanning, 11
Situational cues, 144
Social breakdown syndrome, 145–146
Social environment, 260, 270–271
Social expectations, 91–92
Social role, 147
Social strategies, 91
Social-cognitive model of communication in late life, 89–90
Sociocusis, 51
Solitude, 259
Somatostatin, 30
Space concerns, 265
Speech
　assessment of, 228
　changes in normal aging, 85–86
　evaluation of, 10–11
Speech register, 137
Speech-language pathologist
　as facilitator in group therapy session, 245
　in-service training for, 280
　need to be aware of impact on caregiver, 248
　role of, 128, 238, 240, 250, 279
Spouse caregivers, 158. *See also* Caregivers; Family caregivers
Staggered Spondaic Word Test, 58–59
Stimulation therapy, 246
Stress
　caregiver, 155–157
　communicative, 243
Strial presbycusis, 50, 51
Subcortical dementias, 33
　characteristics of, 22
　differential diagnosis, 108, 189–193
　importance of diagnosing, 71
　language loss in, 25, 27
　memory loss in, 24–25
　motor system in, 71–72, 75
　theories of, 75
　types of, 75–78
Support groups, family, 13, 163

Supranuclear palsy, 191, 193. *See also* Progressive supranuclear palsy (PSP)
Syntactic preservation, 102–104
Syntax
　assessment of, 211
　automatic process, as, 118
　changes in normal aging, 86–87
　studies in, 117
Synthetic Sentence Identification (SSI), 58

## T

Taciturnity, 117
Tangentiality, 117
Telephone enhancement devices, 234
Temporal lobe
　assessment of, 54–58
　impairment of, 58–62
Territoriality, 259–260
Test of Syntactic Complexity, 103
Tests. *See also individual tests*
　for aphasia, 107, 207
　for behavioral assessment, 200
　for language and communication assessment, 206–211
　for neuropsychological assessment, 200–205
　standardized, 143–144
Thalamic dementia, 77–78
Theory of Propositional Control, 285
Title formulation, 126
Token Test, 211
Topographic issues, 259–260
Touch, 269
Transient ischemic attacks, 143
Tympanometry, 228

## V

Validation therapy, 240, 241
Vascular dementia. *See* Multi-infarct dementia (MID)
Verbosity, 87
　as characteristic of DAT, 124
　associated with early dementia, 88, 117
Veterans Administration, 16
Vision changes, 90
Visual environment, 267–268
Visual imagery techniques, 240
Visual impairment, 143
Visual perception deficit, 101
Visual stimuli, 120–121
Visuospatial function, 28, 38–39
Vocabulary, 86
Voice, 85

## W

Wernicke's aphasic patients, 119
Weschler Adult Intelligence Scale Revised (WAIS-R), 200, 202
Weschler Memory Scale, 199, 200
Western Aphasia Battery, 10
Wilson's disease, 191, 193
Word level abilities, 123
Working space, 259

## Y

Yiddish-English speakers, 134–137